CARING FOR THE VULNERABLE

Perspectives in Nursing Theory, Practice, and Research

2ND EDITION

D1304413

EDITORS

Mary de Chesnay, DSN, APRN-BC, FAAN

Acting Dean
N. Jean Bushman Endowed Chair
College of Nursing
Seattle University
Seattle, Washington

Barbara A. Anderson, DrPH, CNM, CHES, FACNM

Associate Dean
College of Nursing
Seattle University
Seattle, Washington

JONES AND BARTLETT PUBLISHERS
Sudbury, Massachusetts
BOSTON   TORONTO   LONDON   SINGAPORE

World Headquarters
Jones and Bartlett Publishers
40 Tall Pine Drive
Sudbury, MA 01776
978-443-5000
info@jbpub.com
www.jbpub.com

Jones and Bartlett Publishers Canada
6339 Ormindale Way
Mississauga, Ontario L5V 1J2
Canada

Jones and Bartlett Publishers International
Barb House, Barb Mews
London W6 7PA
United Kingdom

Jones and Bartlett's books and products are available through most bookstores and online booksellers. To contact Jones and Bartlett Publishers directly, call 800-832-0034, fax 978-443-8000, or visit our website www.jbpub.com.

Substantial discounts on bulk quantities of Jones and Bartlett's publications are available to corporations, professional associations, and other qualified organizations. For details and specific discount information, contact the special sales department at Jones and Bartlett via the above contact information or send an email to specialsales@jbpub.com.

The authors, editor, and publisher have made every effort to provide accurate information. However, they are not responsible for errors, omissions, or for any outcomes related to the use of the contents of this book and take no responsibility for the use of the products and procedures described. Treatments and side effects described in this book may not be applicable to all people; likewise, some people may require a dose or experience a side effect that is not described herein. Drugs and medical devices are discussed that may have limited availability controlled by the Food and Drug Administration (FDA) for use only in a research study or clinical trial. Research, clinical practice, and government regulations often change the accepted standard in this field. When consideration is being given to use of any drug in the clinical setting, the health care provider or reader is responsible for determining FDA status of the drug, reading the package insert, and reviewing prescribing information for the most up-to-date recommendations on dose, precautions, and contraindications, and determining the appropriate usage for the product. This is especially important in the case of drugs that are new or seldom used.

Production Credits
Executive Editor: Kevin Sullivan
Acquisitions Editor: Emily Ekle
Associate Editor: Amy Sibley
Editorial Assistant: Patricia Donnelly
Production Director: Amy Rose
Associate Production Editor: Wendy Swanson
Associate Marketing Manager: Rebecca Wasley
Manufacturing and Inventory Control Supervisor: Amy Bacus

Interactive Technology Manager: Dawn Mahon Priest
Composition: Paw Print Media
Cover Design: Kate Ternullo
Cover Images: © Kevin R. Williams/ShutterStock, Inc., © Ryan McVay/Photodisc/Getty Images, © Photodisc, © EML/ShutterStock, Inc., © jaggat/Shutterstock, Inc., © Photos.com
Printing and Binding: Malloy, Inc.
Cover Printing: Malloy, Inc.

Library of Congress Cataloging-in-Publication Data
Caring for the vulnerable : perspectives in nursing theory, practice, and research / [edited by] Mary de Chesnay, Barbara A. Anderson.— 2nd ed.
   p. ; cm.
   Includes bibliographical references and index.
   ISBN-13: 978-0-7637-5109-8 (pbk. : alk. paper)
   ISBN-10: 0-7637-5109-X (pbk. : alk. paper) 1. Nursing—Social aspects. 2. Transcultural nursing.
3. Nursing—Cross-cultural studies. 4. Nursing—Philosophy.
   [DNLM: 1. Community Health Nursing. 2. Vulnerable Populations. 3. Nursing Theory.
4. Transcultural Nursing. WY 106 C277 2008] I. De Chesnay, Mary. II. Anderson, Barbara A.
   RT86.5.C376 2008
   362.17'3—dc22

                                                2007027287
6048

Printed in the United States of America
12 11 10 09 08   10 9 8 7 6 5 4 3 2

DEDICATION

To my sisters: Ruth, Wendy, Becky, and Sue
—MdC

To the truest of friends: Chris, Helen, Joyce, and Gary
—BA

CONTENTS

| Unit 2 | Nursing Theories | 71 |

CONTRIBUTORS

Heather Andersen, RN
Graduate Student
Seattle University
Seattle, WA

Barbara A. Anderson, DrPH, CNM, CHES
Associate Dean
College of Nursing
Seattle University
Seattle, WA

Anne Watson Bongiorno, PhD, APRN-BC
Associate Professor
SUNY Plattsburgh
Plattsburgh, NY

Doris M. Boutain, PhD, RN
Associate Professor
University of Washington
Seattle, WA

Joyceen Boyle, PhD, RN, FAAN
Associate Dean
University of Arizona
Tucson, AZ

Geraldine R. Britton, RN, FNP, PhD
Assistant Professor
Binghamton University
Binghamton, NY

Angeline Bushy, PhD, RN, FAAN
Professor
University of Central Florida
Daytona Beach, FL

Caroline Cogen, MSN, APRN
Kitsap Nephrology
Bremerton, WA

Pamela M. H. Cone, PhD, RN, CS
Azuza Pacific University
Azuza, CA

Rebecca K. Conte, BSN
Seattle University
Seattle, WA

Mary de Chesnay, DSN, APRN-BC, FAAN
Acting Dean
N. Jean Bushman Endowed Chair
College of Nursing
Seattle University
Seattle, WA

Behice Erci, PhD, RN
Associate Professor
Atatürk University
Hemsirilik Yuksekokulu
Erzurum, Turkey

Linda Frothinger, BSN, RN
Staff Nurse and Swedish Scholar
Swedish Medical Center
Seattle University
Seattle, WA

Amanda B. Frye, RN, BSN, MPh, CHES
Seattle University
Seattle, WA

Elizabeth Furlong, PhD, RN, JD
Associate Professor
Creighton University
Omaha, NE

Elaine Goehner, PhD, RN, CPHQ
Executive Director
Swedish Center for Nursing Excellence
Seattle, WA

Linda Graham, MS, RN
University of Illinois at Chicago
Chicago, IL

Terra Grandmason, MSN, FNP
Family Nurse Practitioner
Seattle, WA

Sarah Hall Gueldner, DSN, RN, FAAN,
FGSA
Arline H. and Curtis F. Garvin Professor
of Nursing
Case Western Reserve University
Cleveland, OH

Lynda Harrison, RN, PhD, FAAN
Professor
University of Alabama at Birmingham
Birmingham, AL

Dena Hassouneh, RN, PhD
Assistant Professor
Oregon Health Science University
Portland, OR

Barbara J. Hatcher, PhD, RN
Director
Center for Learning and Global Public
Health
Secretary General
The World Federation of Public Health
Associations
Washington, DC

David Hibbs, MSN, APRN
Family Nurse Practitioner
Yakima, WA

Gladys L. Husted, PhD, RN
Distinguished Professor
Duquesne University School of Nursing
Pittsburgh, PA

James H. Husted, PhD
Independent Scholar
Pittsburgh, PA

Patricia M. Jergens, RN, MSN, ARNP
VA Medical Center
Seattle, WA

Karen Joines, BSN, RN
Children's Hospital and Regional Medical
Center
Seattle, WA

Andrew R. Kruse, MSN, APRN
Family Nurse Practitioner
Edmonds, WA

Janet L. Larson, PhD, RN, FAAN
Professor and Department Head
University of Illinois at Chicago
Chicago, IL

Andrew Lin, RN
Seattle University
Seattle, WA

Margaret McAllister, RN, BA, EdD
Associate Professor
University of the Sunshine Coast
Maroochydore, Queensland
Australia

Jennifer H. Mercado, RN
Graduate Student
Seattle University
Seattle, WA

Cathy Michaels, PhD, RN, FAAN
Clinical Associate Professor
University of Arizona College of Nursing
Tucson, AZ

Jeri A. Milstead, PhD, RN, FAAN
Dean and Professor
University of Toledo
Toledo, OH

Carol Moffett, PhD, FNP, BC, CDE
Researcher
National Institutes of Health
Sacaton, AZ

Patrick J. M. Murphy, PhD
Assistant Professor
Seattle University
Seattle, WA

Gloria Q. Natividad, MSN, APRN
Family Nurse Practitioner

Lynda P. Nauright, EdD, RN
Professor of Nursing
Kennesaw State University
Kennesaw, GA

Patti Nissley, RN
Seattle University
Seattle, WA

Ellen Olshansky, DNSc, RNC, FAAN
Professor and Director of Nursing
University of California at Irvine
Irvine, CA

Christopher Pamp, MSN, APRN
Nurse Practitioner
Seattle Cardiology
Seattle, WA

Nataly Pasumansky, MSN, ARNP
Nurse Practitioner
Advanced Family Medicine
Bellevue, WA

Rebecca W. Peil, MSN, CFNP
Nurse Practitioner
Children's Oasis Pediatrics
Gilbert, AZ

Jane W. Peterson, PhD, RN
Professor
Seattle University
Seattle, WA

Renee Rassilyer-Bomers, MSN, RN, FNP
Instructor
Seattle University
Seattle, WA

Carl A. Ross, PhD, CRNP, BC, CNE
Professor of Nursing
Robert Morris University
Moon Township, PA

Julia F. Shellhorn, RN
Graduate Student
Seattle University
Seattle, WA

Pamela A. P. Smith, PhD, RN
Director
Clinical Education and Nurse Integration
Swedish Center for Nursing Excellence
Seattle, WA

Justin Speyer, RN
Graduate Student
Seattle University
Seattle, WA

Yvonne M. Sterling, RN, PhD
Professor
Louisiana State University
New Orleans, LA

Charee L. Taccogno, MSN, APRN
Family Nurse Practitioner
Mercer Island, WA

Maile Taualii
Associate Director
Urban Indian Health Institute
Seattle, WA

Susan Terwilliger, EdD(c), RN, PNP
Binghamton University
Binghamton, NY

Lakshmi Thiaragaj, RN
Graduate Student
Seattle University
Seattle, WA

Jenny Hsin-Chun Tsai, PhD, APRN
Assistant Professor
University of Washington
School of Nursing
Seattle, WA

Toni M. Vezeau, PhD, RNC
Associate Professor
Seattle University
Seattle, WA

Carol Vineyard
Senior Nursing Student
Seattle University
Seattle, WA

Mary K. Walker, PhD, RN, FAAN
Dean and Professor
Marcella Niehoff School of Nursing
Loyola University
Chicago, IL
Dean Emerita
College of Nursing
Seattle University
Seattle, WA

Jessica H. Webb, MSN, APRN
Family Nurse Practitioner
Lake Serene Clinic
Lynnwood, WA

JoEllen Wilbur, PhD, APN, FAAN
Professor and Associate Dean
Research Facilitation and Administration
University of Illinois at Chicago
Chicago, IL

Danuta Wojnar, PhD, RN
Assistant Professor
Seattle University
Seattle, WA

Julie Johnson Zerwic, PhD, RN
Associate Professor
University of Illinois at Chicago
Chicago, IL

Rick Zoucha, PhD, APRN, BC, CTN
Associate Professor
Duquesne University School of Nursing
Pittsburgh, PA

FOREWORD

The nursing profession faces many complex challenges in the next few years because we are increasingly providing care to high-risk individuals and groups. As we conceptualize how to frame this care and how our nursing practice will be designed and delivered, the theoretical and practical basis of nursing is shifting dramatically to meet these new societal needs. Mary de Chesnay and her colleagues make a significant contribution to our nursing efforts with the *Second Edition* of *Caring for the Vulnerable*. Traditional nursing roles and care settings are changing in response to the needs of increasingly diverse numbers of vulnerable groups. These changes have tremendous implications for the concepts, theories, ethics, and, ultimately, the practice of nursing.

Health disparities within our culturally diverse populations have become hot-button issues, and there seems to be no single silver bullet to help us address these growing health disparities. Of particular concern to all healthcare providers, as well as to politicians and others, is the growing number of what are termed *vulnerable populations*. This concern has triggered some political response as, finally, healthcare reform is being discussed at state and national levels, although it is not clear what outcomes or solutions will evolve. It is therefore most appropriate that this text focuses broadly on the key concepts of vulnerability and vulnerable populations but, in addition, extends our thinking to theoretical formulations that guide our practice. For example, the label of "vulnerability" can in and of itself be patronizing and, even worse, stigmatizing. Therefore it is important that nurses use the term *vulnerability* after a critical appraisal of how they conceptualize and provide care for both individuals and groups. Vulnerability occurs or is increased from a number of interacting forces and factors, and providing care to vulnerable populations without a clear understanding of the context in which vulnerability occurs is a prelude to disaster. This book sets the stage for understanding vulnerable populations and the context of vulnerability from the perspective of individuals, groups, communities, and populations.

I believe most of us would agree that there are no theories of vulnerability, per se, but that there are many useful, albeit complex, concepts about vulnerability. Vulnerability has a global face, and I applaud the focus of this text on vulnerable populations at home and in international settings. Theoretical frameworks or theories (Watson, Rogers, and Leininger) that were originally developed for other purposes are now being applied to vulnerable populations. They add to our understanding of vulnerability within special groups and settings.

Vulnerability is not limited to issues of patient care because there are significant methodological issues in conducting research with vulnerable populations. Investigators who have worked with vulnerable populations acknowledge that many challenges arise when conducting studies with these populations. These challenges and issues do not arise strictly from methodological problems; they also arise from the theoretical and ethical implications that are inherent with vulnerable populations. Therefore the broadly based content of this textbook is of value to the profession as a whole as we attempt to identify and meet the needs of those vulnerable populations who experience particular health disparities.

This text also addresses practice and educational issues with vulnerable populations, addressing a new emphasis within nursing practice—evidence-based practice—as well as conceptual models for implementing care for communities. I believe there will come a time in nursing when we will move beyond individual patient care that is disease focused, ignoring the context in which care is provided. Instead, we will accept the community/public health challenge of meeting aggregate needs of high-risk and vulnerable groups wherever they are—at home, at work, or in acute care or other settings. This textbook provides an early and firm foundation for nurses who wish to explore the many aspects of vulnerability and the implications of that vulnerability for the care that is provided to clients.

Joyceen Boyle, PhD, RN, FAAN
Associate Dean
College of Nursing
University of Arizona
Tucson, AZ

PREFACE

Caring for the vulnerable members of their society is a function nurses perform without regard for their own ambitions, personal safety, and financial security. They do this work from their desire to help the less fortunate and from their profound commitment to social justice, regardless of religious orientation. *Vulnerability* is a trendy concept, and *vulnerable populations* a term with specific meaning in the present political climate. Both terms are somewhat controversial in the way scholars think about people. Word fashions come and go, but there will always be those who are at risk and nurses will always define their role to care for them.

This book is the *Second Edition* of *Caring for the Vulnerable* and represents an attempt to introduce authors with a variety of unique perspectives. Based on feedback from the faculty and students who used the first edition, the editors have updated chapters from the first edition but have also included much new material to broaden scholarly discussions about vulnerability. With so many content areas that could have been included, the intent here is not to present a comprehensive treatment of the topic but rather to stimulate discussion.

Unit 1 presents key concepts that provide a basic structure for caring for the vulnerable. Unit 2 is an exploration of the relevance of nursing theories to vulnerable populations. In Unit 3, a general overview of issues relating to conducting research and reports of studies shows the kinds of phenomena nurses study and the methods they use to examine questions of interest. In the first edition all the research chapters were qualitative, so we expanded the types of studies for the second edition. Unit 4 consists of a variety of chapters that have practice applicability. A new Unit 5 was added to provide information on program planning. Unit 6 is about the process of learning to work with vulnerable populations and has a new focus on experiential learning, highlighted with a new chapter by Dr. Barbara Anderson, whose help as co-editor has been invaluable. Finally, Unit 7 focuses on policy.

Originally intended as a primary text for undergraduate and graduate nursing courses on vulnerable populations, the book is also appropriate as a supplemental text for courses in community health, nurse practitioner curricula, nursing theory, research methods, and doctoral courses that emphasize vulnerable populations. We are told that the *First Edition* is widely used in Doctor of Nursing Practice (DNP) programs, so we included material on program planning.

Specifically included in the new edition are several short chapters that serve as samples of students' works. These are included in the book because students do not have access to the Instructor's Resources (found online at www.jbpub.com/nursing), and we thought students who use the book might benefit from examples. Finally, by representing the work of nurses in several countries, we hope that the book encourages interest in other cultures and might be appropriate for courses in international nursing.

We are impressed with the breadth of topics that could have been explored and regret that space limitations did not allow for including the work of even more nurse scholars with important things to say about vulnerability. However the book is used, we hope that readers will be inspired to think more about the vulnerable and to publish their ideas about how nurses can better serve people within our own communities, however we may define *community*.

Mary de Chesnay, DSN, APRN-BC, FAAN
Acting Dean
N. Jean Bushman Endowed Chair and Professor
College of Nursing
Seattle University
Seattle, WA

Barbara Anderson, DrPH, CNM, CHES, FACNM
Associate Dean
College of Nursing
Seattle University
Seattle, WA

ACKNOWLEDGMENTS

This book is a reflection of the talents of many people—first among them are the contributing authors. These talented scholars represent a small number of the many nurses around the world who practice and write about social justice. That social justice and care for the vulnerable is a universal phenomenon for nurses is reinforced when we attend professional meetings and when we travel to our own fieldwork sites and see social justice in action in some of the poorest communities of the world. It is inspiring to hear these authors speak and an honor to provide a forum for all who read this book to hear about their work.

Special acknowledgement is given to those students whose work is highlighted in the Instructor's Resources located at www.jbpub.com/nursing. The undergraduate students whose work is included thought carefully about the concepts in the book and care deeply for the people they serve: Christine Aquino, Danielle Berry, Tim Frederickson, Sarah Hillebrand, DoQuyen Huynh, Kate Jansen, Brittany Lyman, Sam Magnotto, Samantha Price, Dorothy Routt, Kerry Sjostedt, Sarah Sjosted, Martin Sullivan, Michael Tampieri, Angela Taylor, Heather Wehmeyer, and Josh Wymer. Megan Peterson did a great job writing slides for the Instructor's Resources.

There are technical support people who labor behind the scenes of any published work and without whose help, manuscripts would look amateurish. Jann Austin was particularly helpful in editing sections of the manuscript. Josh Wymer, Alona Habinsky, Heather Wehmeyer, Lisa Thorson, and Jennipher Jones assisted in preparing the Instructor's Resources and Kathryn Nardozza helped with the clerical side. Dr. Patrick Murphy, author and computer expert, performed miracles with models and figures. The editors and staff at Jones and Bartlett made sure the work was published in a timely manner. We are particularly grateful to Tricia Donnelly who cheerfully answered numerous questions along the way, to Kevin Sullivan and Amy Sibley for their help and encouragement early on, to Wendy Swanson who made the production process run smoothly, to Kate Ternullo for designing the cover, and to Pam Thomson, our wonderful copyeditor.

Finally, and perhaps most importantly, the editors would like to thank all of the vulnerable yet resilient people with whom we have worked during many years of clinical practice and education. Working in every corner of the world, the editors encountered time and time again, the strength of the human spirit and generosity of nature among people who have no reason to welcome strangers, yet who shared what they had and took the time to teach us about their cultures.

Unit One

The world breaks everyone, and afterwards, some are strong at the broken places.

■ ■ ■

Ernest Hemingway
A Farewell to Arms

CONCEPTS

Vulnerable Populations: Vulnerable People

Mary de Chesnay

In this chapter key concepts are introduced to provide a frame of reference for examining healthcare issues related to vulnerability and vulnerable populations. The concepts presented in Unit I, as a whole, form a theoretical perspective on caring for vulnerable populations within a cultural context in which nurses consider not only ethnicity as a cultural factor but also the culture of vulnerability. The goal is to provide culturally competent care.

Vulnerability

There are two aspects related to vulnerability, and it is important to distinguish between them. One aspect focuses on the individual in which the individual is viewed within a system context, whereas the other is an aggregate view of what would be termed "vulnerable populations." Much of the literature on vulnerability is targeted toward the aggregate view, and nurses certainly need to address the needs of groups. However, nurses also treat individuals, and this book is concerned with generating ideas about caring for both individuals and groups. It is critical for practitioners to keep in mind that groups are composed of individuals, and we should not stereotype individuals in terms of their group characteristics. However, working with vulnerable populations is cost-effective because epidemiological patterns can be detected in groups and some standardized interventions can be developed that provide better quality health care to more people.

Vulnerability is a general concept meaning "susceptibility," and its specific connotation in terms of health care is "at risk for health problems." According to Aday (2001), vulnerable populations are those at risk for poor physical, psychological, or social health. Anyone can be vulnerable at any given point in time as a result of life circumstances or response to illness or events. However, the notion of a vulnerable population is a public health concept that refers to vulnerability by virtue of status; that is, some groups are at risk at any given point in time relative to other individuals or groups.

To be a member of a vulnerable population does not necessarily mean one is vulnerable. In fact, many individuals within vulnerable populations would resist the notion that they are vulnerable because they prefer to focus on their strengths rather than their weaknesses. These people might argue that "vulnerable population" is just another label that healthcare professionals use to promote a system of health care that they, the consumers of care, consider patronizing. It is important to distinguish between a state of vulnerability at any given point in time and a labeling process in which groups of people at risk for certain health conditions are further marginalized.

Some members of society who are not members of the culturally defined vulnerable populations described in this book might be vulnerable only in certain contexts. For example, nurses who work in emergency rooms are vulnerable to violence. Hospital employees and visitors are vulnerable to infections. Teachers in preschool and daycare providers are vulnerable to a host of communicable diseases because of their daily contact with young children. People who work with heavy machinery are at risk for certain injuries.

Other examples are people who pick up hitchhikers, drivers who drink, people who travel on airplanes during flu season, college students cramming for exams, and people caught in natural disasters. There is an unfortunate tendency in our culture to judge some vulnerable people as at fault for their own vulnerability and to blame those who place others at risk. For example, rape victims have been blamed for enticing their attackers. People who pick up hitchhikers might be looked upon as foolish while their intentions might have been only kindness and consideration for those stranded by car trouble. Airline passengers who continually sneeze might anger their seatmates, who feel at risk for catching a communicable disease.

Vulnerable Populations

Who are the vulnerable in terms of health care? Vulnerable populations are those with a greater than average risk of developing health problems (Aday, 2001; Sebastian, 1996) by virtue of their marginalized sociocultural status, their limited access to economic resources, or personal characteristics such as age and gender. For example, members of ethnic minority groups have traditionally been marginalized even when they are highly educated and earning good salaries. Immigrants and the poor (including the working poor) have limited access to health care because of the way insurance is obtained. Children, women, and the elderly are vulnerable to a host of healthcare problems, notably violence but also specific health problems associated with development or aging. Developmental examples are susceptibility to poor influenza outcomes for children and the elderly, psychological issues of puberty and menopause, osteoporosis and fractures among older women, and Alzheimer's disease.

Bezruchka (2000, 2001), in his provocative works, addressed the correlation between poverty and illness but also asserted that inequalities in wealth distribution are responsible for the state of health of the American population. Bezruchka argued that the economic structure of a country is the single most powerful determinant of the health of its people. He noted that Japan, with its small gap between rich and poor, has a high percentage of smokers but a low percentage of mortality from smoking. Bezruchka advocated redistribution of wealth as a solution to health disparities.

The controversial prescription drug benefit for Medicare recipients highlights Bezruchka's observations about disparities in the United States. Senior citizens are among the most vulnerable in a society, and Medicare is an attempt to address some of their healthcare costs. However, although practitioners may value a philosophy of social justice (Larkin, 2004), the implementation of social justice is usually balanced with cost. In the case of the Medicare prescription drug benefit, the cost is projected at over $700 billion from 2006 to 2015 (Gellad, Huskamp, Phillips, & Haas, 2006). The difficulties created by attempting to balance social justice with cost illustrate how hard it is to implement the ideal of social justice in the United States.

Concepts and Theories

Aday (2001) published a framework for studying vulnerable populations that incorporated the World Health Organization's (1948) dimensions of health (physical, psychological, and social) into a model of relationships between individual and community on a variety of policy levels. In Aday's framework the variables of access, cost, and quality are critical in understanding the nature of health care for vulnerable populations. Access refers to the ability of people to find, obtain, and pay for health care. Costs can be direct or indirect. Direct costs are the dollars spent by healthcare facilities to provide care. Indirect costs are losses resulting from decreased patient productivity (e.g., absenteeism from work). Quality refers to the relative inadequacy, adequacy, or superiority of services.

Other authors who addressed the conceptual basis of vulnerable populations include Sebastian (1996) and coresearchers (Sebastian et al., 2002), who focused on marginalization as a factor in resource allocation, and Flaskerud and Winslow (1998), who emphasized resource availability in the broad sense of socioeconomic and environmental resources. Karpati, Galea, Awerbuch, and Levins (2002) argued for an ecological approach to understand how social context influences health outcomes. Lessick, Woodring, Naber, and Halstead (1992) described the concept of vulnerability as applied to a person within a system context. Although this study applied the model to maternal–child nursing, the authors argued that the model is appropriate in any clinical setting.

Spiers (2000) argued that epidemiological views of vulnerability are insufficient to explain human experience and offered a new conceptualization based on perceptions that are both etic (externally defined by others) and emic (from the point of view of the person). Etic approaches are helpful in understanding the nature of risk in a quantifiable way. Emic approaches enable one to understand the whole of human experience and, in so doing, help people capitalize on their capacity for action.

Health Disparities

In 1998 President Bill Clinton made a commitment to reduce by the year 2010 health disparities that disproportionately affect racial and ethnic minorities. The Department of Health and Human Services selected six areas to target: infant mortality, cancer screening and management, cardiovascular disease, diabetes, HIV/AIDS, and immunization

(National Institutes of Health [NIH], n.d.). Subsequently, the NIH announced a strategic plan for 2002–2006 that committed funding to three major goals related to research, research infrastructure, and public information/community outreach (NIH, 2002).

Flaskerud et al. (2002) reviewed 79 research reports published in *Nursing Research* and concluded that although nurse researchers have systematically addressed health disparities, they have tended to ignore certain groups, such as indigenous peoples. They also inappropriately lump together as Hispanic members of disparate groups with their own cultural identity (e.g., Puerto Ricans, Mexicans, Cubans, Dominicans).

Aday (2001) emphasized certain groups as vulnerable populations, and the 2010 priorities showcase obvious needs within these groups:

- **High-risk mothers and infants-of-concern.** This population is a result of high rates of teenage pregnancy and poor prenatal care, leading to birth-weight problems and infant mortality. Affected groups include very young women, African-American women, and poorly educated women, all of whom are less likely than middle-class white women to receive adequate prenatal care because of limited access to services.

- **Chronically ill and disabled.** Those in this category not only experience higher death rates than comparable middle-class white women as a result of heart disease, cancer, and stroke, but they are also subject to prevalent chronic conditions such as hypertension, arthritis, and asthma. The debilitating effects of such chronic diseases lead to lost income because of limitations in activities of daily living. African-Americans are more likely to experience ill effects and to die from chronic diseases.

- **Persons living with HIV/AIDS.** Advances in tracing and treating AIDS have resulted in declines in deaths and increases in the number of people living with HIV/AIDS. This increase is also due, in part, to changes in transmission patterns from largely male homosexual or bisexual contact to transmission through heterosexual contact and sharing needles among intravenous drug users.

- **Mentally ill and disabled.** Mental illness is usually broadly defined to include even those with mild anxiety and depression. Prevalence rates are high with age-specific disorders, and severe emotional disorders seriously interfere with activities of daily living and interpersonal relationships.

- **Alcohol and other substance abusers.** The wide array of substances that are abused includes drugs, alcohol, cigarettes, and inhalants (such as glue). Intoxication results in chronic diseases, accidents, and, in some cases, criminal activity. Young male adults in their late teens and early twenties are more likely to smoke, drink, and take drugs.

- **Suicide- or homicide-prone behavior.** Rates differ by age, sex, and race, with elderly white and young Native American men most likely to kill themselves and young African-American, Native American, and Hispanic men most likely to be killed by others.

- **Abusive families.** Children, the elderly, and spouses (overwhelmingly women) are likely targets of violence within the family, and although older children are more likely to be injured, young female children over 3 years old are consistently at risk for sexual abuse.

- **Homeless persons.** Because of problems in identifying this population, it is reasonably certain that the estimated prevalence rates at any given time are low and vary across the country. Generally, more young men are homeless, but all homeless persons are likely to suffer from chronic diseases and are vulnerable to violence.

- **Immigrants/refugees.** Health care for immigrants, refugees, and temporary residents is complicated by the diversity of languages, health practices, food choices, culturally based definitions of health, and previous experiences with American bureaucracies.

Aday (2001) provided much statistical information for these vulnerable groups, but prevalence rates for specific conditions change periodically, and readers are referred to the website of the National Center for Health Statistics at www.cdc.gov/nchs for updated information.

Trends in families over the last five decades (the lifetime of the baby boomers) show marked changes in the demographics of families, and these changes affect health disparities. At present, more men and women are delaying marriage, with more people choosing to live together first. Divorce rates are higher, with a concurrent increase in the single-parent family structure. Out-of-wedlock births have increased, partially due to decreases in marital fertility. There is a sharp and sustained increase in maternal employment (Hofferth, 2003).

Institute of Medicine Study

The U.S. Congress directed the Institute of Medicine (IOM) to study the extent of racial and ethnic differences in health care and to recommend interventions to eliminate health disparities (IOM-National Academy of Sciences, 2003). The IOM found consistent evidence of disparities across a wide range of health services and illnesses, noting that although racial and ethnic disparities occur within a wider historical context, they are unacceptable.

The IOM urged a general public acknowledgment of the problem and specific cross-cultural training for health professionals. They recommended specific legal, regulatory, and policy interventions to increase fairness in access, increase the number of minority health professionals, and better enforce civil rights laws. IOM recommendations with regard to data collection should serve to monitor progress toward the goal of eliminating health disparities based on different treatment for minorities.

Vulnerability to Specific Conditions or Diseases

Much of the research on specific conditions and diseases was generated from psychology data and predates much of the medical and nursing literature on disparities. Researchers focusing on vulnerability to these specific conditions tend to take an individual approach in that conditions or diseases are treated from the point of view of how a particular individual responds to life stressors and how that response can cause the condition to develop or continue.

Researchers have focused on conditions too numerous to report here, but references were found on alcohol consumption in women and vulnerability to sexual aggression (Testa, Livingston, & Collins, 2000), rape myths and vulnerability to sexual assault (Bohner, Danner, Siebler, & Stamson, 2002), self-esteem and unplanned pregnancy (Smith, Gerrard, & Gibbons, 1997), lung transplantation (Kurz, 2002), coronary angioplasty (Edell-Gustafsson & Hetta, 2001), adjustment to lower limb amputation (Behel, Rybarczyk, Elliott, Nicholas, & Nyenhuis, 2002), reaction to natural disasters (Phifer, 1990), reaction to combat stress (Aldwin, Levensen, & Spiro, 1994; Ruef, Litz, & Schlenger, 2000), homelessness (Morrell-Bellai, Goering, & Boydell, 2000; Shinn, Knickman, & Weitzman, 1991), mental retardation (Nettlebeck, Wison, Potter, & Perry, 2000), anxiety (Calvo & Cano-Vindel, 1997; Strauman, 1992), and suicide (Schotte, Cools, & Payvar, 1990).

Depression

Many authors have focused on cognitive variables in an attempt to explain vulnerability to depression (Alloy & Clements, 1992; Alloy, Whitehouse, & Abramson, 2000; Hayes, Castonguay, & Goldfried, 1996; Ingram & Ritter, 2000). Others have explored gender differences (Bromberger & Mathews, 1996; Whiffen, 1988). In a major analysis of the existing literature on depression, Hankin and Abramson (2001) explored the development of gender differences in depression and noted that although both male and female rates rise during middle adolescence, rates in girls rise more sharply after age 13 or puberty. This model of general depression might account for gender differences based on developmentally specific stressors and implies possible treatment options.

Variables related to attitudes present a third area of focus in the literature (Brown, Hammen, Craske, & Wickens, 1995; Joiner, 1995; Zuroff, Blatt, Bondi, & Pilkonis, 1999). In a study of 75 college students researchers found that a high level of "perfectionistic achievement attitudes," as indicated on the Dysfunctional Attitude Scale, correlated with a specific stressor (e.g., poorer than expected performance on a college exam) to predict an increase in symptoms of depression (Brown et al., 1995).

Schizophrenia

Smoking has been observed to be a problem in schizophrenics, and there is some evidence that smokers have a more serious course of mental illness than nonsmokers, the theory being that schizophrenics smoke as a way to self-medicate (Lohr & Flynn, 1992). In a twin study investigating lifetime prevalence of smoking and nicotine withdrawal, Lyons et al. (2002) found that the association between smoking and schizophrenia may be related to familial vulnerability to schizophrenia.

Other authors have examined the relationship between schizophrenia and personality and discovered that this relationship is largely unexplored and might provide a new direction in which to search for knowledge about vulnerability to schizophrenia. In their meta-analysis, Berenbaum and Fujita (1994) found a significant relationship between introversion and schizophrenia and suggested that studies on that relationship might provide new knowledge about the covariation of schizophrenia with mood disorders, particularly depression. In a thoughtful analysis of the literature on the role of the family in schizophrenia, Wuerker (2000) presented evidence for the biological view and concluded that there is a unique vulnerability to stress in schizophrenics and that communication difficulties within families with schizophrenic members may be due to a shared genetic heritage.

Eating Disorders

Acknowledgment of food as a common focus for anxiety has become customary. Canadian researchers refer to "food insecurity" to describe the phenomenon of nutritional vulnerability resulting from food scarcity and insufficient access to food by welfare recipients and low-income people who do not qualify for welfare (McIntyre et al., 2003; Tarasuk, 2003). In the United States, eating disorders are a growing result of body image problems that are particularly prevalent in gay men and heterosexual women (Siever, 1994). In a prospective study of gender and behavioral vulnerabilities related to eating disorders, Leon, Fulkerson, Perry, and Early-Zaid (1995) found significant differences for girls in the variables of weight loss, dieting patterns, vomiting, and use of diet pills. They reported a method for predicting the occurrence of eating disorders based on performance scores on risk-factor status tests early on.

HIV/AIDS

In a meta-analysis of 32 HIV/AIDS studies involving 15,440 participants, Gerrard, Gibbons, and Bushman (1996) found empirical evidence to support the commonly known motivational hypothesis, derived from the Health Belief Model (Becker & Rosenstock, 1987). The authors found that perceived vulnerability was the major force behind prevention behavior in high-risk populations but cautioned that studies were not available for low-risk populations. They also found that risk behavior shapes perceptions of vulnerability; that is, people who engage in high-risk behavior tend to see themselves as more likely to contract HIV than those who engage in low-risk behavior.

Evidence that high-risk men tend to relapse into unsafe sex behaviors was presented in a longitudinal study of results of an intervention in which researchers could successfully predict relapse behavior (Kelly, St. Lawrence, & Brasfield, 1991). In a gender study on emotional distress predictors, Van Servellen, Aguirre, Sarna, and Brecht (2002) found that although all subjects had scores indicating clinical anxiety levels, women had more HIV symptoms and poorer functioning than men.

In a study that used a vulnerable populations framework, Flaskerud and Lee (2001) considered the role that resource availability plays in the health status of informal female caregivers of people with HIV/AIDS (n = 36) and age-related dementias (n = 40). Not surprisingly, the caregivers experienced high levels of both physical and mental health problems. However, the use of the vulnerable populations framework explained the result that the resource variables of income and minority ethnicity contributed the most to understanding health status. In terms of the risk variables, anger was more common in HIV caregivers and was significantly related to depressive mood, which was also high among the HIV caregivers.

Substance Abuse

In a study of 288 undergraduates, Wild, Hinson, Cunningham, and Bacchiochi (2001) examined the inconsistencies between a person's perceived risk of alcohol-related harm and motivation to reduce that risk. They found a general tendency for people to view themselves as less vulnerable than peers regardless of their risk status, but the at-risk group rated themselves more likely to experience harm than the not-at-risk group. The authors concluded that motivational approaches to reducing risk should emphasize not only why people drink but also why they should reduce alcohol consumption. Additional support for the motivational hypothesis—that perceived vulnerability influences prevention behavior—extends to marijuana use (Simons & Carey, 2002) and to early onset of substance abuse among African-American children (Wills, Gibbons, Gerrard, & Brody, 2000).

Finally, in a study of family history of psychopathology in families of the offspring of alcoholics, researchers demonstrated that male college student offspring of these families are a heterogeneous group and that the patterns of heterogeneity are related to familial types in relation to vulnerability to alcoholism (Finn et al., 1997). Three different family types were identified:

1. Low levels of family pathology with moderate levels of alcoholism

2. High levels of family antisocial personality and violence with moderate levels of family drug abuse and depression

3. High levels of familial depression, mania, anxiety disorder, and alcoholism with moderate levels of familial drug abuse

Students as a Vulnerable Population

The April 2007 events at Virginia Tech highlighted for the nation that college students face a new kind of threat as the Columbine tragedy did for high school students. Alienated young people who stalk and kill their classmates, for whatever reasons seem reasonable to them, represent a new type of terrorist. However, the literature has not documented the experience of these alienated students, and we have not found effective ways of treating and preventing violent behavior among them.

Some attempts have been made to document types of violence toward students. The American College Health Association recently published a White Paper on the topic (Carr, 2007). The paper was mostly concerned with the frequent types of violence, such as sexual assault, hazing, suicide, celebratory violence, and racial-gender-homosexual violence. Although spree killings are mentioned, not much attention can be given until more is known about these killers.

Some attention has been given to alcohol use and violence. Marcus and Swett (2003) studied precursors to violence among 451 college students at two sites. They used the Violence Risk Assessment tool to establish the relationship of patterns related to gender, peer pressure, and alcohol use. Nicholson, Maney, Blair, Wamboldt, Mahoney, and Yuan (1998) examined the influence of alcohol use in both sexual and nonsexual violence.

A British study on responding to students' mental health needs illustrates how the previously discussed categories of mental illnesses can be exacerbated in the vulnerable population of college students with mental illnesses. Through surveys and focus groups, Stanley and Manthorpe (2001) studied college students with mental illnesses and identified many issues related to the problems of providing care to students. The authors noted high rates of suicide and need for antidepressant medication strained the National Health Service and that colleges varied widely in their ability to provide effective interventions.

Although these studies document some issues related to campus violence, they do not go far enough to explain and prevent the types of spree killings students have experienced in the last decade. The threat of copycats raises continuing fears among students, parents, and teachers. More research is needed on personal characteristics of these young killers, interventions, and prevention strategies.

Conclusion

There is a growing body of literature pertaining to vulnerability as a key factor of concern to practitioners who work with clients with many different kinds of presenting problems. The concept of vulnerability is explored on two levels in that vulnerability is both an individual and a group concept. In public health the group concept is dominant, and intervention is directed toward aggregates. Other practitioners and researchers focus on individual vulnerabilities to specific conditions or diseases.

References

Aday, L. (2001). *At risk in America*. San Francisco: Jossey-Bass.

Aldwin, C., Levensen, M., & Spiro, A. (1994). Vulnerability and resilience to combat exposure: Can stress have lifelong effects? *Psychology and Aging, 9*, 34–44.

Alloy, L., & Clements, C. (1992). Illusion of control invulnerability to negative affect and depressive symptoms after laboratory and natural stressors. *Journal of Abnormal Psychology, 101*, 234–245.

Alloy, L., Whitehouse, W., & Abramson, J. (2000). The Temple-Wisconsin Cognitive Vulnerability to Depression Project: Lifetime history of axis I psychopathology in individuals at high and low cognitive risk for depression. *Journal of Abnormal Psychology, 109,* 403–418.

Becker, M., & Rosenstock, I. (1987). Comparing social learning theory and the health belief model. In W. B. Ward (Ed.), *Advances in health education and promotion* (Vol. 2, pp. 245–249). Greenwich, CT: JAI Press.

Behel, J., Rybarczyk, B., Elliott, T., Nicholas, J., & Nyenhuis, D. (2002). The role of perceived vulnerability in adjustment to lower extremity amputation: A preliminary investigation. *Rehabilitation Psychology, 47*(1), 92–105.

Berenbaum, H., & Fujita, F. (1994). Schizophrenia and personality: Exploring the boundaries and connections between vulnerability and outcome. *Journal of Abnormal Psychology, 103,* 148–158.

Bezruchka, S. (2000). Culture and medicine: Is globalization dangerous to our health? *Western Journal of Medicine, 172,* 332–334.

Bezruchka, S. (2001). Societal hierarchy and the health Olympics. *Canadian Medical Association Journal, 164,* 1701–1703.

Bohner, G., Danner, U., Siebler, F., & Stamson, G. (2002). Rape myth acceptance and judgments of vulnerability to sexual assault: An Internet experiment. *Experimental Psychology, 49,* 257–269.

Bromberger, J., & Mathews, K. (1996). A "feminine" model of vulnerability to depressive symptoms: A longitudinal investigation of middle-aged women. *Journal of Personality and Social Psychology, 70,* 591–598.

Brown, G., Hammen, C., Craske, M., Wickens, T. (1995). Dimensions of dysfunctional attitudes as vulnerabilities to depressive symptoms. *Journal of Abnormal Psychology, 104,* 431–435.

Calvo, M., & Cano-Vindel, A. (1997). The nature of trait anxiety: Cognitive and biological vulnerability. *European Psychologist, 2,* 301–312.

Carr, J. (2007). Campus violence white paper. *Journal of American College Health, 55*(5), 304–319.

Edell-Gustafsson, U., & Hetta, J. (2001). Fragmented sleep and tiredness in males and females one year after percutaneous transluminal coronary angioplasty (PTCA). *Journal of Advanced Nursing, 34*(2), 203–211.

Finn, P., Sharkansky, E., Viken, R., West, T., Sandy, J., & Bufferd, G. (1997). Heterogeneity in the families of sons of alcoholics: The impact of familial vulnerability type on offspring characteristics. *Journal of Abnormal Psychology, 106,* 26–36.

Flaskerud, J., & Lee, P. (2001). Vulnerability to health problems in female informal caregivers of persons with HIV/AIDS and age-related dementias. *Journal of Advanced Nursing, 33*(1), 60–68.

Flaskerud, J., Lesser, J., Dixon, E., Anderson, N., Conde, F., Kim, S., et al. (2002). Health disparities among vulnerable populations: Evolution of knowledge over five decades in *Nursing Research* publications. *Nursing Research, 51*(2), 74–85.

Flaskerud, J., & Winslow, B. (1998). Conceptualizing vulnerable populations in health-related research. *Nursing Research, 47*(2), 69–78.

Gellad, W., Huskamp, H., Phillips, K., & Haas, J. (2006). How the new Medicare drug benefit could affect vulnerable populations. *Health Affairs, 25*(1), 248–255.

Gerrard, M., Gibbons, F., & Bushman, B. (1996). Relation between perceived vulnerability to HIV and precautionary sexual behavior. *Psychological Bulletin, 119,* 390–409.

Hankin, B., & Abramson, L. (2001). Development of gender differences in depression: An elaborated cognitive vulnerability-transactional stress theory. *Psychological Bulletin, 127,* 773–796.

Hayes, A., Castonguay, L., & Goldfried, M. (1996). Effectiveness of targeting the vulnerability factors of depression in cognitive therapy. *Journal of Consulting and Clinical Psychology, 64,* 623–627.

Hofferth, S. (2003). The American family: Changes and challenges for the 21st century. In H. Wallace, G. Green, & K. Jaros (Eds.). *Health and welfare for families in the 21st century*. Sudbury, MA: Jones and Bartlett.

Ingram, R., & Ritter, J. (2000). Vulnerability to depression: Cognitive reactivity and parental bonding in high-risk individuals. *Journal of Abnormal Psychology, 109*, 588–596.

Institute of Medicine-National Academy of Sciences. (2003). *Unequal treatment: Confronting racial and ethnic disparities in health care*. Washington, DC: The National Academies Press.

Joiner, T. (1995). The price of soliciting and receiving negative feedback: Self-verification theory as a vulnerability to depression. *Journal of Abnormal Psychology, 104*, 364–372.

Karpati, A, Galea, S., Awerbuch, T., & Levins, R. (2002). Variability and vulnerability at the ecological level: Implications for understanding the social determinants of health. *American Journal of Public Health, 92*, 1768–1773.

Kelly, J., St. Lawrence, J., & Brasfield, T. (1991). Predictors of vulnerability to AIDS risk behavior relapse. *Journal of Consulting and Clinical Psychology, 59*(1), 163–166.

Kurz, J. M. (2002). Vulnerability of well spouses involved in lung transplantation. *Journal of Family Nursing, 8*, 353–370.

Larkin, H. (2004). Justice implications of a proposed Medicare prescription drug benefit. *Social Work, 49*(3), 406–414.

Leon, G., Fulkerson, J., Perry, C., & Early-Zaid, M. (1995). Prospective analysis of personality and behavioral vulnerabilities and gender influences in the later development of disordered eating. *Journal of Abnormal Psychology, 104*(1), 140–149.

Lessick, M., Woodring, B., Naber, S., & Halstead, L. (1992). Vulnerability: A conceptual model. *Perinatal and Neonatal Nursing, 6*, 1–14.

Lohr, J., & Flynn, K. (1992). Smoking and schizophrenia. *Schizophrenia Research, 8*, 93–102.

Lyons, M., Bar, J., Kremen, W., Toomey, R., Eisen, S., Goldberg, J., et al. (2002). Nicotine and familial vulnerability to schizophrenia: A discordant twin study. *Journal of Abnormal Psychology, 111*, 687–693.

Marcus, R. & Swett, B. (2003). Multiple precursor scenarios: Predicting and reducing campus violence. *Journal of Interpersonal Violence, 18*(5), 553–571.

McIntyre, L., Glanville, N., Raine, K., Dayle, J., Anderson, B., & Battaglia, N. (2003). Do low-income lone mothers compromise their nutrition to feed their children? *Canadian Medical Association Journal, 168*(6), 686–691.

Morrell-Bellai, T., Goering, P., & Boydell, K. (2000). Becoming and remaining homeless: Qualitative investigation. *Issues in Mental Health Nursing, 21*, 581–604.

National Institutes of Health. (n.d.). *Addressing health disparities: The NIH program of action*. Retrieved December 4, 2003, from http://healthdisparities.nih.gov/whatare.html

National Institutes of Health. (2002). *Strategic research plan and budget to reduce and ultimately eliminate health disparities*. Washington, DC: U.S. Department of Health and Human Services.

Nettlebeck, T., Wison, C., Potter, R., & Perry, C. (2000). The influence of interpersonal competence on personal vulnerability of persons with mental retardation. *Journal of Interpersonal Violence, 15*(1), 46–62.

Nicholson, M., Maney, D., Blair, K., Wamboldt, P., Mahoney, B., & Yuan, J. (1998). Trends in alcohol-related campus violence: Implications for prevention. *Journal of Alcohol and Drug Education, 43*(3), 34–52.

Phifer, J. (1990). Psychological distress and somatic symptoms after natural disaster: Differential vulnerability among older adults. *Psychology and Aging, 5*, 412–420.

Ruef, A., Litz, B., & Schlenger, W. (2000). Hispanic ethnicity and risk for combat-related posttraumatic stress disorder. *Cultural Diversity and Ethnic Minority Psychology, 6*(3), 235–251.

Schotte, D., Cools, J., & Payvar, S. (1990). Problem-solving deficits in suicidal patients: Trait vulnerability or state phenomenon? *Journal of Consulting and Clinical Psychology, 58,* 562–564.

Sebastian, J. (1996). Vulnerability and vulnerable populations. In M. Stanhope & J. Lancaster (Eds.), *Community health nursing: Promoting health of individuals, aggregates and communities* (4th ed.). St. Louis, MO: Mosby.

Sebastian, J., Bolla, C. D., Aretakis, D., Jones, K. J., Schenk, C., Napolitano, M., et al. (2002). Vulnerability and selected vulnerable populations. In M. Stanhope & J. Lancaster (Eds.), *Foundations of community health nursing* (pp. 349–364). St. Louis, MO: Mosby.

Shinn, M., Knickman, J., & Weitzman, B. (1991). Social relationships and vulnerability to becoming homeless among poor families. *American Psychologist, 46,* 1180–1187.

Siever, M. (1994). Sexual orientation and gender as factors in socioculturally acquired vulnerability to body dissatisfaction and eating disorders. *Journal of Consulting and Clinical Psychology, 62*(2), 252–260.

Simons, J., & Carey, K. (2002). Risk and vulnerability for marijuana use: Problems and the role of affect dysregulation. *Psychology of Addictive Behaviors, 16*(1), 72–75.

Smith, G., Gerrard, M., & Gibbons, F. (1997). Self-esteem and the relation between risk behavior and perceptions of vulnerability to unplanned pregnancy in college women. *Health Psychology, 16*(2), 137–146.

Spiers, J. (2000). New perspectives on vulnerability using etic and emic approaches. *Journal of Advanced Nursing, 31*(3), 715–721.

Stanley, N., & Manthorpe, J. (2001). Responding to students' mental health needs: Impermeable systems and diverse users. *Journal of Mental Health, 10,* 41–52.

Strauman, T. (1992). Self-guides, autobiographical memory, and anxiety and dysphoria: Toward a cognitive model of vulnerability to emotional distress. *Journal of Abnormal Psychology, 101,* 87–95.

Tarasuk, V. (2003). Low income, welfare and nutritional vulnerability. *Canadian Medical Association Journal, 168,* 709–710.

Testa, M., Livingston, J., & Collins, R. (2000). The role of women's alcohol consumption in evaluation of vulnerability to sexual aggression. *Experimental and Clinical Psychopharmacology, 8*(2), 185–191.

Van Servellen, G., Aguirre, M., Sarna, L., & Brecht, M. (2002). Differential predictors of emotional distress in HIV-infected men and women. *Western Journal of Nursing Research, 24*(1), 49–72.

Whiffen, V. (1988). Vulnerability to post-partum depression: A prospective multivariate study. *Journal of Abnormal Psychology, 97,* 467–474.

Wild, T. C., Hinson, R., Cunningham, J., & Bacchiochi, J. (2001). Perceived vulnerability to alcohol-related harm in young adults: Independent effects of risky alcohol use and drinking motives. *Experimental and Clinical Psychopharmacology, 9,* 1064–1297.

Wills, T. A., Gibbons, F., Gerrard, M., & Brody, G. (2000). Protection and vulnerability processes relevant for early onset of substance use: A test among African American children. *Health Psychology, 19*(3), 253–263.

World Health Organization. (1948). Constitution of the World Health Organization. In *Handbook of basic documents.* Geneva, Switzerland: Author.

Wuerker, A. (2000). The family and schizophrenia. *Issues in Mental Health Nursing, 21,* 127–141.

Zuroff, D., Blatt, S., Bondi, C., & Pilkonis, P. (1999). Vulnerability to depression: Reexamining state dependence and relative stability. *Journal of Abnormal Psychology, 108,* 76–89.

Rethinking Vulnerability

Cathy Michaels and Carol Moffett

In this chapter we rethink vulnerability as a concept for nursing. Vulnerability implies being at risk for change, change that is usually considered negative and driven by threat or inadequate resource. When applied to health, vulnerability is often related to the risk for negative change in health status, such as acquisition of disease. Nurses have historically focused their services on disease and injury as vulnerable conditions. Being at risk for change (i.e., being vulnerable) can be argued as offering capacity for adaptation.

Vulnerability is essential to personal growth and development related to changes in health. Perception of threat or vulnerability can spur physical and behavioral changes that are adaptive in nature, like changing sedentary life-style practices to ward off heart disease. Change can be produced in broad social systems such as global strategies to counteract avian flu. Viewing vulnerability in different ways acknowledges a process with potential for growth and change and thus has meaning for nursing practice.

Vulnerability is dynamic and relates to all entities. All of humanity and all aspects of the globe and even the universe express vulnerability. Perhaps at the human level, vulnerability is most significant in terms of loss of life, with dimensions of disease, and pain, both psychic and physical. A hurricane, for example, overwhelms the levees in New Orleans and large segments of the population are displaced or perish as a result. Genocide is ongoing in the Sudan and a recent memory in Rwanda. A baby is born to a methamphetamine-addicted mother. An obese child grows into an adult with diabetes and heart disease. An adult manifests schizophrenia. Whether the health of individuals and communities is the result of natural disaster, societal conflict, personal choices, or genetic determinants, vulnerability is the common component. The vulnerable in each of these situations are faced with the necessity of coping with life-altering change. Change may involve grieving over lost lives and life-styles or adjusting to relocation or refugee status. Change entails social system activation to adjust to the impact of disaster, genocide, addiction, obesity, chronic mental illness, or health maintenance within the community. All of us are vulnerable, our degree of vulnerability varying with time and circumstance.

Given that we are all part of a process of change and adaptation, our vulnerability is inseparable from the vulnerabilities of others and the global environment.

Nurses are positioned at the interface of vulnerability and change and are involved in every aspect of the process. They respond to vulnerability and change in their clients as well as in themselves to meet the demands of practice and also the demands of being human in the process. Although the social contract for nursing was initially directed toward addressing vulnerability related to illness, this mandate is maturing, along with science, to address vulnerabilities at any phase in the life process whether at the cellular, individual, organizational, community, or global level. Key to this more recent mandate is a shift in professional mindset related to vulnerability, increasingly viewing nursing as not only doing *to or for* but also *being in partnership with*. To explore different ways of thinking about vulnerability in this chapter we

- Discuss vulnerability in a broad context
- Relate vulnerability to the process of growth through change
- Address implications for nursing

Vulnerability Defined

Vulnerability is defined as "susceptibility to physical or emotional injury, susceptibility to attack, open to censure or criticism; assailable, liable to succumb, as to persuasion or temptation" (*American Heritage Dictionary*, 2000, p. 1). Synonymous terms include exposure, liability, openness, and susceptibility (*Roget's II, Thesaurus*, 1995, p. 1). Semantically, the term has a negative connotation. For the purposes of this chapter vulnerability is viewed from the perspective of openness and a dynamism that fluctuates based on multiple factors, including circumstance and environment. Vulnerability is conceptualized as a quality that is ubiquitous and essential, almost visceral in nature. Triggered by change, vulnerability in turn generates demands for additional change and adaptation to respond.

To live, to exist, means to be vulnerable and to be vulnerable requires ongoing change or evolution, even to stay the same. Hillis (2003) described how cultural practices can lead to evolutionary change. Case in point was the *New York Times* editorial that identified how the culture of cattle raising coevolved with the development of a human enzyme in Africans and Europeans to digest milk ("Milk of Evolution," 2006). Evolution is an " improvised dance of transformation in which ecological balance is worked out again and again" (Sahtouris, 1999, p 15), "a process in which the whole universe is a progression of interrelated phenomena, an unfolding, and a change usually in one direction, and often from simpler forms to more complex forms" (*Merriam-Webster's Online Dictionary*, 2005, p. 1). Evolution, for the purposes of this chapter, relates to change and encompasses aspects that are both animate and inanimate.

Vulnerability is a constant but waxes and wanes in relationship to shifts in the environment, whether inevitable or planned. For humans the environment may be external, like losing one's job or experiencing weather shifts, or internal, such as hosting a replicating virus, experiencing the destruction of alveoli in the lungs from a genetic deficiency of a1-antitrypsin, or losing control of one's anger. Changes in health may not be perceptible to the whole person without technology like laboratory tests or mammograms. Other health changes are easily apparent, such as joint deformities related to arthritis.

Our ability to respond to vulnerability varies like our ability to perceive vulnerability. Most central to systemic response is system capacity to manage change. Capacity is based on a multitude of factors or resources present in the internal or external environment. Nursing functions as a force within the external environment. Facilitating informational access, assisting with institutional or community support, and creating caring relationships are a few of many possible nursing actions that impact the environment for health. Systems theory is useful for examining change and for informing response to change.

Systems Theory

Assuming that vulnerability is linked to evolution, both vulnerability and evolution can be understood from a systems perspective. Every system consists of elements interacting and manifesting as a whole (Wikipedia, 2006). Systems theory can explain the interactions of organisms with their environments and the integration of each part into dynamic wholes, even the consideration of the planet as a system. Systems are operational from the cellular and organism level to the community and ultimately to the planet and the solar system (von Bertalanffy, 1968). Complexity theory adds the following: "complex behavior arises from the interrelationship, interaction, and interconnectivity of elements within a system and between a system and its environment. . . . Complex behavior therefore arises from the *intricate inter-twining or inter-connectivity of elements within a system and between a system and its environment*" (Mitleton-Kelly, 2004, p.2). From complexity theory emerges the notion of coevolution, which proposes that any aspect of evolution in a system depends on the evolution of other aspects of the system. This is the result of connectivity and interdependence.

Ideas integral to systems and to complexity (connectedness, interdependence, communication, information, energy, and patterns) are useful to understanding how evolution is triggered by vulnerability. When vulnerability pushes the entity (person or group) "far from equilibrium," change is forced. The process involves an "exploration of the space of possibilities" where a wide variety of alternatives are considered. "Self-organization with the emergence and creation of new order" is the next step in which ideas, relationships, structures, and forms are created and shape further evolutionary processes (Mitleton-Kelly, 2004).

When Hurricane Katrina struck the gulf coast, an entire region became vulnerable. The imminent threat pushed some to evacuate or to seek shelter, whereas others chose for a variety of reasons to stay in place. When the impact of the hurricane and its aftermath were experienced, the region was pushed "far from equilibrium." Hospitals were debilitated and incapable of dealing with a surge in need. The infrastructure of emergency services was also overwhelmed, and the tragedy compounded over several days. A regional disaster became a national disaster. The "space of possibilities" was explored with evacuation of people to a variety of cities where the inhabitants of those cities scrambled to meet the needs of the displaced who moved into their areas. Further exploration of the space of possibilities expanded to long-term housing and the social service needs of refugees. Eventually over time the rebuilding of the devastated region requires further consideration and alternative possibilities for humans as well as the environment. This process is ongoing and will eventually reveal the "creation of a new order," where some of the displaced never return and where those who reside in the region may not entirely resemble those who left. The healthcare infrastructure will also reflect changes as the demands of the region shift. For example, since Hurricane Katrina hit New Orleans the birth of Latino babies has dramatically increased. In a city characteristically known by black and white, Latino babies change the demographic mix (Porter, 2004) while requiring a shift in cultural and linguistic access to health services.

For a system to evolve and adapt in the face of vulnerability requires the processing and exchange of information. Information contained within energy and matter is exchanged with all aspects of the system and environment through the establishment of connections (networks) (Barbasi, 2003; Morgan, 1997; Schwartz & Russek, 1999). This information is operational from cellular to societal levels and allows for the system to adapt. Often systems are not skilled at interpreting information regarding extreme threat or in the initial assault phase. This was evident in Hurricane Katrina, when segments of the community did not evacuate and the emergency response was mired in chaos. Disasters of all types expose vulnerability, whether economic, physical, emotional, or a combination. The system must respond, but often the response is inefficient. Available information may be misinterpreted or poorly utilized. The success of response is reliant on the speed with which the system can adapt to change. Shifts in perspective or perceptions may be required to maximize the value of information for adaptation. "Adaptability is defined as the use of information to handle environmental uncertainty" (Miller & Miller, 1992, p. 4). Systems that are capable of maximizing the use of informational energy are most likely to survive and thrive (Miller & Miller, 1992). Systems, which seek to maintain status quo, encourage entropy, and this is ultimately the death of the system.

Health care is a service delivered within systems and participates in the environment where humans cope with vulnerability related to health. Health care and the environment interact through the provision of services (flow of energy). Health care is delivered within systems that are vulnerable to changing environments. For example, long-standing hospitals closed, never to reopen, and triage centers were established in tents when Katrina altered the New Orleans environment. In the United States the increasing numbers of uninsured caused a few hospital systems to begin offering free preventive care to the chronically ill in their communities. This strategy was intended to divert care into the less expensive prevention services and away from the expensive emergency care (Ekholm, 2006). The hospital system perceived an increasing threat to their bottom line, which made them vulnerable. Their solution may only temporarily avert the crisis of inadequate resources to meet the healthcare demand, but it has allowed for survival until alternative strategies are developed. For any system to achieve sustainability, informational energy must be evaluated on a continuous basis and the system must adapt to changes in the environment, in this case the burden of the uninsured.

Information and Systems

System behavior is a response to information. Humans, and human systems, experiencing vulnerability interpret information within the context of belief structures framed in a cultural context. Several authors have provided insight into how information is interpreted. Jung (1953–1978) addressed how information is exchanged between conscious thinking and unconscious or psychic process through psychological symbols called archetypes. The tree, for example, is universally recognized as a symbol of life. Archetypes are biologically based and allow people everywhere to express the universality of life through similar thoughts, mythologies, feelings, and patterns of behavior. Archetypes serve the very important purpose of allowing a connection between humans from very diverse cultures; they also carry "genetically transmitted response strategies" (Stevens, 1993, p. 26). This would seem to imply that strategies needed to survive and respond to vulnerability are a part of our DNA.

Archetypes are rich sources of information for ritual. Van Gennep (1909 as cited in O'Neill, 2005) explored rituals of transition, specifically rituals associated with the vulnerability of transitional life events, such as birth and significant maturational transitions of adolescence, adulthood, and marriage (O'Neil, 2005). Cultural life-styles that use rituals or rites serve an essential adaptive function, facilitating the necessary evolutionary process and a shared world view that strengthens the connection of the individual to the group. In the face of uncertainty or danger the collective offers more protection than does a single individual. In systems terms, the whole is more than the sum of its parts, that is, the whole is more than the sum of the individuals in the cultural group.

Conscious thought, as influenced by the archetypes of psychic processes, is at the root of world views and perspectives that are passed back and forth as reality, between people and groups. Bohm (1992) theorized that conscious thought has evolved, in particular with the growth of civilization. Thought is imbedded in ideologies and societal behaviors. He gave an example related to stereotypical thought in which being English and taught that the French are not to be trusted then becomes the logic for many intolerant actions.

Bohm viewed thought as fragmentary in nature, considering only the part and not the whole. Through this fragmentation thought can generate incoherence as well as habitual behavior as it attempts to bring order to incoherence. Thought based on partial information or rigid rules of conformity hobbles possible responses to vulnerability. An example of the limitation of thought is the failure of polio eradication efforts in Nigeria at the beginning of the 21st century. Religious leaders essentially shut down immunization efforts by spreading fear that the vaccine would sterilize children and spread HIV. As a result polio spread throughout Africa (Donnelly, 2004).

Thought that encourages rigid conformity and habitual behavior can be opened up with "thinking," the "exploration of the space of possibilities" as discussed previously. Bohm (1992) theorized that thinking is a process that occurs in the present tense and is best accessed through open dialogue between four or more people. In dialogue, thinking is catalyzed in the process of presenting and responding to the diversity of perspectives offered by members of the dialogue group.

For the nurse to interact successfully with vulnerability requires the ability to use the protective strengthening aspects of culture when appropriate and to identify the limitations imposed by structured thoughts or conforming beliefs that limit envisioning opportunities. Balancing the protective strength and limitations of culture requires great insight and skill. For nurses, fragmentary thought developed as ideologies complicates the environment of care. The nurses and the clients they serve may be committed to ideologies that limit possibilities for adaptation and thus limit response to vulnerability. This implies that thinking that is open to growth and inclusion can ultimately promote a variety of response opportunities. Thinking is an important resource in environments of change (Mitleton-Kelly, 2004).

Health as Expanding Consciousness

Nursing theorist Margaret Newman (1979) conceptualized health as expanding consciousness, a framework that can be considered in terms of Jung's theory of psychic processing as well as systems theory. Newman viewed humans as "Open energy systems; In continual interconnectedness with a universe of open systems (environment); Continuously active in evolving their own pattern of the whole (health); Intuitive as well as affective and cognitive beings; Capable of abstract thinking as well as sensation; More than the sum of their parts." Although Newman does not explicitly identify the unconscious, she does speak to intuiting, feeling, and thinking. Moreover, she does address the connectedness between the conscious and the unconscious by referencing continual activity in evolving their own pattern (Newman, 1979, p. 6 as cited in George, 1995, p. 393).

According to Jung's theory growth begins with a tension of the opposites, one side representing one perspective and the other side, a conflicting perspective. If the individual can tolerate the tension between the two opposites, the inherent goal of the psychic processes is to come up with a new perspective that reflects both opposites. Take, for example, the issue of becoming familiar with and accustomed to a new diagnosis of diabetes. At one end of the continuum is the self-image of a person without diabetes and at the other end, a self-image whose body has lost the ability to automatically control blood sugar. After grappling with this tension of the opposites, the person may reject thinking of self as a "diabetic" or as "normal" but accept thinking of self as a person who has diabetes. Even more difficult is a new diagnosis of metastatic cancer. The tension of the opposites is literally life and death. Through Newman's concept of health as expanding consciousness, the nurse is guided to facilitate the individual in discovering his or her own pattern, to reach the psychic point in which a new and synthesized perspective reflects both life and death. For example, an individual can discover that he or she has lived a full life and can die peacefully. Another individual can come to the realization that he or she will seek all treatment to continue living. The overall pattern is individually unique but influenced by culture and universal dynamics of living. The nurse can gently facilitate awareness of vulnerability related to illness and death and use storytelling, humor, and metaphor to engage the individual's imagination in responding to vulnerability. With this professional nursing support, the individual can respond to death and dying on his or her own terms rather than feeling tossed around by nature.

Interdependence is the foundation for the elements of systems and achieved through the sharing of informational energy. Through the process of sharing information, the system as a whole is created and maintained. The quality of this information and the system's response to it also affects the ability of the whole to meet demands for change and evolution. Jung theorized the system of psychic processes, and Newman conceptualized the process of understanding wholeness of health. In both systems an environmental challenge marks the initial point of vulnerability, a shift in archetypal energy, and a change in pattern. Vulnerability allows for openness to informational energy and growth or integration of the new information is the response. Rethinking vulnerability in this way has tremendous relevance for nursing.

Relevance for Nursing

Nurses encounter vulnerability at all levels (cellular, physiological systems, mind–body, individuals, communities, and societies). Vulnerability is not a license for the nurse to rescue; it is rather an opportunity to encourage growth. In the encounter, nurses can increase relevance in their practice by interacting and responding to human experience of vulnerability as a dynamic and complex process. That is not to say that nurses accept factors like poverty and disease for any individual or group. Nurses can, however, acknowledge both positive and negative factors that are associated with vulnerability and accept vulnerability as inherent to living life and an opening to change that defines individuals and groups. In confronting vulnerability nurses act from acquired skills, available resources, and ultimately on their perspectives and world views related to the vulnerability confronted. This process is facilitated through self-reflection, what Freire (1972) calls praxis or "action in being." Derrida emphasized the importance of a range of perspectives in the reflective process: "It is necessary to recognize the unavoidable limitations and inherent contradictions in the ideas and norms that guide our actions, and do so in a way that keeps them open to constant questioning and continual revision . . ." (Taylor, 2004, p. 8). If vulnerability is conceptualized as an inescapable process, ensconced in tragedy and disparity, nurses could become mired in futility and hopelessness. Alternatively, a rethinking of vulnerability as neutral offers the opportunity for nurses to be in partnership with an adaptive evolutionary process in which an array of possibilities can be envisioned.

Nurses who have a clear grasp of the evolutionary and adaptive perspective understand the ongoing requirement that to live requires change. Change can be driven by internal instructions generated by genetically encoded instructions or mutations, as well as by environmental factors. As described in an educated public discourse, "The interaction of each individual's environmental experience with her/his genome leads to that person's identity" (McCabe & McCabe, 2004, p. 13). Through the explosion of genomics knowledge, there is opportunity for great strides in prevention and treatment options. Nurses are mandated to evolve their body of knowledge and to translate applied scientific data into the practice environment. The environment of encounter includes the biosphere, the psychosociocultural milieu, the world of policy, and technological advancement.

Evolution is informed by systems theory, a familiar theory in nursing. Through understanding that there is an interaction of organisms and that each part is integrated into ever larger dynamic wholes, nurses can perceive vulnerability within a living system context that reflects theories aligned with open systems, such as chaos and complexity theory. Information is essential to maintaining system structures and functions. How that information is conveyed, decoded, and encoded defines the relationships of the parts to the whole. Nurses are enmeshed in life systems and the smaller organizational systems within which they practice. Information management drives their relationships within the practice environment. Access to high-quality appropriate and timely information improves the system's ability to adapt to changes and to respond to vulnerability. System thinking also provides an understanding that change, no matter how small, forces change to the entire system. At a cellular level, for example, change in pancreatic cells can mean diabetes, a disease that redefines a way of living for an individual and family and impacts individual productivity and workplace policies.

The new level of systems thinking, represented by the holosphere, is not as familiar to nursing. This new systems level thinking addresses what Bohm referred to as the connectedness of *matter* and *spirit*, integrated wholes not unlike the hologram, which even when fragmented continue to represent the whole. Integrative medicine addresses this as *mind–body*, and as one example, mounting evidence points to the impact of stress on the immune system and aging. Epel and Blackburn, from the University of California at San Francisco, reported that mothers who provide care for their chronically ill children show evidence of biological aging many years beyond their chronological age, as evidenced by DNA analysis of their white blood cells (Epel & Blackburn cited in Carey, 2004). This has meaning for self-care among nurses and may underlie the popular term "burn-out." Nurses function in roles often steeped with environmental stressors in the provision of care. For nurses to maintain their own health, environments must nurture the nurse as caregiver to maintain the integrity of the system.

Most of nursing is practiced within health systems. Nursing as a profession must not only create and use emerging science but also must adapt to the manner in which the science is made acceptable and understood at the societal level. Vulnerability is generally addressed from an epidemiological perspective of vulnerable populations and health disparity, and health disparities that heighten vulnerability have come to dominate the professional dialogue. Nurses are positioned to facilitate growth in several ways. There are many possibilities for adaptation if thought can be expanded and revised as better information becomes available. Nurses are integral to this process by clarifying information (improving) and facilitating (sharing) access to information for patients and using that information personally and professionally themselves. As described below, this experience of a nurse case manager reflects "tension of the opposites," "information provided through presence," "statements of trust," and "scientific detail":

> I have found that people tend to know their own answers, once they begin to sort out all of who they are today from who they used to be. My trust in their self-knowing engenders self-trust. Certainly, my scientific expertise helps in many situations related to symptom control and the like, but the toughest and most central issues are how to live life given change related to illness, aging, or a turn of events. And, it is those central issues that affect us both; our mutual dialogue facilitates both of us knowing each other and ourselves with growing awareness. There is, in fact, no difference between the mentor and the mentee (personal notes, 1998).

Nursing is enriched by information related to human evolutionary processes over time. This information gives context to evolutionary processes they constantly encounter.

Conclusion

This chapter presents vulnerability as a concept with both positive and negative connotations. Vulnerability was initially presented from the perspective of its importance in allowing change and evolution to occur. Theories of evolution and systems bolster this perspective by noting the adaptation requirements of a living open system. These theories emphasize the importance of interdependence and connectivity as integral to the process of change and evolution in response to alterations in any part of a system.

Individual circumstances may be aligned with heightened and prolonged vulnerability, for example, vulnerability related to poverty. From evolutionary and systems perspectives the creation of effective mechanisms to address the needs of the most at-risk groups is important not only to those at risk but also to the larger society where vulnerability waxes and wanes. The systems perspective allows for an understanding that meeting the needs of the most vulnerable also helps those who are least vulnerable, assuming that holographically a change in one element results in change to the entire system. Honing approaches and techniques to vulnerability among those at greatest risk may improve the outcomes for all. The informational energy of the entire system is allowed to evolve to a higher level of complexity. Nursing is integral to addressing the issues of vulnerability and creating the mechanisms, related to health, that allow for this evolution.

References

The American Heritage dictionary of the English language (4th ed.). (2000). Retrieved July 17, 2007, from http://www.bartleby.com/61/46/V0154600.html

Barbasi, A. (2003). *Linked*. Cambridge, MA: Perseus.

Bohm, D. (1992). *Thought as a system*. New York: Routledge.

Carey, B. (2004, November 30). Too much stress may give genes gray hair. *New York Times*. Retrieved July 17, 2007, from http://www.nytimes.com/2004/11/30/health/30age.html

Donnelly, J. (2004). Africa polio outbreak-feared: Officials blame vaccination refusal by Nigerian state. *Boston Globe*. Retrieved July 17, 2007, from http://www.boston.com/news/world/articles/2004/06/23/africa_polio_outbreak_feared/

Ekholm, E. (10/25/2006). Hospitals try free basic care for uninsured. *New York Times online*. Retrieved October 25, 2006, from http://www.nytimes.com/2006/10/25/health/25insure.html?ex=1166677200&en=70f83c7baabfd8c3&ei=5070

Freire, P. (1972). *The pedagogy of the oppressed*. London: Sheed & Ward.

George, J. (1995). *Nursing theories: The base for professional nursing practice*. Norwalk, CT: Appleton & Lange.

Hillis, D.(2003). *Tree of life*. Retrieved August 22, 2007, from http://www.zo.utexas.edu/faculty/antisense/DownloadfilesToL.html

Jung, C. (1953–1978). *The collected works of C. G. Jung*. London: Routledge and Paul Kegan.

McCabe, E., & McCabe, L. (2004). Act II. *UCLA Magazine*.

Merriam-Webster's online dictionary. (2005). Retrieved July 17, 2007, from http://www.m-w.com/dictionary/evolution

The milk of evolution. (2006, December, 14). *New York Times online*. Retrieved December 14, 2006, from http://www.nytimes.com/2006/12/14/opinion/14thu4.html?pagewanted=all

Miller, J. G., & Miller, J. L. (1992). *Applications of living systems theory*. Retrieved July 17, 2007, from http://www.newciv.org/ISSS_Primer/asem05jm.html

Mitleton-Kelly, E. (2004). *Complexity and information systems*. Retrieved July 17, 2007, from http://www.psych.lse.ac.uk/complexity/ICoSS/Papers/ComplexityandInfoSystems.pdf

Morgan, G. (1997). *Images of organizations*. Thousand Oaks, CA: Sage.

Newman, M. (1979). *Theory development in nursing*. Philadelphia: F. A. Davis.

O'Neil, D., (2005). *Rites of passage*. Retrieved August 22, 2007, from http://anthro.palomar.edu/social/soc_4.htm

Porter, E. (12/11/2004). Katrina begets a baby boom by immigrants. *New York Times online*. Retrieved December 11, 2006, from http://www.nytimes.com/2006/12/11/us/nationalspecial/11babies.html?ex=1166677200&en=431b542013793236&ei=5070

Roget's II: The new thesaurus (3rd ed.). (1995). Retrieved August 22, 2007, from http://www.bartleby.com/62/11/V1681100.html

Sahtouris, E. (1999). *Evidence of evolution. Earthdance: Living systems in evolution*. Retrieved August 22, 2007, from http://www.ratical.org/LifeWeb/Erthdnce/chapter7.html

Schwartz, G., & Russek, L. (1999). *The living energy universe*. Charlottesville, VA: Hampton Roads Publishing.

Stevens, A. (1993). *The two-million-year-old self*. New York: International Publishing.

Talbot, M. (1991) *The holographic universe*. New York: HarperCollins.

Taylor, M. (2004). What Derrida really meant. *University of Chicago Press online*. Retrieved August 22, 2007, from http://www.press.uchicago.edu/books/derrida/taylorderrida.html

von Bertalanffy, L. (1968). *General systems theory*. New York: George Braziller Inc.

Wikipedia. (2006). *Systems theory*. Retrieved July 17, 2007, from http://en.wikipedia.org/wiki/Systems_theory

Chapter 3

Cultural Competence, Resilience, and Advocacy

Mary de Chesnay, Rebecca W. Peil, and Christopher Pamp

The purpose of this chapter is to provide several key concepts particularly useful in caring for people who are vulnerable. Cultural competence is a way of providing care that takes into account cultural differences between the nurse and patient while meeting the health needs of the patient. Resilience is both a characteristic and a desired outcome. Resilience is understood as the capacity for transcending obstacles, present to some degree in all human beings. A goal of nursing is to enhance resilience. Advocacy is presented as a way to take cultural competence to a level beyond the nurse–patient relationship by serving as the patient's surrogate when the patient is incapacitated. The central idea of the chapter is that these three concepts relate in specific ways that enable nurses to frame care within a cultural context, not just for vulnerable populations but for all clients.

Cultural Competence

Cultural competence is a way of practicing one's profession by being sensitive to the differences in cultures of one's constituents and acting in a way that is respectful of the client's values and traditions while performing those activities or procedures necessary for the client's well-being. In nursing, the outcomes are positive changes in health status or life-style changes expected to prevent disease. A social justice view of cultural competence should take into account what Hall (Hall, 1999; Hall, Stevens, & Meleis, 1994) described as marginalization. Marginalized people experience discrimination, poor access to health care, and resultant illnesses and traumas from environmental dangers or violence that make them vulnerable to a wide range of health problems. Culturally competent practitioners, then, would seem to concern themselves not only with superficial skills of learning about other cultures but would view marginalized patients within a wider system context and intervene within that context.

Historically, nursing has moved from a view of cultural sensitivity (focus on awareness) to one of cultural competence (focus on behavior). That is to say that nurses aspire to cultural competence not because the concept is trendy or politically correct as described by Poole (1998), but because nurses are pragmatists who understand that recognizing cultural differences enables them to act with patients and their families in ways that enable them to heal.

Zoucha (2001) urged that we put aside deep-seated feelings of ethnocentrism and accept the value that every health world view is equally valid. Locsin (2000) proposed that cultural blurring might be a technique that bridges the gaps in cultural differences by enabling the practitioner to merge the best of both worlds. Cultural competence then becomes a practice with broad appeal in all the service professions. Teachers, social workers, and physicians understand the usefulness of the concept as not just politically correct but good practice (Bonder, Martin, & Miracle, 2001; Dana & Matheson, 1992; Gutierrez & Alvarez, 1996; Leavitt, 2003; Sutton, 2000).

Models of Cultural Competence

As an exciting theoretical development in nursing, several models have been developed to explore the dimensions of cultural competence. In reference to community health nursing, Kim-Godwin, Clarke, and Barton (2001) constructed a model derived from concept analysis that focuses on the relationship between cultural competence and health outcomes for diverse populations. They suggested that the four dimensions of cultural competence are caring, cultural sensitivity, cultural knowledge, and cultural skills. They developed a cultural competence scale that measures all dimensions except caring. Items include affective and cognitive domains. The authors tested the scale in a sample of 192 senior undergraduate and graduate nursing students and found factors that loaded on two dimensions, sensitivity and skill, explaining 72% of the variance and providing evidence of construct validity.

A second model portrayed cultural competence as a process in which the healthcare provider integrates cultural awareness, cultural knowledge, cultural skill, cultural encounters, and cultural desire (Campinha-Bacote, 2002). This model assumes variation within groups and between groups, an important distinction for those who would treat members of ethnic groups as if they are exactly like everyone else within their group, thereby constructing new stereotypes instead of developing cultural knowledge. Campinha-Bacote (2003, 2005) updated her model to elaborate on several of the key concepts and to suggest the relevance of cultural competence to Christianity and moral reasoning.

Taking a different direction, Purnell (2000, 2002) and Purnell and Paulanka (2003) integrated the concepts of biocultural ecology and workforce issues into his model for cultural competence. Purnell asserted that healthcare providers and recipients of care have a mutual obligation to share information to obtain beneficial outcomes. In this sense the patient is a teacher of culture as well as a client of the provider and the provider becomes a teacher of the culture of health care. Derived from many disciplines and including many domains, the Purnell model might be seen as a diagram encompassing the patient within a series of concentric circles that include family, community, and global society.

A third view of cultural competence is that existing models are insufficient and the term itself is limiting. Wells (2000) argued for extending the concept of cultural competence into *cultural proficiency*. Wells claimed that cultural competence is not adequate and that proficiency is a higher order concept than competence for institutions in that proficiency indicates mastery of a complex set of skills. The process of moving toward proficiency has barriers that are both affective and cognitive. The most serious barrier is the unwillingness to examine one's own assumptions about those who are different from oneself. Wells would say that the most effective way to develop cultural proficiency is to maintain an open attitude and interact with people who are different from oneself, allowing them to become teachers or coaches.

Except for Leininger's (1970, 1995) extensive work, most of the nursing theories do not include cultural competence because they were published long before its emergence as a major concept for nursing. The application of several of the nursing theories to caring for vulnerable populations is discussed elsewhere in Unit II of this book. However, Watson's theory of caring deserves special note. In a theoretical review of Watson's theory, Mendycka (2000) explored the relationship of culture and care, providing a clinical example of how the nurse and patient become more human through their interaction. In his description of a sample case of an American Indian who is HIV positive, Mendycka showed how a nurse practitioner trying to treat the patient with a traditional Western medical approach comes into conflict with the patient's cultural belief system. On one hand, the nurse wants to see the patient more often and suggests pharmacotherapy to prevent full-blown AIDS. On the other, the patient wants to use the healing practices of his tribe: sweat baths, herbs, and prayer. Unless the nurse practitioner can find a way to work with the tribe's medicine man, she is doomed to failure because the patient will place his own cultural belief system above the uncertainties of Western medical practice.

Other authors have recognized the need for institutional change to develop culturally competent models of intervention for the populations served by diverse providers. Home care nurses manage cultural issues with patients (DiCicco-Bloom & Cohen, 2003). Andrews (1998) applied the process of developing cultural competence to administration in an assessment process leading to organizational change in cultural competence. Holistic nursing, which views patients within contexts, has cultural competence as a core value. However, in a review of the concept in the holistic nursing literature, Barnes, Craig, and Chambers (2000) found that only 9.6% of the abstracts made reference to concepts of culture or ethnicity and the authors raised the question as to whether the sample sizes were large enough to address cultural differences or whether the researchers lacked awareness. Finally, authors in psychiatric nursing (Craig, 1999; Kennedy, 1999) and oncology (Kagawa-Singer, 2000) addressed the need for practitioners to develop cultural competence at both an individual and institutional level.

Learning Cultural Competence

Many methods and ideas for developing cultural competence are available in the literature, but there is general agreement that cultural competence happens on affective, cognitive, and behavioral levels and that self-awareness is a critical indicator of success. Campinha-Bacote (2006) suggests that standardization of nursing curricula might be effective.

Simulation activities provide a setting in which participants can practice communication and problem solving as well as develop self-awareness (Meltzof & Lenssen, 2000). Cross-cultural communication exercises for physicians can help develop the skills needed to overcome barriers (Shapiro, Hollingshead, & Morrison, 2002).

Immersion programs are powerful learning experiences at all levels because they enable one to experience different cultures out of one's usual safe context. Immersion programs are probably the best way, although they are costly and time consuming. There are several examples in the Teaching–Learning unit in this book, which also explores in detail how undergraduate students and graduate nursing students can conduct fieldwork that leads to cultural competence. One example of an immersion program used in nutrition studies is a food travel course in which participants learn diverse dietetic preferences and practices (Kuczmarski & Cole, 1999). Another example is a population-based program with the Hutterites of the United States and Canada (Fahrenwald, Boysen, Fischer, & Maurer, 2001).

Didactic materials can be prepared for developing knowledge about groups and are a useful point of reference for practitioners who are under enormous pressure to function with diverse patients in high-acuity settings. An innovative program at the University of Washington used action research as the basis for developing culture clues, which are documents that enable practitioners to see at a glance the dominant preferences of the diverse cultural groups served by the hospital. The documents cover perception of illness, patterns of kinship and decision making, and comfort with touch and were written for a variety of cultures, including Korean, Russian, Latino, Albanian, Vietnamese, and African-American (Abbot et al., 2002).

The didactic approach was also used in Sweden, a country that is becoming more diverse as immigration increases, largely from Eastern Europe and Iraq. The researchers used Leininger's theory to guide development of a curriculum for undergraduate nursing students with specific content areas at all levels (Gebru & Willman, 2003).

Didactic programs are easier and less costly to operate than immersion programs, perhaps because cognitive outcomes are easier to measure than affective outcomes. In a multicultural training course for counseling students, outcomes included development of multicultural knowledge and skill and increased comfort with discussing differing world views, but the program was less successful at getting participants to examine themselves as racial–cultural beings (Tomlinson-Clark, 2000).

Resilience

Resilience has been defined as "the process of adapting well in the face of adversity, trauma, tragedy, or even significant sources of stress such as family and relationship problems, or workplace and financial stressors" (Newman, 2003, p. 42). Other descriptions include "the ability to 'bounce back' in spite of significant stress or adversity" (Place, Reynolds, Cousins, O'Neill, 2002, p. 162) and "spring back" (Place et al., 2002, p. 162). Hope is essential for resilience to exist (Perry, 2002a, 2002b). Resilience is a concept that has been researched in both in qualitative and quantitative studies—across cultures and in many contexts. Frameworks have been developed and campaigns have been launched to help boost this concept of "bouncing back." A common theme in the literature is shifting negatives to positives, that is, figuring out how to rebound from adversity.

The concept of increasing resilience through good coping skills has been researched thoroughly in recent years. Topics include prevention of physical injuries among high school athletes through social support (Smith, Smoll, & Ptacek, 1990), factors that help children overcome the death of a parent (Greeff & Human, 2004), resilience in people with psychiatric disabilities and abuse (Deegan, 2005; Iwaniek, 2006), promoting resilience in asylum seekers (Procter, 2006), and work with military personnel (King, 2006) and the orphans of Quebec (Stein, 2006). In a comprehensive literature review, Bellin and Kovacs (2006) documented a growing body of literature and attention to the problems faced by siblings of children with chronic health problems.

A newly developed family resilience framework encourages a shift from focus on family deficits to family challenges, placing an emphasis on growth from adversity toward hope and strengthened family bonds. This framework utilizes three areas of family resilience: family belief systems, organizational patterns, and communication and problem solving (Walsh, 2003). Newman (2003) describes "The Road to Resilience," a multimedia campaign launched in August 2002 by the American Psychological Association to help Americans bounce back from significant life stressors, hardships, threats, and uncertainty. Its messages focus on the principles that resilience is a journey rather than a single event, each journey is individual, and resilience can be learned by almost anyone (Newman, 2003).

Much current research focuses on the resilience of children—factors that contribute to their resilience and programs that help them to overcome adversity. Though children are not born resilient, many factors contribute to its mastery or lack thereof, including temperament, attentive caregiving, healthy attachments, and opportunities to practice resilience using small stressors that promote flexibility (Perry, 2002a, 2002b). A current intervention program seeks to increase mental health resilience among children of depressed parents by providing them with educational sessions, community resources, and personal skill development (Place et al., 2002). Among victims of childhood cancers, the concept of uncertainty has traditionally been published with reference to its adverse effects (Parry, 2003). However, Parry (2003) found that uncertainty can also foster the development of confidence and resilience, among other positive effects.

Factors that contribute to resilience after the loss of a parent include intrafamilial emotional and practical support, internal strength of the family unit, support from extended family and friends, religious and spiritual beliefs and activities, and individual personality traits such as optimism (Greeff & Human, 2004). Similarly, a study of persons with chronic disabilities found that social support, perseverance, determination, and spiritual beliefs all were protective factors in creating turning points. These factors, along with processes such as transcendence (replacing loss with gain), accommodating (deciding to relinquish), and self-understanding, served to help persons with disabilities gain meaning in their lives (King et al., 2003). Resilience is a key concept in the idea of transformative aging, which emphasizes the importance of transcending the loss, pain, and uncertainty of growing older to create wholeness out of a fragmented life (Walker, 2002). Walker (2002) found that healthcare needs may be better met when mature adults are able to come to a point of "self-transcendence," wherein they have mastered their stress, and also found that women acknowledge and come to terms with their stressors more effectively than men.

Similar factors are found to contribute to resilience across cultural and national boundaries. In a study of several young survivors of the Ethiopian famine of 1984–1985, significant resilience factors were found to be faith and hope, having memories of one's roots, and having a living relative. Not surprisingly, the authors also found that after surviving such horrendous circumstances during childhood, these young adults struggled with depression and anxiety, alternating between hope and depression, dreams and fears (Lothe & Heggen, 2003). A stress-coping model of Native women's health focuses on the moderators of identity, enculturation, spiritual coping, and traditional healing (Walters & Simoni, 2002). Within the U.S. Latino youth population, researchers have described the cultural–community factors of family, *respeto* (respect for the authority of elders), and *personalismo* (the value of relationships for their own merit) as resilience factors against community violence (Clauss-Ehlers & Levi, 2002). An examination highlights the positive influences of farming communities on children, such as family cohesion, being raised by satisfied married couples, participation in community activities, and extended family networks nearby (Larson & Dearmont, 2002).

In a series of semistructured interviews conducted by Peil with a woman who was widowed in her thirties, one may gain further insight into the concept of resilience after the death of a spouse. Nora (not her real name) is a white woman in her early fifties who, after being widowed approximately 15 years ago, has gone on to counsel others who have also suffered the death of partners. These interviews were part of a larger study on success, reported in the first edition of this book (de Chesnay, 2005).

Although Nora does not explicitly mention resilience in her interviews, she does elaborate extensively on the factors that have helped her "successfully overcome grief," which she defines as "the ability to move through the intense part of the pain . . . coping with the situation until the point at which . . . I reinvested in life. . . . Success would mean living a full life again, or having a life that felt . . . full and whole. I'm not living in the pain anymore. I'm happy in my life. I'm fulfilled." Nora's view corresponds well to the following: "to adapt successfully despite the presence of significant adversity" (Place et al., 2002).

Nora credits a wide variety of supports as those that helped her in overcoming her own grief: "I feel like my therapist saved my life. . . . I mean, of course I would've but I didn't—I feel like I couldn't have. . . . I can't even imagine doing it without a support group. . . . I had a wonderful group of friends. . . . I couldn't have gotten through it without them either . . . and I couldn't have gotten through it without [my husband's] family. . . . I could *never* have gotten through without my sense of humor." At least as important as the support of other people, Nora emphasizes spirituality—in a broad sense—as among the most important factors that help widows overcome the death of a spouse. She views spirituality as the belief that, "There's something more than just chaos . . . something greater than just us as individuals. You can see that something greater if two people come together . . . caring about each other or extending love." Spirituality is "people caring about other people. It's loving each other." Many authors have cited the support factors of family, friends, and spirituality, all of which Nora credits for her resilience (Clauss-Ehlers & Levi, 2002; Greeff & Human, 2004; Larson & Dearmont, 2002; Walters & Simoni, 2002).

No matter what the obstacle, protective factors such as social support, spirituality, and effective individual coping mechanisms are factors that increase resilience among people. The implications for nursing are to help clients shift their focus from despair to hope when confronting adversity and, in so doing, develop inner strength.

Advocacy and Advanced Practice Nursing

The focus of this section is primarily concerned with how nurses advocate for their patients in clinical practice and how that might change as they transition into the advanced practice role. A great deal of recent literature, much of it from the United Kingdom, has challenged many of the traditional assumptions of advocacy as an intrinsic part of "the moral art of nursing" (Hewitt, 2002; Mallik, 1997; Willard, 1996). In contrast, there is a paucity of research that examines patient advocacy in advanced practice nursing. However, a key study by Donnelly (2007) used a phenomenological–hermeneutics approach to investigate the essence of advanced nursing practice and found that advocacy emerged as a critical theme.

Emergence of Nursing Advocacy

In the nursing profession's formative years, nursing training was modeled on military training in which there was complete obedience to the physician that ultimately over-arched the interests of the patient (Bernal, 1992; Nelson, 1988; Yarling & McElmurry, 1986). However, as nursing evolved and developed a theoretical base, advocating for patients came to be considered a fundamental and integral part of nursing (Ball, 2006; Mawdsley & Northway, 2007; Nelson, 1988; Newson, 2007; Partin, 2006). The concepts of advocacy, accountability, cooperation, and caring are considered moral and ethical foundations of nursing (Fry, 2001). Accordingly, the American Nurses Association's (2001) *Code of Ethics for Nurses With Interpretive Statements* delineates several advocacy duties of nurses, including protecting the patient's right to self-determination.

As nursing began to distinguish itself from medicine as being more about caring than curing and as having a unique nurse–patient relationship, several theories of nursing advocacy emerged (Mallik, 1997). Gadow (1980) proposed in her theory of existential advocacy that the nurse was "in the ideal position among health providers to experience the patient as a unique human being with individual strengths and complexities—a precondition for advocacy" (p. 81). From this unique position, nurses were enjoined to assist patients in "authentically" exercising their right of self-determination in making healthcare decisions. Curtain (1979) embedded advocacy within the moral art of nursing where advocacy evolves from the shared vulnerability, experience, and humanity of the nurse–patient relationship. Kohnke (1982) defined the role of the nurse advocate as simply to inform the patient and then support whatever decision he or she makes. To better inform the patient. Kohnke's theory of advocacy describes a framework of 10 intersecting areas of knowledge that, taken together, form a "gestalt" for nursing advocacy.

Evidence that nursing students apply the principles of advocacy was reported in a New Zealand study in which fourth-semester nursing students wrote a two-part essay reflecting on their experiences in the previous clinical rotation. Their poignant examples of moral situations demonstrate their deep commitment to their patients' well-being (Beckett, Gilbertson, & Greenwood, 2007).

Reexamination of Advocacy

Recently, critics have argued that many pitfalls exist in the moral concept of nursing advocacy, not the least of which is the danger of paternalism or imposing on patients' autonomy (Melia, 1994). Many assumptions have been challenged: Are nurses uniquely positioned to advocate when other healthcare professionals such as physicians and social workers also have a fiduciary responsibility to the patient (Hyland, 2002)? Do nurses have the autonomy and power to effectively advocate for patients within the healthcare system (Hewitt, 2002; Hyland, 2002; Yarling & McElmurry, 1986)? Is advocacy even possible in today's healthcare environment of short hospital stays, nursing shortages, and nonexistent institutional rewards for performing advocacy (Hamric, 2000)?

Another criticism of advocacy is that it has not been operationalized as a concept and therefore few empirical studies of the role have been done. Because of this inherent complexity, advocacy is not formally taught as a didactic subject in the classroom (Kohnke, 1982; Mallik, 1997). However, the nursing literature has long-standing reference to the idea that experience may be the best teacher, and there are examples of how nurse educators have integrated various "advocacy activities" into clinical experiences where students actually encounter vulnerable patients within the complexity of the healthcare system (Fay, 1978; Namerow, 1982).

The dimensions of nursing advocacy appear to be primarily focused at the individual patient level. Politically, nurses tend not to get involved with consumer advocacy groups or engage in collective legislative action in the cause of patient rights (Mallik, 1997).

Advocacy and the Advanced Nurse Practitioner

A question arises: As nurses move to a more autonomous role as advanced nurse practitioners, how much of their practice is influenced by nursing and how much by medicine? Thrasher (2002) considered the role of the primary care nurse practitioner as an advocate in promoting self-care and clearly chose the nursing model. Supporting her theoretical framework for this role are critical social theory and nursing theories of self-care. Prominently among these theories is Gadow's (1980) philosophy of existential advocacy, including caring and understanding the lived experience of the patient and assisting him or her to self-determination.

To gain an understanding of the meaning and application of advocacy in advanced practice nursing, a semistructured interview was conducted by Pamp with an experienced pediatric nurse practitioner. The informant, whose pseudonym was Star, was an African-American woman of about 30 years of age who practiced in an urban clinic whose patients were predominately lower income and African-American. This interview was part of de Chesnay's (2005) larger study of life histories of successful African-Americans.

Thematically, Star identified responsibility and empowerment as elements that changed when she transitioned from bedside nursing to an independent advanced practice role that enabled her to more effectively advocate for her patients. However, she did not see that the essence of her nursing advocacy, or as she called it "looking out for patients," had changed as a result of being in an expanded role as illustrated by the following: "I think a lot of it was I was trying to get what I wanted from a doctor and at this point I can do those things myself. I don't have to wait for an order to give a med. I just give it. You know, I just write a prescription. I do it myself. And so that way it's very different. I think in terms of just looking out for patients overall, no, there's no difference." Star pointed out how patient advocacy does differ in the advanced practice nursing role in that it is informed by the higher level of responsibility and accountability of being the primary care provider: "I think I feel more responsible for my patients now because they're my patients. In the hospital [where] I worked they were the doctors' patients; they were their responsibility." These statements appear to support views presented earlier that power and autonomy are prerequisites for nurses to effectively advocate for their patients (Hewitt, 2002; Hyland, 2002; Yarling & McElmurry, 1986).

In terms of learning the advocacy role, Star intimated that her hospital experience trained her for her role as patient advocate, as is consistent with other observations (Mallik, 1997). She stated, ". . . you know you do discharge planning in the hospital. You have to connect with outside agencies, home care, do that type of stuff."

Finally, as with most nurses (Mallik, 1997), Star's focus was advocacy at the individual and local level and not directed toward the macro view of consumer advocacy or political health reform: "I'm not so much interested in politics but in the health and well-being of children and the health and well-being of my community."

Conclusion

The ideas presented here have much relevance to nursing practice and the concepts relate in several specific ways. First, cultural competence is a set of behaviors that transcend mere good intentions. Accepting that cultural differences exist reflects an open mind, which in turn leads to exploring the client's own strengths and adaptive capabilities. Using cultural resources at the client's disposal concurrently with "best practices" in nursing and medicine is not only culturally appropriate, it is also likely to develop resilience. Nurses who practice in a culturally competent way serve as better advocates for their clients because they work from a point of view of mobilizing resources in collaboration with others who are knowledgeable about the culture.

References

Abbot, P., Short, E., Dodson, S., Garcia, C., Perkins, J., & Wyant, S. (2002). Improving your cultural awareness with culture clues. *Nurse Practitioner, 27*(2), 44–49.

American Nurses' Association. (2001). *Code of ethics for nurses with interpretive statements.* Washington, DC: American Nurses Publishing.

Andrews, M. (1998). A model for cultural change. *Nursing Management, 29*(10), 62–66.

Ball, S. C. (2006). Nurse-patient advocacy and the right to die. *Psychosocial Nursing and Mental Health Services, 44*(12), 36–42.

Barnes, D., Craig, K., & Chambers, K. (2000). A review of the concept of culture in holistic nursing literature. *Journal of Holistic Nursing, 18*(3), 207–221.

Beckett, A., Gilbertson, S., & Greenwood, S. (2007). Doing the right thing: Nursing students, relational practice and moral agency. *Journal of Nursing Education, 46*(1), 28–32.

Bellin, M. H., & Kovacs, P. J. (2006). Fostering resilience in siblings of youths with a chronic health condition: A review of the literature. *Health and Social Work, 31*(3), 209–216.

Bernal, E. W. (1992). The nurse as patient advocate. *Hastings Center Report, 22*(1), 18–23.

Bonder, B., Martin, L., & Miracle, A. (2001). Achieving cultural competence: The challenge for clients and healthcare workers in a multicultural society. *Generations, 25*(1), 35–43.

Campinha-Bacote, J. (2002). The process of cultural competence in the delivery of health care services: A model of care. *Journal of Transcultural Nursing, 13*(3), 180–184.

Campinha-Bacote, J. (2003). *The process of cultural competence in the delivery of healthcare services: A culturally competent model of care* (4th ed.). Cincinnati, OH: Transcultural CARE Associates.

Campinha-Bacote, J. (2005). A biblically based model of cultural competence in healthcare delivery. *The Journal of Multicultural Nursing and Health, 11*(2), 16–22.

Campinha-Bacote, J. (2006). Cultural competence in nursing curricula: How are we doing 20 years later? *Journal of Nursing Education, 45*(7), 243–244.

Clauss-Ehlers, C. S., & Levi, L. L. (2002). Violence and community, terms in conflict: An ecological approach to resilience. *Journal of Social Distress and the Homeless, 11*(4), 265–278.

Craig, A. B. (1999). Mental health nursing and cultural diversity. *Australian and New Zealand Journal of Mental Health Nursing, 8,* 93–99.

Curtain, L. L. (1979). The nurse as advocate: a philosophical foundation for nursing. *Advances in Nursing Science, 1*(3), 1–10.

Dana, R., & Matheson, L. (1992). An application of the agency cultural competence checklist to a program serving small and diverse ethnic communities. *Psychosocial Rehabilitation Journal, 15*(4), 101–106.

de Chesnay, M. (2005). "Can't keep me down": Life histories of successful African Americans. In M. de Chesnay (Ed.), *Caring for the vulnerable: Perspectives in nursing theory, practice and research* (pp. 221–234). Sudbury, MA: Jones and Bartlett.

Deegan, P. (2005). The importance of personal medicine: A qualitative study of resilience in people with psychiatric disabilities. *Scandinavian Journal of Public Health, 33*, 29–35.

DiCicco-Bloom, B., & Cohen, D. (2003). Home care nurses: A study of the occurrence of culturally competent care. *Journal of Transcultural Nursing, 14*(1), 25–31.

Donnelly, G. (2007). The essence of advanced practice nursing. *Internet Journal of Advanced Practice Nursing, 8*, 1–12.

Fahrenwald, N., Boysen, R., Fischer, C., & Maurer, R. (2001). Developing cultural competence in the baccalaureate nursing student: A populations-based project with the Hutterites. *Journal of Transcultural Nursing, 12*(1), 48–55.

Fay, P. (1978). Sounding board-in support of patient advocacy as a nursing role. *Nursing Outlook, 26*(4), 252–253.

Fry, S. T. (2001). Ethical dimensions of nursing and health care. In J. L. Creasia & B. Parker (Eds.). *The bridge to professional nursing practice* (3rd ed., pp. 272–293). St. Louis, MO: Mosby.

Gadow, S. (1980). Existential advocacy: philosophical foundation of nursing. In S. F. Spicker & S. Gadow (Eds.), *Nursing: Images and ideals* (pp. 79–101). New York: Springer Publishing.

Gebru, K., & Willman, A. (2003). A research-based didactic model for education to promote culturally competent nursing care in Sweden. *Journal of Transcultural Nursing, 14*(1), 55–61.

Greeff, A. P., & Human, B. (2004). Resilience in families in which a parent has died. *American Journal of Family Therapy, 32*(1), 27–42.

Gutierrez, L., & Alvarez, A. (1996). Multicultural community organizing: A strategy for change. *Social Work, 41*(5), 501–509.

Hall, J. M. (1999). Marginalization revisited: Critical, postmodern and liberation perspectives. *Advances in Nursing Science, 22*(1), 88–102.

Hall, J. M., Stevens, P., & Meleis, A. (1994). Marginalization: A guiding concept for valuing diversity in nursing knowledge development. *Advances in Nursing Science, 16*(4), 23–41.

Hamric, A. B. (2000). What is happening to advocacy? *Nursing Outlook, 48*, 103–104.

Hewitt, J. (2002). A critical review of the arguments debating the role of the nurse advocate. *Journal of Advanced Nursing, 37*(5), 439–445.

Hyland, D. (2002). An exploration of the relationship between patient autonomy and patient advocacy: Implications for nursing practice. *Nursing Ethics, 9*(5), 472–482.

Iwaniek, D. (2006). Risk and resilience in cases of emotional abuse. *Child and Family Social Work, 11*(1), 73–82.

Kagawa-Singer, M. (2000). Addressing issues for early detection and screening in ethnic populations. *Oncology Nursing Forum, 27*(9), 55–61.

Kennedy, M. (1999). Cultural competence and psychiatric nursing. *Journal of Transcultural Nursing, 10*(1), 11–18.

Kim-Godwin, Y. S., Clarke, P., & Barton, L. (2001). A model for the delivery of culturally competent care. *Journal of Advanced Nursing, 35*(6), 918–926.

King, G., Cathers, T., Brown, E., Specht, J. A., Willoughby, C., Polgar, J. M., et al. (2003). Turning points and protective processes in the lives of people with chronic disabilities. *Qualitative Health Research, 13*(2), 184–206.

King, L. A. (2006). Deployment risk and resilience inventory: A collection of measures for deployment-related experiences of military personnel and veterans. *Military Psychology, 18*(2), 89–120.

Kohnke, M. F. (1982). *Advocacy: Risk and reality*. St. Louis, MO: C.V. Mosby.

Kuczmarski, M., & Cole, R. (1999). Transcultural food habits travel courses: An interdisciplinary approach to teaching cultural diversity. *Topics in Clinical Nutrition, 15*(1), 59–71.

Larson, N. C., & Dearmont, M. (2002). Strengths of farming communities in fostering resilience in children. *Child Welfare, 81*(5), 821–835.

Leavitt., R. L. (2003). Developing cultural competence in a multicultural world. Part II. *Magazine of Physical Therapy, 11*(1), 56–70.

Leininger, M. (1970). *Nursing and anthropology: Two worlds to blend*. New York: John Wiley & Sons.

Leininger, M. (1995). *Transcultural nursing: Concepts, theories, research and practice*. New York: McGraw-Hill.

Locsin, R. (2000). Building bridges: Affirming culture in health and nursing. *Holistic Nursing Practice, 15*(1), 1–4.

Lothe, E. A., & Heggen, K. (2003). A study of resilience in young Ethiopian famine survivors. *Journal of Transcultural Nursing, 14*(4), 313–320.

Mallik, M. (1997). Advocacy in nursing: A review of the literature. *Journal of Advanced Nursing, 25,* 130–138.

Mawdsley, C., & Northway, T. (2007). The Canadian ICU Collaborative: Patient advocacy at its best. *CCAN, 18*(1), 11–13.

Melia, K. M. (1994). The task of nursing ethics. *Journal of Medical Ethics. 20*(1), 7–11.

Meltzof, N., & Lenssen, J. (2000). Enhancing cultural competence through simulation activities. *Multicultural Perspectives, 2*(1), 29–35.

Mendycka, B. (2000). Exploring culture in nursing: A theory-driven practice. *Holistic Nursing Practice, 15*(1), 32–41.

Namerow, M. J. (1982). Integrating advocacy into the gerontological nursing major. *Journal of Gerontological Nursing, 8*(3), 149–151.

Nelson, M. L. (1988). Advocacy in nursing. *Nursing Outlook, 36*(3), 136–141.

Newman, R. (2003). Providing direction on the road to resilience. *Behavioral Health Management, 23*(4), 42–43.

Newson, P. (2007). The skills of advocacy. *Nursing and Residential Care, 9*(3), 99–102.

Parry, C. (2003). Embracing uncertainty: An exploration of the experiences of childhood cancer survivors. *Qualitative Health Research, 13*(1), 227–246.

Partin, B. (2006). Advocacy in practice: Preventing medication errors: An IOM report. *Nurse Practitioner, 31*(12), 8.

Perry, B. D. (2002a). How children become resilient. *Scholastic Parent & Child, 10*(2), 33–34.

Perry, B. D. (2002b). Resilience: Where does it come, from? *Early Childhood Today, 17*(2), 24–25.

Place, M., Reynolds, J., Cousins, A., & O'Neill, S. (2002). Developing a resilience package for vulnerable children. *Child and Adolescent Mental Health, 7*(4), 162–167.

Poole, D. (1998). Politically correct or culturally competent? *Health and Social Work, 23*(3), 163–167.

Procter, N. (2006). "They first killed his heart (then) he took his own life." Part 2: Practice implications. *International Journal of Nursing Practice, 12*, 42–48.

Purnell, L. (2000). A description of the Purnell model for cultural competence. *Journal of Transcultural Nursing, 11*(1), 40–46.

Purnell, L. (2002). The Purnell model for cultural competence. *Journal of Transcultural Nursing, 13*(3), 193–196.

Purnell, L., & Paulanka, B. (2003). *Transcultural health care: A culturally competent approach* (2nd ed.). Philadelphia: F. A. Davis.

Shapiro, J., Hollingshead, J., & Morrison, E. (2002). Primary care resident, faculty and patient views of barriers to cultural competence and the skills needed to overcome them. *Medical Education, 36,* 749–759.

Smith, R. E., Smoll, F. L., & Ptacek, J. T. (1990). Conjunctive moderator variables in vulnerability and resiliency research life stress, social support and coping skills, and adolescent sport injuries. *Journal of Personality and Social Psychology, 58*(2), 360–370.

Stein, H. (2006). Maltreatment, attachment and resilience in the Orphans of Duplessis. *Psychiatry, 69*(4), 306–313.

Sutton, M. (2000). Cultural competence. *Family Practice Management, 7*(9), 58–61.

Thrasher, C. (2002). The primary care nurse practitioner: Advocate for self care. *Journal of the American Academy of Nurse Practitioners, 14*(3), 113–117.

Tomlinson-Clark, S. (2000). Assessing outcomes in a multicultural training course: A qualitative study. *Counseling Psychology Quarterly, 13*(2), 221–232.

Walker, C. A. (2002). Transformative aging: How mature adults respond to growing older. *Journal of Theory Construction & Testing, 6*(2), 109–116.

Walsh, F. (2003). Family resilience: A framework for clinical practice. *Family Process, 42*(1), 1–18.

Walters, K. L., & Simoni, J. M. (2002). Reconceptualizing Native women's health: An "indigenist" stress-coping model. *American Journal of Public Health, 92,* 520–524.

Wells, M. (2000). Beyond cultural competence: A model for individual and institutional cultural development. *Journal of Community Health Nursing, 17*(4), 189–200.

Willard, C. (1996). The nurse's role of patient advocate: Obligation or imposition? *Journal of Advanced Nursing, 24,* 60–66.

Yarling, R. R., & McElmurry, B. J. (1986). The moral foundation of nursing. *Advances in Nursing Science, 8*(2), 63–73.

Zoucha, R. (2001). President's message. *Journal of Transcultural Nursing, 12*(2), 1.

Social Justice in Nursing: A Review of the Literature

Doris M. Boutain

The purpose of this chapter is to explore how social justice was conceptualized in the nursing literature from 1990 to 2006. Analysis revealed that authors ascribed to social, distributive, and market views of justice. Most authors, however, did not explicitly attend to the differences among these concepts. The three predominant models of justice are reviewed first, and then a framework for how nurses can focus on injustice awareness, amelioration, and transformation as forms of social justice is presented. The multiple methods of promoting a social justice agenda, from consciousness-raising to the re-creation of social policies, are also delineated. Recognizing the many ways to promote social justice can have a transformational impact on how nurses teach, research, and practice.

Although social justice is not a new concept, the nursing literature lacks a coherent and complex understanding of its implications for studying societal health (Drevdahl, Kneipp, Canales, & Dorcy, 2001; Liaschenko, 1999). Social justice is often briefly mentioned after elaborate discussions about ethics. When ethics is defined in the forefront, the concept of social justice is often written in the conclusion section of articles as if it is a related after-thought. Inattention to the subtle variations in how social justice is conceived can inadvertently result in nursing practice, research, and education that are antithetical to a social justice agenda.

Literature Search Methodology

A search of the Cumulative Index of Nursing and Allied Health literature from 1990 to 2006 revealed a total of 211 publications, including journal articles ($n = 200$), dissertations ($n = 7$), and conference abstracts ($n = 4$) categorized with the key words *social justice* and *nursing* as major descriptors. A major descriptor is a term ascribed by the manuscript authors to classify the main focus of their work. Literature using the major descriptors of *social justice* and *nursing* form the basis of this review. The literature reviewed in the sections about views of justice in nursing education, research, and practice is limited to published journal articles written in English-language journals in the stated time frame.

Publications from nursing, sociology, social work, philosophy, public health, and religious studies supplement the literature analysis in the sections about the literature review critique and implications.

Defining Justice in Nursing

The ethical principle of justice was referenced frequently in the nursing literature surveyed. Over 50% of the publications retrieved equated justice with what is fair or what is deserved or "giving to others what is their due" (Lamke, 1996, p. 55). Authors discussed ethics, which is primarily viewed as a framework for understanding how values, duties, principles, and obligations inform people's sense of societal fairness, as the basis for moral decision making (Aroskar, 1995; Harper, 1994). The notion of two orientations to ethics was also highlighted in the literature (Mathes, 2004, 2005). Ethics can be defined by a care orientation or by a justice orientation. For example, ethics can be defined by universal truths (justice orientation) or in relationship to caring for others in context (care orientation) (Mathes, 2004, 2005).

Although many authors mentioned justice, few articles actually defined justice beyond notions of ethical fairness (Drevdahl, 1999; Drevdahl et al., 2001; Harris, 2005; Kneipp & Snider, 2001; Liaschenko, 1999; Thorne, 1999; Vonthron Good & Rodrigues-Fisher, 1993) or ethical relationship formation (Myhrvold, 2003). Liaschenko (1999) outlined the relationship between personal values and justice in an effort to describe how justice can guide nursing practice. Vonthron Good and Rodrigues-Fisher (1993) considered how justice was useful in assessing if vulnerability is compromised or protected in research. Exploring the philosophical underpinning of justice, Drevdahl et al. (2001) compared the concepts of social justice, distributive justice, and market justice. Like other scholars (Sellers & Haag, 1992), they posited that most nurses do not consider the distinction among concepts related to justice (Drevdahl et al., 2001). A few authors broadened the discussion of ethics to globalization (Falk-Rafael, 2006) or structural inequality (Sistrom & Hale, 2006) with implications for social justice.

Without an intricate understanding of the different views of justice, nurses may limit their problem-solving abilities when attempting to understand how unjust social conditions influence health status, access, and delivery. Although concepts like care (Boersma, 2006) and culture (Jackson, 2003) are not mutually exclusive to a justice ideology, inattention to the distinctions between care and justice may result in limited theoretical analysis and thus action. A review of the American Nurses Association *Code of Ethics With Interpretive Statements, Nursing's Social Policy Statement* and *Nursing: Scope and Standards of Practice*, for example, revealed inconsistent and superficial conceptualizations of social justice (Bekemeier & Butterfield, 2005). These points were also a cause for debate in a review of the Canadian Nurses Association 2002 *Revised Code of Ethics* (Hubert, 2004; Kikuchi, 2004). The disjunctions between practice, policy, and politics of justice, however, have a long history in nursing (Murphy, Canales, Norton, & DeFilippis, 2005). It is therefore important to explore the most prominent forms of justice in nursing literature today.

Social, Distributive, and Market Justice

Social, distributive, and market justice are the most common forms of justice referenced in the nursing literature. Social justice is often defined as a concern for "the equitable distribution of benefits and burdens in society" (Redman & Clark, 2002). Social justice is also, but less often, defined as changing social relationships and institutions to promote equitable relationships (Drevdahl et al., 2001). Distributive justice is discussed in reference to the equal distribution of goods and services in society (Schroeder & Ward, 1998; Silva & Ruth, 2003). Market justice posits that people are entitled only to goods and services that they acquire according to guidelines of entitlement (Young, 1990).

Although these forms of justice appear to be similar, there are distinct differences (Beauchamp, 1986; Whitehead, 1992). Social justice is concerned with making equitable the balance between societal benefits and burdens. Social justice posits that there are social rights and collateral responsibilities with those rights (Lebacqz, 1986). Social beings are to both give and receive, using equity as a framework for relating to one another. Equity, derived from the Greek word *epiky*, means that persons must conduct themselves with reasonableness and moderation when exercising their rights (Whitehead, 1992). Distributive justice involves equality more than equity and is used most often to discuss the allocation or distribution of goods and services in society (Young, 1990). Equality focuses on giving the same access and resources to different groups (Sellers & Haag, 1992).

Social justice advocates explore social relationships and how those relationships form the basis for the allocation of goods and services (Young, 1990). Social justice focuses on equity because many theories of social justice assert that equal does not mean just (Lebacqz, 1986). Thus the concepts of social and distributive justice are somewhat parallel yet have different primary foci of study (Drevdahl et al., 2001).

Market justice is also viewed as a form of justice in nursing (Drevdahl, 2002). It is based on honoring the rights of those who have earned entitlement to those privileges. Market justice permits inequality as long as those inequalities result from a fair market system. That is, only those who earn rights are secured their entitled privileges in a market system. Those who earn no rights are not secured privileges.

Critics of the market justice agenda note that using the word *market* as an adjective for justice is itself an oxymoron (Beauchamp, 1986). *Justice* is a word most often used to discuss fairness, equity, or the process of deliberation. The term *market* is most often concerned with the balance between monetary value and goods allocation. The two terms do not work together when discussing equity. Simply "applying the word 'justice' to 'market' does not bring the concept into the realm of justice" (Drevdahl et al., 2001, p. 24). Social justice is not a parallel model to market justice; social justice is antithetical to a market model (Beauchamp, 1986). These two ways of viewing the world, therefore, diametrically oppose each other and simultaneously coexist.

An example may clarify the difference between social, distributive, and market justice. Using a social justice framework, everyone in the United States would be entitled to health care as needed if health care were deemed a right of citizenship. Health care, using a social justice view, is a moral obligation and a right of citizenship. A distributive justice framework would give a certain level of health care to everyone as a result of citizenship. The leveling of health care is needed to ensure enough healthcare services are available for all to receive at least minimal benefit. Using distributive justice, health is a right of citizens but not necessarily a moral responsibility. Persons can receive health care as a result of how much they can pay for those services in a market system. The focus of a market system is not on moral or citizenship rights but on making sure those who want the good of health care, for example, can pay for those services.

All forms of justice, although somewhat distinct, may coexist to varying degrees. There are healthcare services in the United States that are given as needed, such as the care given to children who are orphaned. Then there are incidences when minimal health care is given, such as the medical and dental benefits associated with Medicaid. Persons who can afford more treatment or faster treatment may get those services as well if they can pay a particular price. An example may be healthcare clinics that are designed to give expanded services if clients pay certain access fees. Although these three forms of justice are noted in the nursing literature to varying degrees, seldom is it discussed how these views of justice guide nursing education, research, or practice.

Views of Justice in Nursing Education Articles

Most manuscripts about nursing education and justice focus on the clinical preparation of undergraduate students to meet the needs of a culturally diverse population (Herman & Sassatelli, 2002; Leuning, 2001; Redman & Clark, 2002; Scanlan, Care, & Gessler, 2001). Other publications proclaim the need for a global consciousness (Leuning, 2001; Messias, 2001), critical thinking (Pereira, 2006), culturally sensitive evidence-based practice (McMurray, 2004), and human rights education (Fitzpatrick, 2003) among nurses as the starting point for justice awareness. Also present in the nursing literature are curricular considerations (Fahrenwald et al., 2005; MacIntosh & Wexler, 2005; Myrick, 2005), teaching models (Bond, Mandleco, & Warnick, 2004; Boutain, 2005; Fahrenwald, 2003; Leuning, 2001), case examples (Thompson, 1991), and service-learning experiences (Herman & Sassatelli, 2002; Redman & Clark, 2002) that use justice as a framework to educate undergraduate students. A limited number of articles focus on teaching justice content or processes in graduate education (Shattell, Hogan, & Hernandez, 2006). Few articles use social justice as a theoretical framework for educational scholarship (Kirkham, Hofwegen, and Harwood, 2005; Moule, 2003).

Although some nurse educators discussed the practical application of justice principles, few distinguished between the use of social justice and distributive justice concepts. For instance, authors defined social justice using distributive justice principles of equality (Thompson, 1991) or defined it as working with vulnerable populations (Redman & Clark, 2002). Another manuscript introduced justice in terms of contractual justice, the fair and honest contract between equals (Oddi & Oddi, 2000). In one instance, the words *social justice* were used but never defined (Herman & Sassatelli, 2002). Rarely is social justice used as a framework to critique nursing education models (Sellers & Haag, 1992) and student–faculty relationships (Oddi & Oddi, 2000; Scanlan et al., 2001).

Views of Justice in Nursing Research Articles

Most articles about justice and nursing research focus on the protection of vulnerable populations or working with those who are marginalized in society (Alderson, 2001; Dresden, McElmurry & McCreary, 2003; Guenter et al., 2005; Lamke, 1996; McKane, 2000; Mill & Ogilvie, 2002; Thomas, 2004; Rew, Taylor-Seehafer, & Thomas, 2000; Vonthron Good & Rodrigues-Fisher, 1993). Nurses (Alexis & Vydelingum, 2004; Giddings, 2005a, 2005b; Mantler, Armstrong-Stassen, Horsburgh & Cameron, 2006; Spence Laschinger, 2004) and nursing students (Grant, Giddings, and Beale, 2005) were study participants in six research studies assessing issues of justice in nursing practice accounts. Few articles explicitly stated and defined how social justice was used as a theoretical research framework (Clark, Barton, & Brown, 2002; Blondeau et al., 2000, 2005; Giddings, 2005a, 2005b; Grant et al., 2005), as a measurement parameter for understanding concepts related to nursing (Altun, 2002), or an outcome of a particular methodological approach (Sullivan-Bolyai, Bova, & Harper, 2005).

In the last 5 years, however, more researchers are identifying how the concept of social justice was used in the research process (Guo & Phillips, 2006; Mohammed, 2006; Peterson, Trapp, Fanale, & Kaur, 2003; Racine, 2002; Tee & Lathlean, 2004). Overall, social justice is an infrequently defined framework to guide nursing research. More research articles do address the social justice implications for the research area studied (Andrews & Heath, 2003; Lynam et al., 2003).

Views of Justice in Nursing Practice Articles

Articles about how justice relates to nursing practice focus on how ethics is useful in making moral judgments about care of individuals or populations (Bell, 2003; Lawson, 2005; McMurray, 2006; Stinson, Godkin, & Robinson, 2004; Peter & Morgan, 2001; Phillips & Phillips, 2006; Pieper & Dacher, 2004; Purdy & Wadhwani, 2006; Turkoski, 2005; Williams, 2004). In the last 4 years a growing number of articles focused on using justice as a concept to guide nursing administration and leadership (Curtin & Arnold, 2005a, 2005b; Williams, 2006), nursing practice (Falk-Rafael, 2005; Sutton, 2003), and healthcare management (Williams, 2005). Justice was often defined as "treating people fairly" (Aroskar, 1995) in clinical practice. Other authors view justice as related to fairness but also as a social obligation for nurses to understand how practice is influenced by assumptions and social inequalities that guide the design of health care and society (Benner, 2005; Drevdahl, 2002; Ervin & Bell, 2004; Leung, 2002; Ludwick & Silva, 2000; Russell, 2002). Most authors agree that discussions of justice are needed to assess how the work of individual nurses and the profession at large contribute to the formation of a just healthcare system and society (Haddad, 2002; Schroeder & Ward, 1998).

Despite the recognition that exploring justice is needed, most articles on this topic do not define justice beyond notions about fairness. Or if justice is defined more elaborately in relationship to nursing practice, authors often use a distributive justice framework (Schroeder & Ward, 1998; Silva & Ruth, 2003). Authors using a distributive justice viewpoint assert that "all humans are born with equal opportunities and equal political agency and efficacy" (Schroeder & Ward, 1998, p. 230). The belief that persons are equal forms the basis for the even allocation of goods and services. A main limitation of the distributive view of justice is the lack of acknowledgment that social groups are often regarded unequally on the basis of gender, class, and race; thus the allocation of goods and services is also unequal in U.S. society (Young, 1990).

Acknowledging the limitations of the distributive paradigm, a few authors explore the practice of nurses as embedded in the concept of the just state (Harper, 1994; Kikuchi & Simmons, 1999). The just state is concerned with how laws, public institutions, and communities act to limit or promote social inequalities in society. This view of the just state most closely parallels the concept of social justice.

Social Justice: Definitional Limitations in the Nursing Literature

The main concern with definitions of social justice in nursing is that injustice is viewed as a personal act and justice is seen as an individual response to that act (Liaschenko, 1999; Olsen, 1993). The individualization of social justice is historically related to how nurses conceive the person as the primary site of, and remedy to, unjust conditions (Allen, 1996). Rarely is it highlighted how injustice nationally or globally (Austin, 2001) is created by power imbalances in the distribution of wealth, resources, and access. Seldom is it noted how unequal distribution in resources and access influences healthcare delivery, health status, and health actualization or achievement of optimum health.

Often the articles about health and social justice in nursing limit the focus to underrepresented, vulnerable, or persons of color populations (Herman & Sassatelli, 2002; Redman & Clark, 2002). In the last 5 years, however, there has been more focus on the practices of nurses in terms of enabling or limiting justice. Nevertheless, nursing literature rarely focuses on how inequitable conditions contribute to diminished health actualization in majority groups as well. Deaton and Lubotsky (2003), for example, identified that death rates in U.S. states with more income inequality were higher for all groups than in states with more equal income distributions. After considering the racial and ethnic composition of those U.S. states, it remained unclear why the mortality of the majority group of white Americans was related to racial composition and income inequality (Deaton & Lubotsky, 2003). In part, this is due to the lack of research studying how inequality contributes to poor health outcomes for both minority and majority members of society. Despite this consideration, there is literature suggesting that injustice lessens the presence of optimal health for all (Kawachi & Kennedy, 1999; Subramanian, Blakely, & Kawachi, 2003). Even on a global level, poor environments foster poor health locally and nationally (World Health Organization, 1997).

Considerations such as this remain underdocumented in the nursing literature for several reasons. Nurses have a limited view of social justice (Drevdahl, 2002) and inadequate social policies to guide depth of thinking about social justice (Bekemeier & Butterfield, 2005; Kikuchi, 2004). Because justice is defined in relationship to individual equality and fairness, the social dimensions of justice and injustice are minimized. What is fair, however, does not necessary need to be equal or vice versa (Thorne, 1999). Given the historic disadvantages encountered by underrepresented groups in the United States, for instance, to give equal treatment would not remedy current or past ills.

Social justice asserts that vulnerable persons should be protected from harm and promoted to achieve full status in society. The dynamics of being perceived as privileged or vulnerable would require exploration. Particularly relevant would be an investigation of how nurses themselves are influenced by privilege as they espouse their role as social justice advocates. One question becomes focal: Can nurses really promote a social justice agenda when that promotion will result in the critique and dismantlement of their own advantage?

Social justice critique means, for example, that one must recognize the social factors that construe persons as privileged and/or vulnerable at different points in time. A social justice agenda necessitates transforming systems that promote subordination or disadvantage in the long term and the immediate conditions that limit self-actualization in the short term (Kirkham & Anderson, 2002). It requires a consistent focus on understanding how concepts are conceptualized to limit and/or promote justice (Lutz & Bowers, 2003). The focus on multiple simultaneous sites of social justice action is needed to begin to address the short- and long-term oppressive situations that create social injustice and limit access to health care. A multifocal approach to social justice is needed but is not, as of yet, fully articulated in the nursing literature.

Alternative Views of Social Justice

Definitions of social justice vary across disciplines and over time. Theories about social justice are espoused in philosophy (Young, 1990), public health science (Beauchamp, 1986), and religious studies (Lebacquz, 1986). The use of social justice by nurses as a research framework gained momentum in the early 1990s with the application of womanist, feminist, and social critical theories (Boutain, 1999) and in the late 1990s with the use of postcolonial perspectives (Kirkham & Anderson, 2002). Authors who use critical theories to critique nursing education, research, and practice help guide the nursing profession toward a social justice agenda (Boutain, 1999). However, many of the works were not developed to give explicit attention to the multiple ways to understand social justice as a concept.

One useful framework for nurses to consider is based on the work of Holland (1983). He argued that to be effective in promoting justice, scholars must think of addressing injustice on many fronts. Scholars must deal with the antecedents of injustice, the processes of injustice, and the results of injustice in society. These stages of injustice creation and re-creation help to focus nursing on points of intervention. Nurses can then focus on social justice in terms of social justice awareness, amelioration, or transformation.

Social Justice Awareness, Amelioration, and Transformation

Social justice awareness entails exploring how one conceives others as vulnerable or privileged. Awareness involves asking critical questions about how systems of domination and oppression foster categorizations such as "vulnerability" and "privilege." An example may be helpful in understanding social justice awareness.

Homelessness is a major health and social concern. A focus on social justice awareness may involve conducting a self- and client interview on how housing influences health. Think of what you know about how health is related to housing. Write your thoughts before interviewing clients with and without a home. Talk with clients who have homes and those who do not. Ask them about how having or not having a home influences their health. Record their thoughts.

Conduct a literature review on housing, home ownership, and health. Questions to consider include the following: How does having a home relate to health? What is the health status of those who have homes? What is the health status of those who do not have homes? Compare your initial thoughts with the knowledge gained in the interview and review of relevant literature. You may discover that your awareness of the relationship between housing and health increases.

Social justice awareness is an ongoing process. To alter the analogy as described by Lebacquz (1986), injustice is like a proverbial elephant standing right next to you. You cannot appreciate the entire view. You may not fully recognize how you are affected by or are affecting the elephant. You must continue to move, sensing each part of the elephant at different angles and with different senses. Social justice awareness is temporal and dependent on your frame of reference. Being aware is a start; however, it is not enough.

Social justice amelioration involves addressing the immediate results or antecedents to unjust conditions. To continue with the example of health and homelessness, amelioration entails a direct attempt to address the situation of the clients who are homeless. How that situation is addressed, however, is often to treat the most immediately seen concerns of that person. Getting grants to provide temporary shelter, food, clothing, or health care to the homeless, for example, is an illustration of social justice amelioration. In the short term, amelioration remedies urgent or semiurgent concerns. However, social justice amelioration does not really change the conditions that create others as homeless over and over again.

Social justice transformation also involves critically deliberating about the conditions of home dwelling and homelessness in relationship to health. Who are the most likely to have homes? What conditions were present that allowed them to have homes? Who are the most likely to be homeless? What conditions led them to become known as homeless? How does housing relate to health services allocation, current health status, or future health attainment? Social justice transformation advocates seek to answer these questions in attempts to change or develop just housing and health policies. Their aim is to eliminate or limit the conditions that result in homeless. Social justice transformation is devoted to redressing unjust conditions by changing the structures that foster those unjust situations. Transformation focuses individual actions toward long-range systematic solutions to unjust situations.

The work of Iris Young (1990) is helpful in further understanding social justice transformation. She argues that the distributive justice (similar to social justice amelioration) is based on a false system of distributing services and rights to those who are already marginalized. Thus the rendering of service re-creates the system of privilege by allowing those who give the services (the privileged) to remain in a position of power over those who receive those services (the needy). In the short term it addresses the needs of the most vulnerable, but simultaneously in the long term there is no change in the system because those privileged few in power remain so. Instead, Young believes it is most helpful to restructure systems so that certain services, such as homeless shelters, are no longer needed or are needed infrequently. System restructuring is accomplished by recognizing, confronting, and diminishing entrenched inequalities associated with gender, class, and racial inequalities in society (Young, 1990).

Conclusion

A social justice agenda recognizes that social groups are not treated equally in society. Social justice gives moral privilege to the needs of the most vulnerable group in an effort to promote justice within the society at large. As vulnerability among persons is eliminated or minimized, the moral agency of the privileged can also be elevated. This view of social justice is not clearly articulated in the literature on nursing education, research, and practice, however.

Discussions about social justice remain conceptually limited in most published works in nursing. Without a more complex and nuanced view of social justice, nurses are less able to fully utilize this concept as a framework to redress unjust conditions in healthcare delivery and health attainment. Social justice is regarded as central to the nursing profession despite the need to critically revisit discussions about social justice. Nurses can contribute much to understanding how the interdisciplinary concept of social justice is useful in promoting just health and social relationships in society.

Acknowledgments

Manuscript support for the first edition of this chapter was provided by grants from the National Institute of Child Health and Human Development (HD-41682), the National Institute of Nursing Research (F31 NR07249-01), and the Centers for Disease Control and Prevention (U48/CCU009654-06). Support for the second edition of the chapter was provided by National Institute of Child Health and Human Development (HD-41682), an Intramural Award from the University of Washington School of Nursing, and the March of Dimes Community Award. The author thanks Joseph Fletcher III.

References

Alderson, P. (2001). Prenatal screening, ethics, and Down's syndrome: A literature review. *Nursing Ethics, 8*, 360–374.

Alexis, O., & Vydelingum, V. (2004). The lived experience of overseas black and minority ethnic nurses in the NHS in the south of England. *Diversity in Health and Social Care, 1*(1), 13–20.

Allen, D. (1996). Knowledge, politics, culture, and gender: A discourse perspective. *Canadian Journal of Nursing Research, 28*, 95–102.

Altun, I. (2002). Burnout and nurses' personal and professional values. *Nursing Ethics, 9*, 269–278.

Andrews, J., & Heath, J. (2003). Women and the global tobacco epidemic: Nurses call to action. *International Council of Nurses, 50*, 215–228.

Aroskar, M. (1995). Envisioning nursing as a moral community. *Nursing Outlook, 43*, 134–138.

Austin, W. (2001). Nursing ethics in an era of globalization. *Advances in Nursing Science, 24*, 1–18.

Beauchamp, D. (1986). Public health as social justice: In T. Mappes & J. Zembaty (Eds.), *Biomedical ethics* (pp. 585–593). New York: McGraw-Hill.

Bekemeier, B., & Butterfield, P. (2005). Unreconciled inconsistencies: A critical review of the concept of social justice in three national nursing documents. *Advances in Nursing Science, 28*(2), 152–162.

Bell, S. (2003). Community health nursing, wound care, and . . . ethics? *Journal of Wound, Ostomy and Continence Nurses Society, 30*(5), 259–265.

Benner, P. (2005). Honoring the good behind the rights and justice in healthcare when more than justice is needed. *American Journal of Critical Care, 14*(2), 152–156.

Blondeau, D., Lavoie, M., Valois, P., Keyserlingk, E., Hebert, M., & Martineau, I. (2000). The attitude of Canadian nurses towards advance directives. *Nursing Ethics, 7*, 399–411.

Boersma, R. (2006). Integrating the ethics of care and justice—or are they mutually exclusive? *International Journal for Human Caring, 10, 2.*

Bond, A., Mandleco, B., & Warnick, M. (2004). At the heart of nursing: Stories reflect the professional values in AACN's Essentials Document. *Nurse Educator, 29*(2), 84–88.

Boutain, D. (1999). Critical nursing scholarship: Exploring critical social theory with African-American studies. *Advances in Nursing Science, 21*, 37–47.

Boutain, D. (2005). Social justice as a framework for professional nursing. *Journal of Nursing Education, 44*(9), 404–408.

Clark, L., Barton, J., & Brown, N. (2002). Assessment of community contamination: A critical approach. *Public Health Nursing, 19*, 354–365.

Curtin, L., & Arnold, L. (2005a). A framework for analysis: Part I. *Nursing Administration Quarterly, 29*(2), 183–187.

Curtin, L., & Arnold, L. (2005b). A framework for analysis: Part II. *Nursing Administration Quarterly, 29*(3), 288–291.

Deaton, A., & Lubotsky, D. (2003). Mortality, inequality and race in American cities and states. *Social Science and Medicine, 56*, 1139–1153.

Dresden, E., McElmurry, B., & McCreary, L. (2003). Approaching ethical reasoning in nursing research through a communitarian perspective. *Journal of Professional Nursing, 19*(5), 295–304.

Drevdahl, D. (1999). Sailing beyond: Nursing theory and the person. *Advances in Nursing Science, 21*(4), 1–13.

Drevdahl, D. (2002). Social justice or market justice? The paradoxes of public health partnerships with managed care. *Public Health Nursing, 19*(3), 161–169.

Drevdahl, D., Kneipp, S., Canales, M., & Dorcy, K. (2001). Reinvesting in social justice: A capital idea for public health nursing. *Advances in Nursing Science, 24*, 19–31.

Ervin, N., & Bell, S. (2004). Social justice issues related to uneven distribution of resources. *Journal of the New York State Nurses Association, 35*(1), 8–13.

Fahrenwald, N. (2003). Teaching social justice. *Nurse Educator, 28*(5), 222–226.

Fahrenwald, N., Bassett, S., Tschetter, L., Carson, P., White, L., & Winterboer, V. (2005). Teaching core nursing values. *Journal of Professional Nursing, 21*(1), 46–51.

Falk-Rafael, A. (2005). Advancing nursing theory through theory-guided practice: The emergence of a critical caring perspective. *Advances in Nursing Science, 28*(1), 38–49.

Falk-Rafael, A. (2006). Globalization and global health: Toward nursing praxis in the global community. *Advances in Nursing Science, 29*(1), 2–14.

Fitzpatrick, J. (2003). Social justice, human rights, and nursing education., from the editor. Social justice, human rights, and nursing education. *Nurse Educator, 28*(5), 222–226.

Giddings, L. (2005a). Health disparities, social injustice, and the culture of nursing. *Nursing Research, 54*(5), 304–312.

Giddings, L. (2005b). A theoretical model of social consciousness. *Advances in Nursing Science, 28*(3), 224–239.

Grant, B., Giddings, L., & Beale, J. (2005). Vulnerable bodies: Competing discourses of intimate bodily care. *Journal of Nursing Education, 44*(11), 498–504.

Guenter, D., Majumdar, B., Willms, D., Travers, R., Browne, G., & Robinson, G. (2005). Community-based HIV education and prevention workers respond to a changing environment. *Journal of the Association of Nurses in AIDS Care, 16*(1), 29–36.

Guo, G., & Phillips, L. (2006). Key informants' perceptions of health for elders at the U.S.-Mexico Border. *Public Health Nursing, 23*(3), 224–233.

Haddad, A. (2002). Fairness, respect, and foreign nurses. *RN, 65*(7), 25–28.

Harris, G. (2005). Ethical issues in community care. *Journal of Community Nursing, 19*(11), 12–16.

Herman, C., & Sassatelli, J. (2002). DARING to reach the heartland: A collaborative faith-based partnership in nursing education. *Journal of Nursing Education, 41*(10), 443–445.

Harper, J. (1994). For-profit entities and continuing education: A nursing perspective. *Nursing Outlook, 42*, 217–222.

Holland, J. (1983). *Social analysis: Linking faith and justice.* Maryknoll, NY: Orbis Books.

Hubert, J. (2004). Continuing the dialogue: A response to Kikuchi's critique of the 2002 CNA Code of Ethics. *Canadian Journal of Nursing Leadership, 17*(4), 10–13.

Jackson, D. (2003). Epilogue: Culture, health and social justice. *Contemporary Nurse, 15*(3), 347–348.

Kawachi, I., & Kennedy, B. (1999). Income inequality and health: Pathways and mechanisms. *Health Services Research, 34*(Pt 2), 215–227.

Kikuchi, J. (2004). 2002 CNA Code of Ethics: Some recommendations. *Canadian Journal of Nursing Leadership, 17*(3), 28–33.

Kikuchi, J., & Simmons, H. (1999). Practical nursing judgment: A moderate realist conception. *Scholarly Inquiry in Nursing Practice, 13*(1), 43–55.

Kirkham, S., & Anderson, J. (2002). Postcolonial nursing scholarship:, from epistemology to method. *Advances in Nursing Science, 25*(1), 1–17.

Kirkham, S., Hofwegen, L., & Harwood, C. (2005). Narratives of social justice: Learning in innovative clinical settings. *International Journal of Nursing Education Scholarship, 2*(1).

Kneipp, S., & Snider, M. (2001). Social justice in a market model world. *Journal of Professional Nursing, 17*(3), 113.

Lamke, C. (1996). Distributive justice and HIV disease in intensive care. *Critical Care Nursing Quarterly, 19*(1), 55–64.

Lawson, L. (2005). Furthering the search for truth and justice. *Journal of Forensic Nursing, 1*(4), 149–150.

Lebacqz, K. (1986). *Six theories of justice.* Minneapolis, MN: Augsburg.

Leung, W. (2002). Why the professional-client ethic is inadequate in mental health care. *Nursing Ethics, 9*(1), 51-60.

Leuning, C. (2001). Advancing a global perspective: The world as classroom. *Nursing Science Quarterly, 14*(4), 298-303.

Liaschenko, J. (1999). Can justice coexist with the supremacy of personal values in nursing practice? *Western Journal of Nursing Research, 21*(1), 35-50.

Ludwick, R., & Silva, M. (2000, August). Nursing around the world: Cultural values and ethical conflicts. *Online Journal of Issues in Nursing.* Retrieved January 25, 2007, from http://www.nursingworld.org/#jin/ethical/ethics_4.htm

Lutz, B., & Bowers, B. (2003). Understanding how disability is defined and conceptualized in the literature. *Rehabilitation Nursing, 28*(3), 74-78.

Lynam, M., Henderson, A., Browne, A., Smye, V., Semeniuk, P., Blue, C., & Singh, S. (2003). Healthcare restructuring with a view and efficiency: Reflections on unintended consequences. *Canadian Journal of Nursing Leadership, 16*(1), 112-140.

MacIntosh, J., & Wexler, E. (2005). Interprovincial partnership in nursing education, *Canadian Nurse, 101*(4), 17-20.

Mantler, J., Armstrong-Stassen, M., Horsburgh, M., & Cameron, S. (2006). Reactions of hospital staff nurses to recruitment incentives. *Western Journal of Nursing Research, 28*(1), 70-84.

Mathes, M. (2004). Ethical decision making and nursing. *Medsurg Nursing, 13*(6), 429-431.

Mathes, M. (2005). Ethical decision making and nursing. *Dermatology Nursing, 17*(6), 444-458.

McKane, M. (2000). Research, ethics and the data protection legislation. *Nursing Standard, 2*(14), 36-41.

McMurray, A. (2004). Culturally sensitive evidence-based practice. *Collegian, 11*(4), 14-18.

McMurray, A. (2006). Peace, love and equality: Nurses, interpersonal violence and social justice. *Contemporary Nurse, 21*(2), vii-x.

Messias, D. (2001). Globalization, nursing, and health for all. *Journal of Nursing Scholarship, 33*(1), 9-11.

Mill, J., & Ogilvie, L. (2002). Ethical decision making in international nursing research. *Qualitative Health Research, 12*(6), 807-815.

Mohammed, S. (2006). Moving beyond the "exotic": Applying postcolonial theory in health research. *Advances in Nursing Science, 29*(2), 98-109.

Moule, P. (2003). ICT: A social justice approach to exploring user issues? *Nurse Education Today, 23,* 530-536.

Murphy, N. Canales, M., Norton, S., & DeFilippis, J. (2005). Striving for congruence: The interconnection between values, practice, and political action. *Policy, Politics, & Nursing, 6*(1), 20-29.

Myhrvold, T. (2003). The exclusion of the other: Challenges to the ethics of closeness. *Nursing Philosophy, 4,* 33-43.

Myrick, F. (2005). Educating nurses for the knowledge economy. *International Journal of Nursing Education Scholarship, 2*(1).

Oddi, L., & Oddi, S. (2000). Student-faculty joint authorship: Ethical and legal concerns. *Journal of Professional Nursing, 16*(4), 219-227.

Olsen, D. (1993). Populations vulnerable to the ethics of caring. *Journal of Advanced Nursing, 18,* 1696-1700.

Olsen, D. (2001). Empathetic maturity: Theory of moral point of view in clinical relations. *Advances in Nursing Science, 24*(1), 36-46.

Pereira, A. (2006). Critical thinking. *Dynamics, 17*(3), 4-5.

Peter, E., & Morgan, K. (2001). Explorations of a trust approach to nursing ethics. *Nursing Inquiry, 8,* 3-10.

Petersen, W., Trapp, M., Fanale, M., & Kaur, J. (2003). Evaluating the WEB training program for cancer screening in Native American women. *Holistic Nursing Practice, 17*(5), 262–275.

Phillips, L., & Phillips, W. (2006). Better reproductive healthcare for women with disabilities: A role for nursing leadership. *Advances in Nursing Science, 29*(2), 134–151.

Pieper, B., & Dacher, J. (2004). Looking backward toward our future: Creating the nexus between community health nursing and palliative care. *Journal of the New York State Nurses Association, 35*(1), 20–24.

Purdy, I., & Wadhwani, R. (2006). Embracing bioethics in neonatal intensive care. Part II: Case histories in neonatal ethics. *Neonatal Network, 25*(1), 43–53.

Racine, L. (2002). Implementing a postcolonial feminist perspective in nursing research related to non-Western populations. *Nursing Inquiry, 10*(2), 91–102.

Redman, R., & Clark, L. (2002). Service-learning as a model for integrating social justice in the nursing curriculum. *Journal of Nursing Education, 41*, 446–449.

Rew, L, Taylor-Seehafer, M., & Thomas, N. (2000). Without parental consent: Conducting research with homeless adolescents. *Journal of the Society of Pediatric Nurses, 5*, 131–138.

Russell, K. (2002) Silent voices. *Public Health Nursing, 19*(4), 233–234.

Scanlan, J., Care, W., & Gessler, S. (2001). Dealing with unsafe students in clinical practice. *Nurse Educator, 26*(1), 23–27.

Schroeder, C., & Ward, D. (1998). Women, welfare, and work: One view of the debate, *Nursing Outlook, 46*(5), 226–232.

Sellers, S., & Haag, B. (1992). Achieving equity in nursing education. *Nursing & Health Care, 13*(3), 134–137.

Shattell, M., Hogan, B., & Hernandez, A. (2006). The interpretive research group as an alternative to the interpersonal process recording. *Nurse Educator, 31*(4), 178–182.

Silva, M., & Ruth, L. (2003). Ethics and terrorism: September 11, 2001 and its aftermath. *Online Journal of Issues in Nursing, 8*(1), 21–24.

Sistrom, M., & Hale, P. (2006). Integrative review of population health, income, social capital and structural inequality. *The Journal of Multicultural Nursing & Health, 12*(2), 21–27.

Spence Laschinger, H. (2004). Hospital nurses' perceptions of respect and organizational justice. *Journal of Nursing Administration, 34*(7/8), 354–364.

Stinson, C., Godkin, J., & Robinson, R. (2004). Ethical dilemma: Voluntarily stopping eating and drinking. *Dimensions of Critical Care Nursing, 23*(1), 38–43.

Subramanian, S., Blakely, T., & Kawachi, I. (2003). Income inequality as a public health concern: Where do we stand? *Health Services Research, 38*, 153–167.

Sullivan-Bolyai, S., Bova, C., & Harper, D. (2005). Developing and refining interventions in persons with health disparities: The use of the qualitative description. *Nursing Outlook, 53*, 127–133.

Sutton, J. (2003). The ethics of theatre nurse practice under the microscope. *British Journal of Perioperative Nursing, 13*(10), 405–408.

Tee, S., & Lathlean, J. (2004). The ethics of conducting a co-operative inquiry with vulnerable people. *Journal of Advanced Nursing, 47*(5), 536–543.

Thomas, S. (2004). School connectedness, anger behaviors, and relationship of violent and nonviolent American youth. *Perspectives in Psychiatric Care, 40*(40), 135–148.

Thompson, D. (1991). Ethical case analysis using a hospital bill. *Nurse Educator, 16*(4), 20–23.

Thorne, S. (1999). Are egalitarian relationships a desirable ideal in nursing? *Western Journal of Nursing Research, 21*(1), 16–34.

Turkoski, B. (2005). Culturally sensitive healthcare. *Home Healthcare Nurse, 23*(6), 355–358.

Vonthron Good, B., & Rodrigues-Fisher, L. (1993). Vulnerability: An ethical consideration in research with older adults. *Western Journal of Nursing Research, 15*(6), 780–783.

Whitehead, M. (1992). The concepts and principles of equity and health. *International Journal of Health Services, 22*(3), 429–445.

Williams, A. (2004). Nursing, health and human rights: A framework for international collaboration. *Association of Nurses in AIDS Care, 15*(3), 75–77.

Williams, A. (2005). Thinking about equity in health care. *Journal of Nursing Management, 13,* 397–402.

Williams, L. (2006). The fair factor in matters of trust. *Nursing Administration Quarterly, 30*(1), 30–37.

World Health Organization. (1997). *Health and environments in sustainable development: Five years after the Earth Summit.* Geneva: World Health Organization.

Young, I. (1990). *Justice and the politics of difference.* Princeton, NJ: Princeton University Press.

Chapter 5

Low Literacy and Vulnerable Clients

Toni M. Vezeau

Effective health care requires skills on part of both the providers and the clients. Providers must have a strong knowledge base and successful communication skills that match the needs of their clients. Clients must be able to take in information, make sense of it, apply it to their own situations, and retain the information for future use. These skills are the hallmarks of literacy. Without literacy as a base client skill, there is little chance that healthcare interactions will meet their intended goals. In this chapter we present literacy as a primary driver of vulnerability in health care. The discussion explores the current status of literacy skills in the United States, client and provider aspects of the problem, and recommendations for current practice.

What Is the Status of Literacy in the United States?

The National Adult Literacy Survey (NALS), conducted in 1992, defined literacy as the use of printed information to maneuver in society, meet one's goals, and develop one's knowledge and abilities (Kirsch, Jungeblut, Jenkins, & Kolstad, 1993). Doak, Doak, and Root (2001) modified this definition to include comprehension and retention of verbal and gestural information.

The 1992 NALS is the largest study on adult literacy in the United States ($n = 26{,}000$). This study went far beyond establishing the reading grade level of participants and tested their performance in three areas (Figure 5-1):

1. Prose literacy: printed word in connected sentences and passages; implies skill in finding information and integrating information from several sections of the text.

2. Document literacy: structured prose in arrays of columns and rows, lists, and maps; implies skill in locating information, repeating the search as often as needed, and integrating information.

3. Quantitative literacy: information displayed in graphs, charts, and in numerical form; in addition to locating information, this skill implies that one can infer and apply the needed arithmetic.

Participants were tested on a wide variety of tasks encountered at work, home, and community activities, such as signing a mock Social Security card and filling out personal information on a simple job application.

The original NALS data suggested that one-fourth to one-third of American adults are functionally illiterate and approximately an equal number have marginal literacy skills that disallow full functioning in society. Essentially, half of the adult population in the United States has poor to nonexistent skills in reading, listening, and computation. Minor proportions of the NALS survey were learning disabled (5%) and spoke English as a second language, if at all (15%). However, most were white and born in America. Although education correlated with literacy, generally those adults who had a 10th-grade education read at the 7th- to 8th-grade level. Participants receiving Medicaid had an average of a fifth-grade reading level. One-third of the NALS sample demonstrated basic functionality in understanding and using written information. Only 20% of the sample demonstrated a level of proficiency in handling information to perform complex reading and computation tasks. These data were recomputed using 2003 data and released in 2006 (National Center for Education Statistics, 2006) and showed a slightly worsening trend.

NALS data suggested that certain groups faired much worse in their literacy skills than the general population. Of those adults who tested at the lowest reading level,

- 41–44% were poor
- 33% were over age 65 years
- 25% were immigrants
- 62% did not finish high school (disproportionately represented by Hispanic, African-American, and Asian Pacific participants)

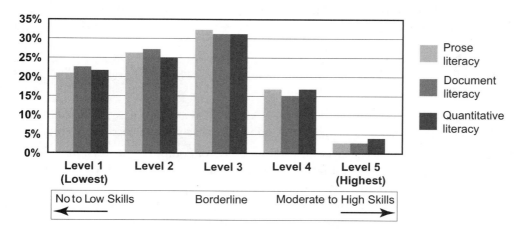

Figure 5-1 Adult Literacy Skills in the United States

Source: Adapted from U.S. Department of Education, Office of Educational Research and Improvement, National Center for Educational Statistics, 1993.

- 12% had physical, mental, or health conditions that disallowed participation in work or school settings
- 75% of the subfunctional group had a mental health problem

Participants in the lowest literacy level had difficulty with performing usual tasks of daily living based on printed information and in performing complex tasks that required following directions and computation. Interestingly, the group considered to have no or minimal functional literacy did not acknowledge themselves as vulnerable, related to their illiteracy. This group noted that they could read "adequately to very well," and less than 25% of these participants stated that they received help with information from family and friends.

A meta-analysis of U.S. studies on literacy in 2005 (Paasche-Orlow, Paker, et al., 2005) reviewed literature from January of 1963 through January 2004 and, based on a pool of 85 articles, essentially upheld the same prevalence rates as stated above, with one exception: Their findings did not show gender to be associated with literacy. Those authors concluded that limited literacy is highly prevalent, negatively affects health, and is consistently associated with education, ethnicity, and age. Could it be true that persons with low literacy are not vulnerable in American society?

What Is the Relationship between Literacy and Health Vulnerability?

Kirsh et al. (1993) discussed literacy as currency in the United States because those with less literacy are much less likely to meet the needs of daily living and to pursue life goals. It is then likely that illiteracy can create health risks and exacerbate existing health conditions.

Literacy as a Predictor of Vulnerability

Aday's (2001) model of vulnerability and health posits that although all humans are vulnerable to illness, segments of the community are much more vulnerable to ill health in terms of initial susceptibility and in their response. Illiteracy is related to each of Aday's (2001) predictors of vulnerability. Persons with poor reading skills who are unable to perform basic literacy functions, such as reading a bus schedule or following directions in completing a task, generally have low social status outside of their immediate social ties. For example, low social status is often related to low-paying jobs with no or minimal healthcare insurance. Low status also can affect a provider's perception of client abilities, creating care that is "edited" based, at times, on misperceptions (Aday, 2001).

Social Status
Social status has been correlated with poor health (Duncan, Daly, McDonough, & Williams, 2002) in that those persons with low status are more likely to use disproportionately more healthcare services, receive substandard care and less information about their illness, and be presented with fewer options. Kirsch et al. (1993) identified that persons with low literacy have much greater difficulty in accessing what Aday calls human capital (jobs, schools,

income, and housing) than those persons with functional literacy skills. Similarly, NALS data are congruent with Aday's third driver of vulnerability, lack of social capital, in that persons who are illiterate are more likely to be single or divorced, live in single-parent homes, and be loosely connected within their own communities.

Access to Care

Additionally, Aday addresses relationships of vulnerability to access to health care, cost of care, and quality of care. Accessing care in the United States most often requires complex language skills, such as

- Identifying and evaluating possible providers of care
- Negotiating appropriate entry points into the system
- Contacting and communicating needs to obtain an appointment
- Successfully traveling to and finding the actual site care
- Skills in interpreting written materials and relating to clock and calendar skills

Access to care is seriously challenged when clients have low literacy skills.

Consequences of Vulnerability

Quality of Care

Literature from the last decade documents well how illiteracy has affected the cost of care and the quality of care (Agency for Healthcare Research and Quality, 2004; Baker, et al., 2002; Institute of Medicine [IOM], 2003). Illiteracy is a significant component to client adherence to care regimens and hospitalizations in numerous health contexts: pregnancy, diabetes, AIDS, asthma, sexually transmitted diseases, women's health, rural residents, immigrants, mental health, advanced age, cardiac surgery, rheumatoid arthritis, prostate cancer, psychiatric clients, older adults, cardiac surgical clients, and payer status.

Without exception, the populations just cited have high prevalence of illiteracy, in proportions that mirror NALS data. These studies noted that persons with literacy problems did not understand instructions and demonstrated less comprehension of their illness or condition.

Costs

Healthy People 2010 (U.S. Department of Health and Human Services, 2000) noted that the consequences of illiteracy are poorer health outcomes and increased healthcare costs, as much as four times greater for those clients who read at or below the second-grade level than for the general populace. Baker et al. (2002) reported that clients with documented low literacy had a 52% higher risk of hospital admission compared with those with functional literacy, even after controlling for age, social and economic factors, and self-reported health. Client illiteracy was the highest predictor of poor asthma knowledge and ineffective use of metered-dose inhalers (Williams, Baker, Honig, Lee, & Nowlan, 1998).

Acknowledging the pervasive influence of illiteracy on the quality of care in the United States, the IOM has identified literacy as one of the top three areas that cut across all other priorities for improvement in our nation's health. The IOM states that literacy is required for self-management and collaborative care, the other two priority cross-cutting areas.

Redefining the Focus

Since the mid-1990s medical literature has used a new term, "health literacy," to address the literacy problem. The Ad Hoc Committee on Health Literacy for the Council on Scientific Affairs of the American Medical Association defined an individual's functional health literacy as "the ability to read and comprehend prescription bottles, appointment slips, and other essential health-related materials required to successfully function as a patient" (American Medical Association, 1999). The National Health Education Standards added the understanding of basic health information, ability to effectively handle the healthcare system, and understand consent forms (Williams, 2000). Health literacy has now become the preferred term for this intersection of health concerns and literacy skills. Williams is articulate in describing the complexity of this nexus: requiring listening, analytical, decision-making, computation, and application skills.

International healthcare work has addressed health literacy in the terms above for a much longer time; related literature exists from the 1960s on. Interestingly, the issues discussed in international literature correspond well to current Western health literature. Watters (2003) summarized well the healthcare implications of no or low literacy in international work: increased use of health system and cost, late entry into care secondary to poor interpretation of symptoms, poor participation in preventative care, shame over literacy status eliminating self-identification of needs to care providers, self-administration medication errors related to literacy errors, and inconsistent shows at appointments. Each of these health concerns related to literacy has been documented in America (American Medical Association, 1999; Baker, 1999; Kefalides, 1999).

In summary, research has supported Aday's theoretical work on health vulnerability. It is clear that, as yet without exception, literacy strongly influences the health of individuals and populations. The problems with literacy, however, are jointly owned and created by clients and providers. It is important to understand specific literacy problems of clients and how providers have contributed to these problems.

How Does Illiteracy Specifically Increase Health Risk of Clients?

Clients with no or low literacy cannot read or interpret pamphlets, directions on prescribed or over-the-counter medications, or diet instructions. A mismatch of vocabulary and skill is just one of the problems. Comprehension of graphics and pictures pose additional and, for many clients, insurmountable challenges (Doak et al., 2001). Literacy is a complex skill requiring much more than the simple reading of words. Literacy has many components, such as decoding, comprehension, and retention of information. The development of literacy involves a series of stages. Finally, literacy is not a "free-standing skill" but involves integration of related life skills to navigate the healthcare system, effectively perform self-care, and make healthcare decisions. This section provides a general overview of literacy components and life skills.

Influence of Illness or Health Condition on Literacy

Health and health care add unique aspects to the concern for client literacy. The effects of health and health care on literacy skills can be temporary or sustained. Such situations as anesthesia due to surgery, blood loss, or acute pain may temporarily impair one's decoding, comprehension, and recall skills. Sustained medical conditions can often interfere with mentation, cognition, and attention. Delayed mental development; neurological conditions, such as Alzheimer's disease; cerebral vascular accidents; and psychological disorders, such as depression or anxiety, may affect literacy skills and the ability of the client to interact effectively with providers. Understandably, clients who have sensory impairments likely have literacy difficulty. Visual difficulties were noted in 20% of the NALS sample that tested in the lowest level of literacy (Kirsch et al., 1993).

Medications may also negatively affect clients' abilities to effectively use their literacy skills, increasing risk for the client. Drug categories such as opiates, anticonvulsants, antidepressives, glucocorticosteroids, some antihypertensives, and thyroid and ovarian hormones are but a few that regularly affect information processing.

Providers need to appreciate how certain therapies and health conditions affect the client's ability to use the literacy skills he or she has. For those clients with low literacy skills, the health situations noted provide serious challenges to a client's ability to use healthcare information.

How Do Healthcare Providers Influence the Literacy Problem?

Clients come to providers with their unique characteristics and abilities related to health literacy. Providers, in their listening, speaking, and written interactions with clients, generally have ignored the literacy variable in care and, in most cases, increased the literacy challenge for their clients (Doak et al., 2001; Hohn, 1998). Literature shows several threads addressing how providers have influenced health literacy: readability of client health education text, measurement of clients' reading levels in specific healthcare settings, and client–provider communications.

Readability of Written Healthcare Education Materials

Since 1988 the literature has documented that the readability of written healthcare instructions, booklets, and informed consent forms have not matched the skills of clients in a general care population (Doak et al., 2001; Forbis & Aligne, 2002). Health educational materials have been tested but often only a few at a time. Doak et al. evaluated 1,234 health education materials and found that over half were written at or above the 10th-grade level. It is important to remember that education levels of clients do not generally match their reading skill levels. The reading skills average four to five grades lower when tested when compared with level of educational attainment. So the news is direr in that even if a client population had a mean of 10th-grade education, most educational materials in current use would outstrip the client skill level (Doak et al., 2001) (Figure 5-2). Studies have documented discharge instructions and client educational materials to be written well above a ninth-grade level of difficulty (Gannon & Hildebrandt, 2002).

Consent forms, contracts, and commonly used self-report diagnostic tools are consistently documented above a ninth-grade level. For example, clients who read at a sixth-grade level and below did not demonstrate comprehension of 54% of the items on the Beck Depression scale; good readers displayed difficulty with a third of the items (Sentell & Ratcliff-Baird, 2003). Similarly, in a study of 1,014 adults completing the Baltimore STD and Behavior Survey, 28% of the adults read at or below the eighth-grade level; this group showed a high error rate in comprehending survey items. The error rate in item comprehension decreased significantly as the literacy level increased ($p < 0.0001$) (Al-Tayyib, Rogers, Gribble, Villarroel, & Turner, 2002).

Studies investigating the literacy challenge of informed consent have consistently rated forms above the 12th-grade level and noted that institutional review boards typically do not take reading difficulty of consent forms into account (Raich, Plomer, & Coyne, 2001). When institutional review boards do, the effect is generally to lower the reading level by one grade (Raich et al., 2001).

Clients with no or low literacy who are given materials that directly affect their understanding of their health condition, who sign written forms that direct care, or who are tested using self-report tools are vulnerable to a host of negative consequences: inadequate understanding of healthcare instructions, agreeing to procedures they do not fully understand, and faulty diagnosis.

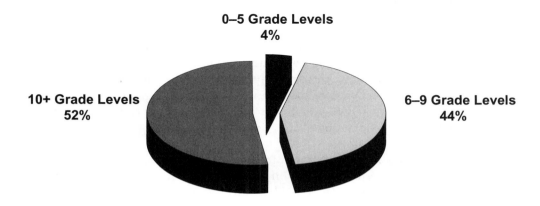

Figure 5-2 Readability of Health Education Materials

Source: Adapted from Doak, Doak, & Root, 2001. Readability levels of 1234 healthcare materials.

Provider–Client Interactions and Communication

Interactions with low literacy clients are just beginning to be studied. Provider–client interactions are influenced by perceptions of both client and provider. As stated previously, the U.S. Census Bureau literacy data and NALS data indicate that persons with low literacy state to others that they read well enough to meet their needs. However, it is important to understand that such clients generally do not self-identify or discuss their literacy status because of stigma associated with illiteracy (Doak et al., 2001; Parikh, Parker, Nurss, Baker, & Wlliams, 1996; Safeer & Keenan, 2005). Not only do low literacy clients not admit to difficulties with literacy to their care providers, significantly, they may also hide their need for help from their spouses and families (Parikh et al., 1996).

Stigma and Shame

Stigma is both self-imposed in the form of shame and evident in how providers interact with clients. Baker et al. (1996) interviewed clients who tested as having no to low literacy. These researchers found that their participants held a deep sense of shame, which was reported as worsened by healthcare providers, who became distressed or irritated when clients had difficulty in filling out forms or reading instructions. Study participants stated that accessing care is daunting because of problems with registration and forms. In many cases these clients avoided seeking care because of poor interactions with their care providers.

Myths and Misidentification

Providers are generally not knowledgeable about illiteracy and interact differentially with clients who admit to literacy problems (Doak et al., 2001; Schillinger, et al., 2003). There are a number of common myths held by providers (Doak, et al., 2001, p. 6):

- "Illiterates are dumb and learn slowly if at all."
- "Most illiterates are poor, immigrants, or minorities."
- "Years of schooling are a good measure of literacy level."

Research refutes each of these myths (Doak et al., 2001). A person's measurement of intelligence does not correlate strongly with literacy skills; correlation with income level is higher. By raw numbers, most persons with illiteracy in the United States are white native-born Americans in all areas of society; minorities and foreign-born in the United States have disproportionately high numbers of persons with no to minimal literacy. Years of schooling show the amount of education the person was exposed to, not the skill level achieved.

Incorrectly, providers may believe they can identify which clients need extra support related to their literacy needs. Bass, Wilson, Griffith, and Barnett (2002) conducted a study to see whether medical residents could correctly identify those with low literacy out of a pool of 182 clients. The residents identified 90% of the clients as having no literacy problem. Of this client group, 36% tested as functionally illiterate. Only 3 of 182 clients were thought to have literacy problems when they did not test as such. This study suggests that providers seriously underestimate the literacy problem in their client group.

Inattention to Literacy Needs

A second study observed senior physicians interacting during several outpatient visits with 74 diabetic clients who spoke only English and tested as having no or low literacy (Schillinger et al., 2003). Even when made aware of the literacy needs of their clients, provider use of language was assessed as well above the literacy level of their clients. The physicians in 80% of encounters did not test comprehension and recall. Those clients whose physicians did test for understanding and short-term recall had significantly greater glycemic control.

Rootman and Ronson (2005) stated the following:

> [W]e are mired in a state of denial over literacy. The immensity of the issue has paralyzed our public institutions, which seem to spend as much energy holding strategy session or denying responsibility as they do actually supporting programs of proven success. . . . It's hardly a promising time for a major national crusade against anything—especially poor literacy, which has no quick fix.

How Can Providers Decrease the Health Risk Due to Illiteracy?

The literature reports a variety of approaches to decrease vulnerability of clients related to literacy problems. Currently, many websites, developed by private and public agencies, exist as clearinghouses to guide clinicians on preferred approaches to working with low literacy clients (Table 5-1).

Identification

Many studies have emphasized a personal approach in discretely asking about literacy status (Feifer, 2003), but considering the breadth of the literacy problem and the reading demand placed on clients in the United States, a systematic approach to address literacy in a client population is indicated. It is now recommended that as part of routine primary care, literacy should be a measured baseline, comparable with many baselines obtained in the course of quality health care.

A first step in intervention for low literacy is to identify those clients with literacy deficits. It has been well validated in research that physicians tend to overestimate clients' literacy levels (Powell & Kripalani, 2005). One study compared physicians who screened for literacy issues with their clients and physicians who did not. It was found that physicians overestimated 62% of the time and voiced more dissatisfaction with the client visit (Seligman, et al., 2005). In contrast, other researchers have found that residents have increased comfort and skill in working with low literacy clients after completing a training program (Rosenthal, Werner, & Dubin, 2004).

TABLE 5-1. Helpful Websites on Health Literacy

- National Adult Literacy Survey (Full Report)
  http://nces.ed.gov/pubs93/93275.pdf

- National Center for Education Statistics
  http://nces.ed.gov/naal/health.asp

- National Institute for Literacy
  http://www.nifl.gov/

- National Cancer Institute, *Clear & Simple: Developing Effective Print Materials for Low-Literate Readers*
  http://www.nci.nih.gov/cancerinformation/clearandsimple

- U.S. Census Bureau Website (Education Statistics)
  http://www.census.gov/population/www/index.html

- *Empowerment Health Education in Adult Literacy: A Guide for Public Health and Adult Literacy Practitioners, Policy Makers and Funders* (White Paper by Marcia Hohn, NIFL)
  http://www.nifl.gov/nifl/fellowship/reports/hohn/HOHN.HTM

- Center for Health Care Strategies: Fact Sheets on Literacy
  http://www.chcs.org/usr_doc/Health_Literacy_Fact_Sheets.pdf

- Partnership for Clear Health Communication (Health Literacy Bibliography, 183 citations)
  http://www.askme3.org/pdfs/bibliography.pdf

- Pfizer Clear Health Communication: Corporate Initiative on Health Literacy
  http://www.pfizerhealthliteracy.com

- Health Literacy Consulting: Corporation Information on Multiple Types of Client Communication
  http://www.healthliteracy.com/articles.asp

- *Healthy People 2010*—Health Communication
  http://www.healthypeople.gov/Document/HTML/Volume1/11HealthCom.htm#_Toc490471353

A few researchers have identified some tools to efficiently screen clients:

- The Rapid Estimate of Adult Literacy in Medicine, or REALM, is a 2-minute test that measures a client's recognition and ability to pronounce common health-care words (Davis, Long, & Jackson, 1993).

- The Test of Functional Health Literacy in Adults (TOFHLA) uses hospital-written materials to test both reading comprehension and basic computational skills. This test takes much longer to administer, about 20–25 minutes. A shortened version of this test (S-TOFHLA) takes about 10–15 minutes to administer. These tests may be useful to assess individual clients with specific needs. Recent testing suggests that using only 3 of the S-TOFHLA 16 questions were effective in identifying low literacy clients ("How often do you have someone help you read hospital materials?" "How confident are you filling out medical forms by yourself?" "How often do you have problems learning about your medical condition because of difficulty understanding written information?") (Chew, Bradley, & Boyko, 2004).

- The Newest Vital Sign is a nutrition label that is accompanied by six questions and takes 3 minutes to give to a client to broadly screen for low literacy (Weiss et al., 2005).

- The most recent test, the Single Item Literacy Screener (SILS) (Morris, MacLean, Chew, & Littenberg, 2006), evaluated 999 adults with diabetes, 169 of whom had low literacy. SILS asks, "How often do you need to have someone help you when you read instructions, pamphlets, or other written material from your doctor or pharmacy?" Sensitivity was reported to be 54%, and specificity was 83%.

Davis et al. (1993) provided an excellent discussion evaluating the pros and cons of multiple screening tools and overcoming obstacles in a primary care setting. Although it takes time and other resources to obtain literacy measures, proper identification of client literacy levels can give clear guidance in effective client education.

For those systems that do not routinely screen, asking blunt questions regarding reading abilities may not yield accurate responses. As discussed earlier, clients with low literacy generally do not disclose their difficulties related to reading. Clients often conceal their literacy problems or may be unaware of their level of difficulty. Schultz (2002) and Doak et al. (2001) identified potential indicators of literacy problems: reading text upside down, difficulty orienting to a brochure, excuses for not reading in front of others (e.g., forgot glasses), mispronouncing words (for English speakers), reluctance to ask questions, missed appointments, difficulty following verbal instructions, relying on family members to fill out forms, and tiring quickly when reading text. When such client behaviors are identified, it is important for the provider to explore the issues.

Education Strategies

Low literacy clients may learn better when multiple modes of information are offered, such as audiovisual materials, pictographs, and small group classes, if they are thoughtfully constructed and pretested (Hahn & Cella, 2003; Houts, Wismer, Egeth, Loscalzo, & Zabora, 2001; Oermann, Webb, & Ashare, 2003). However, it is important to understand that changing the mode of communication alone does not decrease the literacy demand of the message. The decoding, comprehension, and recall components remain the same. However, if there is careful use of language, appropriate use of pictographs and vignettes, client control over the pacing of the information, and provider follow-up to assess comprehension and to individualize the message, then these strategies can be successful

(Doak et al., 2001; Hahn & Cella, 2003; Houts et al., 2001). This combination of strategies is now being tested. DeWalt et al. (2006) included picture-based educational materials, training sessions, a digital scale, and frequent telephone follow-up in a heart-failure management program and found that it reduced hospitalization and death.

Readability of Written Materials

Readability of written materials can be vastly improved. Both the IOM (2003) and *Healthy People 2010* (U.S. Department of Health and Human Services, 2000) lists evidence-based health communication as a high-priority item for the improvement of health care. Multiple tools exist on how to assess the reading level of materials (Doak et al., 2001). SMOG, FOG, Flesch, and Fry and are among the most frequently used readability tools. The formulae are simple and can be done often by hand or by using common software programs, taking only a few minutes (National Cancer Institute, 2003).

However, evaluating the reading demand of text has encountered much criticism in recent years. The tools noted above evaluate aspects of reading demand, such as word familiarity, length of sentences, punctuation, and number of prepositional words. Recently, in the literature new formulae are being developed that address multiple other variables that affect readability. The Singh Readability Assessment Instrument includes handwriting or typography that is legible, interest level of the text, and style of writing (Singh, 2003).

Given the expense and importance of our written materials in today's healthcare environment to our vulnerable clients, written materials need to be tested in a systematic fashion (National Cancer Institute, 2003) before use. Given the NALS data, all systems of health care need to systematize how written materials are evaluated before use (IOM, 2003; U.S. Department of Health and Human Services, 2000).

English as a Second Language

Addressing the needs of English as a second language clients is very complex. Providers generally have taken shortcuts in providing simple English or translated pamphlets that are far above the skill level of such clients, who have significantly longer hospital stays than English-speaking patients (Schillinger & Chen, 2004). Clients with limited English proficiency, even if skilled in their primary language, may be more likely to have children with a fair to poor health status (Flores, Abreu, & Tomany-Korman, 2005). Tools to measure literacy in other languages are just recently being developed (Lee, Bender, Ruiz, & Cho, 2006). Tool development is particularly important, because research suggests that a significant number of clients who report proficiency in English in healthcare settings actually have very limited English literacy (Zun, Sandoun, & Downey, 2006).

Use of Computers and Internet

A number of studies have suggested that technology can be used to address the learning needs of low literacy clients. One primary drawback, however, is that the reading level of most health-related information (83%) in both English and Spanish on the Internet has been found to require a 12th-grade reading level or above to comprehend (Berland et al., 2001). Friedman, Hoffman-Goetz, and Arocha (2004) found cancer information was often written at a college level. This was validated in a 2006 study of websites with colorectal cancer information, noting that not only were the sites at a high reading level, but access and skills in the use of such technology are barriers for those with low literacy. Studies report a high level of client satisfaction with using the Internet but also find that low literacy users greatly overestimate their reading skill in relation to access and comprehension of health information (Birru et al., 2004). Three-fourths of their low literacy subjects did not look past the first page on Google retrievals, stating that the first page always gives them what they need. Seligman et al. (2005) found similar results in a study on diabetic patients with limited literacy. They also found that the Internet education strategy alone did not result in significant changes in weight, hypertension, knowledge, and self-efficacy. Programs that have an adaptive component so that each user had a tailored educational approach yielded more positive results (Nebel et al., 2004).

Improving Literacy through Health Care

Potential strategies to address illiteracy in health care focus on how to identify and work with individual clients so that providers' styles of oral and written communication fit with their clients' skill levels. However, these approaches may essentially be skirting the core issue related to client vulnerability.

As reviewed in this chapter, literacy problems themselves create health risks. By using methods that ignore or accommodate to the literacy deficit, providers essentially perpetuate the illiteracy problem. This approach, in which providers address the consequences of such core problems as illiteracy, perpetuates the predominant tertiary care focus in our system of health care. Literacy affects the lives of our clients in foundational ways: the creation of social stigma and prejudicial attitudes; ability to navigate within complex systems throughout society, including and beyond health care; housing; and money management. Literacy is a core driver of vulnerability in America and needs to be addressed as a foundational aspect of health care.

Healthy People 2010 and the IOM state that providers need to improve their communication related to literacy needs to improve the quality of health care. In addition, health care can and should improve health through literacy. David Baker, a researcher in health literacy, stated the following (Marwick, 1997):

> Millions of Americans cannot achieve health literacy until we can find better ways of communication with them. Rewriting brochures won't get us where we want to go. What we're talking about is a new paradigm, where we change patients' learning capabilities.

The literature review for this chapter found few clinical intervention recommendations that spoke to the need to directly improve client literacy skills. Miles and Davis (1995) recommended that healthcare providers need to partner with community-wide agencies, such as schools and neighborhood settings in which the opportunity to become literate initially foundered. In 2005, Parker evaluated more community approaches to improve literacy by working with libraries to address the long-term nature of low literacy and interventions. Uniquely, she asserted that proper design of all healthcare information, written, verbal, or electronic, aligned with the Plain Language Initiative of the National Institutes of Health is a necessary first step.

Improving provider sensitivity and skills in working with low literacy clients is also required. Providers must be aware of their tendency to overestimate literacy levels, especially in altered health states. Alternative approaches, such as use of pictures, can be useful. Slowing down, using other family members in discussion, and consistent evaluation of learning of all clients is needed. Use of therapeutic relationships and meaningful interactions can change outcomes dramatically. Paasche-Orlow, Reikert, et al. (2005) studied a "teach to goal" strategy that used a multiple method and multiple encounter approach that emphasized effective evaluation of learning, noting that fully one-third of the clients, despite well-planned, focused, and simplified instruction, were unable to demonstrate comprehension of instructions on first evaluation. The authors note that this approach is very time-intensive, but the outcomes were significantly different than the more typical single encounter single method approach in health care.

International literature has already reported programs in which the development of literacy is in tandem with healthcare interventions. Watters (2003) presented a fascinating model that integrates linguistics, literacy, nursing, community partnership, and anthropology that shows potential for use in the United States. Watters reviewed the international programs, citing one in Nepal that noted initially greater costs of a combined maternal nutrition and literacy program, when compared with simply administering vitamin A. However, the combined approach decreased infant and child mortality by one-half. Such programs can help the community first gain the needed tools in literacy, subsequently providing long-term health benefits and decreased vulnerability in the community.

As Baker (1999) stated, in America, this would require a paradigm shift. Rather than compartmentalizing the skills needed to decrease health vulnerability, healthcare providers could actively work to address core issues that lead to clients' need to access care.

Conclusion

Functional illiteracy directly creates health vulnerability in clients. Illiteracy is pervasive in client populations, and clinicians cannot rely on education level or self-disclosure to identify those clients with these needs. Those clients with the greatest health needs are the same clients who do not have the tools to navigate the complex U.S. healthcare system. Current provider communication styles and materials greatly mismatch client literacy skills. Solutions addressing this intersection of healthcare needs and illiteracy have been client-focused and on a micro level. In this chapter we propose that providers need to partner with communities to develop literacy skills in their members to decrease their health risk. International models may provide models for trial in the United States.

References

Aday, L. A. (2001). *At risk in America: The health and health care needs of vulnerable populations in the United States* (2nd ed.). San Francisco: Jossey-Bass.

Agency for Healthcare Research and Quality. (2004). *Literacy and health outcomes.* Evidence Report/Technology Assessment No. 87. Retrieved December 2006, from www.ahrq.gov

Al-Tayyib, A. A., Rogers, S. M., Gribble, J. N., Villarroel, M., & Turner, C. F. (2002). Effect of low medical literacy on health survey measurements. *American Journal of Public Health, 92*(9), 1478–1480.

American Medical Association. (1999). Health literacy report of the Council on Scientific Affairs. Ad Hoc Committee on Health Literacy for the Council on Scientific Affairs. *Journal of the American Medical Association, 10*(6), 552–557.

Baker, D. (1999). Reading between the lines: Deciphering the connections between literacy and health. *Journal of General Internal Medicine, 14,* 315–317.

Baker, D. W., Gazmararian, J. A., Williams, M. V., Scott, T., Parker, R. M., Green, D., Ren, J., & Peel, J. (2002). Functional health literacy and the risk of hospital admission among Medicare managed care enrollees. *American Journal of Public Health, 92*(8), 1278–1283.

Baker, D. W., Parker, R. M., Williams, M. V., Pitkin, K., Parikh, N. S., Coates, W., & Imara, M. (1996). The health care experience of patients with low literacy. *Archives of Family Medicine, 5*(6), 329–334.

Bass, P. F. 3rd, Wilson, J. F., Griffith, C. H., & Barnett, D. R. (2002). Residents' ability to identify patients with low literacy skills. *Academic Medicine, 77*(10), 1039–1041.

Berland, G. K., Elliott, M. N., Morales, L. S., Algazy, J. I., Kravitz, R. L., Broder, M. S., et al. (2001). Health information on the Internet: Accessibility, quality, and readability in English and Spanish. *Journal of the American Medical Association, 285*(20), 2612–2621.

Birru, B. A., Monaco, V. M., Drew, L., Njie, V., Bierria, B. A., Detlefsen, E., et al. (2004). Internet usage by low-literacy adults seeking health information: An observational analysis. *Journal of Medical Internet Research, 6*(3), e25.

Chew, L. D., Bradley, K. A., & Boyko, E. J. (2004). Brief questions to identify patients with inadequate health literacy. *Family Medicine, 36*(8), 588–594.

Davis, T. C., Long, S. W., & Jackson, R. H. (1993). Rapid Estimate of Adult Literacy in Medicine: A shortened screening instrument. *Family Medicine, 25*(6), 391–395.

DeWalt, D. A., Malone, R. M., Bryant, M. E., Kosnar, M. C., Corr, K. E., Rothman, R. L., et al. (2006). A heart failure self-management program for patients of all literacy levels: A randomized, controlled trial. *BMC Health Services Research, 6,* 6–30.

Doak, C. C., Doak, L. G., & Root, J. H. (2001). *Teaching patients with low literacy skills* (2nd ed.). Philadelphia: Lippincott.

Duncan, G. J., Daly, M. C., McDonough, P., & Williams, D. (2002). Optimal indicators of socioeconomic status for health research. *American Journal of Public Health, 92*(7), 1151–1158.

Feifer, R. (2003). How a few simple words improve patient's health. *Managed Care Quarterly, 11*(2), 29–31.

Flores, G., Abreu, M., & Tomany-Korman, S. C. (2005). Limited English proficiency, primary language at home, and disparities in children's health care: How language barriers are measured matters. *Public Health Reports, 120*(4), 418–430.

Forbis, S., & Aligne, C. (2002). Poor readability of asthma management plans found in national guidelines, *Pediatrics, 109,* e52.

Freidman, D. B., Hoffman-Goetz, L. & Arocha, J. F. (2004). Readability of cancer information on the internet. *Journal of Cancer Education, 19*(2), 117–122.

Gannon, W., & Hildebrant, E. (2002). A winning combination: Women, literacy, and participation in health care. *Health Care of Women International, 23*(6–7), 754–760.

Hahn, K. S. (2000). Literacy for health information of adult patients and caregivers in a rural health department. *Clinical Excellence for Nurse Practitioners, 4*(1), 35–40.

Hahn, E. A., & Cella, D. (2003). Health outcomes assessment in vulnerable populations: Measurement challenges and recommendations. *Archives of Physical Medicine and Rehabilitation, 84*(4 Suppl 2), S35–S42.

Hohn, M. D. (1998). *Empowerment health education in adult literature: A guide for public health and adult literacy practitioners, policy makers, and funders.* Retrieved August 22, 2007, from http://www.nifl.gov/nifl/fellowship/reports/hohn/HOHN.HTM

Houts, P. S., Wismer, J. T., Egeth, H. E., Loscalzo, M. J., & Zabora, J. R. (2001). Using pictographs to enhance recall of spoken medical instruction. *Patient Education and Counseling, 43*(3), 231–242.

Institute of Medicine of the National Academies. (2003). Priority areas for national action: Transforming health care quality. Washington, DC: The National Academies Press.

Kefalides, P. (1999). Illiteracy: The silent barrier to health care. *Annals of Internal Medicine, 130*(4), 333–336.

Kirsch, I. S., Jungeblut, A., Jenkins, L., & Kolstad, A. (1993). *Executive summary of adult literacy in America: A first look at the results of the National Adult Literacy Survey.* Retrieved August 22, 2007, from http://nces.ed.gov/pubs93/93275.pdf

Lee, S. Y., Bender, D. E., Ruiz, R. E., & Cho, Y. I. (2006). Development of an easy-to-use Spanish health literacy test. *Health Services Research, 41*(4 Pt 1), 1392–1412.

Marwick, D. (1997). Patients' lack of literacy may contribute to billions of dollars in higher hospital costs. *Journal of the American Medical Association, 278*(12), 971–972.

Miles, S., & Davis, T. (1995). Patients who can't read. Implications for the health care system. *Journal of the American Medical Association, 274*(21), 1677–1682.

Morris, N. S., MacLean, C. D., Chew, L. D., & Littenberg, B. (2006). The Single Item Literacy Screener: Evaluation of a brief instrument to identify limited reading ability. *BMC Family Practice, 7*(21), 107.

National Cancer Institute. (2003). *Clear & simple: Developing effective print materials for low-literate clients.* Retrieved August 22, 2007, from http://www.nci.nih.gov/cancerinformation/clearandsimple

National Center for Health Statistics. (2006). *National assessment of adult literacy.* Retrieved August 22, 2007, from http://nces.ed.gov/NAAL/index.asp?file=AssessmentOf/HealthLiteracy/Health LiteracyResults.asp&PageID=158

Nebel, I. T., Klemm, T., Fasshauer, M., Muller, J., Verlohren, H. J., Klaiberg, A., et al. (2004). Comparative analysis of conventional and an adaptive computer-based hypoglycaemia education programs. *Patient Education and Counseling, 53*(3), 315–318.

Oermann, M. H., Webb, S. A., & Ashare, J. A. (2003). Outcomes of videotape instruction in clinic waiting area. *Orthopedic Nursing, 22*(2),102–105.

Paasche-Orlow, M., Parker, R., Gazmararian, J., Neilsen-Bohlman, L., & Rudd, R. R. (2005a). The prevalence of limited health literacy. *Journal of General Internal Medicine, 20*, 175–184.

Paasche-Orlow, M., Reikert, K. A., Bilderback, A., Chanmugam, A., Hill, P., Rand, C., et al. (2005b). Tailored education may reduce health literacy disparities in asthma self-management. *American Journal of Respiratory and Critical Care Medicine, 172*(8), 980–986.

Parikh, N. S., Parker, R. M., Nurss, J. R., Baker, D. W., & Williams, M. V. (1996). Shame and health literacy: The unspoken connection. *Patient Education and Counseling, 27*(1), 33–39.

Parker, R. (2005). Library outreach: Overcoming health literacy challenges. *Journal of the Medical Library Association, 93*(3), S81–S85.

Parker, R. M., Ratzan, S. C., & Lurie, N. (2003). Health literacy: A policy challenge for advancing high-quality health care. *Health Affairs (Project Hope), 22*(4), 147–153.

Powell, C., & Kripalani, S. (2005). Resident recognition of low literacy as a risk factor in hospital readmission. *Journal of General Internal Medicine, 20*(11), 1042–1044.

Raich, P. C., Plomer, K. D., & Coyne, C. A. (2001). Literacy, comprehension, and informed consent in clinical research. *Cancer Investigation, 19*(4), 437–445.

Rootman, I., & Ronson, B. (2005). Literacy and health research in Canada: Where have we been and where have we gone? *Canadian Journal of Public Health, 96*(Suppl 2), S62–S77.

Rosenthal, M. S., Werner, M. J. & Dubin, N. H. (2004). The effect of a literacy training program on family medicine residents. *Family Medicine, 36*(8), 582–587.

Safeer, R. S., & Keenan, J. (2005). Health literacy: The gap between physicians and patients. *American Family Physician, 72*(3), 463–468.

Schillinger, D., & Chen, A. (2004). Literacy and language: Disentangling measures of access. *Journal of General Internal Medicine, 19,* 288–290.

Schillinger, D., Piette, J., Grumbach, K., Wang, F., Willson, C., Daher, C., et al. (2003). Physician communication with diabetic patients who have low literacy. *Archives of Internal Medicine, 163*(1), 83–90.

Schultz, M. (2002). Low literacy skills needn't hinder care. *RN, 65*(4), 45–48.

Seligman, H. K., Wang, F. F., Palacios, J. L., Wilson, C. L., Haher, C., Piette, J. D., et al. (2005). Physician notification of their diabetes patients' limited health literacy: A randomized controlled study. *Journal of General Internal Medicine, 20,* 1001–1007.

Sentell, T., & Ratcliff-Baird, B. (2003). Literacy and comprehension of Beck Depression Inventory response alternatives. *Community Mental Health Journal, 39*(4), 323–331.

Singh, J. (2003). Research briefs reading grade level and readability of printed cancer education materials. *Oncology Nursing Forum, 30*(5), 867–870.

U.S. Department of Health and Human Services. (2000). *Healthy People 2010: Understanding and improving health.* Washington, DC: The National Academies Press.

Watters, E. K. (2003). Literacy for health: An interdisciplinary model. *Journal of Transcultural Nursing, 14*(1), 48–54.

Weiss, B. D., Mays, M. Z., Martz, W., Castro, K. M., DeWalt, D., Pignone, M., et al. (2005). Quick assessment of literacy in primary health care: The Newest Vital Sign. *Annals of Family Medicine, 31*(6), 514–522.

Williams, M. V. (2000). *Definition of "health literacy."* Message posted to National Institute for Literacy list server. Retrieved August 23, 2007, from http://www.nifl.gov/nifl-health/2000/0439.html

Williams, M. V., Baker, D., Honig, E. G., Lee, T. M., & Nowlan, A. (1998). Inadequate literacy as a barrier to asthma knowledge and self-care. *Chest, 114,* 1008–1015.

Zun, L. S., Sadoun, T. A., & Downey, L. (2006). English-language competency of self-declared English-speaking Hispanic patients using written tests of health literacy. *Journal of the National Medical Association, 98*(6), 912–919.

Unit Two

The obvious is that which is never seen until someone expresses it simply.

■ ■ ■

Kahlil Gibran

NURSING THEORIES

Chapter 6

Nursing Theories Applied to Vulnerable Populations: Examples from Turkey

Behice Erci

In this chapter we present the areas in which nursing models and theories guide nursing practice related to vulnerable populations. Nine nursing theories are presented with detailed clinical examples for several of those theories believed to be more applicable. Readers are referred to the primary sources for complete description and explanation of the theoretical concepts.

Importance of Theories in Advanced Nursing Practice

The dilemma for nurse educators is how best to prepare nurses for advanced practice roles. Is nursing theory important? Does it contribute to clinical practice? Which theories form sound foundations for advanced practice? Theories exist to challenge existing practice, create new approaches to practice, and remodel the structure of rules and principles. Furthermore, theories should ultimately improve nursing practice. Usually, this goal is achieved by using theory or portions of theory to guide practice.

Defining the scope of advanced practice requires that the role of nurses be considered unique. For nursing practice to be viewed as professional, it is essential that practice is based on theory. Theory and theoretical frameworks are intended to provide guidance and rationale for professional practice, but as advanced practice roles evolve in nursing, the incorporation of nursing theory becomes problematic. It has been suggested that the wide variety of definitions and concepts discussed in most nursing theories do not explain or predict anything. Therefore they cannot practically be applied to clinical situations and are of little use to nurses in advanced practice.

Orem's General Theory of Nursing

The self-care theory (Berbiglia, 1997; Orem, 1995) linked patient assessments with nursing diagnosis, expected patient outcomes, discharge planning, quality assurance, clinical research, and external agency reports. There are three subtheories within Orem's theory. The *theory of self-care deficit* details how individuals can benefit from nursing because they are subject to health-related or self-derived limitations. The *theory of self-care* states that care is a learned behavior that purposely regulates human structural integrity, functioning, and development. The *theory of nursing systems describes* how nurses use their abilities to prescribe, design, and provide nursing care.

Application to Vulnerable Populations

To provide nursing care, Orem identifies operations that are specifically professional–technological, including diagnostic, prescriptive, treatment or regulatory, and case management. The application of Orem's theory to nursing practice is relevant as a framework in a variety of settings, including acute care units, ambulatory clinics, community health programs, high-rise senior centers, nursing homes, hospices, and rehabilitation centers. The theory is applied to patients with specific diseases or conditions, including adolescents with chronic disease, alcoholics, the chronically ill, head and neck surgery, rheumatoid arthritis, and cardiac conditions (Conway, McMillan, & Solman, 2006). The theory is also applied to selected age groups, including the aged, children, and mothers with newborns.

Example
Yeliz is 29 years old, married, and 5 months pregnant. She has anemia, is underweight, and is under the care of a primary healthcare center. Complete data have been compiled from the client's records and a home visit. The nurses are concerned that her self-care requisites (or requirements) are not being met. These are food, healthy activity, and rest. She requires assistance in food preparation but can eat on her own. Her priority diagnoses are inadequate food intake, low activity level, and fatigue due to inadequate rest.

Diagnostic and Prescriptive Operations All three priority diagnoses previously listed are related to preventing health deterioration. In this client's case the self-care deficit theory of nursing proposes a supportive educational nursing system that is designed to individualize her care. The individualization of the nursing system is accomplished through the overlay of basic conditioning factors and developmental self-care requisites (or requirements for life and health) on the therapeutic self-care demands (those processes necessary to maintain life or health). The expected outcome is health status maintenance, health promotion, and prevention of further health deterioration through the strengthening of the self-care agency. Unless expected outcomes are provided, the nursing system design will change.

Regulatory Operations The self-care deficit theory of nursing is especially useful with this client. The theory changes the focus away from disease to the strengths and/or weaknesses of the self-care agent. It is evident that the client does seek to prevent and/or manage the conditions threatening her health, yet she requires assistance in this area. The most significant self-care deficit is in the area of nutrition. Guided by the theory, the nurse analyzed the self-care agency from the perspective of the basic conditioning factors. Cultural variety should be considered in reaching for the expected outcome.

Data collection for the client in terms of self-care requisites led to the following proposed outcomes: maintenance of the healthy environment, ability of the client to feed herself, and discussion of her condition and medical regimen with the home health nurse and aide and the client's family. The nursing diagnosis showed a potential for anemic complications such as falls and decreased mobility. Methods of help and/or intervention included teaching, guiding, and providing and/or maintaining direction in an environment that supported personal development. Self-care agency is inadequate and implies the necessity to gain better understanding of the cause and subsequent prevention of problems. The nursing diagnosis is "potential for exacerbation and increased disability related to knowledge deficits concerning problems." Teaching, guiding, and directing are methods of helping. For the nursing diagnosis, "inability to maintain ideal body weight related to cultural attitudes toward eating and weight gain and meal preparation by aide," the methods of helping are to provide and maintain an environment that supports personal development.

Roy's Adaptation Model

Roy drew upon expanded insights in relating spirituality and science to present a new definition of adaptation and related scientific and philosophical assumptions (Connerley, Ristau, Lindberg, & McFarland, 1999; Roy, 1976). Her philosophical stance articulates that nurses see persons as coextensive with their physical and social environments. Furthermore, nurse scholars take a value-based stance rooted in beliefs and hopes about the human person, and they develop a discipline that participates in enhancing the well-being of persons and of the earth. Roy viewed persons and groups as adaptive systems with cognator and regulator subsystems acting to maintain adaptation in the four adaptive modes: physiological–physical, self-concept–group identity, role function, and interdependence.

Application to Vulnerable Populations

Roy used a problem-solving approach for gathering data, identifying the capacities and needs of the human adaptive system, selecting and implementing approaches for nursing care, and evaluating the outcome of the care provided. The approach includes assessment of behavior and stimuli and is consistent with the nursing process of assessment, diagnosis, planning, implementation, and evaluation.

Example
Hasan is a 35-year-old man recently admitted to the oncology nursing unit for evaluation after undergoing surgery for class IV prostate cancer. He has smoked approximately two packs of cigarettes a day for the past 9 years. He is married and lives with his wife. He has done well after surgery except for being unable to completely empty his urinary bladder.

Hasan is having continued postoperative pain. When he goes home, it will be necessary for him to perform intermittent self-catheterization. His home medications are an antibiotic and an analgesic as needed. In addition, he will be receiving radiation therapy on an outpatient basis. Hasan is extremely tearful. He expresses great concern over his future. He believes that this illness is a punishment for his past life.

Physiological Adaptive Mode The client's health problems are complex. It is impossible to develop interventions for all his health problems within this chapter. Therefore only representative examples are given. Physiological adaptive mode refers to the basic and complex biological processes necessary to maintain life.

Assessment of Behavior Postoperatively, the patient is unable to completely empty his urinary bladder. He states that he is "numb" and unable to tell when he needs to void. Catheterization for residual urine has revealed that he is retaining 300 ml of urine after voiding. It is necessary for him to perform intermittent self-catheterization at home. Unsanitary conditions at Hasan's home place him at high risk for developing a urinary tract infection. He states that he is scared about performing self-catheterization.

Assessment of Stimuli In this phase of the nursing process, the nurse searches for the stimuli responsible for certain observed behaviors. After the stimuli are identified, they are classified as focal, contextual, or residual. The focal stimulus for the client's urinary retention is the disease process. Contextual stimuli include tissue trauma resulting from surgery and radiation therapy. Anxiety is a residual stimulus. Infection is a potential problem. The focal stimulus is the need for intermittent self-catheterization. Contextual stimuli include altered skin integrity related to surgical incision, poor understanding of aseptic principles, and unsanitary conditions at Hasan's home.

Nursing Diagnosis From the assessment of behaviors and the assessment of stimuli, the following nursing diagnoses are made:

1. Altered elimination: urinary retention related to surgical trauma, radiation therapy, and anxiety
2. Potential for infection related to intermittent self-catheterization, altered skin integrity resulting from surgical incision, poor understanding of aseptic principles, and unsanitary conditions at the client's home

Goal Setting Goals are set mutually between the nurse and the client for each of the nursing diagnoses. The goals are (1) complete urinary elimination every 4 hours as evidenced by correct demonstration of the procedure for intermittent self-catheterization and (2) continued absence of signs of infection of the surgical incision and urinary tract.

Implementation To help the client attain these goals, the following nursing interventions were implemented:

1. To address the issue of incomplete elimination, the client is taught the importance of performing intermittent self-catheterization every 4 hours to prevent damage to the urinary bladder. He is taught to assess his abdomen for bladder distention and the proper procedure for intermittent self-catheterization. He is instructed to keep a record of the exact time and amount of voiding and catheterizations. In addition, the client is taught relaxation techniques to facilitate voiding so it will not be necessary for him to catheterize himself as often.

2. To address the potential for infection, the client is taught the importance of washing hands before touching the surgical incision or doing incision care. After the procedure for incision care is demonstrated by the nursing staff, and the client is asked to perform a return demonstration. After the intermittent self-catheterization procedure is explained and demonstrated, the client is asked to perform a return demonstration.

Evaluation An evaluation of the client's adaptive level is performed each shift.

Self-Concept Adaptive Mode

Assessment of Behavior The client is extremely tearful. He expresses great concern over his future. Exploration of the client's tearfulness revealed that the client is afraid of dying. Also, the client has not asked the nurse any questions about sexuality. His hesitancy to introduce the subject may be related to his cultural background. In this case the nurse introduces the topic. Salient findings are as follows: (1) the client recently learned of a diagnosis of prostate cancer, (2) he has undergone a recent operation, (3) he is receiving radiation therapy in the hospital and this therapy will continue when he leaves the hospital, and (4) the client has a lack of information about the impact of prostate cancer and chemotherapy on sexuality.

Assessment of Stimuli The client is an adult, married, and has a fifth grade education. He is in an emotionally distant and sometimes abusive relationship. Being diagnosed with prostate cancer at an early age has resulted in a maturational crisis for the client. This is complicated by the fact that several of his relatives have died of cancer. It is important for the nurse to assess coping strategies. One coping strategy that is mentioned is that the client is frequently tearful.

Nursing Diagnosis The following nursing diagnoses are made:

1. Fear and anxiety of dying related to medical diagnosis and witnessing other family members' deaths as a result of cancer

2. Spiritual distress related to severe life-threatening illness and perception of moral–ethical–spiritual self

3. Sexual dysfunction related to the disease process, need for radiation therapy at home, weakness, fatigue, pain, anxiety, and a lack of information about the impact of prostate cancer and chemotherapy on sexuality

4. Grieving related to body image disturbance, lack of self-ideal, and potential for premature death

Goal Setting To help the client achieve adaptation in the self-concept adaptive mode, the following goals are set:

1. Decrease fear and anxiety of dying as evidenced by less tearfulness, relaxed facial expression, relaxed body movements, verbalization of new coping strategies, and fewer verbalizations of fear and anxiety

2. Decrease spiritual distress as evidenced by verbalization of positive feelings about self-verbalization about the value and meaning of his life, and less tearfulness

3. Resume sexual relationship that is satisfying to both partners and evidenced by verbalization of self as sexually capable and acceptable, verbalization of alternative methods of sexual expression during the first 10 weeks after surgery

4. Progression through the grieving process as evidenced by verbalization of feelings regarding body image, self-ideal, and potential for premature death

Implementation The following nursing interventions are implemented to help achieve these goals in the self-concept adaptive mode:

1. *Fear and anxiety of dying related to medical diagnosis and witnessing other family members' deaths as a result of cancer*

   Although the client's prognosis appeared to be good, he remained fearful of dying. Time is taken to sit with the client, make eye contact, and actively listen. The client is asked to share an extremely difficult experience he encountered in the past. He is asked how he coped with that experience. Once his present coping strategies are assessed, new coping strategies are suggested.

   He is encouraged to express his feelings openly. After allowing the client adequate time to express his feelings, truthful and realistic hope based on the client medical history is offered. A cancer support group meets each week in the hospital where the client is a patient. The client is given a schedule of the meeting times and topics. He and his partner are encouraged to attend the cancer support group meetings.

2. *Spiritual distress related to severe life-threatening illness and perception of moral–ethical–spiritual self*

The client is encouraged to express his feelings openly about his illness. It is suggested that times of illness are good times to renew spiritual ties. The client is supported in positive aspects of his life.

3. *Sexual dysfunction related to the disease process, need for radiation therapy at home, weakness, fatigue, pain, anxiety, and a lack of information about the impact of prostate cancer and chemotherapy on sexuality*

    A complete sexual assessment is conducted to evaluate the perceived adequacy of the client's sexual relationship and to elicit concerns or issues about sexuality before his diagnosis with prostate cancer. A private conversation is initiated with the client to gain an understanding of his sexual concerns resulting from his therapy and his beliefs about the effects of prostate in regard to sexual functioning. The client is instructed regarding possible changes in sexual functioning, such as a temporary inability to achieve or sustain an erection, for up to several months.

4. *Grieving related to body image disturbance, loss of self-ideal, and potential for premature death*

    The client's perceptions regarding the impact of the diagnosis of prostate cancer on his body image, self-ideal, roles, and his future are explored. Hasan is encouraged to verbally acknowledge the losses he is experiencing. The client is observed to determine which stage of the grief process he currently experiences. The grieving process is explained to the client and to his family, and they are assured that grieving is a normal process. The nursing staff should offer realistic reassurance about the client prognosis. The client is encouraged to attend the cancer support group so he can talk to others who better understand his grief.

Evaluation Behavior change is expected.

King's Theory

The focus of King's theory (1971) is on individuals whose interactions in groups within social systems influence behavior within the systems (Gonot, 1989). In other words, the perceptions that people experience as a result of their surroundings influence their own behavior. King's theory is system based. Concepts of self-growth and development and body image are important (Frey & Norris, 1997; Gonot, 1989). The goal of nursing is to help individuals maintain their health so they can function in their roles.

Application to Vulnerable Populations

It is within this interpersonal system of nurse–client that the traditional steps of the nursing process are carried out. Nurse and client meet in some situation, perceive each other, make judgments about the other, take some mental action, and react to each one's perceptions of the other. Because these behaviors cannot be directly observed, one can only draw inferences from them. The next step in the process is interaction that can be directly observed. When interactions lead to transactions, goal attainment behaviors are exhibited. An assumption underlying the interaction process is that of reciprocally contingent behavior in which the behavior of one person influences the behavior of the other and vice versa (Gonot, 1989).

Example

Elif is 50 years old and has heart failure. She is married and lives with her husband. She describes him as emotionally distant and abusive at times. She is having continued cardiac pain and palpitation. She will be receiving cardiac therapy on an outpatient basis. Elif is extremely tearful and anxious. She expresses great concern over her future.

From King's framework, Elif is conceptualized as a personal system in interaction with other systems. Many of these interactions influence her health. In addition, her recent diagnosis of heart failure influences her health. Together Elif and the nurse communicate, engage in mutual goal setting, and make decisions about the means to achieve goals.

Nursing care for Elif begins with assessment, which includes collection, interpretation, and verification of data. Sources of data are Elif herself, primarily perception, behavior, and past experiences; knowledge of concepts in the systems framework; critical thinking skills; ability to use nursing process; and medical knowledge about the treatment and prognosis of heart failure. Care should well cover the full range of nursing practice: maintenance and restoration of health, care of the sick, and promotion of health.

The nurse forms an interpersonal system with Elif. The transaction process includes perception, judgments, mental actions, and reactions of both individuals. The nurse assesses and applies knowledge of concepts and processes. Critical concepts are perception, self-coping, interaction, role, stress, power, and decision making. The nurse's perception serves as a basis for gathering and interpreting information. Elif's perceptions influence her thoughts and actions and are assessed through verbal and nonverbal behaviors. Because perceptual accuracy is important to the interaction process, the nurse analyzes her own perceptions and her interpretation of Elif's perceptions with Elif. It is expected that perceptions might be influenced by her emotional state, stress, or pain.

According to King, self is the conception of who and what one is and includes one's subjective totality of attitudes, values, experiences, commitments, and awareness of individual existence. Elif reveals important information about herself. She is tearful and expresses fear and concern. Her past behavior provides some basis for her present feeling in that Elif has not taken actions to promote and maintain her own health. Clearly, feelings about self and situation are psychological stressors.

Elif has physical and interpersonal stressors as well. Physical stressors are a result of the illness. Cardiac function, pain, and palpitation are identified as immediate problems. In the interpersonal system, Elif identifies a distant and abusive relationship with her husband. There is a major lack of emotional support during this very difficult time. Her husband's inability to provide basic emotional support is likely to change Elif's physical status.

An additional stressor is the living situation. It is also possible that the lack of personal and perhaps family space contributes to stress. Coping with personal and interpersonal stressors is likely to influence both health and illness outcomes. Elif may need additional resources to help her cope with the immediate situation and the future.

Communication is the key to establishing mutuality and trust between Elif and the nurse and the means to establish patient priorities and move the interaction process toward goal setting. Elif is expected to participate in identifying goals. However, direction from the nurse will likely be necessary because of Elif's overwhelming needs and lack of resources.

Nurses can find direction for assisting patients to identifying goals based on the assumptions that underlie King's systems framework. Nurses assist patients to adjust to changes in their health status. Decisions about goals must be based on the capabilities, limitations, priorities of the patient, and situation. In this situation the immediate goals seem to be controlled by cardiac pain and palpitation, although this needs validation by Elif.

The first nursing action is to perform psychological assessment and provide crisis intervention. Other important goals and actions will be directed toward mobilizing resources, especially husband support. However, it is possible that nursing goals and client goals may be incongruent. Continuous analysis, synthesis, and validation are critical to keep on track.

In addition to decisions about goals, Elif is expected to be involved in decisions about actions to meet goals. Involving Elif in decision making may be a challenge because of her sense of powerlessness over the illness, treatment, and ability to contribute to family functioning. Yet empowering Elif is likely to increase her sense of self, which in turn can reduce stress, improve coping, change perceptions, and lead to changes in her physical state.

Goal attainment needs ongoing evaluation. For Elif, follow-up on pain, palpitation, and cardiac function after discharge is necessary. An option might be to arrange for in-home nursing services. Having a professional in the home would also contribute to further assessment of the family, validation of progress toward goals, and modifications in plans to achieve goals. According to King, if transactions are made, goals will be attained. Goal attainment can improve or maintain health, control illness, or lead to a peaceful death. If goals are not attained, the nurse needs to reexamine the nursing process, critical thinking process, and transaction process.

Leininger's Theory of Culture Care

Leininger's interest in cultural dimensions of human care and caring led to the development of her theory (Leininger, 1995). She subscribed to the central tenet that "care is the essence of nursing and the central, dominant, and unifying focus of nursing" (Leininger, 1991, p. 35). The unique focus of Leininger's theory is care, which she believes to be inextricably linked with culture. She defines culture as "the learned, shared, and transmitted values, beliefs, norms, and life ways of a particular group that guides their thinking, decisions, and actions in patterned ways" (Leininger, 1991, p. 47). The ultimate purpose of care is to provide culturally congruent care to people of different or similar cultures to "maintain or regain their well-being and health or face death in a culturally appropriate way" (Leininger, 1991, p. 39).

Example

A group of Iraqi refugees fled to a city in southeastern Turkey to seek refuge from political unrest, persecution, and extreme poverty. Providing culturally congruent nursing care to this group of people is difficult because of differences in language. This leads to difficulty in understanding the lifeways of this group. The children have diarrhea, and it is difficult for the nurse to observe, interview, and collect data related to cultural practices that might explain the diarrhea. The nurse helps the group to preserve favorable health and caring life-styles about poverty and diarrhea. The nurse provides help for cultural adaptation, negotiation, or adjustment to the refugees' health and life-styles. The nurse can reconstruct or alter designs to help clients change health or life patterns in ways meaningful to them.

Watson's Theory of Human Caring

The caring model or theory can also be considered a philosophical and moral–ethical foundation for professional nursing and part of the central focus for nursing at the disciplinary level. Watson's model of caring is both art and science; it offers a framework that embraces and intersects with art, science, humanities, spirituality, and new dimensions of mind–body–spirit. Concepts of the theory include nursing, person, health, human care, and environment. Watson's relevance to nursing ethics is particularly appropriate (Watson, 2005).

Application to Vulnerable Populations

Watson emphasizes that it is possible to read, study, learn about, even teach and research the caring theory; however, to truly "get it," one has to personally experience it. Thus the model is both an invitation and an opportunity to interact with the ideas, experiment with, and grow. If one chooses to use the caring perspective as theory, model, philosophy, ethic, or ethos for transforming self and practice or self and system, then a variety of questions related to one's view of caring and what it means to be human might help (McCance, McKenna, & Boore, 1999; Watson, 1996; Watson & Smith, 2002).

Example

Nesim is 60 years old, married, and lives with his family. His primary diagnosis is hypertension. Under older models of care the patient might be convinced that he would simply overcome his hypertension—that it would "go away." In the Watson model, however, the nurse should aim to sustain a helping–trusting, authentic, caring relationship to develop the capacity of the patient to problem solve and to teach him and his family proper care. The nurse educates the patient about hypertension and about improving self-health,

thereby enabling and authenticating the deep belief system of the patient. The nu
portive of the expression of positive and negative feelings by the patient. Nesim
as the nurse creates a healing environment at all levels (physical as well as nonpl

The patient should be assisted in the creative use of self and all ways of knowing as part
of the caring process. The nurse must engage Nesim in the artistry of caring–healing practices that are "human care essentials," which potentate alignment of mind–body–spirit,
wholeness, and unity of being in all aspects of care (Watson, 1996, p. 157). The patient
should be followed to evaluate the medical and dietary treatment of hypertension.

Rogers' Science of Unitary Human Beings

Rogers formulated a theory to describe humans and the life process in humans (Daily et
al., 1994; Rogers, 1990, 1992, 1994). Over the ensuing years four critical elements emerged
that are basic to the proposed system: energy fields, open systems, pattern, and pandimensionality (Rogers, 1992). The final concept, pandimensionality, was previously known
as multidimensionality and four-dimensionality. Though Rogers never updated her work,
the theory still provides much that is useful (Malinski, 2006).

Application to Vulnerable Populations

Within Rogers' model the critical-thinking process can be divided into three components:
pattern appraisal, mutual patterning, and evaluation. The critical-thinking process begins
with a comprehensive pattern appraisal. The life process possesses its own unity and is
inseparable from the environment. This holistic appraisal requires the identification of
patterns that reflect the whole. The pattern appraisal is a comprehensive assessment.

Knowledge gained in the appraisal process is via cognitive input, sensory input, intu-
ition, and language. The nurse gains a great deal of appraisal knowledge during the interview with the client by using the feeling or sensing level of knowing. Often described as
instinctual, intuitive knowledge is best realized through reflection. Reflection assists in
appraising patterns. Manifestations of patterns are not static but partial perceptions of
the synthesis of the past, present, and future. These perceptions provide the basis for intuitive knowing. Manifestation, patterns, and rhythms are an indication of evolutionary
emergence of the human field. Pattern appraisal and rhythm identification, along with
reflection, provide the content for appraisal validation with the patient.

Once the client and nurse have consensus with respect to the appraisal, then nursing
action is centered on mutual patterning of the client human–environmental field. The goal
of the nursing action is to bring and promote symphonic interaction between human and
environment. This is done to strengthen the coherence and integrity of the human field and
to "direct and redirect patterning of the human and environmental fields" (Rogers, 1990, p.
122). Patterning activities can be devised with respect to the initial pattern appraisal.

The evaluation process is ongoing and fluid as the nurse reflects on his or her intuitive
knowing. During the evaluation phase the nurse repeats the pattern appraisal process to

determine the level of dissonance perceived. The perceptions are then shared with the client and family and friends. Further mutual patterning is directed by the perceptions found during the evaluation process. This process continues as long as the nurse–client relationship continues (Bultmeier, 1997).

Example
Ayse is a 32-year-old woman recently admitted to the infection-nursing unit for evaluation after experiencing urinary infection and late-stage AIDS. Her weight is 58 kilograms, down from her usual weight of about 80 kilograms. She has smoked approximately one pack of cigarettes a day for the past 16 years. She has two children and is married and lives with her husband in conditions she describes as less than sanitary. She describes her husband as emotionally distant and abusive at times. She is having continued pain and nausea. It will be necessary for her to perform intermittent self-catheterization at home. Her home medications are an antibiotic, an analgesic, and an antiemetic. She will soon be receiving radiation therapy on an outpatient basis. Ayse is extremely tearful. She expresses great concern over her future and the future of her two children. She believes that this illness is a punishment for her past life.

Within the Rogerian model, the process of caring for Ayse begins with pattern appraisal, the most important component of the nursing process. The nurse must engage in caring–healing practices that are human care essentials. The purpose is to potentiate alignment followed by mutual patterning and evaluation.

Pattern Appraisal The history provides a major portion of the pattern appraisal. Ayse has a pattern of smoking, which has been associated with poor health. This visible rhythmical pattern is a manifestation of evolution toward dissonance. In addition, Ayse has a pattern manifestation that has been labeled AIDS. This emergent pattern manifests as dissonant. Ayse has a low educational level, which is relevant as patterning activities are introduced. The nurse has reported that Ayse has a manifestation of fear. Ayse reports the fear of dealing with her life after this illness, and the nurse senses this manifestation of fear. Ayse's self-knowledge links the illness to her personal belief of "being punished" for past mistakes. History and focusing on the "relative present" to explore the pattern of punishment is imperative. It is important that the nurse appraise the environment of the hospital and of the others who share her existence. The pain and fear are dissonant manifestations. Dissonance can be perceived in many aspects of Ayse's appraisal: her unsanitary living conditions and her relationship with her husband, the manifestations of AIDS, weight loss, pain, nausea, and tobacco use. Finally, dissonance is also conceptualized as fear and is manifested in the emotional distance that she feels.

On completion of the pattern appraisal, the nurse presents the analysis to the patient. Emphasis can be placed on areas in which dissonance and harmony are noted in the personal and environmental field manifestations. Consensus needs to be reached with Ayse before patterning activities can be suggested and implemented.

Mutual Patterning Patterning can be approached from many directions. The process is mutual between nurse and patient. Medications are patterning modalities. Ayse is receiving medications. Decisions are made in conjunction with Ayse regarding the use of the medications and the patterning that emerges with the introduction of these modalities. Personal knowledge regarding the medications empowers Ayse to be a vital agent in the selection of modalities. Ayse possesses freedom and involvement in the selection of modalities. Options include therapeutic touch, humor, meditation, visualization, and imagery.

Therapeutic touch can be introduced to Ayse, particularly to reduce her pain. Touch in combination with medications provides patterning that Ayse can direct. The nurse can introduce the process of touch to Ayse's husband and teach him how to incorporate touch into her care. Another option would be to teach Ayse how to center her energy and channel it to the area that is experiencing pain.

Patterning directed at the manifestation of fear is critical. Options include imagery, music, light, and meditation. Fear manifests as her apprehension about self-catheterization. Emphasis needs to be placed on having Ayse direct how, where, when, and with whom the self-catheterization is taught. Establishing a rhythm to the catheterization schedule that is harmonious with Ayse's life would reduce dissonance. Patterning of nutrition and catheterization based on the pattern appraisal can assist in empowering Ayse to learn self-catheterization. A rhythm will evolve that is harmonious with Ayse and her energy field rhythm and that empower Ayse to direct this phase of her treatment.

Human-environment patterning needs to involve the other individuals who share Ayse's environment, including her husband and children. Options relate to increased communication and sanitation patterns. The nurse talks with the family and Ayse to determine what Ayse would prefer to change in her environment to improve sanitation. Options are introduced that allow pattern evolution integral with her environment that is not perceived as dissonant.

Evaluation The evaluation process centers on the perceptions of dissonance that exist after the mutual patterning activities are implemented, to determine whether they were successful. Specific emphasis is placed on emergent patterns of dissonance that are still evident. Manifestations of pain, fear, and tension with family members are appraised. The nurse continually evaluates the amount of dissonance that is apparent with respect to Ayse as he or she cares for her. A summary of the dissonance and/or harmony that the nurse perceives is then shared with Ayse, and mutual patterning is modified or instituted as indicated based on the evaluation.

Roper, Logan, and Tierney's Model of Nursing

In the United Kingdom the model of nursing used most predominantly is that of Roper, Logan, and Tierney (2002) that bases its principles on a model of living. The model is made up of five components: activities of daily living, lifespan, dependence/independence continuum, factors influencing activities of daily living, and individuality in living. Roper et al. suggest that these five components are as applicable to a model of living as they are to a model of nursing. Their work has applicability to a variety of clinical situations (Mooney & O'Brien, 2006; Timmins, 2006).

Example
Hatice is 55 years old. She has difficult respiration and constipation. She cannot do her own cleaning. First, considering 12 activities of daily living and affecting factors, the nurse collects data about the client and sets nursing diagnoses, goals, and activities.

Diagnosis:	Difficult breathing
Goal setting:	Effective breathing
Activity:	The nurse monitors breathing patterns and respirations and provides clean and normal temperature of the client's room.
Diagnosis:	Constipation
Goal setting:	Normal defecation
Activity:	The nurse provides warm water for the client every morning and encourages appropriate exercise. After these activities, the nurse should evaluate the results.

Peplau's Interpersonal Model

Peplau's interpersonal relations model relates to the meta-paradigm of the discipline of nursing (Forchuk, 1993). These concepts are the view of the person, health, nursing, and environment. Peplau's model describes the individual as a system with components of the physiological, psychological, and social. The individual is an unstable system where equilibrium is a desirable state but occurs only through death. This is supported by Peplau's statement that "man is an organism that lives in an unstable equilibrium (i.e., physiological, psychological, and social fluidity) and life is the process of striving in the direction of stable equilibrium (i.e., a fixed pattern that is never reached except in death)" (Peplau, 1992, p. 82). Despite the early publication of the model, Peplaus's work continues to have high applicability (McCamant, 2006; Moraes, Lopes, & Brage, 2006; Stockmann, 2005; Vandemark, 2006).

Application to Vulnerable Populations

The interpersonal relationship between the nurse and the client as described by Peplau (1992) has four clearly discernible phases: orientation, identification, exploitation, and resolution. These phases are interlocking and require overlapping roles and functions as the nurse and the client learn to work together to resolve difficulties in relation to health problems. During the orientation phase of the relationship, the client and nurse come together as strangers meeting for the first time. During this phase the development of trust and empowerment of the client are primary considerations. This is best achieved by encouraging the client to participate in identifying the problem and allowing the client to be an active participant. By asking for and receiving help, the client will feel more at ease expressing needs, knowing that the nurse will take care of those needs. Once orientation has been accomplished, the relationship is ready to enter the next phase.

During the identification phase of the relationship, the client in partnership with the nurse identifies problems. Once the client has identified the nurse as a person willing and able to provide the necessary help, the main problem and other related problems can then be worked on, in the context of the nurse–client relationship. Throughout the identification phase both the nurse and the client must clarify each other's perceptions and expectations. The perceptions and expectations of the nurse and the client affect the ability of both to identify problems and the necessary solutions. When clarity of perceptions and expectations is achieved, the client will learn how to make use of the nurse–client relationship. In turn, the nurse will establish a trusting relationship. Once identification has occurred, the relationship enters the next phase.

During the phase of exploitation the client takes full advantage of all available services. The degree to which these services are used is based on the needs and the interest of the client. During this time the client begins to feel like an integral part of the helping environment and starts to take control of the situation by using the help available from the services offered. Within this phase clients begin to develop responsibility and become more independent. From this sense of self-determination, clients develop an inner strength that allows them to face new challenges. This is best described by Peplau: "Exploiting what a situation offers gives rise to new differentiations of the problem and to the development and improvement of skill in interpersonal relations" (Peplau, 1992, pp. 41–42). As the relationship passes through all the aforementioned phases and the needs of the client have been met, the relationship passes to closure or the phase of resolution.

The strength of the model is the focus on the nurse–client relationship. The focus on this relationship allows for the nurse and the client to work together as partners in problem solving. The model encourages and supports empowerment of the client by encouraging the client to accept responsibility for well-being. The focus on the partnership of the nurse and the client and the emphasis on meeting the identified needs of the client make the model ideal for short-term crisis intervention. Although focusing on getting sick people well, the model is also applicable to health promotion. The focus of the Peplau model on the nurse–client relationship provides a foundation for many types of interactions between the nurse and the client that enhance health.

Example
Tarkan is a 46-year-old married man scheduled for a heart operation next week. The client has had a few hospitalizations and is anxious about the operation. The first phase of Peplau's model is orientation. Because the client has previously been cared for at the hospital, he is familiar with the layout of the facility as well as the general rules and regulations

of the facility and orientation is quickly established. In the next phase of the relationship, identification, the nurse and Tarkan identify problems that require attention, including his feelings about the operation and potential to die as a result. The nurse should also identify that the client is experiencing mixed emotions about the operation because he understands it is necessary. Then the nurse also identifies that the client requires additional support because he has been relatively stable for a time and yet requires this operation. In the next phase, exploitation, Tarkan quickly begins making use of the available resources and services at his disposal and talks with the nurse about his fears and hopes. He expresses feelings of mixed emotions, and the nurse comforts him by reminding him that his feelings are normal. In turn, he expresses relief.

Because the client had been hospitalized twice within a 1-year period, the client was provided with information on services that could be accessed to assist him further should the need arise. With the client making full use of the available services, the nurse–client relationship then entered the final phase, resolution. During resolution the client becomes less dependent on the nurse for one-on-one interactions and no longer seeks further assistance.

Neuman's Health Care Systems Model

The Neuman Health Care Systems Model (Neuman, 1995) is related here to the meta-paradigm of the discipline of nursing. Like other models of nursing the major concepts are person, health, nursing, and the environment, but Neuman uses a systems approach to explain how these elements interact in ways that provide nurses with guidance to intervene with patients, families, or communities. Her view of health seems to be that of a continuum rather than a dichotomy of health and illness (Ross, 1985). Not much is found in the current nursing literature on Neuman's model as newer models have developed, but her legacy should be honored.

Example

Dilek is a 25-year-old woman experiencing violence from her husband and auditory and visual hallucinations. An intrapersonal stressor for Dilek is the limited effect the current medication regime is having on her acute symptoms, including difficulty sleeping. Both interpersonal and extrapersonal stressors exacerbate these intrapersonal stressors. The interpersonal stressors are the strained relationship with her husband related to the charges brought against him for sexual and physical abuse. The extrapersonal stressor is identified as inadequate community resources that could help her stay in her home. Once the stressors have been identified, a determination of the level of prevention required to strengthen the flexible line of defense is made.

In Dilek's situation the identified stressors have penetrated the line of defense. Therefore the goal is to prevent further regression. This is a tertiary level of intervention. As tertiary prevention is concerned with maintaining and supporting existing strengths of the client, this is best achieved through intensive conversations of the nurse with the client to emphasize her existing strengths. Dilek is encouraged to express her mixed feelings of relief and sadness about her relationship with her husband, and her feelings are validated as normal. The alleviation of her psychiatric symptoms is achieved without alteration to her established medication regime.

The primary level of intervention is aimed at health promotion. One of the identified stressors is inadequate community resources. The client attends the local mental health center on a regular basis. However, these appointments with the mental health center occur only once a month. The client should be provided with information related to crisis centers, emergency support, and grief counseling. The nurse follows up to ensure that client makes contact with these resources to strengthen the flexible line of defense.

Conclusion

In this chapter we reviewed of some of the major nursing theories. Although the examples are from Turkey, the elements of these models are global and timeless.

References

Berbiglia, V. A. (1997). Orem's self-care deficit theory in nursing practice. In M. Alligood & A. Marriner-Tomey (Eds.), *Nursing theory utilization & application.* St. Louis, MO: Mosby-Year Book.

Bultmeier, K. (1997). Rogers' science of unitary human being in nursing practice. In M. Alligood & A. Marriner-Tomey (Eds.), *Nursing theory utilization & application.* St. Louis, MO: Mosby-Year Book.

Connerley, K., Ristau, S., Lindberg, C., & McFarland, M. (1999). *The Roy Model in nursing practice: The Roy Adaptation Model* (2nd ed., pp. 515–534). Stamford, CT: Appleton & Lange.

Conway, J., McMillan, M., & Solman, A. (2006). Enhancing cardiac rehabilitation nursing through aligning practice to theory: Implications for nursing education. *Journal of Continuing Education in Nursing, 37*(5), 233–238.

Daily, I. S., Maupin, J. S., Murray, C. A., Satterly, M. C., Schnell, D. L., & Wallace, T. L. (1994). Martha E. Roger: Unitary human beings. In A. Marriner-Tomey (Ed.), *Nursing theorists and their work* (3rd ed., pp. 211–230). St. Louis, MO: C. V. Mosby.

Forchuk, C. (1993). *Hildegarde E. Peplau: Interpersonal nursing theory.* Newbury Park, CA: Sage.

Frey, M. A., & Norris, D. (1997). King's System framework and theory in nursing practice. In M. Alligood & A. Marriner-Tomey (Eds.), *Nursing theory utilization & application.* St. Louis, MO: Mosby-Year Book.

Gonot, P. J. (1989). Imogene M. King's conceptual framework of nursing. In J. J. Fitzpatrick & A. L. Whall (Eds.), *Conceptual models of nursing analysis and application* (2nd ed.). California: Appleton & Lange.

King, I. M. (1971). *Toward a theory for nursing.* New York: John Wiley & Sons.

Leininger, M. M. (1991). *Culture care diversity and universality: A theory of nursing.* New York: National League of Nursing Press.

Leininger, M. M. (1995). *Transcultual nursing: Concepts, theories, research & practice* (2nd ed.). New York: McGraw-Hill.

Malinski, V. (2006). Rogerian science-based nursing theories. *Nursing Science Quarterly, 19*(1), 7–12.

McCamant, K. (2006). Humanistic nursing, interpersonal relations theory and the empathy-altruism hypothesis. *Nursing Science Quarterly, 19*(4), 334–338.

McCance, T., McKenna, H., & Boore, J. (1999). Caring: Theoretical perspectives of relevance to nursing. *Journal of Advanced Nursing, 30,* 1388–1395.

Mooney, M., & O'Brien, F. (2006). Developing a plan of care using the Roper, Logan and Tierney model. *British Journal of Nursing, 15*(16), 887–892.

Moraes, L., Lopes, M., & Brage, V. (2006). Analysis of the functional components of Peplau's theory and its confluence with the group reference. *Acta Paulista de Enfermagen, 19*(2), 228–233.

Neuman, B. (1995). *The Neuman Systems Model* (3rd. ed.). Stamford, CT: Appleton & Lange.

Orem, D. E. (1995). *Nursing concepts of practice* (5th ed.). St. Louis, MO: Mosby.

Peplau, H. E. (1992). *Interpersonal relations in nursing.* New York: Springer.

Rogers, M. E. (1990). Nursing: Science of unitary, irreducible, human beings: Update 1990. In E. A. M. Barrett (Ed.), *Visions of Rogers' science-based nursing* (pp. 5–11). New York: National League for Nursing.

Rogers, M. E. (1992). Window on science of unitary human beings. In M. O'Toole (Ed.), *Miller-Keane encyclopedia and dictionary of medicine, nursing, and allied health* (p. 1339). Philadelphia: W. B. Saunders.

Rogers, M. E. (1994). The science of unitary human beings: Current perspectives. *Nursing Science Quarterly, 7*(1), 33–35.

Roper, N., Logan, W., & Tierney, A., (2002). *The elements of nursing* (4th ed.). Edinburgh: Churchill Livingstone.

Ross, M. (1985). The Betty Neuman Systems Model in nursing practice: A case study approach. *Journal of Advanced Nursing, 10,* 199–207.

Roy, C. (1976). *Introduction to nursing: An adaptation model.* Englewood Cliffs, NJ: Prentice-Hall.

Stockmann, C. (2005). A literature review of the progress of the psychiatric nurse-patient relationship as described by Peplau. *Issues in Mental Health Nursing, 26,* 911–919.

Timmins, F. (2006). Conceptual models used by nurses working in coronary care units: A discussion paper. *European Journal of Cardiovascular Nursing, 5*(4), 253–257.

Vandemark, L. (2006). Awareness of self and expanding consciousness: Using nursing theories to prepare nurse therapists. *Issues in Mental Health Nursing, 27*(6), 605–615.

Watson, J. (1996). Watson's theory of transpersonal caring. In P. H. Walker & B. Neuman (Eds.), *Blueprint for use of nursing models: Education, research, practice, & administration* (pp. 141–184). New York: NLN Press.

Watson, J. (2005). Caring science: Belonging before being as ethical cosmology. *Nursing Science Quarterly, 18*(4), 304–305.

Watson, J., & Smith, M. (2002). Caring science and the science of unitary human beings: A trans-theoretical discourse for nursing knowledge development. *Journal of Advanced Nursing, 37,* 452.

Chapter 7

Culturally Competent Care for Sa

Karen Joines and Mary de Chesnay

The purpose of this chapter is to discuss how Samoan beliefs might be considered in designing culturally competent nursing interventions for Samoan patients using Watson's Theory of Human Care. Though the focus here is on Samoans in America, the principles also apply to Samoans who have settled in other countries. The principles of providing culturally competent care are relevant globally as world immigration patterns challenge nurses in many countries to meet the needs of their newest citizens.

Emigrating from the South Pacific during the past few decades, Samoans have contributed to the cultural diversity of the United States, particularly along the West Coast. Americans often view the territories of the Pacific Islands in terms of exotic tourism to this tropical paradise. However, many Samoans in their native land live in impoverished conditions, and although they might view their homeland as paradise, they are limited in the degree to which they can advance economically. According to McGrath (2002), over 60% of American Samoans have moved to the continental United States in recent decades in search of better educational and economic opportunities.

Dietary patterns are particularly relevant to nursing practice among Samoan immigrants, particularly to New Zealand and the United States, because the high-fat low-fiber diet of many Samoans is related to increased risk of cardiovascular disease. In a New Zealand study, Galanis, McGarvey, Quested, Sio, and Amuli (1999) found differences in dietary patterns among western Samoans and American Samoans, with westerners tending toward a diet high in fat primarily from coconut cream. American Samoans tended to eat more processed foods and had higher blood levels of cholesterol, protein, and sodium.

Similarly, diabetes is of concern to Samoans, and a unique partnership among Pacific Islanders has led to the development of coalitions to educate people about the risks of the disease. Braun et.al. (2003) described a coalition-sponsored training program in the South Pacific. Among the outcomes of the project for American Samoans has been the creation of community-building efforts to sponsor programs in diabetes awareness, education, and screening. Designing such programs will hopefully facilitate prevention and early intervention.

Fritsch (1992) identified the need for nurses of the South Pacific to take the lead in efforts to improve the health of their people. In a speech to the South Pacific Nurses Forum, she urged nurses to become actively involved in formulating health policy. As nurses and Samoans, they are in a particularly powerful position to develop policy for Samoans. For example, researchers in preventing suicide argue that Western models of health promotion and suicide prevention are not appropriate and argue that resilience strategies must be culturally relevant, that is, "developed by the people for the people" (Stewart-Withers & O'Brien, 2006, p. 209). These authors point out that despite Western influence and governance, Samoans retain their culture and traditions and maintain political power at the tribal level.

Samoan views on health often conflict with those held by practitioners in the American health care delivery system, so to provide appropriate care to Samoans, American health-care providers must learn how to integrate Samoan culture into care plans in a culturally competent way. In particular, there are three Samoan beliefs that primarily influence their health perception and practices: holistic view of self, collective involvement, and spirituality. Though the Samoans' views are different from Americans' views, it is not impossible to incorporate Samoan beliefs into quality health care. Watson's Theory of Human Care provides direction for how nurses might design interventions that are culturally based (Watson, 2002, 2005; Watson & Smith 2002).

Watson's Theory of Human Care

Watson's Theory of Human Care is one of many models and theories created to help nurses understand how culture influences well-being. Watson described a central focus of her theory as addressing the "ontological questions of what it means to be, to be ill, healed, caring and humane" (as cited in Bernick, 2004). With this focus at the forefront of their practice, nurses create a healing environment for their patients that reach deep facets of the human experience, encompassing the soul, mind, and body. Watson developed 10 carative factors to aid nurses in using the theory in nursing practice:

1. Humanistic–altruistic system of values
2. Faith–hope
3. Sensitivity to self and to others
4. Helping–trusting, human care relationship
5. Expressing positive and negative feelings
6. Creative problem-solving caring processes
7. Transpersonal teaching–learning
8. Supportive, protective, and/or corrective mental, physical, societal, and spiritual environment
9. Human-needs assistance
10. Existential–phenomenological–spiritual forces (as cited in Bernick, 2004)

Using these 10 carative factors, the healing–caring model serves as an appropriate guideline in creating culturally competent interventions because of its inherent focus on what is meaningful to the individual. In applying Watson's theory, the work of Mendycka is particularly relevant.

Mendycka (2000) explored Watson's theory in a case study in which he provided a strong rationale for the applicability of Watson's work to culturally competent practice and identified three reasons. First, Watson utilized a phenomenological approach to understand what health and illness means to the patient. When nurses work with clients of a different ethnicity or culture, it is essential for the nurse to understand the clients' perceptions and meanings of health and illness before performing any care or teaching. Without a basic understanding of the client's culture, the client and nurse may experience cultural conflict and confusion, and the client may not return for care. Second, the theory involves an intersubjective process that teaches the nurse how to identify with himself or herself and with others by engaging with clients in their experiences. This promotes an environment in which a therapeutic relationship can develop and also assists nurses in developing care plans in concert with patients and families rather than for them. Third, the goal of the theory is to establish holistic harmony within mind, body, and soul.

In particular, the third aspect of holism is relevant to Samoans and has been discussed in regard to other cultures. Erci (2005), in reviewing Watson's theory, noted that the healing environment is key. That Erci applied the theory to a patient from Turkey reinforces the universality of the model. Irish nurses also validated the theory in terms of individual healing processes that are strengthened through authentic relationships defined by caring practices (McCance, McKenna, & Boore 1999).

Because Samoans view care holistically and value collective family involvement, Watson's theory provides a useful basis for interventions with Samoans:

- Develops a helping and trusting relationship with the patient (carative factor 4);

- Develops a capacity to problem solve with the patient and family (carative factor 6);

- Educates, enables, and empowers the client while authenticating his or her beliefs (carative factors 3, 7, and 10);

- Creates a healing environment on all levels to reach harmony (carative factor 8).

These interventions capture the essence of Watson's theory and are consistent with Samoan beliefs. Indeed, one might argue that Watson's principles are universal.

Samoan Perceptions on Health and Traditional Treatments

One of the issues related to providing culturally competent care to populations from small countries or isolated regions of the world is that data-based literature is not available to guide practice. As more studies are conducted, the state of the art of literature will evolve and more sophisticated approaches can be designed. One key study was conducted by a team of Samoan and Japanese nurses and involved qualitative interviews with

Samoan caregivers and family members. The philosophy underlying the research was to develop culturally based ways in which nurses could conduct workshops to help caregivers of Samoan elderly provide better care and relieve their own stress (Mulatilo, Taupau, & Enoka, 2000).

Holistic View of Self

The Samoan concept of self is holistic in that each person has three parts—physical, mental, and spiritual—that together make the person complete. Based on the belief in holism, Samoans assert that a person is healthy when all elements are in balance and harmony. When a patient is not well in one part, all other parts are affected. Therefore when illness affects a person, Samoans believe treatment should be aimed at all three parts, with the goal of reaching harmony and balance (Tamasese, Peteru, Waldegrave, & Bush, 2005). The family is key to successful intervention with Samoan patients (Mulatilo et al., 2000).

Rather than focusing on cures, traditional Samoan healing emphasizes achieving balance and wellness. Traditional remedies use medicinal plants in a variety of ways. Samoans boil leaves or bark to create a drinkable tea and cook roots into a healing meal. In addition to plants, Samoans use oils, massage, and hot and cool applications as treatments (Rogers, n.d.; Saau, 1996). For example, a common approach used by elderly Samoan women to heal headaches is heating tea leaves with water and massaging them into the forehead (Saau, 1996).

Contrast with Western Medicine

Holistic views regarding health and treatment are in sharp contrast with traditional American health care, which is aimed primarily at curing physical ailments and disease. Conventional treatments focus on alleviating biological or physical symptoms using modern technologies and treatments established through scientific research. To accommodate their beliefs in America, many Samoans continue to practice traditional healing as adjuncts to American treatments, rather than as replacements (Rogers, n.d.).

Issues Contributing to Vulnerability

Many Samoans attempt to find traditional healers who have knowledge of ancient healing practices. In Seattle, few Samoan healers are available to elderly clients, and as a result many families perform traditional healing practices to the best of their knowledge with the supplies that are available to them (Saau, 1996). This may cause emotional stress and feelings of cultural isolation if they attempt to create the remedies themselves and feel unsuccessful and limited by resource constraints. The homemade remedies may also be harmful if the client is not fully knowledgeable of what plants to use and how to use them properly. In addition, elderly Samoans may feel alienated or not respected by American healthcare providers who discourage their traditional practices. As a result, many choose not to access American health care.

Interventions

In applying Watson's theory, several carative factors are used. Carative factor 3 is used when nurses approach elderly Samoans in a nonjudgmental and unbiased manner. Beginning with a comprehensive assessment, the nurse converses with the client to elicit the client's perspective on the meaning of the ailment, using carative factor 10 in discovering the patient's phenomenological beliefs regarding health. By asking for information concerning his or her perceptions and cultural practices, the nurse conveys genuine appreciation and interest in the client's priorities. Thus a door opens in the nurse–patient relationship that enables the nurse to establish trust (carative factor 4). Demonstrating respect is critical to success in working with vulnerable clients (de Chesnay, Wharton, & Pamp, 2005).

There are several practical interventions in achieving a trusting and partnering relationship with culturally diverse patients. When assessing alternative health treatments, the nurse should ask clients about their health practices and assess the knowledge they have regarding the treatment being used (i.e., What plant is used? How is it used?). Efficacy and safety are two important topics to address when confronted with a client who uses alternative methods. It is important not to reduce the meaning of the client's experience by placing judgment on cultural healing methods. It is more effective to encourage the client to use complementary healing methods as supplementary treatments to conventional treatments. Safety is a concern when patients use combinations of treatments, and if the nurse does not know whether the practice is safe, she or he will have to research the treatment and discuss it with the healthcare team. While teaching, the nurse should authenticate the client's beliefs and avoid discounting the beliefs.

It is essential that the nurse document and inform the physician regarding all alternative treatments, which has the additional benefit of developing a positive relationship between the physician and the client. The nurse can advocate for the patient's needs by creating a care plan that integrates a holistic approach. By asking the cultural questions and conducting a thorough meaningful assessment of the client's perspective, the nurse fosters cultural identity, the client's sense of control, and partnership in care.

Collective Involvement

Samoans believe that every human exists in the context of an interrelated network of family and community and that the interdependence and harmony created within the relationships contribute to health and well-being (Tamasese et al., 2005). They believe each relationship is defined by specific roles and responsibilities, and if a person cannot fulfill his or her roles, disharmony occurs within the relationship. This disharmony can impair the health of the individual (Management Science for Health, n.d.). Therefore when illness affects a person, one element of healing involves reconnecting and strengthening relationships that are unbalanced. One method is through a ritual called *ho'oponopono*, which includes a method of family counseling, conflict resolution, self-reflection, and a formal session of apology and forgiveness (Management Science for Health, n.d.).

Because Samoan patients maintain an existence within a collective context, families are included in all aspects of health care, including the decision-making process. McLaughlin and Braun (1998) conducted a study on healthcare decision-making processes within Samoan families and discovered the following principles regarding the elderly and decision making. Samoans do not prefer to have a choice in major healthcare decisions because they rely on a physician's paternalistic judgment to decide the best course of action. If they must make a decision, the Samoan family collectively decides the best course of action. In addition, elderly patients often do not want physicians to inform them if they have a terminal illness because the family prefers to be informed first to protect the patient from troubling information regarding his or her health.

Contrast with Western Medicine

The Samoan value of collective involvement comes in direct conflict with values in Western health care, primarily the values of personal autonomy, self-reliance, and independence. In America there is a strong focus on protecting an individual's right to privacy, right to refuse treatment, and right to autonomous choice. Based on these values, it is unethical and illegal for a physician to perform or provide treatments to a client without informed consent, even if the client requests otherwise (Lundy & Janes, 2001). American healthcare providers do acknowledge the effects relationships have on a patient's health and claim to practice family-centered care, but always within the parameters of individualism.

Issues Contributing to Vulnerability

The difference in how decisions are made can delay treatment and create a frustrating experience for both the family and healthcare providers. If a Samoan experiences resistance from physicians in allowing the family to make the decision, he or she may choose not to participate in any treatment. Language barriers, unclear communication, and lack of knowledge of American health policy can contribute to the conflicts between Samoans and healthcare providers. Most importantly, in situations in which the client is most vulnerable, such as in an incapacitated state, his or her preference to have the family make decisions will not be honored without legal recourse. If there is no durable power of attorney, the family does not have the authority to decide what is in the best interests of the patient.

Interventions

As is highlighted in Watson's Theory of Human Care, nurses must strive to develop a capacity to problem solve with the patient and family (Erci, 2005; Mendycka, 2000). In using carative factor 6 while working with Samoans, essential tasks for the nurse are to maintain flexibility, establish a partnership, ensure clear communications, and ensure appropriate legal action. Partnership with the family is an essential aspect of providing care to elderly Samoans. Therefore it is critical to use a true family-centered approach while creating the care plan. The nurse should view the family as a positive influence and include them in the treatment strategy. Family members can help keep the patient adherent with treatment and can increase the patient's resilience by providing support and encouragement. The nurse can provide education and information to all members of the family. To do this, however, the nurse must ensure that all information is handled with confidentiality unless permitted by the patient. Therefore it is important to determine who is legally permitted to receive the information without formal permission by the patient. Having the family elect a spokesperson can streamline the communication process.

Conflict may arise if the client is asked directly to make a decision among treatment options. The nurse should discuss all options with the family and allow adequate time for them to make a decision. If the patient does not want to know the diagnosis but wishes to receive treatment, the nurse can discuss the importance of completing an informed consent with the family. Their involvement will make the process easier for the client to cope. Before planning health teaching, the nurse must assess the need for an interpreter because this indicates to the client and family that the nurse values their involvement and wishes to make it easier for them to participate.

The most difficult conflict may arise in situations where the patient is incapacitated and the family wishes to make all decisions regarding end-of-life treatments. The nurse can assist in preventing ethical and legal conflict by providing information to the patient (while he or she is competent) and the family on advance directives. By explaining the role of a durable power of attorney, the patient has the option of legally designating a person to serve as a surrogate decision maker in end-of-life decisions. This ensures that the patient and family are prepared, and adequate preparation prevents insult to the family, who would otherwise have limited decision-making authority in what treatments their family member would receive.

Spirituality and Health

Religion and spirituality are highly valued in Samoan culture. Faith in God transcends into all areas of life, including perception on health. Samoans believe that deceased family members exist as spirits, actively influencing and participating in their lives. If unresolved conflict existed while the family member was alive, the deceased person can return as a spirit to "curse" an individual (Saau, 1996). For this reason many Samoans assert that two forms of illness exist: one that involves "Samoan spirits" and another identified as "European illnesses" (Rogers, n.d.). They base their healthcare decisions on the belief that traditional Samoan healers can treat spiritual illnesses and American doctors can treat European illnesses (Rogers, n.d.). In addition, Samoans believe that through prayer intervention, God manifests His healing powers by granting positive outcomes of medical treatment (traditional or Western) (Saau, 1996). Furthermore, medical treatment can only be effective if the family has faith that God can manifest His healing powers through the treatment. They ultimately believe that everything occurs in accordance with God's will; thus there is a strong belief in fate (Saau, 1996).

Contrast with Western Medicine

Western healthcare providers do not generally view spiritual conflicts as causative factors for disease and illness. The "superstitions" described by the client are often undervalued and ignored as the medical team focuses on finding biological and physical causes. For example, although we incorporate spirituality into nursing curricula, we do not fully explore what this means in practice and how nurses might use spiritual techniques with patients. In fact, many settings seem to have a cultural norm in which prayer and spiritual comfort are to be provided only by the chaplain. However, prayer is a recognized source of strength among many healthcare providers, and studies have been conducted in which a key finding is that prayer is associated with better patient outcomes (Bormann et al., 2005; DiJoseph & Cavendish, 2005; Flannelly et al., 2005; Meraviglia, 2006; Tracy et al., 2005; Tzeng & Yin, 2006). DiJoseph and Cavendish (2005) drew the connection of prayer to nursing theories, including Watson.

However, many nurses and physicians do not use prayer as an effective method for treatment for a variety of reasons. In some cases they have not received formal training that prepares them to provide spiritual care. They may not view spiritual care as an important aspect of nursing or medical care. They may have their own spiritual conflicts and may not be comfortable talking with others about issues of spirituality. There can be time constraints, need to focus on technology, or misdiagnosis of spiritual issues as manifestations of anxiety and depression (E. Weeg, personal communication, 2007).

Issues Contributing to Vulnerability

Many Samoans may be reluctant to use Western healthcare providers because of the lack of spiritual acknowledgment and appreciation in treatment modalities. In addition, Samoans underutilize treatment that may be beneficial if they believe they have a Samoan illness that can only be healed through traditional methods. In these cases Samoans delay seeking treatment and their illnesses are complicated by waiting to determine whether it is a Samoan or European illness.

Interventions

It is important for nurses to wait to discuss spiritual practices until after establishing rapport, because Samoan clients may view spirituality as a sensitive topic and may be reluctant to share information. The nurse should explain the purpose of gathering the information so that the patient is aware that the nurse values spiritual needs and wants to incorporate the patient's needs into the care plan. The client will be more open to the discussion if the nurse is honest, nonjudgmental, and respectful.

The nurse should assess what the client perceives to be the cause and meaning of the illness and whether the illness is "Samoan" or "European," followed by an assessment of the spiritual practices in which the patient participates (carative factor 10). In addition, providing clients an opportunity to disclose their spiritual journey or experience may help them reflect on the impact their spirituality has on the meaning of past and present life experiences. Identifying and validating their spiritual practices and beliefs as strengths that promote positive coping methods conveys that the nurse is open to ideas held by the client (carative factor 5). Nurses can also assist in connecting patients with spiritual resources, such as chaplains. Christian Samoans might appreciate knowing the chaplain and visiting the chapel, but it should not be assumed that all Samoans want to see the chaplain.

At any rate, the nurse should not dismiss the importance of spiritual care, because it is a primary strength in Samoan life that provides clients with hope. Meeting the spiritual needs of patients promotes resilience. For elderly Samoans who maintain spiritual practices developed over a lifetime, it is critical to respect their need to pray in their own way (carative factor 8).

Case Study

A young Samoan woman was admitted with encephalopathy of unknown etiology to a local Seattle hospital. Although physically recognizable, her incoherent speech and violent attacks were a shock to her family and friends. The healthcare team conducted many tests to reach a diagnosis, but they could not find a cause for her behavior. Because the doctors had no physical explanation for the behavior, the Samoan family members diagnosed her with a spiritual curse: The young woman had been possessed by the spirits of several deceased family members. The woman's grandmother made a homemade lotion with native plants and oils, and in an emotional routine the family rubbed the lotion on the woman's body, surrounding her in a tight circle of prayer for over 2 hours. In several occasions they called out to the deceased family members, asking them to remove themselves from the woman's body.

This case study is an example of two cultures and perspectives meeting in a hospital setting: Samoan tradition and American health care. The situation in the case study is not uncommon, especially in regional or inner-city hospitals. The following discussion is aimed at providing the acute care nurse with practical interventions to handle the situation described in the case study with culturally competent care.

In the acute care setting, the goal for nursing personnel is to develop collaboration and partnership with the patient and family so that the health care, spiritual, and cultural needs of the patient are met. This is not to say that the nurse is only responsible for managing his or her basic nursing tasks; the nurse is the mediator and the connector between the healthcare team and the patient and family, responsible for overseeing that the patient is having his or her holistic needs met.

To begin a collaborative relationship with the patient and family, the nurse coming on shift must first establish rapport. Establishing rapport is a process of communication laced with veracity and compassion. Upon entering the room it is as simple as asking, "how are you doing?" to as complex as asking, "how do you interpret your daughters behavior?" In the case study above, the nurse should take the time to address the family's feelings regarding the tests being performed. She or he should spend 10 to 15 minutes speaking with the family to address their frustrations and questions, keeping in mind that it is most important to listen and not to speak. At this point if it were unknown, the nurse could find out the family's perspective on what the illness means to them and if there are any cultural beliefs that reflect their understanding on how it is caused and treated. If the nurse encounters a time constraint, he or she should tell the family they would like to come back to gather more information or would like to request a multifaith chaplain who could get more information for the healthcare team. When mentioning the request for a chaplain, the nurse should explain that a multifaith chaplain is used to provide spiritual support and to gather information that can be passed to the healthcare team so they can provide the best care for the patient in accordance with her cultural and spiritual needs.

After establishing rapport the nurse can assess the patient's holistic needs by communicating with the family, "How can we support her cultural and spiritual needs?" Nursing personnel should discuss the plan of care with the family and develop a schedule, highlighting the need for clustering care to ensure the family has privacy. In the most desired circumstance the nurse involved in this case study should have been aware of the spiritual routine before its occurrence so that maximal time and privacy is given to the patient and her family. If the routine was being performed without the nurse's knowledge and she or he happened to interrupt the routine, the nurse should then prioritize which care tasks need to be performed to interrupt as little as possible, if at all.

Conclusion

Here we focused on the nurse's pivotal role in promoting the integration of cultural diversity and holistic care into care plans for Samoans. Watson's Theory of Human Care was applied to the analysis in forming culturally competent interventions. The primary interventions include conducting thorough and meaningful assessments to evaluate the patient's perspectives, developing a trusting relationship, and collaborating with the patient and family to integrate their beliefs and practices into the care plan. In particular, spiritual practices need to be incorporated into the care plan.

There are many issues involved in providing effective care for the elderly within this population, but it is crucial to note that healthcare workers are most effective if they have an appreciation for cultural diversity and ways in which they can integrate their cultural sensitivity in practice. Although it might appear that these techniques are useful with clients who are not Samoan, it is important to stress that the specific techniques are based on what the literature says about Samoan culture and should be validated with individuals and families. The world is becoming increasingly smaller and more diverse. Our healthcare systems should reflect a caring orientation that reflects competence in nursing with diverse vulnerable populations.

Acknowledgment

The authors are indebted to Eileen Weeg, a nurse expert in spirituality, for her helpful comments regarding the draft of this chapter.

References

Bernick, L. (2004). Caring for older adults: Practice guided by Watson's caring-healing model. *Nursing Science Quarterly, 17*(2), 128–134.

Braun, K., Ichiho, H., Kuhaulua, R., Aitaoto, N., Tsark, J., Spegal, R., et al. (2003). Empowerment through community building: Diabetes today in the Pacific. *Journal of Public Health Management Practice, 9*(Suppl), S19–S25.

de Chesnay, M., Wharton, R., & Pamp, C. (2005). Cultural competence, resilience, and advocacy. In M. de Chesnay (Ed.), *Caring for the vulnerable: Perspectives in nursing theory, practice, and research,* (pp. 31–41). Sudbury, MA: Jones and Bartlett.

DiJoseph, J., & Cavendish, R. (2005). Expanding the dialogue on prayer relevant to holistic care. *Holistic Nursing Practice, 19*(4), 147–155.

Erci, B. (2005). Nursing theories applied to vulnerable populations: Examples from Turkey. In M. de Chesnay (Ed.), *Caring for the vulnerable: Perspectives in nursing theory, practice, and research,* (pp. 43–60). Sudbury, MA: Jones and Bartlett.

Fritsch, K. L. (1992). South Pacific nursing education: Visions of the future. *International Nursing Review, 39*(1), 19.

Galanis, D., McGarvey, S., Quested, C., Sio, B., & Amuli, S.A. (1999). Dietary intake of modernizing Samoans: Implications for risk of cardiovascular disease. *Journal of the American Dietetic Association, 99*(2), 184–191.

Lundy, K. S., & Janes, S. (2001). *Community health nursing: Caring for the public's health.* Sudbury, MA: Jones and Bartlett.

Management Science for Health. (n.d.). *The provider's guide to quality and culture: Pacific Islanders.* Retrieved August 23, 2007, from http://erc.msh.org/mainpage.cfm?file=5.4.8.htm&module=provider&language=English&ggroup=culture

McCance, T., McKenna, H., & Boore, J. (1999). Caring: Theoretical perspectives of relevance to nursing. *Journal of Advanced Nursing, 30*(6), 1388–1395.

McGrath, B. B. (2002). Seattle fa'a Samoa. *The Contemporary Pacific, 14,* 307–340.

McLaughlin, L. A., & Braun, K. L. (1998). Asian and Pacific Islander cultural values: Considerations for health care decision-making. *Health and Social Work, 2,* 116–122.

Mendycka, B. (2000). Exploring culture in nursing: A theory-driven practice. *Holistic Nursing Practice, 15,* 32–41.

Meraviglia, M. (2006). Effects of spirituality in breast cancer survivors. *Oncology Nursing Forum, 33,* 1–7.

Mulatilo, M., Taupau, T., & Enoka, I. (2000). Teaching families to be caregivers for the elderly. *Nursing and Health Sciences, 2,* 51–58.

Rogers, N. (n.d.). Creating balance: Samoa struggles to find and equilibrium between ancient healing techniques and modern medical practices. *A Broad View Magazine: South Pacific Region.* Retrieved August 23, 2007, from http://www.abroadviewmagazine.com/regions/so_pac/creat_bal.html

Saau, L. (1996). *Voices of the Samoan community.* Retrieved August 23, 2007, from http://www.xculture.org/resource/library/download/samoan.pdf

Stewart-Withers, R. R., & O'Brien, A. P. (2006). Suicide prevention and social capital: A Samoan perspective. *Health Sociology Review, 15,* 209–220.

Tamasese, K., Peteru, C., Waldegrave, C., & Bush, A.(2005). Ole taeao afua, the new morning: A qualitative investigation into Samoan perspectives on mental health and culturally appropriate services. *Australian and New Zealand Journal of Psychiatry, 39,* 300–309.

Tracy, M., Lindquist, R., Savik, K., Watanuki, S., Sendelbach, S., Kreitzer, M., & Berman, B. (2005). Use of complementary and alternative therapies: A national survey of critical care nurses. *American Journal of Critical Care, 14*(5), 404–416.

Tzeng, H., & Yin, C. (2006). Learning to respect a patient's spiritual needs concerning an unknown infectious disease. *Nursing Ethics, 13*, 17–28.

Watson, J. (2002). Intentionality and caring-healing consciousness: A practice of transpersonal nursing. *Holistic Nursing Practice, 16*(4), 12–19.

Watson, J. (2005). Caring science: Belonging before being as ethical cosmology. *Nursing Science Quarterly, 18*(4), 304–305.

Watson, J., & Smith, M. C. (2002). Caring science and the science of unitary human beings: A trans-theoretical discourse for nursing knowledge development. *Journal of Advanced Nursing, 37*(5), 452–461.

The Ethical Experience of Caring for Vulnerable Populations: The Symphonological Approach

Gladys L. Husted and James H. Husted

As members of humankind we share with other animals the fact that our nature and relationship to the world makes us vulnerable. We are all prone to encounter, in one way or another, which blocks our efficient functioning as the kind of being we are. Our vulnerability is an inescapable part of our nature and of the influence of the world in which we live.

This is true not only of animals and humans but of everything that exists. Rocks, rose bushes, and rainbows come into and go out of existence. But to us as humans, and in fact to every animal, there is a noteworthy difference between the alternatives of staying in existence and going out of existence. This is not true of rocks, rose bushes, and rainbows. Animals act to avoid various perils to which they are vulnerable. As rational animals we (sometimes) use our powers of reason to initiate actions to oppose the loss of our well-being.

One of the ways we can do this is through ethical awareness, extending the time frame of our actions and making them more intelligible. Another is by establishing healthcare systems. The motivation for each of these is a reasoned desire to escape the consequences of various aspects of our vulnerability.

Healthcare systems are far more efficient in achieving this than are contemporary ethical systems. Ethical systems can conflict with the purposes of the healthcare setting and the rational expectations of patients. When these systems (e.g., deontology and utilitarianism) are dominant in a healthcare setting they expose patients to a virulent form of vulnerability.

Perhaps only in the court system are the benefits of an appropriate[1] ethic, insightfully applied, greater than in the healthcare system. And only in the court system are the harms of an inappropriate ethic or its inappropriate application greater. At all odds, the healthcare setting is among the most complex of ethical arenas.

Patients in the healthcare system suffer a vast multitude of disabilities through injury or illness. This makes the pursuit of a spectrum of individual values, which various patients hold, vulnerable. "Illness creates a range of negative emotions in patients including anxiety, fear, powerlessness, and vulnerability. . . . Patients might feel vulnerable because they are aware that there is potential to be hurt both physically and emotionally. Feelings of fear and powerlessness will perhaps contribute to a general sense of feeling vulnerable: being wide open to harm" (Armstrong, 2006, pp. 110 and 112).

Agency

For bioethics, one disability defines and sets apart every patient regardless of the nature of his[2] affliction. This is the loss of agency—the power of an individual person to initiate and sustain action, the power to act on his purposes. Every patient suffers an impaired ability to take the actions that further his life and his flourishing. This is the overall object of the healthcare sciences. All of bioethics, properly so-called, is directed against this general disability. There cannot be an ethic for every sort of disability. The onset of disability and loss of well-being and agency sets the standard for the healthcare setting in terms of ethical awareness in relation to the disabled.

Every patient[3] needs someone to take actions for him. Every patient needs someone to help him regain his lost agency. This is true even of the dying patient. The vulnerability of a patient is the central concern of bioethics, the concern that he may fail to gain a foreseeable increase in, or even to lose a part of, his agency through the actions or interactions of healthcare professionals.

The fact that patients are vulnerable is established by the fact that they are patients. As patients they remain vulnerable—more vulnerable than they were before they became patients. Healthcare professionals possess an undesirable degree of power over patients (Husted & Husted, 2007).

The more acute the potential for the loss of agency is, the greater the vulnerability. The measure of success for a practice-based bioethic is a patient's vital objective that he shall retain or regain his power to initiate and sustain actions. To achieve this purpose, symphonology interweaves professional (therapeutic) practice and ethical interaction. By weaving them together in parsimonious temporal interactions, emphasis can easily be shifted from therapeutic to ethical concerns and back again. It is here that ethics connects and interweaves with health care and with human life and purposes. It is here that bioethics steps in to overcome the harm that can be done by the whims of healthcare personnel or reliance on the contemporary ethical systems.

The Nurse as a Second Self

According to Aristotle (McKeon, trans. 1941), a friend is, in his famous phrase, "another self" to his friend. Likewise, a nurse whose profession can be defined as consisting in acting as "the agent of a patient doing for a patient what he would do for himself if he were able" is another self to her patients (Husted & Husted, 2007). In filling the defining responsibilities of her profession, such a nurse significantly reduces the vulnerability of a patient. However, paradoxically, currently fashionable ethical beliefs imparted by her formal education may produce a willingness to aggress against the agency of her patient. The obvious impracticality of the contemporary systems results in ethical decision-making processes constituted by a string of empty associations. The attempt to interweave utilitarianism, deontology, or subjectivism, individual or social, within the nurse–patient relationship and a nurse's responsibility eventually instills an indifference or a blend of resentment and self-righteousness that places a patient in a subsidiary, irrelevant, or even adversarial ethical status.

At the same time, no patient ever came into the healthcare setting for the purpose of losing his right to self-determination. The great majority of patients assume that a nurse's ethical responsibilities consist of filling her role as a nurse. However, a patient may assume a misplaced trust in a healthcare professional. This simply involves the false assumption that the stable goal of the professional is to help him regain his lost agency. Probably no patient suspects, and none would be comforted by, the knowledge that nurses consider it their ethical responsibility to

- Act on assumed duties with no concern for the nature of their consequences and whose relevance would be unconnected to him and whose nature is completely unknown to a patient (the ethic of deontology)
- Bring about, in any dilemma, the greatest good for the greatest number; a goal that becomes a nurse's ethical fantasy, alienating a nurse from her patient, her profession, and herself (the ethic of utilitarianism)
- Follow her subjective (emotional) state of the moment, however whimsical, or the subjective sentiments of her culture or society, however irrelevant to the life and well-being of her individual patient

A patient is seldom more imperiled than when he is vulnerable to the intentional misdirected self-righteousness of a nurse (as ethic of subjectivism).

Being "a second self," a concerned nurse does not seek to gain dominion over a vulnerable friend but accepts his right to retain his individual identity. She makes it, as far as she can, unnecessary for a patient to defend himself. When appropriate, she defends him. A concerned nurse has no interest in choosing the values or determining the fate of even the most vulnerable patient.

If a nurse were to be shorn of all her out-of-context ethical preconceptions, all that would be left are the ethical demands of her profession. If she is guided by this, her ethical concern is her relation to her patient as an independent ethical equal, deserving of her understanding and empathy.

Relationship of Nurse and Patient

A patient is one who has lost or suffered a decrease in agency; one who is unable to take the actions his survival or well-being requires (Husted & Husted, 2007). Because she is defined as the agent of her patient, it is appropriate that the center of a nurse's professional concern should be her patient. When the center of her attention is not her patient, a nurse is practicing a perverse form of nursing. This perverseness arises through the choice of a flawed and irrelevant standard for nursing practice. There is nothing in the theory or practice of any healthcare profession to justify the professional using preconceptions or emotional ideas as inspiration. Nothing other than the well-being of the patient can serve as an objective standard of professional judgment. No other standard will allow an intelligible interweaving of the practice of nursing and an ethic appropriate to that practice.

A patient must exercise the resources of his character that enable him to achieve greater well-being through his power to take independent action. A nurse's standard of success is met when she strengthens these resources and increases the opportunity of her patient to exercise them. For a professional ethic, one defined by a nurse's practice, this is the standard by which she measures her practice. It is the reason for being and the ethical guidepost of her profession.

Ethics of Professional Practice

The ethic of a committed nurse must be practice based. This is any ethical system in which the nature and ends of professional practice determine the nature, application, and general purposes of the profession's ethical standards. Its purpose is to enhance the benefits available to patients through the healthcare system. An ethic that is not skillfully exercised and harmoniously interwoven with practice cannot justifiably be the ethic of a healthcare professional. It is the ethic of a nurse who is merely "going through the motions." Every form of a practice-based bioethic is derived from, and is intended to be appropriate to, the self-determination of a patient, the purposes of a healthcare setting, and the role of a healthcare professional. Most nurses eventually adopt some form of a practice-based system. It is a significant benefit to them if they recognize this. It is a significant benefit to their patients if this recognition allows their system to be sufficiently complete, cohesive, and coherent to be predictable. An ethic not derived from the practice of the healthcare professions and the purposes of the healthcare setting must fail to meet the needs of a patient. Ethical decisions and actions guided by a nurse's feelings or the demands she attributes to her duty often fail. If they succeed, they succeed only by accident. To the extent that a patient is vulnerable, these decisions and actions create a greater vulnerability. The standard of a nurse's practice by which its competence is to be measured is not the nurse and the way she happens to practice. It is practice itself, as it can be and should be.

A practice-based ethical system places a nurse in harmony with the promise of the healthcare system and the trust of her patients. Such a system produces positive pride in her profession and in herself as a practitioner of this profession. And, as a corollary, it increases the confidence that each of her patients can appropriately place in her. It reduces or eliminates her patients' vulnerability, at least in their relation to her.

Nature of the Nurse–Patient Agreement

Of necessity, a practice-based system is symphonological, a term derived from *symphonia*, a Greek word meaning agreement. This is an approach to ethical interaction from professional responsibility, the responsibility encoded in a nurse's professional agreement with her patient. A practice-based bioethic aims to relate professionals and patients internally, to bring them into the same ethical context. It makes human values its focus and ensures that the healthcare setting is minimally arbitrary and maximally purposeful. This context influences directly or indirectly the way in which a nurse performs (Gastmans, 1998).

Bioethics places particular emphasis on situations where one person is extremely vulnerable, where the goals pursued are crucial, or where the dilemmas to be resolved are extraordinarily complex (Husted & Husted, 2007). A practice-based bioethic is based on interaction between a professional and a patient who relate to each other through understanding and agreement. One engages with a nurse assuming that she has agreed to act in her role as a healthcare professional. In engaging her, one agrees to be a patient, one willing for her to act for him. Logically and ethically there is an inescapable implication that the ethical interactions between nurse and patient will conform to this agreement.

Necessity of the Nurse–Patient Agreement

"How can two walk together lest they agree?" (1 *Kings* 3:16–28). The simple action of two people walking together is an interaction and is therefore, necessarily, the product of an agreement. Much more so, the complex and vital actions that take place in a healthcare system are interactions and are therefore products of a complex and vital agreement.

An agreement is a shared state of awareness established by a decision on the part of each party to the agreement. Where a patient is not able to take part in the forming of an agreement or actively participate in it, it is an implicit agreement based on a high probability that, if the patient were able, it would be formed. The agreement between nurse and patient is the foundation of the ethical interaction between them. It is structured by the expectations of each and the commitments that each makes to the other. Each agrees to satisfy these reasonable expectations and to live up to the commitment. The agreement makes their interaction intelligible. It helps each to understand what is expected and what is committed to in their interaction. Whenever a nurse fails to be guided by her professional agreement, her profession becomes, in effect, a hobby. She may believe that ethically she succeeds, but in relation to her patients and her profession she fails.

Nursing Interactions

Every action that a nurse takes is an interaction. There are no isolated actions, actions without a recipient, in the healthcare system. Isolated actions would neither be nursing nor of any consequence. A nurse's profession implies that her agreement is to interact. Even in the cases of a patient who cannot actively participate in his care, professional practice remains an interaction. A nurse interacts with the vital functions of her patients. The less a patient can participate in his care, the weaker he is in their interactions, the more vulnerable he is. A concerned nurse does, even for the most vulnerable, precisely what she does for every patient: She acts to overcome his vulnerability, his inability to take action, his patiency. Although with the more vulnerable, her actions may need to be more powerful and more precise. "The core of ethical behaviour between staff and patients may reside in the seeming minutiae of small social exchanges" (Grant and Briscoe, 2002, para. 7). In the context of a practice-based ethic, interaction begins with support for a patient's right to self-determination

Rights

One evening, strolling across a field in a deserted park, Tom sees Dick approaching from the other side. Tom has recently lost his financial shirt. He is broke and has no bright prospects for the future. Dick is a rich recluse in ill health. He is known to carry large sums of money with him. Tom is aware of this. Tom could rob Dick, solve his financial problems, and no one would be the wiser. Dick, for his part, is unacquainted with Tom. Tom, in common with everyone in town, knows that Dick is subject to hallucinations. On this day everyone from this small town except Tom and Dick has taken a bus to the county fair. Every circumstance seems to invite Tom to rob Dick. The odds on Tom being caught are minuscule. None of this enters Tom's mind. As they pass, Dick speaks a conventional pleasantry to him and Tom replies in kind. Tom never conceives of robbing Dick. Without thinking about it, Tom has recognized Dick's rights. If you had seen this event, you would have seen the operation of an individual's rights, Dick's right not to be aggressed against.

Now what is it you have seen? You have seen the product of a spontaneous and unnoticed agreement. This agreement holds between every noncriminal member of the human species. One instance of this is the agreement existing between Tom and Dick.

Rights[4] is defined as "The product of an implicit agreement among rational beings, made and held by virtue of their rationality, not to obtain actions from one another, nor to put one another in any circumstance except through voluntary consent, objectively gained" (Husted & Husted, 2007).

Imagine, if you can, a healthcare setting devoid of this agreement. Without the recognition of individual rights, this system would never have come into being. No one would conceive of something as intricate as a healthcare system. Human existence would be, in the words of philosopher Thomas Hobbes (1588–1679), "solitary, poore, nastie, brutish, and short" (Oakeshott, 1957, p. 47). To the extent that the recognition of individual rights does not guide interaction, human life must be and is right now solitary, poore, nastie, brutish, and short.

Individual rights belong to each human individual by virtue of his or her membership in the human species. In becoming a patient, an individual does not lose this membership. His rights are not increased—this is not necessary—but neither are his rights decreased—this is not permissible. He is a rational being ethically equal to all other rational beings. The nature of every interpersonal ethical system arises from the attitude of that system toward individual rights. The nature of the ethical practice of every nurse is shaped by her attitude toward the individual rights of her patient. As there is a decrease in the recognition of human rights, there is an increase in the vulnerability of the patient and vice versa.

Ethical practice does not allow a professional to violate the rights of a patient. A dedication to human values is internal to the nature of the healthcare setting. This dedication presupposes respect for the individual rights of patients. Only when an individual has reason to be confident that he will not be the victim of aggression can he exercise his human virtues in the pursuit of his individual values.

The rights agreement is the ethical foundation for explicit agreements. It is the already established agreement that explicit agreements will be objective, voluntary, and honored. Harmony is a state wherein each person can interact without fear of aggression and betrayal. When rights encompass an agreement to nonaggression and nothing besides this, then the rights agreement creates a state of harmony among rational beings. Reliance on rights is possible and productive, even though crime is possible in the same way that reliance on health is reasonable despite the possibility of injury or illness. The practice of nursing, ideally, goes beyond respect for rights, but a professional practice-based ethic must begin with a nurse's undaunted pride in her profession and the recognition of the dignity of her patients (Hardt, 2001).

Paradox of Group Purpose

A bioethical view of rights must be concerned with individual human purposes. Nurses and patients are defined in terms of human purposes. The healthcare system is inspired by a concern for individual purposes. In the healthcare setting individual rights are manifested in the view that a patient's pursuit of his purposes should not be aggressed against. Individual purposes are the precondition and motivation of the healthcare setting and of rights. If people did not act on purposes, rights would have no relevance to ethics, and ethics would have no relevance to human life. Without the protection of rights, human individuals could not act on their purposes. Every moment of their lives would be spent defending themselves. Rights and purposes are intricately interwoven.

Much of the literature about vulnerable patients deals with vulnerable patient populations. As nurses we have to differentiate between vulnerable populations and the vulnerable patient as a unique individual requiring attention to his own specific characteristics. The concept of populations assists our understanding and communication with others; however, it does not create another entity. Populations have no purposes and no rights. No population ever occupied a hospital bed.

Nurses and patients disagree. Patients and patients disagree. Nurses disagree with each other. It is to the advantage of every individual to accept these differences in opinions and motivations as relevant to and defended by individual rights. The right to different motivations is the reason for being of ethics. Any defense of the idea that differences in motivations as such are unjustified would involve an individual in arguing that the motivation of his individual and different point of view is justified while, at the same time, that the motivation behind individual and different points of view are unjustified.

Agreement, Bioethical Standards, and the Vulnerable Patient

Virtues are the standards of a practice-based bioethic. Whatever actions a nurse takes to defend and strengthen them are justifiable ethical actions. The nurse's virtues, to the extent that she is virtuous, sharpen her attention to her patient. The patients' virtues, to the extent that he is able to act on his virtues, sharpen his attention to his life, health, and well-being. Any actions that a nurse takes that weaken virtues are unethical and unjustifiable actions. The rights agreement is the sanction of the virtues. The nurse–patient agreement is an interaction taken in service of the virtues. The virtues, by their nature, are instruments of human purpose, and this nature structures the nature of individual purposes and human persons. Their nature is the inspiration for agreement making. The bioethical standards, the measuring rods of success, are the virtues of autonomy, freedom, objectivity, self-assertion, beneficence, and fidelity.[5]

Autonomy is the uniqueness of a person, that which makes a person the individual he or she is. It is the right to be who he or she is and act on that basis. If a nurse can strengthen and nurture her patients' autonomy, then she helps them make their purposes and actions their own. She can help them gain a better understanding and acceptance of themselves. This is her ethical means of meeting her agreement.

Freedom is the power (and right) to take long-term action based on one's own evaluation of a situation. A patient who is less able to exercise his ability to take free action is more vulnerable than one who is more able. This is because he is at a greater risk of harm, less able to know, to make known, or to defend what his free action would be. Therefore nurses or other healthcare professionals act as the agent through whom patients are able to regain their power to exercise free choice. If she can strengthen and nurture her patients' freedom, she helps them to have a clear vision of what their long-term motivations and values are and what these demand of them in their present situation. She helps them achieve the endurance to take long-term actions toward the pursuit of their values.

Objectivity is the ability to know something and interact with it as it is in itself apart from one's preconceived ideas of it. It is a patient's need to achieve and sustain the exercise of his objective awareness. A patient who is able to contribute information about himself and understand the information given to him in light of available alternatives and his own uniqueness is less vulnerable than one who cannot. All actions that involve the pursuit of benefits and the avoidance of harm occur among the physical realities in which one acts. The loss of objective awareness is a radical form of vulnerability. It makes one vulnerable to the loss of the other virtues. If the nurse can strengthen and nurture the objectivity of her patient, she enables a patient to act appropriately on his autonomous and objective awareness of his circumstances. The strength of mind necessary to maintain objective awareness of facts outside of his mind and a stable awareness of items of knowledge that are relevant to his actions are necessary to his endurance and success.

Self-assertion is an agent's self-ownership, the power and right of an agent to control his time and effort, the right to initiate his own actions. A patient who is able to control his time and effort is less vulnerable than a patient who must rely on others to do this for him. A nurse, as the agent of a patient, assists him in regaining and exercising his power of self-assertion.

Beneficence means competence in acting to acquire what is beneficial in accordance with one's desires and values, the ability to pursue benefits and to avoid harms. A patient who is able to define benefit and harm for himself and according to his unique values is less vulnerable than one who cannot. A nurse must exert great care not to view benefit and harm for a patient according to her own idea of benefit and harm. The determination of benefit and harm is very individual. If she can strengthen and nurture his benefit seeking, she helps motivate her patient to retain his values and achieve his goals according to his long-term purposes. His courage to accept his own desires for himself, his pursuit of benefit, and his ability to avoid harm will be strengthened.

Fidelity denotes a nurse's commitment to her professional role and a patient's commitment to his life and values.[6] All that a patient endures when he suffers through his vulnerability can be summed up by the fact that he loses his integrity and his power to be faithful to himself and the values he has chosen for his life. A nurse can exert her virtues as codified in the bioethical standards to help a patient regain and/or exert his virtues to achieve an active future. If she can strengthen and nurture his fidelity to himself, she can help him to retain a clear understanding of himself in relation to his ambitions. This will assist him in being faithful to his life and flourishing.

Justified Ethical Activity

No virtue a nurse can offer a patient is more productive to his life, health, and well-being than her knowledge of who she is both individually and as a healthcare professional. This is the virtue that enables her to feel and express empathy for her patient. It also is a virtue that enables her to intend to do good, to intend to benefit her patient.

A practice-based bioethic is an outline of the appropriate ways to interpret the healthcare professional–patient agreement. The bioethical standards, as virtues to be exercised, are preconditions of each and every agreement. The bioethical standards, as virtues to be strengthened, are the standards of ethical decision making in the healthcare system. They are standards because as virtues they are the purpose that brings a person into the healthcare setting to regain or strengthen them. His agency is constituted by these virtues.

A Patient's Agency

A nurse's most obvious standard or measure of ethical justification is the agency of her patient. According to this standard, failing to take action or acting to frustrate a patient's rightful efforts undercuts the ability of a nurse to objectively justify her actions. The standards of a patient's success in the healthcare system are the virtues he seeks to strengthen and regain. If he succeeds in this purpose, his interactions are successful. Insofar as a nurse assists him in this, nurse and patient are equally successful. Insofar as her actions are oriented to this goal, they are justifiable. A committed nurse, through observation and communication, can come to understand how these virtues are expressed (or fail to be expressed) in the actions of her patient. She can discover whether they function and how they function in motivating him. Her understanding can guide and justify her actions.

All these virtues, by their presence or absence, form the unique character structures of a human individual. The human values that individuals pursue are made possible by these character structures exercised in successful action. They are themselves human values. The social condition necessary to this pursuit is freedom from aggression. This necessary condition of the achievement of human values is the right of every human individual that is established by the species-wide and unspoken agreement that establishes these rights. If a nurse maintains respect for her patient's rights, any action she takes is justifiable.

To the extent that rights can be violated, nothing and no one is secure. Because there are no dependable intelligible sequences to interaction, foresight and predictability are illusory. Under these circumstances a patient cannot function as a rational being, an individual who possesses purposes and rights. A patient will have a right to do and to depend on nothing. The professional will have a right, derived from coercion, to do anything, to be unpredictable. Under these conditions interactions are impossible. To the extent that events are guided by the unexpected "agreements" that are secured through deception or force, a patient's rights are violated. The recognition of a patient's rights is the only defense he has in the healthcare system.

Conclusion

"Although ethical issues in health care receive much publicity, attention is rarely given to the non-dramatic, everyday ethics of health care" (Smith, 2005, para. 1). This would include the day-to-day care of vulnerable patients who may not present an actual dilemma but whose care must be diligent because of their fragile condition. When the role of a nurse is not set by a clear and logically comprehensive definition, any action or omission on her part is allowable. This state of affairs is a violation of her profession. The professional cannot agree to act as the agent of a patient if something within the profession itself prevents this. To the extent that the definition and the nature of her role are, actually or potentially, in conflict, no agreement is possible.

Rights are not routinely violated in the healthcare system. If this were the case there would be a revolt and a reformation of the system. When rights are violated, it is usually the rights of the most vulnerable, those who have no voice and cannot defend themselves against the self-righteous irrationality of healthcare professionals.

Two factors are necessary, and almost sufficient, for a nurse's justifiable ethical inter-actions: her unwavering recognition of a patient's rights and her unimpeachable adher-ence to the essence of her profession. In a healthcare setting that is governed by a practice-based ethic, some patients are more vulnerable than others but not vulnerable in relation to a nurse. To a great extent, the degree of a patient's vulnerability is a function of a healthcare professional's character. Sometimes a patient is completely vulnerable, but the right agreement holds by virtue of his nature and her nature, and ethically, a patient's rights are always and absolutely invulnerable.

Endnotes

[1] "Appropriate" means according to the internal purposes of the setting.

[2] The pronouns *she* and *her* are used to designate the healthcare professional and *he* and *him* to des-ignate the patient. This is, in part, for the reader's ease of understanding. More importantly, the singular is preferred to the plural or indeterminate because professionals and patients are indi-viduals and a practice-based ethic is, necessarily, an individualistic ethic.

[3] The word "patient" is derived from the Greek word *pathos* meaning experiences, suffering, or pas-sivity. Other words with the same root are "pathos" itself (that in experience which evokes empathy or compassion), "pathetic" (evoking tenderness, pity, or sorrow), and "passive" (inca-pable of action).

[4] "Rights" is used in this chapter as a singular concept denoting an overarching agreement.

[5] "Autonomy" is not used here in its customary dictionary definition of independence. We use autonomy to denote the uniqueness of each individual person. The definition of "freedom" includes everything relevant to a person's independence.

[6] All definitions are taken, from husted and Husted (2007).

References

Armstrong, A. E. (2006). Towards a strong virtue ethic for nursing practice. *Nursing Philosophy, 7,* 110–124.

Gastmans, C. (1998). Challenges to nursing values in a changing nursing environment. *Nursing Ethics, 5,* 236–245.

Grant, V. J., & Briscoe, J. (2002). Everyday ethics in an acute psychiatric unit. *Journal of Medical Ethics, 28,* 173–176.

Hardt, M. (2001). Core then care: The nurse leader's role in "caring." *Nursing Administration Quarterly, 25*(3), 37–45.

Husted, G. L., & Husted, H. (2007, forthcoming). *Ethical decision making in nursing and health care: The symphonological approach* (4th ed.). New York: Springer.

McKeon, R. (Ed.), (1941). *The basic works of Aristotle.* New York: Random House.

Oakeshott, M. (Ed.), (1957). *Leviathan.* Oxford: Basil Blackwell.

Smith, K. V. (2005). Ethical issues related to health care: The older adult's perspective. *Journal of Gerontological Nursing, 31,* 32–39.

Giving Voice to Vulnerable Populations: Rogerian Theory

Sarah Hall Gueldner, Geraldine R. Britton, and Susan Terwilliger

The human condition of vulnerability is a concept of vital concern to nurses in that a large portion of nursing practice is spent either helping individuals who find themselves in a vulnerable position or helping them avoid vulnerability. However, nursing has been slow in developing theoretical constructs of vulnerability within a nursing perspective (Spiers, 2000). Traditional definitions of vulnerability are framed within an epidemiological approach to identify individuals and groups at risk for harm. Groups most often labeled as vulnerable include the elderly, children, the poor, people with disability or chronic illness, people from minority cultures, and captive populations such as prisoners and refugees (Saunders & Valente, 1992). Labels of vulnerability are customarily applied in relation to socioeconomic, minority, or other stigmatizing status (Demi & Warren, 1995) and reflect a tendency to blame the victim rather than the prevailing social structures. The generally accepted marker for vulnerability has been the inability to function independently in accord with the values of a particular society. Fortunately, there is growing dialogue about vulnerability from the perspective of the person experiencing it, a view that is more congruent with the philosophical stance of nursing (Morse, 1997; Spiers, 2000).

The Rogerian conceptual system (Rogers, 1992), which focuses on the person as integral with and inseparable from his or her environment, holds considerable relevance as an innovative nursing framework to use in addressing the problem of vulnerability. Accordingly, the remainder of this discussion is directed toward application of the theoretical base of Rogerian nursing science to the human condition of vulnerability. Because persons who are vulnerable are at greater risk for not being heard, the last part of the chapter describes the Wellbeing Picture Scale (WPS), a 10-item innovative picture-based tool that offers a menu of paired pictures rather than words, giving people who may not be able to read English text an alternative more user-friendly way of expressing their sense of well-being.

A Rogerian Perspective of Vulnerability

According to Martha Rogers, energy fields are the fundamental unit of everything, both living and nonliving. The fields are without boundary and dynamic, changing continuously. Two energy fields are identified: the human field and the environmental field. Rogers emphasized that humans and environments do not *have* energy fields; rather, they *are* energy fields. Likewise, she insisted that the human field is unitary and cannot be reduced to a biological field, a physical field, or a psychosocial field. As postulated by Rogers, human and environmental fields flow together in a constant mutual process that is unitary rather than separate. Within this world view humans are energy fields that exist in constant mutual process with their immediate and extended environmental energy field, which includes, and cannot be separated from, other living and nonliving fields. She also postulated that both human and environmental energy patterns change continually during this process. The inseparability of the human energy field from its immediate and extended environmental energy field is perhaps the most central feature of the Rogerian conceptual system.

Phillips and Bramlett (1994) asserted that the mutual human–environmental field process can be harmonious or dissonant. Resonant with Rogers' science, these researchers posit vulnerability as an emergent condition that arises when there is dissonance within the mutual human–environmental field process. This view is consistent with Rogerian scholar Barrett's (1990) theory of power, which associates power with individuals' knowing participation in change within their mutual human–environmental process for the betterment of the whole, including themselves. These authors perceive vulnerability as the opposite condition of power, a condition that may occur when an individual is unable or does not choose to participate in an informed and purposeful way in change. Persons in this situation essentially have no voice and may be intentionally or unintentionally left behind in a compromised position. Within this line of thinking, an individual's sense of dissonance or disharmony within the mutual human–environmental field process would be viewed as a manifestation of vulnerability, placing individuals or groups at risk. Barrett developed the text-based tool, Power as Knowing Participation in Change (PKPC), to measure this concept; a subscale of the tool addresses awareness as an essential feature of knowing participation.

Lack of knowing participation may be associated with a number of scenarios. Individuals may be uninformed or misinformed about situations involving their unique human–environmental field process, or they may be unable to participate due to one or more specific circumstances such as illness (e.g., stroke or dementia) or injury (e.g., hip fracture). Common situations that may limit or prevent knowing participation include compromised vision or hearing, aphasia, difficulty with mobility, and confusion or dementia. Other circumstances that may limit knowing participation include any situation that hinders a person from engaging in sufficient communication within the community; examples might include lack of transportation or limited language facility.

Insufficient means or the inability to move about freely may diminish presence, making it more difficult, if not impossible, to be "at the table," to achieve representation. Stigmatized individuals or groups such as single mothers, persons who are homeless, and persons perceived as unattractive or different are also at risk for a lack of information or misinformation that may lead to inappropriate participation based on misjudgment. Indeed, information may actually be withheld if participation is not welcome.

Parse's (2003) theory of community becoming, also an extension of Rogers' nursing science, is particularly applicable to the theoretical tenet of vulnerability. She defines community in terms of the relational experience of being "in community" and describes it as a resource, dynamic and continuously changing to represent the good of the individual to achieve the best for all. According to her definition, community is not a location or a group of people who have similar interests; rather, community is the human connectedness with the universe, including connectedness with what she terms "yet-to-be possibles." This view represents a paradigm shift, wherein vulnerability is an emergent characteristic of the community in process that occurs when an individual or group becomes disconnected from the group and therefore from needed resources. Parse describes a nontraditional model of health service for individuals and families who have become disconnected from resources. The process involves imaging the vision of possibilities and inviting others to capture the vision, thus energizing the community to build partnerships to overcome the disconnect.

Within this conceptualization, vulnerability arises as an emergent characteristic when connectedness is compromised by a lack of communication or flawed communication that leads to exclusion from resources. Vulnerability might be seen as an unfortunate estrangement from the process of community. Within this view persons who are at particular risk for vulnerability are those who for some reason are unable to call enough attention to their needs to garner the support of their community.

Based on Parse's (1997) "human becoming" perspective, her view of nursing practice also differs from traditional nursing practice in that the nurse does not offer standardized professional advice or opinions stemming from the nurse's own value system. Rather, according to Parse, nursing involves a "true presence with and respect for the other" wherein the nurse dwells with the person or family to enhance their perceived "possibles." Parse points out that it is essential to go with vulnerable persons to where they are rather than to attempt to judge, change, or control them. It is in dwelling with the individual in discussion that meanings emerge, and it is in this process of illuminating meaning that possibilities for transcendence are seen.

In Parse's words, "The nurse in true presence with person or family is not a guide or a beacon, but rather an inspiring attentive presence that calls the other to shed light on the meaning moments of his or her life. It is the person or family in the presence of the nurse that illuminates the meaning and mobilizes the capacity to transcend and move beyond. The person is coauthor of his or her own health . . . choosing rhythmical patterns of relating while reaching for personal hopes and dreams" (Parse, 1997, p. 40). She continues,

"True presence is a special way of *being with* in which the nurse bears witness to the person's or family's own living of value priorities. True presence is an interpersonal art grounded in a strong knowledge base 'reflecting the belief that each person knows *the way* somewhere within self'" (Parse, 1997, p. 40). Certainly, nowhere is it more important to respect the person as he or she is than when working with those who are vulnerable.

Parse describes a humanitarian model of nursing practice based on true presence and profound respect. Use of this model enables people to find actions that increase their ability to knowingly participate in change to improve their position, thus becoming less vulnerable. Parse refers to this process as the search for the possible beyond the now.

However, in even this overall positive system some are likely to find themselves in vulnerable circumstances. Some individuals and groups (such as young children) are placed at risk because they cannot speak for themselves and depend on others to advocate for them. Likewise, sick or frail members of the community may be too weak or impaired to participate knowingly (or sufficiently) in the change process to advance their betterment. They may not be mobile enough, think clearly enough, or be articulate enough to capture community attention and garner the resources they need.

Individuals or families at special risk for vulnerability include those who

- Have energy-draining illnesses or conditions such as stroke, heart attack, cancer, or depression

- Are not included in the dominant culture

- Have compromised language facility, making them at greater risk for being unheard

- Are out of their familiar turf (i.e., new in the community and do not know the "rules" or avenues for help)

- Are unable to comprehend information (i.e., never learned to read, have diminished vision or hearing, are unconscious or have dementia, or are unable to comprehend English)

- Have illness or injury that limits independence (i.e., broken hips that make it more difficult to stay physically connected with the community)

- Lack the ability to access services needed for everyday life (i.e., means for obtaining food, place to live, health services)

- Are in a position of diminished visibility (e.g., live in a remote area or are homebound, becoming disconnected from community notice)

Viewed from Parse's theory of community becoming, the approach to overcoming vulnerability is a matter of reconnecting the person or group to the community. This sometimes happens naturally through family and friends or through social institutions and/or programs such as churches and civic organizations. But it may take the focused attention and time of individuals, such as nurses, to help the person or family as they gain insight about the possibilities that are available to them.

Giving Voice: An Application of Rogerian Nursing Science

To address the lack of voice that is so intricately associated with the experience of vulnerability, this section describes a simple picture tool, the WPS, developed within the Rogerian conceptual system to amplify the voice of persons who otherwise might not be heard (Gueldner et al., 2005).

The WPS is a 10-item non-language-based pictorial scale that measures general sense of well-being as a reflection of the mutual human–environmental field process. It was originally designed as an easy-to-administer tool for use with the broadest possible range of adult populations, including persons who have limited formal education, do not speak English as their first language, may not be able to see well, or may be too sick or frail to respond to lengthier or more complex measures. Ten pairs of 1-inch drawings depicting a sense of high or low well-being are arranged at opposite ends of a seven-choice, unnumbered, semantic differential scale. The 10 items included are eyes open and closed, shoes sitting still and running, butterfly and turtle, candle lit and not lit, faucet running full and dripping, puzzle pieces together and separated, pencil sharp and dull, sun full and partially cloud covered, balloons inflated and partially deflated, and lion and mouse. Individuals are asked to view each of the 10 picture pairs and mark the point along the scale between the pictures to indicate which they feel most like, for example, a lighted candle or an unlit candle. The brief instructions for the WPS are translated and administered in Taiwanese, Japanese, Korean, Egyptian, and Spanish. Psychometric properties for the tool were established in a sample of 1,027 individuals in the United States, Taiwan, and Japan; the sample was 56% Asian, 34% white, and 10% African-American or Hispanic. The overall Cronbach's alpha was found to be 0.8795 across the three countries. Five of the 10 items were completely consistent across countries (puzzle, balloon, sun, eyes, and lion), and all others were consistent across two of the three countries.

Conceptual Formulation of Well-Being

Rogers maintained that, "the purpose of nursing is to promote health and well-being for all persons wherever they are" (1992, p. 258). According to Hills (1998), well-being is generally defined as a relative sense of harmony and satisfaction in one's life. Smith (1981) and Todaro-Franceschi (1999) defined health as movement toward self-fulfillment or realization of one's potential, a view that is congruent with Parse's (1997) theory of human becoming. Newman (1994) does not distinguish health from well-being but singularly defines it as a manifestation of expanding consciousness that may occur during, but is not separate from, the experience of illness. This view is supported by the work of Hills (1998), who demonstrated a relationship between well-being and awareness.

Conceptually, the WPS assesses the energy field in regard to four characteristics judged to be associated with well-being: frequency of movement (i.e., intensity) within the energy field, awareness of one's self as energy, action emanating from the energy field, and power as knowing participation in change within the mutual human–environmental energy field process.

Frequency
The term *frequency* denotes the intensity of motion within the energy field(s). It is postulated that higher frequency is associated with a greater sense of well-being and that it is experienced as a sense of vitality.

Awareness
Awareness refers to the sense an individual has of his or her potential for change within the mutual human–environmental field. It signals readiness for moving toward one's potential and is postulated to be positively associated with a sense of well-being. The concept of awareness is congruent with Newman's (1994) theory of health as expanding consciousness and Parse's (1997) theory of human becoming (unfolding). Barrett (1990) included a subscale of awareness in her PKPC tool, and Hills (1998) discussed enlightenment as a manifestation of expanded awareness, higher level field motion, and well-being. Awareness is postulated to be a positive manifestation of the dynamics of the mutual human–environmental field process.

Action
Action is conceptualized as an emergent of the "continuous mutual human-environmental field process" (Rogers, 1992), reflecting the frequency of the human energy field. Action is viewed as an expression of field energy associated with well-being. Examples of action include activities associated with daily living, such as preparing food, eating, personal grooming, participating in social events, exercising, or doing chores, as well as actively engaging in innovative thinking or the creation of art forms.

Power
As described by Barrett (1990), power is the capacity of an individual to engage knowingly in change. Barrett defined it as the degree to which an individual is able to express energy as power to create desired change within his or her human-environmental energy field process. When power is prominent, it is postulated that one would have a sense of confidence; conversely, it would follow that powerlessness is associated with a sense of vulnerability. Power might also be conceptualized as the capacity of an individual to commute the three aforementioned conditions (energy expressed as frequency, awareness, and action) into an emergent sense of well-being.

WPS Development

The more than 10 years of developmental work and field testing of early versions of the WPS revealed a correlation with several other tools designed to measure aspects of well-being within the Rogerian framework (Gueldner, Bramlett, Johnston, & Guillory, 1996). Johnston (1994), in a sample of nursing home residents and community-dwelling elders, reported a highly significant correlation ($r = 0.6647$) between the WPS tool and her Human Field Image Metaphor Scale, which uses two- or three-word metaphors to measure image. Gueldner et al. (1996) found an even greater correlation ($r = 0.7841$) between the WPS and Barrett's (1990) PKPC tool, which measures an individual's capacity for awareness, choices, freedom to act intentionally, and involvement to bring about harmony in the human–environmental field process.

Davis (1989), in a matched sample of 30 men 19–51 years of age who had been hospitalized for traumatic injuries and 30 noninjured men, demonstrated positive significant correlations between the score on the WPS and scores on the PKPC tool ($p = 0.002$) and Rosenberg's self-esteem scale ($p = 0.02$). She also found a difference in the between-group mean scores that approached significance ($p = 0.059$), warranting further consideration in a larger sample.

Hindman (1993), in a sample of 40 nursing home residents and 40 community-dwelling older adults, demonstrated a significant correlation ($p = 0.001$) between the mean score on the WPS and humor as measured by the Situational Humor Response Questionnaire. She also found that the mean score was higher for the community-dwelling group of older adults ($p = 0.001$) than for their counterparts who lived in the nursing home and that individuals who perceived their income as adequate scored higher ($p = 0.05$) than those who perceived their income to be less than adequate. Older participants scored lower ($p = 0.05$) on the WPS.

Hills (1998), in a study of 874 mothers of 6-month-old infants, found that mothers who scored higher on the picture tool also reported higher levels of awareness ($p = 0.001$) as measured by the awareness subscale of Barrett's (1990) PKPC tool and well-being ($p < 0.001$) as measured by Cantril's Ladder for Well-Being.

Gueldner et al. (2005) administered the WPS and the Geriatric Depression Scale (GDS) to 200 older adults who were attending lunch events at six senior centers in upstate New York and reported a significant correlation ($p < 0.05$) between the WPS and the GDS. One-fifth (20%) of those who participated in the study scored above the cut-off of 5 (indicating concern for depression) on the GDS; 10% scored above 8 on the GDS, and three individuals scored an alarming 13–14 on the GDS. These findings support the ability of the more user-friendly WPS to screen for depression in community-dwelling elders.

Use of the WPS with Children

Because of their dependent status, children are at particular risk for vulnerability and their voices may not be heard; others tend to speak for them. Thus the developers of the tool believe that the WPS holds potential for giving voice to children as well as to adults. The WPS was used by two researchers to measure well-being in children.

Abbate (1990) used the early 18-item version of the tool as a pre- and posttest measure of well-being in eight school-aged children (aged 5–16 years) with cerebral palsy who participated in a 10-week therapeutic horsemanship program. The mean of the pretest scores was 82.75 and the mean of the posttest scores, 86.38. The scores of four children increased over the 10-week period, one did not change, and the scores of three decreased. All the children in the study had already been riding horses for several years, leading Abbate to suggest that some of the children may have already achieved the most significant gain from their participation in the riding program before the onset of the study. Abbate noted that even the most impaired children seemed comfortable and confident in placing their mark along the seven-point scoring line between the picture pairs (the younger ones used crayons), supporting its utility with children. This was the first study that used the WPS tool with children, and the sample was small. However, the findings provided impetus and direction for developing a children's version of the instrument.

More recently, Terwilliger (2007) modified the format of the 10-item WPS for use with a sample of 20 fourth- and fifth-grade elementary school children. The original seven-point Likert Scale between each pair of pictures was reconfigured and abbreviated to four boxes (two boxes were placed closer to the picture on the left of the page and the other two boxes were placed closer to the picture pair on the right side of the page). For each item the investigator asked the child to point to the picture they "felt most like." Then they were each asked to place a mark in one of the two boxes to indicate whether they felt "a little bit" like the picture they had chosen or "a lot" like it. The investigator repeated each item and pointed out the designated boxes as many times as necessary if the child seemed to have difficulty understanding the scoring instructions. The scoring mechanism was adjusted so that the children's scores retained the range from 7 to 70, with higher scores indicating a higher sense of well-being. The mean scores of the children were significantly higher ($p < 0.05$) at postintervention than at preintervention. Although the sample size for this study was modest, the findings lend support for the use of the WPS with children.

In summary, work by Gueldner et al. (1996), Hills (1998), and Johnston (1994) confirmed a high correlation between scores on the WPS and other measures of well-being developed within the Rogerian conceptual system. Additionally, the work of Davis (1989), Hills (1998), and Hindman (1993) demonstrated a high correlation between the WPS tool and a number of established measures of well-being developed by other disciplines. Although both were limited in sample size, the studies of Abbate (1990) and Terwilliger (2007) demonstrated the potential usability of the tool in children. Given these findings, the WPS is offered as a general measure of well-being mediated through frequency, awareness, action, and power emanating within an individual's mutual human–environmental field process.

Conclusion

Given these findings the WPS is offered as a general index of well-being and for use with international populations who might have difficulty reading English text. The instrument is seen as having the potential to give voice to those who are too sick or weak to participate in studies that require lengthy measures of well-being and, perhaps, even to persons with mild to moderate cognitive impairment. A secondary purpose of the tool rests in its potential for use as an easy-to-administer clinical indicator of well-being across a wide sector of clinical settings. Based on the work of Abbate (1990) and Terwilliger (2007), a children's version of the tool is presently being developed and tested.

References

Abbate, M. F. (1990). *The relationship of therapeutic horsemanship and human field motion in children with cerebral palsy.* Unpublished master's thesis, Georgia State University, Atlanta.

Barrett, E. A. M. (1990). A measure of power as knowing participation in change. In O. L. Strickland & C. F. Waltz (Eds.), *The measurement of nursing outcomes: Measuring client self-care and coping skills* (Vol. 4). New York: Springer.

Davis, A. E. (1989). *The relationship between the phenomenon of traumatic injury and the patterns of power, human field motion, esteem and risk taking.* Unpublished doctoral dissertation, Georgia State University, Atlanta.

Demi, A. S., & Warren, N. A. (1995). Issues in conducting research with vulnerable families. *Western Journal of Nursing Research, 17,* 188–202.

Gueldner, S. H., Bramlett, M. H., Johnston, L. W., & Guillory, J. A. (1996). Index of Field Energy. *Rogerian Nursing Science News, 8*(4), 6.

Gueldner, S. H., Michel, Y., Bramlett, M. H., Liu, C. F., Johnston, L. W., Endo, E., et al. (2005). The Wellbeing Picture Scale: A refined version of the Index of Field Energy. *Nursing Science Quarterly, 18*(1), 42–50.

Hills, R. (1998). *Maternal field patterning of awareness, wakefulness, human field motion and well-being in mothers with 6 month old infants: A Rogerian science perspective.* Unpublished doctoral dissertation, Wayne State University, Detroit, Michigan.

Hindman, M. (1993). *Humor and field energy in older adults.* Unpublished doctoral dissertation, Medical College of Georgia, Augusta.

Johnston, L. W. (1994). Psychometric analysis of Johnston's Human Field Image Metaphor Scale. *Visions: Journal of Rogerian Nursing Science, 2,* 7–11.

Morse, J. M. (1997). Responding to threats to integrity of self. *Advances in Nursing Science, 19,* 21–36.

Newman, M. A. (1994). *Health as expanding consciousness.* New York: National League for Nursing.

Parse, R. R. (1997). The human becoming theory: The was, is, and will be. *Nursing Science Quarterly, 10*(1), 32–38.

Parse, R. R. (2003). *Community: A human becoming perspective.* Sudbury, MA: Jones and Bartlett.

Phillips, B. B., & Bramlett, M. H. (1994). Integrated awareness: A key to the pattern of mutual process. *Visions, 2,* 7–12.

Rogers, M. E. (1992). Nursing science and the space age. *Nursing Science Quarterly, 5,* 27–34.

Saunders, J. M., & Valente, S. M. (1992). Overview. *Western Journal of Nursing Research, 14,* 700–702.

Smith, J. A. (1981) The idea of health: A philosophical inquiry. *Advances in Nursing Science, 4,* 43–49.

Spiers, J. (2000). New perspectives on vulnerability using emic and etic approaches. *Journal of Advanced Nursing, 31,* 715–721.

Terwilliger, S. (2007). *A study of children enrolled in a school-based physical activity program with attention to overweight and depression.* Unpublished doctoral dissertation, Binghamton University, Binghamton, NY.

Todaro-Franceschi, V. (1999). *The enigma of energy.* New York: Crossroad.

Application of the Barnard Parent/ Caregiver–Child Interaction Model to Care of Premature Infants

Danuta Wojnar

Parent–infant interaction is the context in which most infants initially experience the world. Under normal circumstances it is within the parent–infant relationship that the infant learns about the environment. It is the parent who teaches the infant basic principles of communication while mediating the amount of sensory input the infant receives. Yet over 10% of infants are born prematurely each year and require hospitalization in the newborn intensive care unit (NICU) (Hamilton et al., 2007). Highly specialized care available in the NICU enhances preterm infants' chance for survival; however, complications of prematurity, such as acute and chronic illness (Guzzetta et al., 2006; Roy et al., 2006), developmental delays (Casey, Whiteside-Mansell, Barrett, Bradley, & Gargus, 2006; Raju, Higgins, Stark, & Leveno, 2006), and deprivation of quality parent–child interactions (Als, 1997; Barnard, 1997; Lindrea & Stainton, 2000), pose serious threats to long-term infant outcomes.

The purpose of this chapter is to discuss the Barnard (1976) Parent/Caregiver–Child Interaction Model as a framework for delivering relationship-based developmentally supportive interventions to preterm infants and their parents. Examples are provided from research and practice that demonstrate clinical applicability of the Barnard model.

Barnard Parent/Caregiver–Child Interaction Model

In the early 1970s Dr. Kathryn Barnard was contracted by the U.S. Public Health Service to study ways of measuring the health and caregiving environments of infants and young children (Barnard, 1994). Before Barnard's work, research findings of the time indicated that the primary focus of caregiving in the early months of an infant's life was to establish routines and positive patterns of interaction to support the infant's optimal growth and development (Brazelton, 1973; Sameroff & Chandler, 1975). Barnard's research with mothers and infants indicated that all dimensions of child development (physical, emotional, intellectual, and social development) interact with each other in complex ways. Deficit in one of the domains affects the others.

Another insight Barnard and her research team gained from this work was that infants and young children undergo behavioral changes and internal reorganization in response to their caregiving and environmental stimuli. This suggests that one cannot understand early child development without taking into consideration interactions between the child, caregiver, and environment (Barnard, 1994). As a result of Barnard's early work, she developed the Parent/Caregiver–Child Interaction Model to depict strengths and weaknesses in interactions between infants and parents/caregivers and to direct behavior-specific interventions to foster children's social–emotional and cognitive growth and development (Barnard, 1976).

The Parent/Caregiver–Child Interaction Model uses the language of systems and developmental theories in the introduction of ideas. She calls the elements of her model "an interactive system" (Barnard, 1994, p. 6). In contrast to reductionist theories, system theory focuses on understanding how the parts of the system are arranged, what they do, how they are related, how as a whole they interact with the environment, and how they evolve and acquire new properties (von Bertalanffy, 1968).

An influence of developmental theory is also evident in Barnard's model. According to developmental theory, learning occurs when individuals interact with their environment. The learner actively constructs understanding from processing his or her behavior and making meaning of every new experience (Rowe, 1966). Barnard asserts that it is within the interactive system with the environment that the child's emotional, intellectual, and physical needs are met or not met (Barnard, 1994, p. 6).

The model expands on existing knowledge by focusing on the parent/caregiver–child environment interactive process, reflecting the fact that infants and young children influence the parent and the environment while simultaneously depending on parents to mediate their life experiences and create learning opportunities. The central focus of Barnard's model is to assess the child's health in the context of interpersonal interaction and adaptation that occurs between the child and caregiver in any given environment.

Major Concepts and Definitions

The integral component of the Barnard Parent/Caregiver–Child Interaction Model is the interactive system consisting of the parent/caregiver, the child, and the environment (Barnard, 1994). The concepts in Barnard's model are directly observable and include the infant's behaviors, the parent/caregiver's behaviors, and the parent/caregiver's and child's environment.

Parent/Caregiver Behavior

The parent/caregiver refers to the child's mother, father, or a primary caregiver and his or her characteristics, including psychosocial skills, concern about the child, physical and mental health, expectations of the child, parenting style, and ability to adapt to new situations (Barnard, 1994).

- *Sensitivity to cues* refers to the caregiver's ability to accurately interpret and respond sensitively to the infant needs and wants.

- *Alleviation of distress* refers to the effectiveness of the parent/caregiver to respond to the infant distress, which depends on the ability to recognize that the distress has occurred and have the repertoire of soothing actions to calm the child.

- *Social–emotional growth fostering* activities refer to the ability to initiate age-appropriate affectionate play and to provide appropriate verbal and nonverbal reinforcement for desirable child behavior.

Infant or Child Behavior

- *Clarity of cues* refers to the infant's ability to communicate his or her needs and wants through changes in facial expressions, alertness, fussiness, and body posture, to name a few. Cues that are inconsistent can cause difficulties in the parent/caregiver's adaptation process (Barnard, 1994).

- The *responsiveness* to the parent/caregiver refers to the child's ability to reciprocate the caregiver's efforts, such as smiling, rocking, or soothing activities.

The lack of the child responsiveness to the caregiver's efforts is assumed to make the parental adaptation to the child difficult or even impossible (Barnard, 1994).

Environment

The *environment* refers to the environment of both the parent/caregiver and the child. The characteristics of the environment include animate (people) and inanimate (physical environment of the family including objects, sounds, and visual and tactile stimulation) elements (Barnard, 1994).

Schematic Representation

Barnard (1976) depicted the parent/caregiver–child interactive system as a diagram with the arrows moving in circular motion from the child to the parent/caregiver and from the parent/caregiver to the child. Barnard defined the break drawn in each arrow as interference in the adaptive process, which can be caused by the caregiver, the infant, or the environment. The model has been discussed widely in the nursing literature (Margolis et al., 2001; Marriner Tomey, 2006; Sumner & Spietz, 1994). The Barnard Parent/Caregiver–Child Interaction Model is based on 10 theoretical propositions:

1. In the child health assessment the goal is to identify problems at a point before they develop and when intervention would be most effective.

2. Social–environmental factors are important for determining child health outcomes.

3. The caregiver–infant interaction provides information that reflects the nature of the child's ongoing environment.

4. Each parent brings to caregiving a basic personality and skill level that is the foundation on which caregiving skill is built. The enactment of caregiving depends on these characteristics as well as characteristics of the child and environment.

5. Through interaction, caregivers and children modify each other's behavior. That is, the caregiver's behavior influences the child and in turn the child influences the caregiver so that both are changed.

6. The adaptation process of the parent/caregiver and child is more modifiable than the child's' and the parent/caregiver's characteristics; therefore intervention should be aimed at supporting the parent's sensitivity and responsiveness to the infant's needs.

7. An important way to promote learning is to respond to child-initiated behaviors and to reinforce the child's attempts to try new things.

8. A major task for the helping professions is to promote a positive early learning environment that includes a nurturing relationship.

9. Assessing the child's social environment, including the quality of caregiver–child interaction, is important in any comprehensive child health assessment model.

10. Assessing the child's physical environment is equally important in any child health assessment model (Barnard, 1994).

Evaluation of the Barnard Model

According to Meleis (1997), evaluation is the cornerstone of further theory development, education, research, practice, administration, and daily decision-making process. Criteria used to evaluate Barnard's model include clarity, consistency, simplicity/complexity, usefulness, and generalizability. Meleis states that, "precision of boundaries, a communication of a sense of orderliness, vividness, and consistency through theory" (1997, p. 262) are indicators of a theoretical model's clarity. Although Barnard (1976) did not clearly define theoretical concepts in her model, she described them and thus implied the definitions. The concepts in the Barnard model are interconnected and form an interactive system. Because of the ongoing interaction, they influence each other and acquire new properties. The model articulates only some concepts consistent with the domain of nursing as proposed by Meleis (1997). For example, Barnard clearly addresses the concepts of environment (the physical and social environment of the child), client (parent/caregiver and the child), and the interaction (between the parent–child dyad and environment). Health is treated indirectly (interactive system provides the basis for assessing optimal child growth and development). Client transitions, nursing therapeutics, and health are not articulated and require further development.

Simplicity refers to a theory with a minimal number of concepts. On the other hand, complexity refers to the explanations and relationships among variables (Chinn & Kramer, 1991; Meleis, 1997). The appropriateness of the level of complexity within a theory depends on the nature of the concepts and relationships they are set to explain or predict (Meleis, 1997). The Barnard model at first glance is a relatively simple and elegant framework that relates to the parent–child interaction and its important elements. However, the many propositions made by Barnard about the nature of relationships between parent/caregiver, child, and environment imply high-level abstraction and complexity. According to Meleis (1997), consistency of a theoretical model depends on the level of congruency and the fit between different components of theory, for example, the fit between assumptions and concept definitions, the fit between concept definitions and their use in propositions, and the fit between concepts and exemplars (Meleis, 1997).

The theoretical basis of the Barnard model is assessed using NCAST Feeding and Teaching Scales (Barnard, 1994). The scales were developed to examine parent–infant interaction. Barnard's team and others tested the scales for reliability. The scales were established as reliable by studies of internal consistency and test–retest procedures (Barnard, 1994). The validity of the scales to evaluate quality of parent/caregiver–child interaction has also been assessed (Barnard, 1994). Researchers, nurses, and other clinicians interested in using the scales to assess parent–child interaction are required to receive certification by NCAST programs at the University of Washington and to achieve reliability of at least 85% in using these scales.

Research Applications with Preterm Infants

Considerable amount of research has been conducted over the past 20 years to assess and test parent/caregiver–child interactions. Using prospective longitudinal designs, researchers have consistently demonstrated important links between the quality of parent/caregiver–child interaction, environmental influences, and child development outcomes (Barnard & Kelly, 1990; Diehl, 1997; Farel, Freeman, Keenan, & Huber, 1991; Lewis & Coates, 1980; Leitch, 1999; Nakamura, Stewart, & Tatarka, 2000). Few published studies tested early NICU interventions designed to prevent the development of negative parent–infant interaction trajectories or to reduce hospital length of stay. In one of the earliest intervention studies, Parker, Zahr, Cole, and Brecht (1992) tested the efficacy of maternal education, training, and support in premature infants' behavioral and developmental functioning. Random assignment was made to intervention ($n = 26$) and control ($n = 15$) groups. Follow-up assessment took place at 4 and 8 months to determine the quality of infant stimulation in the home environment. There were no statistically significant differences either in maternal affective behavior or in infant social behavior between the groups. However, mothers in the intervention group scored significantly higher on the quality of stimulation value of the child's home environment using the Home Observation for Measurement of the Environment Inventory.

Likewise, Harrison, Sherrod, Dunn, and Olivet (1991) reported encouraging findings from a pilot intervention study to measure effectiveness of teaching parents about preterm infants' cues. The participants were assigned to two intervention groups and one control group. Mothers in the first intervention group (*n* = 10) received demonstration and verbal and written instruction that focused on understanding preterm infants cues. The second intervention group (*n* = 10) received brief instruction about the mothers' assessment of infant behavior and was asked to rate their infants' behavior. The control group (*n* = 10) received routine NICU care and support. A feeding episode was scored approximately 6 weeks after discharge using the Barnard Feeding Scale (Barnard, 1976). The total highest parent score was reported for the mothers who received the most intense preparation.

In a subsequent study, Lawhon (1994) provided individualized interventions focused on enhancing parental and newborn competence in interaction to parents and their infants born before 32 weeks of gestation. At approximately 1 month after discharge, a trained observer rated feeding interaction using the Barnard (1976) NCAST Feeding Scale. The scores in the intervention group were comparable with scores previously reported for full-term infants, suggesting that the intervention designed for the study was quite effective.

Most recent investigations focused on two areas: (1) testing early NICU interventions with parents to prevent the development of negative parent–infant interaction trajectories to reduce hospital length of stay and (2) reducing parenting stress after preterm birth. Using a randomized controlled design, a Norwegian team (Kaaresen, Rønning, Ulvund, & Dahl, 2006) tested the effects of an early intervention program on parenting stress after a preterm birth until 1 year corrected age with a sample of 140 infants and their parents. The intervention consisted of eight sessions shortly before discharge and four home visits by specially trained nurses focusing on the infant's unique characteristics, temperament, and developmental potential and the interaction between the infant and the parents. Seventy-one infants were included in the preterm intervention group, and 69 were included in the preterm control group. Fathers and mothers in the intervention group reported consistently lower scores within the distractibility and hyperactivity behavior and higher scores on parenting competence and attachment subscales compared with the preterm control group. There were no differences in mean summary stress scores between the mothers and fathers in the two groups at 12 months, suggesting that parenting programs may reduce parents' stress among both mothers and fathers of preterm infants to a level comparable with their term peers.

Melnyk et al. (2006) investigated the efficacy of an educational–behavioral intervention program called Creating Opportunities for Parent Empowerment (COPE) designed to enhance parent–infant interactions and parent mental health outcomes for the ultimate purpose of improving child developmental and behavior outcomes. A sample of 260 families participated in the intervention from 2001 to 2004 in two NICUs in the northeast United States. Parents completed self-administered instruments during hospitalization, within 7 days after infant discharge, and at 2 months' corrected age. Blinded observers rated parent–infant interactions in the NICU. All participants received four intervention sessions of audio-taped and written materials. Parents in the COPE program received information and behavioral activities about the appearance and behavioral characteristics of preterm infants and how best to parent them. The comparison intervention contained information regarding hospital services and policies. Mothers in the COPE program reported significantly less stress in the NICU and less depression and anxiety at 2 months' corrected infant age than did comparison mothers. Blinded observers rated mothers and fathers in the COPE program as more positive in interactions with their infants. Mothers and fathers also reported stronger beliefs about their parental role and what behaviors and characteristics to expect of their infants during hospitalization. Infants in the COPE program had a 3.8-day shorter NICU length of stay (mean, 31.86 vs. 35.63 days) and 3.9-day shorter total hospital length of stay (mean, 35.29 vs. 39.19 days) than did comparison infants, suggesting that a reproducible educational–behavioral intervention program for parents that begins soon after infant's admission to NICU can improve parent mental health outcomes, enhance parent–infant interaction, and reduce hospital length of stay.

Collectively, lessons learned from the intervention studies with preterm infants and their parents indicate that relatively simple interventions can be a powerful way of improving the quality of parent–child interaction and parent and child outcomes. Findings also suggest that the parent–child interaction can be modified to meet the preterm infants' capacity to interact, and this therapeutic aim can be an integral part of everyday clinical practice in the NICU. In addition, it appears that the most effective interventions involved multiple parent teaching modalities and time points.

Barnard Model: Practice Application to Preterm Infants

The usefulness of Barnard's model has been demonstrated in research, education, and clinical practice. Barnard's (1976) original research led to the development of the NCAST Feeding and Teaching Scales, which have been standardized for use with several ethnic groups and different infant age groups. These outcome measures are now used as a standardized assessment tool of parent–infant feeding and teaching interactions in more than 10 countries by over 10,000 researchers and health professionals and are reliable at 85% or higher in using the scales. Barnard's model has an international appeal to educators and appears in maternity nursing courses at the baccalaureate, master's, and doctoral levels. It has also been used as a framework for nursing practice with childbearing families (Early Head Start Programs in Washington State and Public Health Services across the United States).

One specific case of applying Barnard's model in clinical practice is facilitating the parent–infant interaction that occurs during feeding. For example, during the past decade nurses at the IWK Health Center in Halifax, Nova Scotia, have effectively used Barnard's principles to facilitate individualized guidance for parents learning to interact with both their term and preterm newborns. In the NICU, caregivers routinely discuss the strengths and gaps in feeding interaction using the model as a framework for feedback after feeding.

Specific NCAST Feeding Scale items are used in an effort to explain and help mothers to recognize infant cues that would signal them to respond in ways that promote more effective feeding. Staff members encourage mothers to pay attention to how they sustain eye contact, their facial expressions, gentle talking and stroking, and recognizing satiation cues, such as slow-down in feeding. They are encouraged to maintain a relaxed posture and to note disengagement cues such as crying, back arching, or falling asleep as a signal to terminate the feeding. Recognizing that the preterm infant's cues are not as clear as in term infants, the teaching strategies may require focusing on one cluster of cues at a time and setting small measurable goals to promote positive parent–child relationship and positive feeding interactions in the future.

Conclusion

Barnard's Parent/Caregiver–Child Interaction Model has been used in education, research, and clinical practice for over two decades. The results of the research review and evaluation of the model suggest that it effectively describes child development within the context of the infant's interaction with the caregiver and environment.

The process of model development is consistent with the inductive form of logic in that the theorist formulates concepts and relationships based on existing theory, research, and clinical observations. Barnard provides evidence of the applicability of her model in health education, research, and clinical practice. The model has been used internationally as a theoretical framework for maternity nursing practice. The NCAST Feeding and Teaching Scales to assess parent/caregiver–child interactions in clinical practice and research have a high level of precision and reliability. The information presented in this chapter suggests that the model offers a useful framework for designing and testing clinical interventions with preterm infants and their parents. Intervention research findings suggest that timing of the clinical interventions should occur early in the parent–child relationship and be sustained over time for maximal effects.

However, Barnard's model is limited to early child development within the context of relationships with caregiver and environment. The model is applicable to all disciplines that are concerned with parent–child relationships. There has been little recent effort to test the model. In its current state the model does not fulfill criteria for theory set forth by Meleis (1997). Therefore the model should be refined and further developed. However, the model does offer an excellent framework for use in clinical practice and research with preterm infants and their parents.

References

Als, H. (1997). Earliest intervention for preterm infants in newborn intensive care unit. In M. J. Guralnick (Ed.), *The effectiveness of early intervention* (pp. 23–47). Baltimore: Brooks Publishing.

Barnard, K. E. (1976). The Barnard Model. In G. Sumner & A. Spietz (Eds.), *NCAST caregiver/parent–child interaction feeding manual* (pp. 8–14). Seattle: NCAST Publications, University of Washington School of Nursing.

Barnard, K. E. (1994). Development of feeding and teaching scales. In G. Sumner & A. Spietz (Eds.), *NCAST caregiver/parent–child interaction feeding manual* (pp. 3–7). Seattle: NCAST Publications, University of Washington School of Nursing.

Barnard, K. E. (1997). Influencing parent-child interaction for children at risk. In M. J. Guralnick (Ed.), *The effectiveness of early intervention* (pp. 249–271). Baltimore: Brooks Publishing.

Barnard, K. E., & Kelly, J. F. (1990). Assessment of parent child interaction. In S. J. Meleis & J. P. Shonkoff (Eds.), *Handbook of early childhood intervention* (pp. 278–302). New York: Cambridge University Press.

Brazelton, T. B. (1973). Neonatal behavioral assessment scale. *Clinics in Developmental Medicine.* London: Spastics International Medical Publications.

Casey, P. H., Whiteside-Mansell, L., Barrett, K., Bradley, R. H., & Gargus, R. (2006). Impact of prenatal and/or postnatal growth problems in low birth weight preterm infants on school age outcomes: An 8-year longitudinal evaluation. *Pediatrics, 118*(3), 1078–1086.

Chinn, P. L., & Kramer, M. K. (1991). *Theory and nursing: A systematic approach* (3rd ed.). St. Louis. MO: Mosby.

Diehl, K. (1997). Adolescent mothers: What produces positive mother-infant interaction? *The American Journal of Maternal Child Nursing, 22,* 89–95.

Farel, A. M., Freeman, V. A., Keenan, N. L., & Huber, C. J. (1991). Interaction between high-risk infants and their mothers: The NCAST as an assessment tool. *Research in Nursing and Health, 14*(2), 109–118.

Guzetta, A., Mazotti, S., Tinelli, F., Bancale, A., Ferretti, G., Battini, R., et al. (2006). Early assessment of visual information processing and neurological outcome for preterm infants. *Neuropediatrics, 37*(5), 278–285.

Hamilton, B. E., Minino, A. M., Martin, J. A., Kochanek, K. D., Strobino, D. M., & Guyer, B. (2007). Annual summary of vital statistics: 2005. *Pediatrics, 11*(20), 345–360.

Harrison, L., Sherrod, R. A., Dunn, L., & Olivet, L. (1991). Effects of hospital based instruction on interactions between parents and preterm infants. *Neonatal Network, 9,* 27–33.

Kaaresen, P. I., Rønning, J. A., Ulvund, S. E., & Dahl, L. B. (2006). A randomized, controlled trial of the effectiveness of an early intervention program in reducing parenting stress after preterm birth. *Pediatrics, 118*(1), e9–e19.

Lawhon, G. (1994). *Facilitation of parenting within the newborn intensive care unit.* Unpublished doctoral dissertation, University of Washington, Seattle.

Leitch, D. B. (1999). Mother-infant: achieving synchrony. *Nursing Research, 48,* 55–58.

Lewis, M., & Coates, D. L. (1980). Mother-infant interaction and cognitive development in 12-week-old infants. *Infant Behavior and Development, 3,* 95–105.

Lindrea, K. B., & Stainton, C. M. (2000). Infant massage outcomes. *Journal of Maternal Child Nursing, 25,* 95–98.

Margolis, P. A., Stevens, R., Bordley, W. C., Stuart, J., Harlan, C., Keyes-Elstein, L., et al. (2001). From concept to application: the impact of a community-wide intervention to improve the delivery of preventive services to children. *Pediatrics, 108*(3), E:42.

Marriner Tomey, A. (2006). Nursing theorists of historical significance. In A. Marriner Tomey & M. Raile Alligood (Eds.), *Nursing theorists and their work* (6th ed., pp. 62–64). St. Louis, MO: Mosby.

Meleis, A. I. (1997). A model for evaluation of theories: Description, analysis, critique, testing, and support. In M. Zuccarini, E. Cotlier, & T. Gibbons (Eds.), *Theoretical nursing: Development and progress.* Philadelphia: Lippincott-Raven.

Melnyk, B. M., Feinstein, N. F., Alpert-Gillis, L., Fairbanks, E., Crean, H. F., Sinkin, R. A., et al. (2006). Reducing premature infants' length of stay and improving parents' mental health outcomes with Creating Opportunities for Parent Empowerment (COPE) neonatal intensive care unit program: A randomized, controlled trial. *Pediatrics, 118*(5), e1414–e1427.

Nakamura, W. M., Stewart, K. B., & Tatarka, M. E. (2000). Assessing father-infant interactions using the NCAST teaching scale: a pilot study. *American Journal of Occupational Therapy, 54*(1), 44–51.

Parker, S. J., Zahr, L. K., Cole, J. G., & Brecht, M. L. (1992). Outcome after developmental intervention in the neonatal intensive care unit for mothers of preterm infants with low socioeconomic status. *Journal of Pediatrics, 120,* 780–785.

Raju, T. N., Higgins, R. D., Stark, A. R., & Leveno, K. J. (2006). Optimizing care and outcomes for late preterm (near-term) infants: a summary of the workshop sponsored by the National Institute of Child Health and Human Development. *Pediatrics, 118*(3), 1207–1214.

Roy, K. K., Baruah, J., Kumar, S., Malhorta, N., Deorari, A. K., & Sharma J. B. (2006). Maternal antenatal profile and immediate neonatal outcome in VLBW and ELBW babies. *Indian Journal of Pediatrics, 73*(8), 669–673.

Rowe, P. G. (1966). The developmental conceptual framework to the study of the family. In F. I. Nye & F. M. Berardo (Eds.), *Emerging conceptual frameworks in family analysis.* New York: Praeger.

Sameroff, A. J., & Chandler, M. J. (1975). Reproductive risk and the continuum of caretaker casualty. In F. D. Horowitz (Ed.), *Review of child development research* (pp. 187–245). Chicago: University of Chicago Press.

Sumner, G., & Spietz, A. (Eds.) (1994). *NCAST caregiver/parent-child interaction teaching manual* (pp. 3–6). Seattle: NCAST Publications, University of Washington School of Nursing.

von Bertalanffy, L. (1968). *General system theory: Foundations, development application.* New York: George Braziller.

The Utility of Leininger's Culture Care Theory with Vulnerable Populations

Rick Zoucha

In the ever-evolving healthcare environment in the United States a multitude of people have access to services that promote health and well-being and reduce the effects of illness. Similarly, there are people who are not afforded the same access to healthcare services as others based on the distinction of vulnerability. According to Campos-Outcalt et al. (1994), vulnerable populations can be defined as groups of people who experience physical disabilities, mental disabilities, cultural differences, geographical separation, limited economic resources, and, due to barriers, might be unable to integrate into the mainstream health services and delivery system. The authors include as vulnerable the urban and rural poor (especially ethnic and racial minorities), Native Americans, chronically disabled children and adults, frail elderly, people who are homeless, and undocumented immigrants. Shi and Stevens (2005) define vulnerable populations as racial and ethnic minorities, uninsured, children, elderly, poor, chronically ill, people with AIDS, alcohol or substance abusers, people who are homeless, underserved rural and urban groups, people who do not speak English or have difficulties in communicating in healthcare settings, those who are poorly educated or illiterate, those with low incomes, and members of minority groups. In addition, victims of violence are at risk of being vulnerable (Zoucha, 2006).

Leininger (1996a) contends that regardless of economic, political, and even genetic differences, everyone has a culture. This chapter discusses Leininger's Culture Care Theory and the utility of the theory in working with vulnerable populations related to cultural differences in the research and practice settings.

Leininger's Theory of Culture Care Diversity and Universality

Leininger and McFarland (2006) define cultural care as the "subjectively and objectively learned and transmitted values, beliefs, and patterned lifeways that assist, support, facilitate, or enable another individual or group to maintain health and well-being, to improve their human condition and lifeways, or to deal with illnesses, handicaps, or death." Leininger (1996b) describes culture as learned values, beliefs, rules of behavior, and life-style practices of a particular group of people. Andrews and Boyle (2003) found culture to contain four basic characteristics: it is learned, shared, dynamic, and able to adapt to specific conditions. Culture involves all types of behavior that are socially acquired and transmitted by means such as customs, techniques, beliefs, institutions, and material objects (Locke, 1998). According to Leininger (1991b) and Andrews and Boyle (1999), humans exist within culture and culture is viewed as a universal phenomena. Leininger has taken the concept of culture and an ethical orientation of caring and developed a theory appropriate for nursing practice, research, and education (Zoucha & Husted, 2000). She also contends that individuals, families, and communities must be viewed in the context of culture (Zoucha & Husted, 2002)

Leininger and McFarland's (2006) theory of culture care diversity and universality is the product of over 50 years of research and development in which they studied over 60 cultures and identified 172 care constructs for use by nursing and other healthcare professionals. The Sunrise Model (Leininger & McFarland, 2002) depicts Leininger's theory and presents seven cultural and social structure dimensions of technological, religious and philosophical, kinship and social, political and legal, economic, and educational factors as well as cultural values beliefs and lifeways. The theory describes the diverse healthcare systems ranging from folk beliefs and practices to nursing and other heath care professional systems often used by people around the world. Leininger and McFarland (2006) describe two systems of caring that exist in every culture they studied. The first system of caring is generic and is considered the oldest form of caring or nurturing. Generic caring consists of culturally derived interpersonal practices and is considered essential for health, growth, and survival of humans (Reynolds & Leininger, 1993). Generic caring is often referred to as folk practices and is defined culturally (Leininger, 1996b).

According to Leininger and McFarland (2006), the second type of caring is considered therapeutic, cognitively learned, practiced, and transmitted through formal and informal professional education such as schools of nursing, medicine, and dentistry. Professional learning can and does include concepts and techniques to enhance professional practices as well as interpersonal communication techniques and holistic aspects of care. Historically, professional care has not always included ideas about folk care because that may not have been valued by nurses and other healthcare professionals (Leininger & McFarland, 2002).

In their theory, Leininger and McFarland (2006) contend that if professional and generic care practices do not fit together, this might affect client/patient recovery, health, and well-being and result in care that is not culturally congruent with the beliefs of the person, family, or community. To provide culturally congruent care, Leininger and McFarland (2002) assert that professionals must link and synthesize generic and professional care knowledge to benefit the client. This link is a bridge, where a bridge is appropriate, between the professional and folk healthcare systems (Leininger & McFarland, 2002).

Leininger and McFarland (2006) contend that three predictive modes of care are derived and based on the use of generic (emic) care knowledge and professional (etic) care knowledge obtained from research and experience using the sunrise model. The three modes of action are cultural care preservation/maintenance, cultural care accommodation/negotiation, and, cultural care repatterning/restructuring.

Cultural care preservation/maintenance (Leininger & McFarland, 2006) refers to assistive, supportive, facilitative, or enabling professional actions and decisions that help individuals, families, and communities from a particular culture retain and preserve care values so that they can maintain well-being, recover from illness, or face possible handicap or death. Leininger and McFarland (2002) describe cultural care accommodation/negotiation as assistive, facilitative, or enabling creative professional actions and potential decisions that can help individuals, families, and communities of a particular culture to adapt to or to negotiate with others for satisfying healthcare outcomes with professional caregivers. Cultural care repatterning/restructuring is described as the assistive, supportive, facilitative, and enabling by nurses and other healthcare professionals to promote actions and decisions that may help the person, family, and or community change or modify behaviors affecting their lifeways for a new and different health pattern. This repatterning/restructuring (Leininger, 2002b) is done while respecting the individual, family, and community cultural values and beliefs while still providing and promoting a healthier life-style than before the changes were coestablished with the person, family, and community. Leininger (2002a) asserts in her theory that the predicted three modes of action serve to guide judgments, decisions, and actions culminating in the promotion of culturally congruent care.

Leininger (2002) describes culturally congruent care as beneficial, satisfying, and meaningful to the individuals, families, and communities served by nurses. Cultural imposition occurs when nurses and other healthcare professionals impose their beliefs, practices, and values on another culture because they believe their ideas are superior to those of the other person or group (Leininger, 2002a). Leininger uses the concepts of cultural congruence and cultural imposition to focus on acceptable (caring) and unacceptable (noncaring) behavior by nurses in the practice, education, and research arena.

Utility of the Theory in Nursing Research and Practice

In addition to the development of the theory of cultural care, Leininger (1991a) developed a research method that is very useful in understanding the phenomena of culture care for vulnerable populations. As described earlier, vulnerability includes culture differences. Leininger's qualitative "ethnonursing" research method was created to work in conjunction with the theory (Sunrise Model) as a guide for research. The ethnonursing research method involves description and analysis of the lifeways of a people from the emic point of view (the viewpoint of the person being studied) with the ultimate goal of generating nursing knowledge to help those people (Leininger, 2002). Leininger (2002) suggests the method be used in conjunction with research enablers such as Leininger's observation-participation-reflection enabler, Leininger's stranger to trusted friend enabler, Sunrise Model enabler, specific domain of inquiry enabler, and Leininger's acculturation enabler.

The enabler guides can also be used in the clinical setting in an attempt to move from stranger to trusted friend between the nurse and client. The notion of being viewed as a friend can promote culturally congruent care in many cultures (Zoucha & Reeves, 1999). This friend-like or personal relationship between the nurse and client/patient can decrease the cultural difference vulnerability of the person because the cultural care needs of the client are known to the nurse. The nurse is then able to promote care that is congruent with the person's culture and essentially promote the health and well-being needs of the person, family, and community.

The connection between the theory, research, and practice is addressed by using the identified enablers to promote a deeper understanding of the cultural phenomena of interest regardless of the context (research or clinical practice). This allows for a holistic and comprehensive view of the domain of inquiry and the particular culture being studied. As transcultural nurse researchers and clinicians seek to understand the phenomena of interest for vulnerable populations, it is possible to decreases one aspect of vulnerability described as cultural differences. If indeed transcultural nurses use the finding of studies in actual clinical practice, then an understanding of the person, family, and community can be viewed from a cultural care perspective, therefore increasing the understanding of not only the cultural care needs but exposing the vulnerability related to being culturally different.

The concern of personal, family, and community vulnerability regarding cultural difference is that if nurses pursue an understanding of culture in relation to health and well-being, then there is an ethical motivation to promote care that is culturally congruent. This motivation can possibly decrease the vulnerability for the individual, family, and community. Zoucha and Husted (2000) contend that cultural caring should consider the person, family, and community in the context of their culture and result in the promotion of ethical and culturally congruent care. In agreement with Leininger's theory, Zoucha and Husted (2000) believe that it is the ethical responsibility and duty of the nurse to promote, provide, and encourage care that is culturally based and congruent with the values, beliefs, and traditions of the individual, family, and community.

Leininger's theory does provide a holistic and emic view of factors that describe culture and those cultural values and beliefs that are meaningful to individuals, families, and communities. However, in critiquing Leininger's theory it does not explicitly state in the context of the Sunrise Model or theory the related factors of racism, poverty, and history of oppression that are common for people other than the dominant culture in the United States. Leininger does consider these issues in her writing and presentations but does not make it clear in the explication of the theory and Sunrise Model in relationship to research and clinical practice. Adding the factors of racism, poverty, and history of oppression to the Sunrise Model as part of the experience for people of different cultures (from the dominant culture) may assist nurses and other healthcare professionals in understanding the meaning of vulnerability. Through the use of the theory nurses and other healthcare professionals can promote health and well-being while decreasing the experience of being vulnerable.

Conclusion

Individuals, families, and communities identified as vulnerable due to cultural differences can be understood in a manner that seeks to expose the vulnerability and focus on the cultural care needs. Leininger's Theory of Culture Care Diversity and Universality promotes a deep and clear understanding of the individual, family, and community from a unique cultural perspective. Using the theory and the identified enablers for research and clinical practice allow for the nurse to view the individual, family, and community from the perspective of the seven cultural factors identified in the Sunrise Model as religion, kinship, technology, education, economic, political and legal, and cultural lifeways. In using this view, nurses and other healthcare professionals can decrease the vulnerability of the individual, family, and community by uncovering the concern of cultural difference and promoting ethical practice that is congruent with the cultural beliefs of those in the caring relationship with nurses and other healthcare professionals.

References

Andrews, M. M., & Boyle., J. S. (1999). *Transcultural concepts in nursing care* (3rd ed.). Philadelphia: Lippincott.

Andrews, M. M., & Boyle., J. S. (2003). *Transcultural concepts in nursing care* (4th ed.). Philadelphia: Lippincott Williams & Wilkins.

Campos-Outcalt, D., Fernandez, R., Hollow, W., Lundeen, S., Nelson, K., Schuster, B., et al. (1994). *Providing quality health care to vulnerable populations*. Retrieved August 23, 2007, from http://www.primarycaresociety.org/1994d.htm

Leininger, M. (1996a). Culture care theory, research, and practice. *Nursing Science Quarterly, 9*(2), 71–78.

Leininger, M. (1996b). Response to Swendson and Windsor: rethinking cultural sensitivity. *Nursing Inquiry, , 3*(4), 238–241.

Leininger, M. (2002a). Culture care theory: A major contribution to advance transcultural nursing knowledge and practices. *Journal of Transcultural Nursing, 13*(3), 189–192; discussion 200–181.

Leininger, M. (2002b). Madeleine Leininger on transcultural nursing and culturally competent care. Interview by Mary Agnes Seisser. *Journal of Healthcare Quality, 24*(2), 18–21.

Leininger, M. M. (1991a). Ethnonursing: A research method with enablers to study the theory of Culture Care. *NLN Publication*(15-2402), 73–117.

Leininger, M. M. (1991b). The theory of culture care diversity and universality. *NLN Publication* (15-2402), 5–68.

Leininger, M., & McFarland, M. (2006). *Culture care diversity and universality: A worldwide nursing theory* (2nd ed.). Sudbury, MA: Jones and Bartlett.

Leininger, M. M., & McFarland, M. R. (2002). *Transcultural nursing: Concepts, theories, research and practice* (3rd ed.). New York: McGraw-Hill.

Locke, D. (1998). *Increasing multicultural understanding: A comprehensive model* (2nd ed.). Newbury Park, CA: Sage.

Reynolds, C. L., & Leininger, M. M. (1993). *Madeline Leininger, culture care diversity and universality theory*. Newbury Park, CA: Sage.

Shi, L., & Stevens, G. (2005). *Vulnerable populations in the United States*. San Francisco: Jossey-Bass

Zoucha, R. (2006). Considering culture in understanding interpersonal violence. *Journal of Forensic Nursing, 2*(4), 195–196.

Zoucha, R., & Husted, G. L. (2000). The ethical dimensions of delivering culturally congruent nursing and health care. *Issues of Mental Health Nursing, 21*(3), 325–340.

Zoucha, R., & Husted, G. L. (2002). The ethical dimensions of delivering culturally congruent nursing and health care. *Review Series Psychiatry, 3*, 10–11.

Zoucha, R. D., & Reeves, J. (1999). A view of professional caring as personal for Mexican Americans. *International Journal of Human Caring, 3*(3), 14–20.

Positive Skills, Positive Strategies: Solution-Focused Nursing

Margaret McAllister

In my 25 years of experience in nursing and in teaching nurses for 16 years, I am frequently made aware of a need, a frustration, and a sense of powerlessness in nurses, especially when working with clients who have multilayered and enduring problems. In working with this population it is hard to know how one can be recovery oriented, empowering, and retain optimism for change. This chapter outlines a practical philosophy for being strategic, forward looking, and positive with clients. Called solution-focused nursing, it derives from critical social theory and positive psychology ideas.

The chapter begins with a client's experience with emergency health care. The narrative is analyzed, drawing from it key lessons, before moving on to a philosophical framework for nursing that helps clinicians be solution focused and strategic rather than reactive and overwhelmed.

Zara's Experience

The following narrative relates the experience of a client, Zara, who went to the emergency department for treatment:

> A while ago I had an experience that I don't ever want to repeat. I had developed a headache that just wouldn't go away. The pain had become so bad that I was throwing up and beginning to have panic attacks. I'd had headaches before, but never this bad. I'd also had long-standing anxiety, treated with medications, that developed as a consequence of childhood abuse issues that I considered pretty much resolved after quite a few years of therapy.
>
> After about 6 hours of trying to relieve the headache with paracetamol, cold compresses, and resting, the pain was just not easing. When I began vomiting, I knew I needed help. I called an ambulance and was taken to the public emergency department.

I was placed on a gurney and wheeled into a room away from the nurse's station. No one told me what was happening, whether I'd be okay, or even if they'd be watching me. Some time later a nurse came to take my temperature and blood pressure. He also asked me to rate the severity of my pain.

Then a doctor came in. She seemed kind and sympathetic at first—holding my hand, gently asking me questions, and reassuring me that the pain would subside with IV medications. She said she wanted me to stay overnight, but I told her that I felt panicky in hospitals and if the pain subsided, I'd be better off at home.

The nurse asked me why I felt panicky and I told them both that I had a lot of experience with hospitals—the last being a year ago when I was in the psychiatric unit. The doctor asked me about the reason for this stay, and I told her that it was to prevent any risks of problems that might arise after gynecological surgery. My psychiatrist had been concerned that the surgery could be triggering, because I had a history with dissociation disorder.

Revealing this information seemed to cause a sudden change in the doctor's attitude. She stopped asking me questions and just pushed up my shirt to examine my body. She saw some old scars and asked me how they were caused. Again, I was honest and told her I used to self-harm. That's when she pulled away immediately. It seemed like she was disgusted and I felt terribly ashamed.

Without a word of explanation the doctor left the room. At this point I had not been given anything for my headache and was still feeling panicky and nauseous. I looked toward the nurse. In that moment I really needed him.

Reflective Activity

Imagine you were that nurse with a client, like Zara, in pain and distress. Your colleague has acted in a way that led the person to feel ashamed. Now you must provide physical and psychological safety and minimize risks of mounting anxiety and panic.

And what of the longer term? Two issues of concern come to mind: The client's future well-being and health service utilization and promoting more effective clinician–client interactions.

Analysis of the Narrative

In generating a satisfactory complete response to these questions and in suggesting an effective care pathway for this nurse, it is helpful to reflect on what some of the significant elements within this story might mean for practice. First, the experience of ill-health can be fundamentally disempowering. Second, people who come to health services are vulnerable and need nursing support. And finally, nursing work not only frequently involves change-oriented work with clients but also with the healthcare culture.

The experience of illness is not comfortable or pleasant at the best of times, but when a client presents to a health service expecting timely quality care and they are not helped to feel safe and secure, and indeed are made to feel worse, the experience can be traumatizing (Arnold, 1994; Hartman, 1995).

Too often, clients complain of substandard care in Australian health services (SANE Australia, 2004). A significant number of clients, especially young people, who present for emergency care do not stay for treatment (Ryan, Parle, & Babidge, 1998). Additionally, when they have preexisting mental health problems, they commonly feel labeled, judged, objectified, and ashamed (Johnstone, 1997). This is a fundamentally disempowering experience that can have long-term negative health and social consequences. Many clients do not have adequate psychosocial assessments completed and are lost to follow-up (Bennowith et al., 2002). Clients may be unwilling to use the health service again, they may later act out their negative feelings on to others with hostility or violence, or they may act inwardly and allow shame and guilty feelings to spill into a vicious cycle, such as the cycle of self-harm (Figure 12-1).

Similarly, nurses required to work in such an environment frequently find that they themselves are oppressed and become disempowered (Jackson, Clare, & Mannix, 2002). Without adequate strategies to effectively intervene in situations such as these, nurses become disillusioned, disaffected, and demoralized.

In a study examining everyday conversations of nurses working with clients who self-injure (Estefan, McAllister, & Rowe, 2004), it was found that only the outward acts of injury tended to be the focus of care by nurses, so that most did not focus on events that might trigger the urge to self-harm. They did not discuss the need to empathize with the

Figure 12-1 The Cycle of Self-Harm

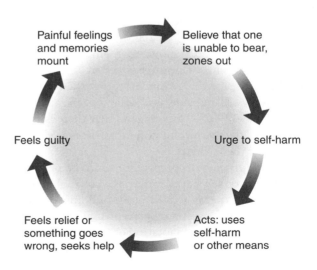

Painful feelings and memories mount

Believe that one is unable to bear, zones out

Urge to self-harm

Acts: uses self-harm or other means

Feels relief or something goes wrong, seeks help

Feels guilty

individual's specific and present concerns, and they did not reveal a concern for helping the clients address issues of self-injury or work with them to find safer ways to express distress and communicate their needs. The study also revealed that nurses frequently felt unprepared, lacked clear frameworks for practice, and were vulnerable to subtle tensions in practice that led to managing before caring, valuing diagnosis before understanding, and focusing on behaviors rather than personal meanings and the client. The effects for patients and for care are that alienating, unhelpful, diagnostic, and socially loaded labels are attributed to people. In the story above the fact that the client had been a past psychiatric patient led to substandard health care and a negative experience. The patient was passive and alienated. The caregiving experience was also burdensome for the doctor.

As many have argued, a model of care that is problem-centered is unlikely to offer inspiring or sustainable positive outcomes for clinicians or patients (Hall, 1996; White & Epston, 1990). This is true for virtually all healthcare contexts (Hedtke & Winslade, 2004; Wade, 1997). Yet this problem orientation remains dominant (McAllister, 2003).

A problem orientation may be useful in helping to isolate problems, target areas of change, and apply interventions dispassionately and rationally, but these actions are not always appropriate. Constantly searching for problems may prevent appreciating things that are going right for a person. It may also be that some problems may never be resolved completely, and a focus on the negative is inherently pessimistic. Problems and difficulties become the main concern rather than feats and achievements. Problems are seen as something to be overcome rather than to be tolerated and perhaps integrated.

Positive and protective client outcomes are unlikely to be developed and achieved. These include feelings of distress manageability, social supports, health-seeking behavior, optimism, and self-belief in managing feelings (Resnick et al., 1997). For nurses, there is the risk of anxiety and frustration from lack of strategies and skills, a sense of low professional self-efficacy, and feeling vicariously traumatized through dealing with these clients (Hartman, 1995; McAllister, 2003).

Yet clinicians who respond with empathy, a nonjudgmental stance, and supportive counseling skills have a positive effect on outcomes for clients (Webber, 2002). Clients are more likely to stay for treatment, to use the health service again rather than attempt to inadequately self-manage, and to accept organized follow-up care under such circumstances (Shaw, 2002). This suggests that there is much nurses can do to instill hope and to facilitate effective meaningful experiences, and, importantly, to provide supportive connections for these clients.

It is not sufficient to prepare nurses to be proficient in technical procedures in a situation such as this. What they need is a collaborative way of working with both clients and colleagues, one that is actively peace-building, so that the negative emotions generated in an encounter such as this are prevented and/or contained. It is crucial that nurses be part of the solution, as this adaptation of Bell Hooks's words (1994) reflects: "When those who know, oppress, and dominate others and continue to discriminate and attempt to disempower, then they become part of the problem."

Toward a Power-Building Practice

I believe at some level nurses who are complicit in allowing a disempowering environment to persist are unhappy and unfulfilled and that this accounts for why so many become disenchanted with their work and leave the profession. That is why it is crucial that we as nurses find a way to circumvent this situation, by inventing a way of working that gives nurses responsibility for engendering a supportive environment. In this framework of care, it is not just technical skills that are important, but the psychosocial health and well-being of all players must be paramount.

Solution-focused nursing is a philosophy of care that I developed after years of being confronted with the reality that nurses do tend to take a reactive approach with patients. There is a tendency to be concerned with problems and problem resolution rather than an approach that is preventative, strategic, and proactive. This perhaps is why the nurse in the story was very efficient in responding to the client's pain at least in the beginning. He assessed the person's physiological status and gathered some baseline data on the severity and nature of the discomfort, but he wasn't very adept at engendering a comfortable comforting environment for the person. His clinical colleague behaved in a tactless and damaging way, yet the nurse did not feel in a position to act, either in reaction or preemptively.

This is not surprising because in most health service cultures the dominant philosophy is one that favors a problem orientation and a medical model. In this world view, it is the person's presenting problems or illnesses that take priority, and the concern is to stabilize the body, be it the physical or psychological parts of that body. Further, in this model the nurse's role is primarily that of assistant to medical practitioners and to ameliorate suffering and promote restoration of health and well-being.

Consider this quotation (Harrison, 1994, p. 4) about why it is that clinicians negatively label and ostracize clients such as these: "When time and resources are limited and no one really knows how best to help, it's easier to make judgments and use labels than to spend time looking for possible causes of distress."

Yet health services will always have limited resources, and clients who present for emergency care will always have more concerns than just their physical ailment. As human service workers it is a health professional's responsibility to know how to act in compassionate yet effective ways.

Toward Empowerment

So let's take a different approach, one drawn from critical social theory and the positive psychology movement to see what other possibilities emerge for nursing practice. Critical social theory alerts us to the reality that people in society who are in submissive or marginalized positions, in this situation patients, are likely to have power removed from them, to not be free to speak their mind, and to experience further effects of being oppressed and alienated. These typically include self-directed hostility and violence, anger, and avoidance toward the disempowering other (Freire, 1972; Roberts, 1994).

Critical social theory suggests that power needs to be shifted so that it is shared between the people in positions of authority and those who are subordinate. Given that in health services there is a desire to encourage clients to take a more active role in their own health care and to be more responsible service users, such an approach makes perfect sense. Clinicians who share power with clients and who are explanatory, consultative, and collaborative are working closer to achieving their service goals. This does, by its nature, offer a proactive role for clinicians such as nurses (Hopton, 1997).

Positive psychology says that people are more likely to become healthy when their strengths and capacities are being tapped, because when there is over-focus on the person's vulnerabilities and deficiencies, then the client and the caregiver can begin to lose hope, become helpless, and give up (Peterson, Maier, & Seligman, 1995; Seligman, 1995). In such cases chronicity, depression, and a self-fulfilling prophecy of doom and gloom can set in.

Models of care are subtle and can become deeply embedded in clinicians' daily working life so that they can be reproduced unconsciously, without thought. But when they are critically reflected on, they can be challenged and replaced. I believe that nurses do feel uncomfortable with the degree of influence the medical model has over their professional practice. Yet because the medical model is the most familiar world view in health services, it is also the one that people tend to resort to when they lack an alternative. But critical social theory would also urge that the alternative world view needs to be brought in from the margins and consciously used so that it does begin to compete with that which has been taken for granted.

One effective way that we can challenge ourselves to not unconsciously reproduce the medical model in our day-to-day interactions with clients is to exercise our abstract creative brain and rethink practice. This process has been coined "conscientization" (Freire, 1972; Martin & Younger, 2000). Harden (1996) argues that such a process is crucial for all groups seeking emancipation. She states that only when oppression in nursing has been recognized and a critical consciousness achieved can true humanistic care be given. Try this consciousness-raising activity as an example:

> Go to a collection of paintings by Frida Kahlo (Herrera, 1991) and find the picture entitled, "The little deer." Complete a surface level reading of this picture by writing down all of the elements you see within the frame.
>
> Now try to look more deeply and make an attempt to answer these questions: Imagine this "person" is the client in the story just recounted. How might she be feeling? What factors are contributing to this feeling state?
>
> Where is the light coming from in this painting? What might this signify? If the role of the nurse is to take the person from a position of darkness and fear to a position of light and comfort, what could a nurse do if she or he was painted into this frame?

Frida Kahlo, the Mexican artist, provides many vivid evocative expressions, many of them autobiographical, of the experience of pain and vulnerability. But also in this and other paintings of hers one gets a sense of strength, endurance, and resilience. Through all this pain and loneliness, there's a power to her spirit. Recently at a conference on nursing practice development, I showed this image to try to promote thought on reframing care by thinking about the lived experience of being a patient and being in pain. I asked participants to tell me what they saw in this image, what it meant to them.

The following insights, drawn from the audience, remain with me and perhaps they resonate for you: that people can be wounded, in pain, dehumanized, lost, vulnerable, and at risk, but that good nursing care and good health care comes when clinicians are able to be with clients and perhaps reorient them. Just by turning around and facing a new direction we can help to show people ways out of their dilemmas. To me good health care is about finding ways to turn crises into turning points.

To think about this image and the role of nursing whenever nurses find themselves in a difficult position with clients or colleagues I believe is illuminating. It suggests a way forward and that way emphasizes shared humanity and noticing people's inherent strengths that can be enduring even within hardships and challenges.

Solution-Focused Nursing

Many nursing scholars argue for a model of practice that is antioppressive but do not clearly show how that may be done (Harden, 1996; Hopton, 1997; Martin & Younger, 2000). Solution-focused nursing attempts to fill this gap by stating a simple philosophy and clarifying practices nurses can use in a range of different healthcare situations. Solution-focused nursing comprises six principles:

1. The person, not the problem, is at the center of inquiry.

2. Problems and strengths may be present at all times. Looking for and then developing inner strengths and resources will be affirming and will assist in coping and adaptation. By working with what's going right with a client, one can be enhancing their hope, optimism, and self-belief, thus maximizing their health capacity.

3. Resilience is as important as vulnerability.

4. The nurse's role moves beyond illness care toward adaptation and recovery.

5. The goal is to create change at three levels: in the client, nursing, and society.

6. The way of being with clients is proactive rather than reactive.

This model of care is very much focused on achieving empowerment for clients and emancipation for nursing. Where clients may have been overlooked, patronized, and marginalized in the healthcare relationship, nurses have similarly had their power constrained and their potential reduced. In addition to principles and phases of the working relationship, several concepts inherent to empowerment need close analysis and perhaps reframing: power, skill, awareness, and language (Table 12-1).

TABLE 12-1	Elements of Empowerment
Element	**Characteristics**
Power	Rather than avoid power, nurses can see power as having positive influence, as a resource to be shared, and as a tool to use "softly."
Nursing skill	The skill of nursing is neither just about technical proficiency nor is it something that remains within the individual nurse's sphere of ownership. Skill also refers to being with a patient supportively, knowing what not to say as well as how best to communicate. Skill is something to be shared with clients and with colleagues. It is in the sharing where sustainable development and advancements are made.
Awareness	Awareness is a state of being as well as a goal within the nurse–client relationship. Being aware means not being unconscious to the practices that keep groups disempowered. Achieving awareness as a goal refers to the sharing of knowledge, skills, and understanding.
Language	Language provides the codes through which we talk about and understand the world in which we live. Language transmits powerful messages. Unconscious use of language can lead to oppression and ongoing marginalization. Conscious usage can be the tool by which nurses move toward an alternative to dominating practices.

It is not uncommon for clinicians working in a deficit model to feel disempowered, out of their depth, and directionless. Bowles, Mackintosh, and Torn (2001) conducted a pretest–posttest study to evaluate the impact of solution-focused communication training. Before training they found that nurses commonly believed they were inadequate, illustrated in the comment, "I really didn't feel like I was offering anything in terms of solutions." Nurses also believed they had no direction with patients. One nurse, for example, said that there was, "Lots of waffling going on, I let people waffle. . . . I was a good listener, I can listen for weeks with no solution in sight."

Yet after training nurses said they had new tools to work with. Participants said things like, "I know where I'm going now with something. I mean, the listening's still there, but it's different now. . . . I feel as if I'm listening more intently." Also, the quality of interactions that nurses had with patients changed. One nurse said, "I think it's empowered me. It's released me from this awful feeling that as the nurse I have to put a plaster on and sort of send them away." Significantly, nurses were also able to transfer the skills learned in one context to other situations, and these interactions used optimism and change-based strategies.

Solution-focused nursing involves three phases: joining, building, and extending.

Joining

In the joining phase effort is made to get to know who the person is, what their strengths and vulnerabilities are, and what the nature of there condition is, physically as well as psychosocially. It is important to notice and develop areas in the person that are healthy and adaptive because this leads to appropriate behavior.

In Zara's case the nurse could have used the time when he was measuring her vital signs to spend just a few moments engaging Zara. This requires a conscious stance wherein you move away from the position of detached dispassionate expert to one who is, to put it simply, human. In this way a connection is made based on what is shared between a client and a clinician rather than what keeps them separate. Note the following example:

> Zara, my name is Paul. I'm your nurse. You must be feeling awful (wait and listen), being in pain, being here alone. You have made a good decision getting help now. I need to tell you that there will be a wait ahead as the team is really busy here.
>
> By trying to relax, you may help to contain the pain. Have you found, in the past, effective ways to be calm? How would you feel about using those strategies or some that I could suggest?

Even if answers are not forthcoming, the nurse has made an effort to show his or her concern and opened up a pathway to collaborate. It sets a respectful tone and invites the person to become active in his or her own health care.

Building

In the building phase the aim is to be educative and supportive. Empowerment is all about giving the skills to clients so they can better understand health and well-being and better self-manage. It aims to develop in the client a sense of capability and inner strength and motivation to get through the present health challenge.

Solution-focused nursing is not about a forced optimism. It is not about being solution forced, because it involves appreciation for the fact that people have vulnerabilities and strengths. Thus in a respectful empowering relationship, the person feels supported and also motivated. Skill deficits (such as ways to relax and relieve head tension) and excesses (such as the mechanism of self-injury, which can be very effective in managing pent-up distress) can be discussed.

In emergency health care, such as in Zara's case, the building phase may be brief, perhaps taking only a couple of minutes, but it is nonetheless the heart of the nurse–client relationship. Without the building phase nursing work has no purpose. It may be as simple as conveying the value of optimism in change or as complex as showing a client ways to self-manage a chronic debilitating disease. The following example illustrates this point:

> Zara, this kind of headache is something that, with effort, you could minimize and even prevent. Would you like to learn more about factors that influence headaches?

Together, the nurse and client might work on building a repertoire of coping skills to deal with the immediate situation, talking through issues such as relationships, tension management, and being both capable and strong at the same time as sometimes feeling vulnerable and emotional. This may help to build up in the client feelings of optimism, so that the client can adapt, recover, and get stronger in the longer term.

In this phase too the work may not be exclusively focused on the nurse–client relationship. Indeed, nurses may find that the change that is needed rests within their own workplace culture and not within the client. Solution-focused nursing sees that the possibilities for change rest equally within the cultural and social sphere as they do within the client relationship. This notion is quite a departure from the medical model, and even from other nursing models that emphasize and centralize concern for the individual client (Gordon, 1994; Roper, Logan, & Tierney, 1980). The implication is that the profession of nursing plays no part in creating and sustaining ill health when what we so often see is that it patently does.

Zara's experience emphasizes this notion clearly. The nurse in this story, by failing to intervene tactfully and assertively with the doctor, is being complicit in harmful care. On the other hand, in being ethical and empowering nurses have a duty and a moral obligation to protect the person's dignity. But how does one act in a delicate situation such as this? Again, the answers rest in simply being human, thinking of a way to be empathic and respectful yet advocating for better care for clients:

> Sue, got a few minutes? I noticed back there with Zara that you looked uncomfortable and you didn't speak much to her. (Waits and listens) . . . It's a challenge sometimes to be nonjudgmental. Yet it's so important. Want to talk some more about this?

Therefore the solution-focused nursing model values moving beyond individual-focused care to valuing the role of social and cultural care. It involves noticing discourses, practices, actions, and inactions that constrain, obscure, or mislead our aim to be empowering and enabling, and it requires nurses to suggest more enabling ways of thinking about and practicing nursing and health care.

Extending

In the extending phase the emphasis is on encouraging the person to transfer the skills learned in the nurse–patient relationship so they can be used in other contexts such as when they are faced with social situations that are upsetting. It also involves setting the client up with social supports that can be used in place of the clinician–client relationship and therefore be more enduring and sustainable.

Again, in Zara's case this phase would be brief, perhaps a matter of seconds. Time and duration are not important but conveying the belief that change has been made and that the way ahead is positive are

> If you need help again, Zara, you know what to do and you know more about ways to self-manage, right? (Waits for confirmation.)

Note that all these examples of being solution focused are not unidirectional, which is often the case in expert-care models, but rather this model emphasizes working alongside the client and negotiating care with them. The nurse relies on the client giving feedback that the message has been received. The nurse makes an effort to engage in conversation and real dialogue. The belief is that in a partnership model, the person is more likely to feel understood, cared for, and motivated to resume self-caring work.

Conclusion

Positive nursing strategies are about taking action, knowing that small steps in the right direction can have a huge impact. It is about nurturing the things you want to grow—in clients, in the relationship, and in the health service culture. It is about encouraging innovation, creativity, and bright ideas. It is about moving beyond the routine and mechanical in the knowledge that technical competence is only half the story to nursing practice. It is about making a commitment to collaborate, to question, to practice humanism in the everyday and having the courage to do things differently.

References

Arnold, L. (1994). *Understanding self-injury.* Bristol, UK: Bristol Crisis Service for Women.

Bennowith, O., Stocks, M., Gunnell, D., Peters, J., Evans, M., & Sharp, D. (2002). General practice based interventions to prevent repeat episodes of deliberate self harm: Cluster randomized controlled trial. *British Medical Journal, 324,* 1254–1257.

Bowles, N., Mackintosh, C., & Torn, A. (2001). Nurses' communication skills: an evaluation of the impact of solution-focused communication training. *Journal of Advanced Nursing, 36*(3), 347–354.

Estefan, A., McAllister, M., & Rowe, J. (2004). Difference, dialogue, dialectics: A study of caring and self-harm. In K. Kavanagh & V. Knowlden (Eds.), *Interpretive studies in healthcare and the human sciences: Vol. III. Many voices: Toward caring culture in healthcare and healing* (pp. 21–61). Madison: University of Wisconsin Press.

Freire, P. (1972). *Pedagogy of the oppressed.* Harmondsworth, UK: Penguin.

Gordon, M. (1994). *Nursing diagnosis: Process and application* (3rd ed.). St. Louis, MO: Mosby.

Hall, B. (1996). The psychiatric model: A critical analysis of its undermining effects on nursing in chronic mental illness. *Advanced Nursing Science, 18*(3), 16–26.

Harden, J. (1996). Enlightenment, empowerment and emancipation: The case for critical pedagogy in nurse education. *Nurse Education Today, 16*(1), 32–37.

Harrison, D. (1994). *Understanding self-harm.* London: Mind Publications.

Hartman, C. (1995). The nurse-patient relationship and victims of violence. *Scholarly Inquiry for Nursing Practice, 9*(2), 175–192.

Hedtke, L., & Winslade, J. (2004). *Remembering lives: Conversations with the dying and the bereaved.* New York: Baywood.

Herrera, H. (1991). The little deer. In *Frida Kahlo: The paintings* (p. 189). London: Bloomsbury.

Hooks, B. (1994). *Teaching to transgress: Education as the practice of freedom.* New York: Routledge.

Hopton, J. (1997). Towards anti-oppressive practice in mental health nursing. *British Journal of Nursing, 6*(15), 874–878.

Jackson, D., Clare, J., & Mannix, J . (2002). Who would want to be a nurse? Violence in the workplace—a factor in recruitment and retention. *Journal of Nursing Management, 10,* 13–20.

Johnstone, L. (1997). Self-injury and the psychiatric response. *Feminism and Psychology, 7*(3), 421–426.

McAllister, M. (2003). Doing practice differently: Solution focused nursing. *Journal of Advanced Nursing, 41*(6), 528–535.

Martin, G., & Younger, D. (2000). Anti oppressive practice: A route to the empowerment of people with dementia through communication and choice *Journal of Psychiatric & Mental Health Nursing, 7*(1), 59–67.

Petersen, C., Maier, S., & Seligman, M. (1995). *Learned helplessness: A theory for the age of personal control.* New York: Oxford University Press.

Resnick, M., Bearman, P., Blum, R., Bauman, K., Harris, K, Jones, J., et al. (1997). Protecting adolescents from harm: Findings from the National Longitudinal Study on Adolescent Health. *Journal of the American Medical Association, 278*, 823–832.

Roberts, S. (1994, Fall). Oppressed group behaviour: Implications for nursing, *Revolution: the Journal of Nurse Empowerment, 4*(3), 29–35.

Roper N., Logan W., & Tierney A. (1980). *The elements of nursing.* New York: Churchill Livingstone.

Ryan, M., Parle, M., & Babidge, N. (1998). What precipitates deliberate self-harm? A cognitive behavioural formulation of attempted suicide presentations at an inner city hospital. *Australian Health Review, 21*(3), 194–211.

SANE Australia. (2004). *Dare to care! SANE mental health report,* 2004. South Melbourne: Sane Australia.

Seligman, M. (1995). *The optimistic child.* Boston: Houghton.

Shaw, N. (2002). Shifting conversations on girls' and women's self-injury: An analysis of the clinical literature in historical context. *Feminism and Psychology, 12*(2), 191–219.

Wade, A. (1997). Small acts of living: Everyday resistance to violence and other forms of oppression. *Contemporary Family Therapy, 19*(1), 23–39.

Webber, R. (2002). Young people and their quest for meaning. *Youth Studies Australia, 21*(1), 40–43.

White, M., & Epston, D. (1990). *Narrative means to therapeutic ends.* New York: Norton.

Unit Three

"Everything that is done in the world is done by hope."

■ ■ ■

Martin Luther

RESEARCH

Methodological and Ethical Issues in Research with Vulnerable Populations

Mary de Chesnay, Patrick J. M. Murphy, Lynda Harrison, and Maile Taualii

The purpose of the research unit is to explore ways to study phenomena of interest to nurses who study vulnerable populations. Particular attention is given to differences and similarities between qualitative and quantitative designs and methods of data collection, analysis, issues of informed consent, and use of data. Following this overview chapter are several research chapters that report studies with participants who might be considered vulnerable.

Developing the Proposal

The following guidelines represent one way of developing a thesis or dissertation research proposal and can be adapted for other purposes. In terms of writing a proposal for funding, the guidelines of the sponsor must be followed, but the outline presented here covers all the aspects that would generally be found in a funding proposal, except budget, though the formats vary. These guidelines are presented with the expectation that readers can adapt the outline for their own preferences and institutional requirements. Much of the work of developing a research proposal is universal and appropriate to all types of research with all kinds of populations, but our focus in this chapter is research issues with vulnerable populations. Some proposals have fewer or more chapters or headings, but basically the content covered here is appropriate for most research proposals.

At the heart of all good research proposals is a meaningful question that the researcher, and subsequently the proposal reviewer, feels a compelling need to answer. Although one can quite literally investigate anything under the sun, research involving vulnerable populations should take care to identify questions that will likely have a beneficial impact on the populations being studied. It is becoming increasingly common for institutional review boards (IRBs) who are charged with protecting human subjects to decline research proposals based on the writer's failure to demonstrate the significance of the proposed study (Olsen & Mahrenholz, 2000). Considering the significance of a proposed research question early in the process helps to ensure that the best question is addressed and the most meaningful proposal is written.

It might be helpful to think of the process of preparing a research proposal as having two main phases: the *conceptualization phase,* in which the researcher thinks through the basic problem and reviews the literature, and the *methodological phase,* in which the researcher describes the detailed plan for conducting the study. After the work has been completed the investigator enters the *dissemination phase,* in which the study's findings are reported to the scientific community. This chapter is a discussion of the first two phases. In most disciplines research reports in peer-reviewed journals are the gold standard, but presentations at professional meetings are also appropriate and are particularly helpful for obtaining feedback before publishing. In nursing it is also useful to the general public to present results in nonscientific literature when there are important clinical implications. Nurses can be particularly effective in writing columns and addressing health issues on radio and television programs because they have credibility with the general public.

Although one might be tempted to view proceeding from the conceptualization phase to the design phase as the shortest possible distance from point A to point B, preparing a scientifically rigorous research proposal is rarely a linear process. Indeed, the question the researcher initially intends to ask may not be the one ultimately pursued. At each step in the proposal preparation process the writer becomes more knowledgeable about the subject matter. This permits a greater understanding of the population being studied and a more in-depth analysis of the literature on the topic. If the researcher is willing to be reflective during this process, modifications (or quite possibly an entirely new research question) may arise as a result of considering the information uncovered at this stage in the proposal process. Although this makes for a more cyclical path, it is an important mechanism to ensure the researcher is investigating a significant question.

Conceptualization Phase

During the conceptualization phase of developing a proposal, the researcher commits to a problem to study, finds a way to ask the question so that the problem can be studied, and describes the theoretical underpinnings of the study. So many people are affected by disparities in health care at so many levels that researchers should have no difficulty identifying researchable problems. The challenge is to design studies that benefit vulnerable populations and reduce health disparities. Even seemingly small proposals have the potential to provide enormous benefits and long-lasting effects to a local community.

Usually, the conceptualization phase starts with the basic idea or problem. Some researchers refer to the idea as an "itch" that grabs their attention from some observation in the real world. For example, a nurse might question a practice or policy that the institution maintains out of habit. One might think of these practices as "cherished delusions" because they are rooted in institutional folklore rather than in science, but people in authority in institutions in which they have a long vested interest in the status quo tend to hold onto them.

For example, in the 1960s, although the concept of vulnerable populations was not in use, obstetrical units were quite protective of newborns as vulnerable to infection. Rightly so, but the best practice was limited to minimizing contact with newborns. Nursing students of this generation were taught not to let new fathers hold their newborn infants because of the risk of infection. Even though aseptic techniques were known and could have been applied equally to new fathers as to the newborn nursery staff, it was a sacred belief among the nursery staff that fathers would contaminate their infants. Hence, the policy was developed not to let the newborns leave the nursery except for brief and reluctantly granted visits to mothers. Fortunately, a large body of research was generated on family-centered care and this particular policy was relegated to history.

It is hoped that many other nursing processes based on folklore, "rules of thumb," and tradition will follow suit and become things of the past, and there is reason for encouragement. Evidence-based medicine and evidence-based nursing practice have increasingly become the standard of care in the United States. Evidence-based nursing practice requires scientific justification for clinical decisions and follows the same general principles as a well-conducted research proposal, requiring that decisions are grounded in empirical observations that are based on reproducible data (McAlister, Straus, Guyatt, & Haynes, 2000). To ensure the best research outcome, one must develop a hypothesis that predicts the answer to the studied research question. The more commonplace evidence-based practice and hypothesis-directed research become in providing care to vulnerable populations, the less need there is for cherished delusions.

The act of articulating a research question as a problem that can be studied is no small task. Fortunately, it is possible to develop a research proposal that builds on the work of others. Nursing science and vulnerable populations research can be viewed as an ongoing dialogue conducted through thousands of peer-reviewed research articles in dozens (if not hundreds) of reputable journals. This is one reason conducting a thorough literature review is essential for developing the best proposal possible.

There are numerous approaches for successfully undertaking a comprehensive literature review (Oxman & Guyatt, 1993). As the researcher begins reading through published articles related to the vulnerable population and research question of interest, it is advisable to take note of the questions that appear to have been asked, which seem to remain unanswered, and what approaches have been used to answering those questions. Conducting a thorough literature review helps to hone a research question and assists in developing the best methodology.

Special Considerations with Vulnerable Populations: The Significance of the Study
As a clinical discipline, nursing should describe the significance of research to the population. The following section provides an example of ethical issues related to research with indigenous populations as well as the need for studies that can actually be useful to the population. Indigenous people are a particularly vulnerable population (Liao, 2004). Experiencing the worst health disparities in the country, the first inhabitants of the

United States are often targeted for research projects (Norton & Manson, 1996). Research in American Indian, Alaska Native, and Native Hawaiian communities must be conducted with respect and sensitivity. In the past indigenous people have been subjected to immoral treatment by researchers (Udall, Brugge, Benally, & Yazzie-Lewis, 2006). The mistreatment by the scientific community has contributed to the distrust of researchers, and therefore an increased sensitivity must be implemented when working with indigenous communities (Wolf, 1989).

This chapter thoughtfully outlines the importance of designing a meaningful research proposal that both contributes to the scientific knowledge and is beneficial to the community in which the research is conducted. This is especially true for research in indigenous communities, and there are a number of reasons why designing a meaningful research proposal is imperative. The first is related to the severity of health disparities among indigenous populations. Indigenous communities are facing epidemics of disease and cannot afford to focus on issues that will not benefit their communities. Second, indigenous communities are under constant political threat. Examples of these threats include the 1954 Termination Bills that eliminated the existence of six tribes, the 2007 and 2008 President's budget proposal to eliminate health programs for the 61% of American Indians and Alaska Natives who happen to reside in cities, and the denial of federal recognition of Native Hawaiians. Producing meaningful research for indigenous communities assists them in describing the burden of disease and advocating for continued efforts to reduce that burden. Third, conducting meaningful research in indigenous communities contributes to scientific knowledge. Effective and meaningful research can assist in identifying the true rate of disease and correct the inaccuracies reported in health statistics. Finally, conducting meaningful research in indigenous communities helps to restore trust by helping to heal some of the pain and suffering caused by past criminal research studies. By criminal research, we mean unethical treatment of research subjects and lack of respect for the rights of communities.

Methodological Phase

In the methodological phase of developing a research proposal, it is important to make all the decisions related to designing the study, recruiting the sample, collecting data, and analyzing data. The methodological phase is a natural extension of the groundwork laid during the conceptual development. Deciding the details of the study enables the researcher to direct the concepts and ideas that have been swirling around into a plan of action that can answer the central research question and test the proposed hypothesis.

Special Methodological Considerations with Vulnerable Populations

Appropriate Designs Scholars can debate the relative merits of qualitative and quantitative designs, but the question of which designs are better is misdirected. The point of research is to answer questions. Some questions lend themselves to generating emic (from the participant's point of view) data, and usually qualitative designs are best. Qualitative designs generate rich data that may or may not be generalizable. At some point, in a discipline such as nursing, it becomes useful to generate data that provide the basis for predicting and controlling. These data are usually quantitative and etic (from the researcher's point of view) and form the basis for evidence-based practice. Both types of designs are useful for different purposes.

Qualitative designs lend themselves to research with vulnerable populations because these designs by nature are implemented with great attention to respecting the autonomy of those who participate in the study. Indeed, the terms *participant, coresearcher, respondent,* or *cultural informant* are used in place of the term *subject.* Quantitative designs can be implemented effectively as well, provided there is particular attention paid to the rights of subjects.

Protecting the Rights of the Population It is the job of the IRB to ensure that the rights of all human subjects are protected, and the federal guidelines mandate full reviews for those considered vulnerable. For example, full IRB reviews are required when subjects are children, pregnant women, prisoners, mentally disabled, and frail elderly people. IRBs have great latitude in interpreting the federal guidelines, and some might designate other groups as vulnerable.

Chapter 21 describes the advantages of participatory action research, which is a way of involving the community in the decision making about the research. The detailed account of the processes involved in participatory action research is applicable to both qualitative and quantitative research. Examples of participatory action research studies can be found in the first edition of this book as well as in the nursing and social studies literature (Colvin, de Chesnay, Mercado, & Benavides, 2005; Crandall, Senturia, Sullivan, & Shiu-Thornton, 2005; Evans et al., 2005; Kelly, 2005; McAllister, 2005; Sullivan, 2005; Young, 2006).

Another technique for protecting the rights of vulnerable populations in research is to name an advisory board that includes members of the target population. These individuals are helpful in speaking on behalf of the population and also are valuable consultants on a variety of cultural and language problems that occur in the course of conducting research. One of the decisions that advisory board members from the target population can help make is resolving the issue of intellectual property rights. Increasingly, communities are insisting on their rights to own the data.

Incentives Whether to offer incentives is controversial. Some believe any incentive to poor subjects represents undue coercion. However, most authors believe incentives are acceptable if balanced with degree of deprivation of subjects. For example, small food gifts, telephone calling cards, small amounts of cash, and bus passes are minor gifts that would usually not be seen as coercive (Ensign, 2003).

A more insidious form of coercion concerns research on prisoners. In the mid-20th century abuses of prisoners were rampant. They were unknowing and ill-informed participants in many clinical trials for drugs and cosmetics. Today, prisoners often enroll in clinical trials from desperation to obtain medical care at crowded understaffed prisons.

Informed Consent With the increase in regulations about research with human subjects, special attention is being given to informed consent, a sticky issue when people cannot speak for themselves that is resolved by having someone else speak for them. Yet over-protectiveness can lead to denial of consent on behalf of vulnerable persons, placing them in the position of not benefiting from the research. For example, research with the developmentally disabled requires consent by a legal guardian, and there must be provision for the disabled person to participate to his or her capacity (Weisstub & Arboleda-Florez, 1997). If the guardian does not consent, the person does not receive the benefit of the study.

Cultural issues can also affect informed consent. Rashad, Phipps, and Haith-Cooper (2004) discuss the difficulties of obtaining informed consent of Egyptian women. Although poor Egyptian women are often research subjects, their low literacy level prevents full understanding if British or American consent forms are used. Although personal autonomy and accountability to God is a key concept of Islam, culturally, Egyptian women tend to defer to the male authority figures in their families. Signing a consent form is a major commitment in many cultures, and obtaining signed consents (preferred in Western research) is often difficult or impossible (Davison, Brown, & Moffitt, 2006).

Outline of a Research Proposal

The following outline is offered to assist nurses who are developing research proposals to think through the decisions involved in research, particularly with regard to vulnerable populations. For novice researchers it might be helpful to write the first draft in the first person, a technique not acceptable in final drafts and most scientific writing. However, writing in the first person helps the novice to "own" the study by picturing each step in a logical order. The elements of a final research report are shown below, with the first three chapters considered in the proposal.

Chapter I: Overview of the Study (or Preview of Coming Attractions)

- What are you going to investigate (purpose or statement of the problem and research questions or hypotheses, including null hypotheses)?

  Qualitative Example: What is the lived experience of currently pregnant women whose pregnancy is a result of rape?

  Quantitative Example: The research question is this: Are there significant differences between men and women on a stress scale that measures reaction to the diagnosis of cancer?

  Null Hypothesis: There is no significant difference or the mean of the male group equals the mean of the female group.

  Research Hypothesis: The female group will score significantly higher than the male group or the means will not be equal.

- What theoretical support does the idea have (conceptual framework or theoretical support)?

  Qualitative Example: Often, qualitative researchers do not specify a theoretical framework before conducting the study. The rationale is that the researcher might become biased and not view the data with adequate scientific objectivity.

  Quantitative Example: In quantitative research it is customary to consider the research to be theory testing, even if one is conducting descriptive research as a "fishing expedition" to see whether any interesting relationships appear. The researcher often used theory to support the logic of the study, if not to test a particular theory.

- What assumptions underlie the problem? It is useful to think of this section as statements that you must accept as true to do the work. For qualitative interviews (and quantitative surveys) you must be able to trust what people tell you.

  Qualitative Example: Participants tell the truth as they see it.

  Quantitative Example: The sphygmomanometer is calibrated accurately for the purposes of the study.

- What definitions of terms are important to state? Typically, these definitions in quantitative research are called *operational definitions* because they describe how you know the item when you see it. (An operational definition usually starts with the phrase: "a score of . . . or above on the [name of instrument]. You may also want to include a conceptual definition, which is the usual meaning of the concept of interest or a definition according to a specific author. In contrast, qualitative research usually does not include measurements, so operational definitions are not appropriate, but conceptual definitions may be important to state.)

  Qualitative Example: Bereavement is defined as the process of grieving the loss of a loved one through death of the loved one.

  Quantitative Example: In a study involving adolescent pregnancy, *adolescents* are defined as males and females between the ages of 13 and 18 years.

- Are there any expected limitations to your design (not delimitations, which are intentional decisions about how to narrow the scope of your population or focus)?

  Qualitative Example: For the interview with the third participant, there were distractions present at the setting (e.g., children running around the room).

  Quantitative Example: Sample size may not have been sufficient to capture meaningful differences between groups.

- How important is the study (significance) to nursing? In vulnerable populations research, will the study contribute to reducing health disparities?

  For both qualitative and quantitative designs, it is critical to discuss the importance of conducting the study in specific terms. It is not enough to make a sweeping pronouncement that the study is significant; rather, say *how* it is significant. How will it benefit the population if not the subjects in the study? How will the study enable nurses in the clinical setting to provide better care? How will the study increase knowledge about a little-known or understudied phenomenon? How can the results help to reduce health disparities? How can the study results be used to benefit the community being studied?

Special Considerations for Vulnerable Populations in Stating the Problem

The statement of the problem is critical in defining your approach to the problem. Have the research questions or hypotheses been stated in ways that are appropriate to the design and will the research question advance understanding of health disparities or interventions with vulnerable populations? We are not advocating that all research needs to address the needs of vulnerable populations, but it does seem appropriate that nurse researchers pay more attention to conducting studies that are likely to lead to improved nursing interventions. Both quantitative and qualitative designs are needed and should be logically related to the statement of the problem.

The assumptions of the study are particularly relevant to research with vulnerable populations and worthy of special mention. Although researchers attempt to control bias in quantitative research and acknowledge bias in qualitative research, there is a particular type of bias that occurs when the researcher is not of the same population as the subjects or participants. In this sense bias refers to the concept of ethnocentric bias, an anthropological concept that means the researcher might assume things about the study population or about how the conceptual framework of the study works for the population based on ideas derived from his or her own culture.

This kind of bias may also be a limiting factor in studies of populations within one's own culture. There could be a tendency for the investigator to accept as true for all people those ideas held to be true within one's own narrow circle of family and friends and to disregard ideas in conflict with those of one's own circles.

Ethnocentric bias is not necessarily malicious, as when individuals express racial prejudices, but it does affect the investigator's ability to interpret data from the emic (participant's) point of view rather than from preconceived ideas about how people "should" behave or think. For example, one of the critical assumptions in qualitative research is that the participants will tell the truth as they see it. If they feel antagonized by comments that reflect ethnocentric bias on the part of the researcher, they may be inclined either to mislead the investigator or to simply not answer questions. This is similar to the dynamic in which subjects try to please the researcher by responding as they believe the researcher wishes them to respond.

From the researcher's perspective, the danger lies in misinterpreting data. If the investigator cannot bracket his or her biases, then it becomes highly likely that he or she will miss the point of what participants were trying to say.

Chapter II: The Review of Research Literature (or Why You Are Not Reinventing the Wheel)

During the conceptual phase of preparing a research proposal, the researcher first surveys the literature for a general sense of what has been previously done and what questions have already been asked. This is then followed by a more detailed examination of the literature examining how specific research questions have been articulated and what methods have been used. Once the researcher makes any necessary revisions to the proposed research question, it is then possible to thoroughly scour the literature for the most crucial articles relating to the anticipated research. The literature describing vulnerable populations is large and complicated. The explosion of vulnerable population studies and research publications, although clearly reason to celebrate, makes sorting through an exponentially growing body of knowledge a bit of challenge (Dixon-Woods et al., 2006). For this reason, a variety of search strategies may need to be used.

Literature searching contains elements of both science and art. Like the development and redevelopment of the research question itself, a successful literature search often requires multiple iterations as the researcher crafts a specific hypothesis and devises a research plan. As the number of articles in the researcher's possession accumulates, it is particularly worthwhile to identify apparent gaps in the literature. This can be useful for helping revise a literature search strategy as well as for potentially identifying an unexplored area of research within the field. The next challenge for the researcher is to selectively and succinctly summarize the current state of the literature in the literature review section of the research proposal.

In this section the researcher frames the problem within the context of knowledge in the discipline. For quantitative studies the main literature review is conducted before the study, but for qualitative studies the major part of the literature review might be done after the study and would be based on the concepts that emerged from the data.

This chapter is organized according to the concepts in the conceptual framework in chapter I and describes the studies in the literature review first, followed by the state of the art of the literature and how the study fills gaps in the existing literature:

- Concepts: A brief description is written of each study reviewed that supports the concepts within the conceptual framework. The brief description should include the highlights of the study such as sample size and type, design, key findings, and anything important to the point you are trying to make. Repeat this step for as many concepts as are included in the conceptual framework.

- Areas of agreement in literature: A paragraph or two summarizes the main points on which authors agree.

- Areas of disagreement: A paragraph or two summarizes where authors disagree.

- State of the art on the topic: A few paragraphs clearly articulate where the literature is strong and where the gaps are.

- How your study fills gaps in the existing literature: A brief statement is written of how your study fills the gaps or why your study needs to be done to replicate what someone else has done.

Research Examples Illustrating Special Considerations for Vulnerable Populations
Examples of special considerations in conceptualizing and planning research with vulnerable populations are presented from two separate studies: one study that focused on examining the effects of a gentle touch intervention for preterm infants in the neonatal intensive care unit (Harrison, Williams, Berbaum, Stem, & Leeper, 2000) and a second study that involved focus groups with Latino immigrant parents to identify parents' perceptions of their children's health needs (Harrison & Scarinci, in press). Preterm infants are considered vulnerable because of their physiological fragility, and Latino immigrant parents are considered vulnerable because of their status as ethnic minorities and also because of economic, cultural, and language barriers to healthcare services.

Because of the physical vulnerability of preterm infants, it was essential to carefully review previous research during the conceptualization phase to ensure that there were no reports of risks that might arise from the proposed tactile intervention and that the significance of the proposed study justified any potential risks that might ensue during the study. It was also critical to identify a conceptual framework to provide support for the proposed intervention and to identify potential extraneous variables that should be considered to minimize any unnecessary risks to the infants who were assigned to the intervention group. The authors developed the following conceptual framework based on a thorough review of previous research and discussions with other researchers who had conducted studies evaluating preterm infants' responses to touch and massage and briefly summarized the framework in one of the publications that presented the findings from this study (Harrison et al., 2000, p. 438):

> The conceptual framework for this study was based on the premise that gentle human touch (GHT) would stimulate tactile and pressure receptors promoting infant comfort and reducing stress, resulting in positive immediate and longer-term outcomes. Immediate outcomes would be reflected in physiologic indicators of reduced stress and of maintenance of comfort during the GHT intervention, including maintenance of heart rate and levels of oxygen saturation (O_2 sat) within normal ranges. Immediate outcomes would also be reflected by reduced levels of stress during the GHT intervention as evidenced by decreased levels of behavioral distress cues. Immediate outcomes would also be reflected by decreased energy expenditure as evidenced by decreased levels of motor activity and maintenance of a sleep state as opposed to an active awake or fuss/cry state during and after the GHT intervention. By reducing stress and energy expendi-

ture during the early weeks in the NICU, it was predicted that the GHT intervention would result in longer-term benefits including reduced levels of morbidity and increased weight gain during the infant's hospitalization, and reduced levels of motor activity and increased quiet sleep when the infants were 17–20 days of age. It was also predicted that providing supplemental tactile stimulation would enhance sensory maturation and thereby promote more optimal behavioral organization at the time of hospital discharge among infants in the GHT group as compared to infants in the control group.

Because of the vulnerability of preterm infants, any type of supplemental stimulation poses some risk of adverse physiological and behavioral response, and thus it was also important to identify procedures to identify and respond to any such adverse responses that might arise during the course of the study. To minimize any potential adverse effects of the GHT intervention, the researchers used a "decision tree" protocol throughout the study. This protocol involved establishing criteria that would be considered indicators of adverse physiologic responses to the GHT and specifying procedures that would be followed if the infants demonstrated any of these indicators (Harrison et al., p. 440):

> The GHT lasted for up to 10 minutes but was discontinued if the infant demonstrated signs of physiological distress (heart rate " 100 or $\geq$ 200 beats per minute [bpm] for 12 seconds or more; or arterial O_2 saturation levels < 90% for longer than 30 seconds). If the touch had to be discontinued early due to changes in either heart rate or oxygen saturation levels, the researcher waited at least 30 minutes before instituting another GHT intervention. The decision to provide the GHT for 10 minutes was based on findings from previous studies of gentle touch and massage in which positive outcomes were noted following supplemental tactile interventions that lasted from 10–15 minutes.

In a study that involved focus groups with 82 Latino immigrant parents, special issues were considered when conceptualizing and planning the study (Harrison & Scarinci, 2007). Of particular importance in this study was identifying and minimizing potential sources of ethnocentric bias in planning the study and in collecting and analyzing the data. One strategy that was used was to involve members of the community where the research was conducted in planning the study, including plans for recruitment of focus group participants as well as the format of the questions that would guide the focus groups. Native Spanish speakers led the focus groups and participated in training to help them learn to maintain objectivity during the sessions and respond to themes and concerns that arose during the groups. Each focus group was tape recorded, and following each session the principal investigator met with the group leaders to review the sessions and share concerns and perceptions about the sessions. These "debriefing" sessions provided important guidance and learning opportunities for both the focus group facilitators and the principal investigator and helped to minimize problems with bias.

There were many instances during the focus groups in which it appeared that group participants were trying to please the researcher by responding as they thought the researcher wanted them to respond, and it was important to help the group facilitators learn to identify these situations and appropriately respond to them. For example, in one of the groups mothers were sharing diverse opinions about whether it was appropriate to spank their children. After several mothers had expressed differing opinions on this topic, one asked the group leader what she thought, as though seeking reinforcement for her own opinion. The leader stated that her role was to listen and facilitate discussion, not to provide her own view or opinion.

Another consideration in planning this study was planning procedures for obtaining informed consent. All consent forms were translated and available in Spanish, although the researchers recognized that there were some Guatemalan immigrants in the study community who did not speak Spanish and were not able to read their Mayan language. Special approval was obtained from the IRB to have the consent forms read to these participants in their native language (Canjobal) by a bilingual translator.

Design Phase
During the design phase of developing a proposal, the researcher presents the detailed plan of the activities in the study with rationale for each methodological decision and the approach to be used for data collection and analysis. It is also helpful to the reader of the proposal for the investigator to present not only what is planned, but why alternative decisions might be less desirable. For example, certain design decisions might be particularly appropriate in research with vulnerable populations.

Chapter III: Methodology (or Plan for the Study)

Design
The type of design to be used is described (e.g., ethnographic, experimental, survey, cross-sectional, phenomenological, etc.). One of the fundamental decisions the researcher needs to make at this stage of the proposal development is whether to collect quantitative data, qualitative data, or a combination of the two. All three approaches have been successfully used in conducting nursing research studying vulnerable populations (Carr, 1994). However, each has distinct advantages and drawbacks that should be considered.

Qualitative research aims to provide a robust description of the data that cannot be readily reduced to a numerical format. *Quantitative research* involves the examination of numerical data and the construction of mathematical models to describe the events that are observed.

Qualitative data are collected directly by the researcher and may include quoted words, pictures, or objects. *Quantitative data* are collected by using a research instrument that translates the researcher's observations into numerical data. Although qualitative data may be regarded as more robust and paint a more contextualized picture of the researcher's observations, quantitative data may be regarded as substantially more efficient for analyzing large data sets and enables the researcher to be more removed from data collection and interpretation (Corner, 1991).

One increasing trend in vulnerable populations research is to conduct studies that include both quantitative and qualitative research components, referred to as "triangulation" by Halcomb and Andrew (2005). One major benefit to collecting both quantitative and qualitative data for the same sample set is that it may increase the researcher's confidence in the collected data and provide for a more complete data analysis and interpretation.

Whereas the collection of qualitative and quantitative may be an added encumbrance for the researcher, it may be the approach that enables a researcher to produce the most inclusive results on a complex and multifaceted population.

Sample

The number of people who will serve as the sample and the sampling method (where and how the sample will be recruited) are described. The sample inclusion and exclusion criteria (delimitations) are decided. The rationale for the sample, including statements about inclusion of women and minorities, is provided. The IRB statement is included stating how the rights of subjects or participants will be protected, including how you will obtain informed consent, code the data, and store the data. The IRB statement is usually a sentence that simply states that approval will be sought from the institution's IRB before the study is initiated. Other elements of the study are described as well:

- *Setting:* Describe where data collection will take place and how any potential distractions will be controlled.

- *Incentives:* Discuss whether incentives will be offered (e.g., bus fare to site of data collection, reimbursement, free lab tests). Incentives should not be so great that people feel coerced or feel they cannot pass up the incentive.

- *Tools:* Describe instruments and data analysis, how the variables of interest will be measured, and how you will make sense of the data (i.e., analyze the data).

- *Validity and reliability:* Decide how you will know whether you have good data (in qualitative research, these terms are *accuracy* and *replicability*).

- *Procedures:* Describe a step-by-step plan for procedures for data collection and analysis.

- *Timeline:* Provide a chart that lists the activities in the research plan month by month.

The three-chapter plan constitutes a proposal for a thesis or dissertation. (For grants, the same decisions have to be made but the format varies by sponsor.)

Chapter IV: Results (or What Happened? Presentation of the Raw Data)

The results section of a thesis or dissertation can be summarized by the intentional dryness of a 1950s TV police officer who only has one thing on his mind: "Just the facts, ma'am." Whereas the preceding chapters walk the reader through the development of the research question and act as a scholarly tour guide of the literature, the results section should be written in a way that allows the reader to interpret the data directly. Graphs, figures, and tables may aid in the visual presentation and organization of the data, but the researcher's own interpretation of what the data mean are intentionally and conspicuously absent. By this point in the proposal the reviewer is aware of the researcher's question, hypothesis, and methodology for attempting to answer the problem. One can consider this lack of commentary in the results section as an academic courtesy to the reviewer, allowing him or her to arrive at his or her own conclusions as to what the researcher's data are saying.

Some researchers like to describe the sample in this section as a way to lead off the discussion of findings. A simple chart that shows the demographics of the sample can help the reader frame the results for the population.

In the order of each hypothesis or research question, describe the data that addressed that question. Use raw data only, do not conclude anything about the data and make no interpretations.

Chapter V: Discussion (or What Sense Do You Make of What You Learned and What Are You Going to Do for an Encore?)

The elements of the discussion are as follows:

- *Conclusions:* This is a concise statement of the answer to each research question or hypothesis. Some people like to interpret here, that is, to say how confident the investigator is in each conclusion. The thorough discussion that follows each conclusion incorporates the investigator's interpretation of data and should tie the data back to the literature. If the study has extended over a long time period, it is advisable to conduct a new literature search to capture any recent studies.

- *Implications:* Describe here how each conclusion can be used to help address the needs of vulnerable populations or nursing practice, education, administration, or health policy.

- *Recommendations:* These are statements that indicate what further research should be conducted based on the findings.

Conclusion

This chapter provided a framework readers might use to develop research proposals. Potential sponsors may have different guidelines, but the authors have attempted to include the most important considerations of designing research involving vulnerable populations. In the following two chapters, sample proposals are presented to illustrate some of the key points of this chapter.

References

Carr, L. T. (1994). The strengths and weaknesses of quantitative and qualitative research: What method for nursing? *Journal of Advanced Nursing, 20*(4), 716–721.

Colvin, S., de Chesnay, M., Mercado, T., & Benavides, C. (2005). Child health in a barrio of Managua. In M. de Chesnay (Ed.), *Caring for the vulnerable: Perspectives in nursing theory, practice, and research* (pp. 161–170). Sudbury, MA: Jones and Bartlett.

Corner, J. (1991). In search of more complete answers to research questions. Quantitative versus qualitative research methods: Is there a way forward? *Journal of Advanced Nursing, 16*(6), 718–727.

Crandall, M. Senturia, K., Sullivan, M., & Shiu-Thornton, S. (2005). Latina survivors of domestic violence: Understanding through qualitative analysis. *Hispanic Health Care International, 3*(3), 179–187.

Davison, C., Brown, M., & Moffitt, P. (2006). Student researchers negotiating consent in northern aboriginal communities. *International Journal of Qualitative Methods, 5*(2), 1–10.

Dixon-Woods, M., Cavers, D., Agarwal, S., Annandale, E., Arthur, A., Harvey, J., et al. (2006). Conducting a critical interpretive synthesis of the literature on access to healthcare by vulnerable groups. *BMC Medical Research Methodology, 26*(6), 35.

Ensign, J. (2003). Ethical issues in qualitative health research with homeless youths. *Journal of Advanced Nursing, 43*(1), 43–50.

Evans, J., Butler, L., Etowa, J., Crawley, I., Rayson, D., & Bell, D. (2005). Gendered and cultural relations: Exploring African Nova Scotians' perceptions of breast and prostate cancer. *Research and Theory for Nursing Practice, 19*(3), 257–273.

Halcomb, E., & Andrew, S. (2005). Triangulation as a method for contemporary nursing research. *Nurse Researcher, 13*(2), 71–82.

Harrison, L., & Scarinci, I. (2007). Child health needs of rural Alabama Latino families. *Journal of Community Health Nursing, 24*(1), 31–47.

Harrison, L. L., Williams, A. K., Berbaum, M. L., Stem, J. T., & Leepr, J. (2000). Physiologic and behavioral effects of gentle human touch on preterm infants. *Research in Nursing & Health, 23*, 435–446.

Kelly, P. (2005). Practical suggestions for community interventions using participatory action research. *Public Health Nursing, 22*(1), 65–73.

Liao, Y. (2004). REACH 2010 Surveillance for health status in minority communities—United States, 2001–2002. *MMWR Surveillance Summary, 53*, 1–36.

McAlister, F. A., Straus, S. E., Guyatt, G. H., & Haynes, R. B. (2000). Users' guides to the medical literature: XX. Integrating research evidence with the care of the individual patient. Evidence-Based Medicine Working Group. *Journal of the American Medical Association, 283*(21), 2829–2836.

McAllister, M. (2005). Women with dissociative identity disorder: Solution-focused nursing. In M. de Chesnay (Ed.), *Caring for the vulnerable: Perspectives in nursing theory, practice, and research* (pp. 181–188). Sudbury, MA: Jones and Bartlett.

Norton, I. M., & Manson, S. M. (1996). Research in American Indian and Alaska Native communities: Navigating the cultural universe of values and process. *Journal of Consulting Clinical Psychology, 64*(5), 856–860.

Olsen, D. P., & Mahrenholz, D. (2000). IRB-identified ethical issues in nursing research. *Journal of Professional Nursing, 16*(3), 140–148.

Oxman, A. D., & Guyatt, G. H. (1993). The science of reviewing research. *Annals of the New York Academy of Science, 31*(703), 125–133.

Rashad, A., Phipps, F. M., & Haith-Cooper, M. (2004). Obtaining informed consent in an Egyptian research study. *Nursing Ethics, 11*(4), 394–399.

Sutton, L. B., Erlen, J. A., Glad, J. M., & Siminoff, L. A. (2003). Recruiting vulnerable populations for research: Revisiting the ethical issues. *Journal of Professional Nursing, 19*(2), 106–112.

Udall, S., Brugge, D., Benally, T., & Yazzie-Lewis, E. (2006). *The Navajo people and uranium mining.* Albuquerque: University of New Mexico Press.

Weisstub, D., & Arboledo-Florez, J. (1997). Ethical research with the developmentally disabled. *Canadian Journal of Psychiatry, 42*, 492–496.

Wolf, A. S. (1989). The Barrow studies: An Alaskan's perspective. *American Indian and Alaska Native Mental Health Research, 2*, 35–40.

Young, L. (2006) Participatory action research: A research strategy for nursing? *Western Journal of Nursing Research, 28*(5), 499–504.

Sample Qualitative Research Proposal: The Lived Experiences of Taiwanese-Americans with Pre-Diabetes Type 2

Andrew Lin

The following is a shortened version of a sample research proposal for qualitative designs. The study has not been conducted.

Chapter I: Study Overview

Research Question

What are the lived experiences of Taiwanese-Americans with pre-diabetes type 2 (non–insulin-dependent diabetes mellitus) in the Seattle area?

Theoretical Support

Pre-diabetes is a collection of health risks that increase the chances of developing heart disease, stroke, and diabetes. According to a national health survey, more than one in five Americans has metabolic syndrome (Diabetes Prevention Program Research Group, 2005). The number of people with metabolic syndrome increases with age and affects more than 40% of people in their sixties and seventies (National Institute of Diabetes and Digestive and Kidney Diseases [NIDDK], 2005). Pre-diabetes is characterized by a series of biochemical changes. Over time, these changes lead to the development of one or more associated medical conditions. The sequence begins when insulin, a hormone excreted from the pancreas, loses its ability to make the body's cells absorb glucose from the blood. When this happens, glucose levels remain high after eating. The pancreas, sensing a high glucose level in the blood, continues to excrete insulin. Loss of insulin production may be genetic or secondary to high fat levels with fatty deposits in the pancreas (Hillestrom, 2006).

Consistently high levels of insulin and glucose are linked to many harmful changes to the body, including damage to the lining of coronary and other arteries, a key step toward the development of heart disease or stroke; changes in the kidneys' ability to remove salt, which leads to high blood pressure, heart disease, and stroke; an increase in triglyceride levels, resulting in an increased risk of developing cardiovascular disease; an increased risk of blood clot formation, which can block arteries and cause heart attacks and strokes; and a slowing of insulin production, which can signal the start of type 2 diabetes, a disease that can increase the risk for a heart attack or stroke and may damage the eyes, nerves, or kidneys. Because physical inactivity and excess weight are the main underlying contributors to the development of metabolic syndrome (pre-diabetes), getting more exercise and losing weight can help reduce or prevent the complications associated with this condition.

Conceptual Framework

The proposed qualitative study consists of generating emic data. To maximize the chance of interpreting data correctly, the literature is reviewed after the study and consists of examining the literature on the concepts that emerge from the data.

Assumption

The main assumption for this study is that people will tell the truth as they see it.

Definitions

Diabetes mellitus is a disorder of carbohydrate metabolism that occurs in genetically predisposed individuals, characterized by inadequate production or utilization of insulin and resulting in excessive amounts of glucose in the blood and urine, excessive thirst, weight loss, and in some cases progressive destruction of small blood vessels, leading to such complications as infections and gangrene of the limbs or blindness. *Type 2 diabetes,* a mild sometimes asymptomatic form of diabetes mellitus, is characterized by diminished tissue sensitivity to insulin and sometimes by impaired beta cell function, which is exacerbated by obesity and often treatable by diet and exercise. *Pre-diabetes type 2* (also called *metabolic syndrome, insulin resistance syndrome, syndrome X,* and *dysmetabolic syndrome*) is a condition in which carbohydrate metabolism is mildly abnormal but other criteria indicating diabetes mellitus are absent; in these cases, development of diabetes mellitus is expected.

Clinically, pre-diabetes type 2 is a syndrome marked by the presence of usually three or more of a group of factors, such as high blood pressure (130/85 mm Hg or higher), abdominal obesity (a waistline of 40 inches or more for men and 35 inches or more for women, measured across the belly), high triglyceride levels (150 mg/dl or higher), low high-density lipoprotein levels (less than 40 mg/dl for men or under 50 mg/dl for women), and insulin resistance (fasting blood sugar level greater than 100 mg/dl). These factors are linked to increased risk of cardiovascular disease and type 2 diabetes.

Limitations

Generalizability is not a concern because the study is designed to provide rich detail for each participant. However, medical records are not available to the researcher, which could give a better picture of the clinical care received.

Significance to Advanced Practice Nursing with Vulnerable Populations

Diet, exercise, and disease prevention education are hallmarks of nursing and should be used by advanced practice nurses. The incidence of type 2 diabetes among minorities in the United States and abroad has been increasing at above-expected rates, especially among Asian-Americans, African-Americans, Hispanics, and Native American (NIDDK, 2001). These groups of people have traditionally had less access to health care for a variety of reasons: socioeconomic status, fear, misunderstanding, lack of representation or culturally sensitive protocols, lower quality of care, and immigration status. The amount of funds spent as well as the attitude toward health, family, and aging are vastly different among Asian-Americans versus non-Hispanic whites (Aday, 2001).

Being aware of culture-specific incidence and the lack of obesity in many Asian-Americans with type 2 diabetes or pre-diabetes allow these populations to take better care of themselves. In addition to this, implementing more sensitive screening tools and staying current on literature regarding the incidence and characteristics of type 2 diabetes in minority populations not only increases quality of care, but also increases the appropriateness and efficiency of care by providing insight into the importance of factors that are related to type 2 diabetes.

Chapter II: Review of Research Literature

The literature is reviewed to provide background for the study, but the primary literature review occurs after the concepts emerge from the data.

Prevalence

The global burden of type 2 diabetes is both significant and rising, with most of the increase registered in the last two decades (NIDDK, 2005). From 2003 to 2025 the worldwide prevalence of diabetes in adults is expected to increase from 5.0% to 6.2%, or to 328 million (NIDDK, 2005). The largest proportional and absolute increase will occur in developing countries, where the prevalence will rise from 4.2% to 5.6%. In India and China the adult diabetic population is expected to double by 2025 to about 73 million and 46 million, respectively (Wong & Wang, 2006). All minorities, except natives of Alaska, have a prevalence of non–insulin-dependent diabetes mellitus that is two to six times greater than that of white persons. The United States spends $132 billion on diabetes care per year (NIDDK, 2005).

The number of Asians in the United States has increased rapidly in recent years, a nearly 2.5-fold increase from 1970 to 1980 and another nearly 2-fold increase from 1980 to 1990 (Fujimoto, 1994). According to U.S. Census data (2000), Asians comprised 4.2% of the nation's population, with 49% living in the West. Incidence and prevalence data indicate that non–insulin-dependent diabetes mellitus is higher in migrant Asians versus native nonimmigrant Asians (NIDDK, 2005). In Hawaii and California, Asians 20 years or older are 2 and 1.5 times (respectively) as likely to be diagnosed with diabetes as whites after adjusting for population age differences. Because type 2 diabetes is considered to be one of the diseases associated with life-style changes seen with westernization, researching these populations will lead to a better understanding of factors mediating this association.

Asian Populations

Studies in Asian populations have suggested that dietary changes and reduction in physical activity are life-style changes that are important in the etiology of diabetes type 2 (Fujimoto, 1994). The relative importance of genetic heritage, diet, exercise, socioeconomic status, culture, language, and access to health care in the prevalence, incidence, and mortality of diabetes is unclear. In the United States, 8.2% of the population over 20 years of age have diabetes type 2, with a 25% diabetes type 2 rate in older adults (65 or greater); this rate will increase as more are diagnosed at an earlier age and are expected to live longer (NIDDK, 2005). The risk for development of diabetes, however, is not uniform among populations. Research has shown that minority populations living in industrialized countries are at greatest risk (Kenny, Aubert, & Geiss, 1994). This increase is troubling because high-risk migrant populations were believed to have low diabetes prevalence in their homelands.

State of the Art

Several researchers have proposed that the increase of type 2 diabetes among minorities is due to a genotype that was a survival advantage to those populations that experienced food shortages and were able to store energy as fat (the "thrifty" genotype hypothesis) (Fujimoto, 1994). Proponents contend that this trait is detrimental in times of abundance, such as in westernization, namely increased amounts of protein and fat consumption. This is based on the observation that type 2 diabetes occurs more frequently among ethnic groups, immigrants, and families (Fujimoto, 1994).

The exact pathogenic mechanism of type 2 diabetes is not clearly understood and is heterogeneous (Rewers and Hamman, 1994). Most type 2 diabetes cases are believed to have initial insulin resistance and hyperinsulinemia followed by B-cell failure. Increased amounts of adipose tissue in the body have been shown to affect insulin response. Both insulin resistance and B-cell failure have multiple genetic and nongenetic factors (Rewers & Hamman, 1994). Some newer data suggest that B-cell defect may be concurrent, or even preceding, the development of insulin resistance (Hillestrom, 2006). In addition, B-cell autoimmunity, characteristic of type 1 diabetes, is present in 10–33% of patients clinically diagnosed with type 2 diabetes (Rewers & Hamman, 1994).

Although many treatments are available for adults with diabetes, as used in routine clinical practice, such treatments are only partially effective in reducing the risk of serious complications (Oldroyd, Unwin, White, Mathers, & Alberti, 2005). Primary prevention of type 2 diabetes, through interventions and the development of more sensitive screening tools, thus represents an attractive strategy for reducing diabetes-related morbidity and mortality. Some of the risk factors for the development of type 2 diabetes, such as obesity, physical inactivity, and high-fat diet, can potentially be modified. Weight loss with life-style modification seems to be the most effective way so far, given that it addresses other cardiovascular disease risk factors as well (Diabetes Prevention Program Research Group, 2005). The challenge is to try to implement these findings in our society or among high-risk patients, taking into consideration the great difficulties involved in changing and maintaining life-style modifications.

There is debate about the efficacy of type 2 diabetes screening and intervention for the Asian-American population, due to the lack of correlation between body mass index and diabetes type 2 incidence (Wong & Wang, 2006). This issue needs to be resolved to be able to sensitively detect high-risk Asian-Americans. The Diabetes Prevention Program is an ongoing nationwide, multicenter, multipractice research collaboration that is addressing the utility of screening tools for Asian-American populations with type 2 diabetes, insulin resistance, and impaired glucose tolerance. The Diabetes Prevention Program has implemented several exercise, diet, and social programs emphasizing healthy aging, with the specific goals of disease prevention, symptom management, and, in the case of pre-diabetes, symptom reversal. The intensity of life-style modifications necessary to reach these goals is not clear, and several of these types of programs have found minimal improvement between treatment groups, arguing against the utility of these programs (Oldroyd et al., 2005). Further research is needed to delineate effective screening, prevention, and treatment practices for Asian-Americans at risk of getting type 2 diabetes.

Areas of Agreement and Disagreement

The relative importance of genetic heritage, diet, exercise, socioeconomic status, culture, language, and access to health care in the prevalence, incidence, and mortality of diabetes is unclear. These risk factors are currently being studied. Researchers agree that a combination of these factors contribute to the development of diabetes, yet most disagree on the importance of each and also to the specific pathways that result in insulin resistance.

Gaps

Why does this study need to be done? This study is designed to hear the voices and perspectives of a racial minority group who is at high risk of developing serious disease. The results of this study can assist both clinicians and patients on the effectiveness of treatment modalities, and the results could serve as an indication of the types of interventions that are successful. This kind of study is necessary to discover how effective screening and treatment protocols are on a first-hand basis. Identifying and understanding the obstacles and issues that are faced on a personal basis are the most important in developing a realistic and effective treatment regimen when working with Taiwanese-Americans with type 2 diabetes.

Chapter III: Methodology

Design

This study will be a phenomenological study derived from the qualitative–naturalistic design. Contextual information will be obtained from individual interviews of participants who are Taiwanese-American men and women aged 50 to 75 living in the Seattle area who have been diagnosed with pre-diabetes type 2 (non–insulin-dependent diabetes mellitus). To assist my search for potential coresearchers, my race and upbringing will aid me. Both of my Taiwanese parents raised me in the Northwest, and I speak fluent Taiwanese. I am actively connected to the Taiwanese community, and this will be useful in establishing rapport with interviewees.

Sample

Ten people will be interviewed via a combination of purposive and snowball sampling. Purposive participants will be identified primarily through personal connections and through local programs that focus on the prevention of diabetes in the Asian-American community, such as the Health Promotions Research Center, which has an office in the School of Public Health at the University of Washington (UWSPH). I have some connections with UWSPH because I was a research study coordinator for the University of Washington and collaborated with one of the main investigators for quite a few research studies before becoming a full-time graduate student at Seattle University.

Semistructured interviews will consist of several open-ended questions. Specific data demographic data collected will be name, age, gender, occupation, marital status, children, date diagnosed with pre-diabetes, and other pertinent medical history. Topics covered during the interviews will be culture, family and friends, healthcare experiences, diet, and exercise (Appendix 14.1). In-depth interviewing of individuals is a means of obtaining rich detail that cannot be gotten by other means. Asking questions that foster the development of this rich detail are of utmost importance. The careful examination, analyses, and contextualization of content are necessary to coming to any conclusion of the content and its processes and concepts.

Setting

Data collection will take place in the participants' homes or at a public place, such as a restaurant or café. The goal of the setting is to ensure privacy and convenience for the interviewee. A tape recorder will be used during interviews.

Institutional Review Board Statement

This study proposal will be submitted to the university institutional review board for approval. Forms will be locked in a secure area, and identifying information will be blacked out after data analysis. Electronic files will have two levels of security: password protection and information not used as identifiers. Potential participants will be given a consent form that explains the purpose, procedures, confidentiality, benefits, risks, and voluntary nature of the study. Those who opt to be part of the study will return a signed copy of the consent form and a copy will be given to them for their keeping. Contact information will be given to potential participants in case of any concerns, questions, or desire to withdraw from the study.

Data Analysis

Data will be analyzed using de Chesnay's (personal communication, 2006) method of delineating content, processes/themes, and concepts. Content is the transcription of the interview in its entirety, without censorship. Content will be organized into categories as defined by topic. The processes/themes portion will entail the interviewers' thoughts and input into the content. After thoroughly examining both the content and processes/themes, certain concepts will become apparent. This analysis will be revisited several times to ensure the best categorization and description of processes and concepts. If data saturation is reached earlier fewer people will be interviewed. This will not be evident until some data analysis is performed. Once the concepts and subconcepts are clearly defined, a typology will be created that will serve as the basis of the conceptual framework that describes the living experiences of Taiwanese-American immigrants with pre-diabetes in the Seattle area.

Procedures

1. Institutional review board applications will be submitted to the university institutional review board.

2. Once approval is obtained, recording and data collection equipment will be purchased.

3. Data entry files will be created using Microsoft Word and Microsoft Excel. Security keys will be made and only accessible to the researcher.

4. Potential study participants will be identified through community sources.

5. Contact with potential participants will be made. Contact will entail introducing myself, explaining the study, explaining study participant rights (using the consent form as a guideline), obtaining informed consent, and scheduling interviews.

6. Interviews will be audio-taped.

7. Tapes will be transcribed into Microsoft Word during the same several months that interviews take place. Data analysis will be performed concurrent with data entry.

8. Once data collection is finished (when 10 participants have been interviewed or data saturation has been reached), a final report will be generated summarizing findings.

9. The final report will be reviewed and modified, and then submitted for publication.

Timeline

It is expected that the study can be completed in 1 year (Table 14-1), but this will depend largely on the availability of participants to end the study with 10 interviewees. When responses to interview questions are similar to several other interviewers', data saturation will have been reached; if this happens, fewer than 10 interviewees may be needed.

TABLE 14-1 Projected Timeline

Research Activities	Month									
	1	2	3	4	5	6	7	8	9	10
IRB approval			X	X	X					
Purchase equipment		X	X	X						
Set up data entry files			X	X						
Identify study participants			X	X	X	X				
Interviews/data collection			X	X	X	X	X			
Data analysis						X	X	X	X	X
Final report writing								X	X	X
Submission for publication							X	X	X	

References

Aday, L. (2001). *At risk in America.* San Francisco: Jossey-Bass.

Diabetes Prevention Program Research Group. (2005). Strategies to identify adults at high risk for type 2 diabetes. *Diabetes Care, 28,* 138–144.

Fujimoto, W. Y. (1994). Diabetes in Asian and Pacific Islander Americans. In National Diabetes Data Group (Ed.), *Diabetes in America* (pp. 661–682). Bethesda, MD: National Institutes of Health.

Hillestrom, K. (2006). Oxidative stress may be a consequence of diabetes, not a pathogenic factor. *Scandinavian Journal of Clinical & Laboratory Investigation, 66*(5), 363–370.

Kenny, S. J., Aubert, R. E., & Geiss, L. S. (1994). Prevalence and incidence of non-insulin-dependent diabetes. In NIDDK *Diabetes in America* (pp. 47–68). Bethesda, MD: National Institutes of Health.

National Institute of Diabetes and Digestive and Kidney Diseases (NIDDK), National Institutes of Health. (2001). *Changing the way diabetes is treated: A progress report from the National Diabetes Education Program.* Bethesda, MD: National Diabetes Clearing House.

National Institute of Diabetes and Digestive and Kidney Diseases (NIDDK), National Institutes of Health. (2005). *National diabetes statistics.* Bethesda, MD: National Diabetes Clearing House.

Oldroyd, J., Unwin, N. C., White, M., Mathers, J. C., & Alberti, K. (2005). Randomised control trial evaluating lifestyle interactions in people with impaired glucose tolerance. *Diabetes Research and Clinical Practice, 72,* 117–127.

Rewers, M., & Hamman, R. (1994). Risk factors for non-insulin-dependent diabetes. In NIDDK, *Diabetes in America* (pp. 179–220). Bethesda, MD: National Institutes of Health.

Wong, K. C., & Wang, Z. (2006). Prevalence of type 2 diabetes mellitus of Chinese populations in Mainland China, Hong Kong, and Taiwan. *Diabetes Research & Clinical Practice, 43,* 126–134.

Appendix 14-1   Semistructured Interview Guide

Background closed-ended questions:

- What is your name? American name?
- How old are you?
- Are you married?
- Do you have children? Grandchildren?
- Where did you live in Taiwan?
- Do you still have family in Taiwan?
- How long have you been in the United States?
- Do you have family in the United States?
- Did anyone come to the United States with you?
- How often do you go back to Taiwan?
- What kind of work do you, or did you, do?
- What kinds of hobbies do you have?

Background open-ended questions:

- Why did you move to the United States?
- What do you like about living in the United States?
- What do you dislike about living in the United States?
- What sorts of communities are you involved in?
- How would you describe yourself?
- Has anything changed since being diagnosed?

Closed-ended questions related to pre-diabetes:

- When were you diagnosed with pre-diabetes?
- Who diagnosed you?
- Is this your regular physician?
- How often do you get medical checkups?
- Do you see any other practitioners?
- Do you discuss healthcare issues with others?
- What medications are you taking to manage pre-diabetes?

(continues)

Appendix 14-1 Semistructured Interview Guide (continued)

Open-ended questions related to pre-diabetes:

- How do you hear about health-related issues?
- What are your concerns regarding diabetes?
- How did you react to being diagnosed?
- How did your family and friends react?
- How likely do you think you are to develop diabetes?
- What is your understanding of pre-diabetes?
- Tell me about any natural remedies you are taking to manage pre-diabetes.

Open-ended questions related to diet and exercise:

- Tell me about your typical diet and your food taste (likes and dislikes).
- What kinds of foods should you eat more of, what should you avoid? Is this hard to do?
- Describe kinds of physical activities you regularly engage in.

Sample Quantitative Research Proposal: The Effects of Relaxation Exercises on Anxiety and Discomfort Associated with Pelvic Examinations

Patricia Nissley

This chapter is a shortened version of a sample outline of a quantitative research proposal. The study has not been conducted.

Chapter I: Overview of the Study

Purpose and Hypothesis

The purpose of the study is to determine the effects of relaxation exercises on anxiety and discomfort associated with pelvic examinations. It is hypothesized that relaxation exercises will decrease anxiety and discomfort during pelvic examinations.

Research Questions

What are the effects of relaxation exercises on the anxiety and pain associated with the pelvic examination? What is the effect of relaxation exercises on discomfort during pelvic examinations? Does giving patient control during a pelvic examination increase comfort? Does comfort level of the patient during pelvic examinations play a role in making future appointments?

Theoretical Support

The theoretical basis for the study includes three main concepts: relaxation exercises, anxiety with pelvic examinations, and discomfort with pelvic examinations. Relaxation exercises, in particular belly breathing, are used to enhance relaxation by providing a focus for several senses (S. Jones, personal communication, April 2006). Belly breathing involves the combination of touch, sight, and mental imagery, which can distract from other stimuli

(S. Jones, personal communication, April 2006). Pelvic examinations have been well documented as a source of anxiety and discomfort, which may play a role in adherence to annual pelvic examinations (Fiddes, Scott, Fletcher, & Glasier, 2003; Kahn et al., 1999; Wright, Fenwick, Stephenson, & Monterosso, 2005).

Assumptions

Several assumptions will be made concerning the study:

1. Subjects will complete the questionnaire to the best of their knowledge.

2. Subjects will listen and respond to instructions from provider regarding comfort measures.

3. The principle investigator (PI) will read the instructions correctly.

Definitions

Anxiety is defined as subjective, transitory, and conscious feelings of apprehension and tension (Johnson & Spielberger, 1968). *High anxiety* is defined as a score of 40 or higher on the State-Trait Anxiety Inventory (STAI) (Barnett & Parker, 1986; Spielberger, Gorsuch, & Lushene, 1970). A score of 3 or higher on the 10-point Likert pain scale will be considered painful for this study, which reflects a smaller amount of pain. Belly breathing consists of placing hands on abdomen and watching hands rise and fall with each deep breath (S. Jones, personal communication, April 2006). The pelvic examination consists of a Papanicolaou (Pap) smear and sexually transmitted infection testing with insertion of a speculum into the vagina and a bimanual examination to palpate reproductive organs.

Limitations

1. The participants may be nonrandom in that those who elect to participate in the study may be more comfortable with pelvic examinations than nonparticipants.

2. The study is nonblinded so the provider knows the subject's study group.

3. The participants are taken from only one medical clinic so generalizability may be limited to that population.

Significance

Researching ways to decrease anxiety associated with pelvic examinations may provide benefits for both healthcare providers and women seeking gynecological care. Kohen (1980) described the importance of the first pelvic examination on future examinations. A positive experience may encourage a woman to have regular examinations and give positive feedback to her peers (Kahn et al., 1999). Regularly scheduled examinations can help detect abnormal changes in the cervix associated with cervical cancer; cervical cancer when detected and treated early has a high cure rate (Centers for Disease Control and Prevention, 2003).

The study has particular significance to vulnerable populations in that the results will help design better ways to decrease the negative experience of pelvic examinations. Although middle-class women may have been educated as to the benefits and can access prevention services through insurance plans, low-income women may have not received access and may not be aware of the importance of these examinations in prevention or early diagnosis. Furthermore, if they receive care primarily in crowded public clinics, they may not have received appropriate and culturally sensitive treatment by healthcare providers. Finally, in a large metropolitan area there is great diversity with numerous immigrants and refugees from cultures in which pelvic examinations are not regularly performed. Examinations can be particularly frightening to women who undergo them for the first time.

Feasibility and Application

The effect of relaxation exercises on discomfort during pelvic examinations appears to be a feasible research option. It can be measured quantitatively or qualitatively and is easily implemented. Exploring this research question may provide information useful to nurse practitioners who regularly perform pelvic and cervical examinations. If relaxation exercises improve the quality of the examination, it is possible that patients may be more likely to continue with regular examinations and associate examinations with a positive experience.

The research question is applicable to all women seeking pelvic and cervical examinations and may be particularly useful for adolescent females. This specific age group may not have had prior pelvic examinations and may fear or dread them. Because annual examinations are important for sexually active women, the proposed exercises may decrease discomfort associated with the examinations and improve compliance.

Chapter II: Review of Research Literature

Discomfort during Examinations

A qualitative study involving adolescent females found that 13 of 15 participants considered a Pap smear to be painful, uncomfortable, and an overall negative experience (Kahn et al., 1999). The adolescent females interviewed in the previous study received most of their information about the examination from peers. The most common descriptions given by peers were that the examinations were painful and uncomfortable (Kahn et al., 1999).

A second study about pelvic examinations revealed similar misgivings about the examination, but this time from women of all ages (Fiddes et al., 2003). Sixty-eight percent had some reservations about the Pap smear, whereas 81% under age 25 and 78% over age 25 had similar feelings about the pelvic examination (Fiddes et al., 2003) Additionally, the presence or absence of previous pelvic examinations did not change the outlook on the pelvic examination (Fiddes et al., 2003).

Perceived barriers to the Pap smear include pain and discomfort, peer advice, and provider style (Kahn et al., 1999). Adolescents interviewed believed that part of the pain and discomfort of the pelvic examination is associated with the style of a provider, indicating that more gentle providers mean less pain. The relationship with a provider can be important, especially in developing trust, being gentle, and relieving some anxiety (Kahn et al., 1999).

Anxiety

Williams, Park, and Kline (1992) researched the effects of a newly designed gown on anxiety during pelvic examinations. The results of the study indicated reduced distress before beginning the examination by increasing physical and emotional comfort. This intervention was a cost-effective way to alleviate some stress associated with pelvic examinations. However, researchers acknowledge that the gown did not have effects on other aspects of the examination, including the anxiety and pain felt during the actual pelvic examination (Williams et al., 1992).

Relaxation

Positive mental imagery and/or self-hypnosis are two types of relaxation exercises that may help to relieve anxiety during pelvic examinations (Faymonville et al., 2000; Kwekkeboom, Huseby-Moore, & Ward, 1998). A hypnotic state has been shown to lead to a decrease in heart and respiratory rate and muscle relaxation (Faymonville et al., 2000). A hypnotic state is also associated with a statistically significant decrease in pain (Faymonville et al., 2000).

Most people find symptom relief with mental imagery; however, it depends on the patient (Kwekkeboom et al., 1998). In other words, if a person does not want it to work, it probably will not. Mental imagery is more effective with better concentration. The amount of concentration given is more important in determining symptom relief than the ability to generate any imagery (Kwekkeboom et al., 1998).

In addition to mental imagery, a method to cope with anxiety and discomfort may be to take control of the situation (Kohen, 1980; Wright et al., 2005). A pilot study involving self-insertion of the speculum returned positive results. Wright et al. (2005) found that self-insertion turned out to be a good option and a positive experience for women. Fifty-five percent of the time, self-inserted speculums led to a clear view of the cervix on the first attempt and 39% with only minor adjustments (Wright et al., 2005). However, women who prefer to dissociate, or pretend as if the examination is not happening, did not prefer to self-insert the speculum (Wright et al., 2005). It is possible that these women will more greatly benefit from mental imagery or self-hypnosis.

State of the Art

It is generally agreed on in the literature that pelvic examinations are uncomfortable (Fiddes et al., 2003; Kahn et al., 1999; Wright et al., 2005). It is also agreed on that uncomfortable situations can lead to anxiety and may affect adherence to regularly scheduled pelvic examinations, especially in adolescents (Fiddes et al., 2003; Kahn et al., 1999; Wright et al., 2005).

Some disagreements in the literature reflect the amount and type of discomfort that is experienced during a pelvic examination. Wright et al. (2005) concluded that much of the anxiety and discomfort surrounding pelvic examinations could be eased with greater patient involvement during the examination. Kahn et al. (1999) interviewed a younger population and found that some of the discomfort was from fear of the unknown and dread in anticipation of the examination. Fiddes et al. (2003) found that many women found the examination uncomfortable but acknowledged the usefulness of the examination.

An area of agreement in the literature is that mental imagery or self-hypnosis can improve discomfort and reduce anxiety (Faymonville et al., 2000; Kwekkeboom et al., 1998). Disagreement in the literature involves worsening of symptoms. Kwekkeboom et al. (1998) found that if the patient was not in favor of mental imagery, then the process may be considered tedious and cumbersome and may perpetuate negative feelings. Faymonville et al. (2000) found that a hypnotic state can decrease the perception of pain.

Gaps

There are several gaps in the literature. First, many of the studies on relaxation exercises and pelvic examinations were done more than 10 years ago. There is a critical need for more current studies. Second, few studies were replicated, leaving open questions about designs, validity, and reliability. There is literature about relaxation and mental imagery effects on other types of treatment or examinations but little data specific to pelvic examinations. The need for research in this area is great, especially considering the widespread agreement that pelvic examinations may be uncomfortable and the frequency with which pelvic examinations are performed.

Chapter III: Methodology

Design

A classic experimental design will be used, with a pretest–posttest comparison group design.

Sample

A convenience sample of 30–50 women aged 18–30 years will be obtained by inviting all regularly scheduled appointments for annual pelvic examinations and Pap smear at a local clinic. Informed consent forms from university and clinic will be given as each patient checks in for her appointment and will be stored separately from the surveys to ensure confidentiality. The consent form will include the following information: (1) information about the experiment testing comfort measures during pelvic examinations, (2) statements about risks and benefits, (3) description of the experiment, (4) how confidentiality will be assured, and (5) contact information for the primary researcher and the institutional review board.

For the intervention group the examining nurse will read the following statement right before beginning the examination: "Rest your hands on your lower stomach, right below your belly button. Watch your hands rise with each breath, and feel yourself relax while I am performing the examination." For the comparison group, the nurse will read the following statement right before beginning the examination: "Try to relax while I am performing the examination." The previous statement will be consistent with the typical comfort measure the nurse uses for pelvic examinations outside of the present study.

Setting

The same nurse at the clinic will perform all examinations over a period of 4 or 6 days, with the number of days dependent on the number of participants obtained each day. The provider will perform examinations with the intervention on days 1, 3, and 5 and the comparison group examinations on days 2, 4, and 6. The informed consent forms will be collected and surveys given while in the examination room.

Instrumentation

One survey will be given before the examination, consisting of demographic information and the STAI (Spielberger et al., 1970). The demographic information will be used to look for possible trends and will include age, ethnicity, years of education, previous pelvic examination, and experience with previous pelvic examination. The STAI measures the transitory emotional response to a stressful situation with 20 phrases using the four-point Likert scale, with a score of 40 or higher regarded as high anxiety (Barnett & Parker, 1986; Spielberger, et al., 1970). After the examination participants will be given a survey including the STAI and 10-point pain Likert scale.

Data Analysis

Before analysis, all data will be checked for data file errors. Within-group comparisons of pretests and posttests will be analyzed by t-tests for related samples. The pain scale will be analyzed using frequency distributions for each group. Demographic information and STAI scores will be compared using frequency distributions and measures of central tendency. If the PI is able to assess a change between pretest and posttest scores, then a Wilcoxon matched-pairs signed-ranks test, along with the Mann-Whitney U test, will be used to analyze between group measures of pretest–posttest differences.

Validity and Reliability

Research has shown that the STAI is a reliable and valid instrument with strong internal consistency (Sesti, 2000). However, the STAI does not have test–retest reliability due to the test's transient nature.

Procedures

1. University institutional review board and clinic approval will be obtained for this study.
2. Cooperation will be obtained from the clinic.
3. Information, expectations, and requirements will be discussed with the nurse who is to perform the examinations.
4. The sample will be recruited.
5. Appointments will be scheduled for explaining the study and data collection.
6. Data will be collected.
    a. Informed consent form will be given at time of check-in.
    b. PI will collect signed informed consent forms and place in file folder 1.
    c. PI will give pretest survey and copy of informed consent form for subjects to take home.
    d. PI will collect pretest survey and store in examination room temporarily.
    d. The nurse will perform examination.
    e. PI will give posttest survey.
    f. PI will collect posttest survey, attach to pretest survey, and place in file folder 2.
7. Data will be input into SPSS computer software by researcher.
8. Data will be analyzed by researcher and statistician.
9. Literature review will be expanded and completed.
10. Final report will be written.

References

Barnett, B., & Parker, G. (1986). Possible determinants, correlates, and consequences of high levels of anxiety in primiparous mothers. *Psychological Medicine, 16,* 177–185.

Centers for Disease Control and Prevention. (2003, October). *Cervical cancer: Basic facts on screening and the Pap test.* [CDC pub. no. 99-6949]. Atlanta: Centers for Disease Control.

Faymonville, M. E., Laureys, S., Degueldre, C., Del Fiore, G., Luxen, A., Franck, G., et al. (2000). Neural mechanisms of antinociceptive effects of hypnosis. *Anesthesiology, 92,* 1257–1267.

Fiddes, P., Scott, A., Fletcher, J., & Glasier, A. (2003). Attitudes towards pelvic examination and chaperones: A questionnaire survey of patients and providers. *Contraception, 67,* 313–317.

Johnson, D. T., & Spielberger, C. D. (1968). The effects of relaxation training and the passage of time on measures of state and trait anxiety. *Journal of Clinical Psychology, 24*(1), 20–23.

Kahn, J. A., Chiou, V., Allen, J. D., Goodman, E., Perlman, S. E., & Emans, S. J. (1999). Beliefs about the Papanicolaou smears and compliance with Papanicolaou smear follow-up in adolescents. *Archives of Pediatric & Adolescent Medicine, 153,* 1046–1054.

Kohen, D. P. (1980). Relaxation/mental imagery (self-hypnosis) and pelvic examinations in adolescents. *Journal of Developmental and Behavioral Pediatrics, 1*(4), 180–186.

Kwekkeboom, K., Huseby-Moore, K., & Ward, S. (1998). Imaging ability and effective use of guided imagery. *Research in Nursing and Health, 21,* 189–198.

Sesti, A. (2000). State trait anxiety inventory (STAI) in medication clinical trials. *QOL Newsletter, 25,* 15–16.

Spielberger, C. D., Gorsuch, R. L., & Lushene, R. E. (1970). *State-Trait Anxiety Inventory Test Manual.* Palo Alto, CA: Consulting Psychologist Press.

Williams, J. G., Park, L. I., & Kline, J. (1992). Reducing distress associated with pelvic examinations: A stimulus control intervention. *Women & Health, 18*(2), 41–53.

Wright, D., Fenwick, J., Stephenson, P., & Monterosso, L. (2005). Speculum "self insertion": A pilot study. *Journal of Clinical Nursing, 14,* 1098–1111.

African-American Families Having Children with Asthma: A Critical Review

Yvonne M. Sterling and Jane W. Peterson

Revisited here is the issue of family responses, ethnicity, and culture as well as the methods used to study African-Americans having chronically ill children. Extending the information given in an earlier article (Sterling, Peterson, & Weekes, 1997), we describe the current state of knowledge about African-American childhood asthma and the involved families.

A comprehensive report of the state of childhood asthma in the United States (Akinbami, 2006) reveals that asthma is the most common childhood chronic disease, with African-American and Puerto Rican children having the highest prevalence. Furthermore, although asthma deaths have decreased, African-American children have higher mortality than do white children. Akinbami presents an alarming national portrait of children with asthma, warranting a priority for more research, evidence-based practice guidelines, and policy development. Particular attention is being given to minority children, especially African-Americans, for important reasons. In two editorials that discuss findings of the landmark National Cooperative Inner City Asthma Study of preponderantly African-American children, Klinnert (1997) and Platt-Mills (1997) noted the identification of factors that may have contributed to the understanding of increased asthma prevalence and morbidity in that population. Key and pertinent questions remain, however, as to how to improve asthma outcomes in African-American children.

Epidemiological data depict the high prevalence (Quinn, Shalowitz, Berry, Mijanovich, & Wolf, 2006; Smith, Hatcher-Ross, Wertheimer, & Kahn, 2005; Yeats & Shy, 2001) and asthma-related risk factors among African-American children (Grischkan et al., 2004; Higgins, Wakefield, & Cloutier, 2005; Klinnert et al., 2005; Koinis & Murdock, 2005; von Maffei et al., 2001; Meuer, George, Subichin, Malloy, & Gehring, 2000; Oliveti, Keresmar, & Redline, 1996), the possible impact of infant birth weight (Brooks, Byrd, Weitzman, Auinger, & McBride, 2001; Joseph, Ownby, Peterson, & Johnson, 2002), health service use (Cohen et al., 2006; Murray, Stang, & Tierney, 1997; Ortega et al., 2001), and the effect of race/racial disparities (Chan, Keeler, Schonlau, Rosen, & Mangione-Smith, 2005; McDaniel, Paxson, & Waldfogel, 2006; Pearlman et al., 2006; Quinn et al., 2006; Stingone & Claudio, 2006).

Various risk factors, such as socioeconomic status, have been examined to determine whether they influence asthma diagnosis, severity, and other outcomes. Higgins et al. (2005) in a sample of more than 19,000 children found that asthma frequency was related to ethnicity, socioeconomic status, and several home environmental factors. They also found that asthma among African-American children was more severe than among their white counterparts. von Maffei et al. (2001) interviewed more than 300 African-American mothers and found that 16% had at least one child at home with physician-diagnosed asthma. Risk factors associated with the child's asthma included maternal smoking and maternal asthma or allergies.

Wheezing in infants and toddlers may not mean the child has asthma, and the diagnosis of asthma in this age group is difficult to make (Sterling & El Dahr, 2006). Using the National Infant Health Survey and longitudinal follow-up survey, Brooks et al. (2001) estimated the independent contribution of birth weight to asthma prevalence in young children, comparing African-American and white children. Finding prevalence variations according to birth weight, those authors concluded that the increased contribution to asthma in African-American population correlated with the increased prevalence of low birth weight in this group. In other studies birth weight was also found to account for the increased prevalence of asthma (Joseph et al., 2002; McDaniel et al., 2006).

Oliveti et al. (1996) investigated prenatal and perinatal risk factors for asthma in 262 inner-city African-American children, finding that maternal smoking during pregnancy, no prenatal care, and lower birth weights may have increased those children's susceptibility to asthma. In a sample of 251 children who were preterm infants, among whom 97 were diagnosed as having asthma, Grischkan et al. (2004) investigated the role of perinatal exposures with regard to being at risk for asthma. Interestingly, they found that asthma was associated with children who were former preterm infants, had chronic lung disease, and were treated with mechanical lung ventilation and corticosteroids. The children with asthma in this study were mostly African-American males with impaired lung function. Regarding perinatal exposures, the investigators found that the history of maternal asthma was significantly higher in the asthma group but found no significant group differences with regard to maternal smoking during pregnancy and education.

In a comparative study of risk factors among three ethnic groups of families with infants or toddlers having multiple wheezing episodes, Klinnert et al. (2002) found risk patterns were different and distinct in each group. For example, African-American infant birth weights were lowest, yet no differences among groups were found in gestational age or mean IgE levels.

Disparities, Race, and Use of Health Services

African-American patterns of health care and the effect of racial disparities on asthma outcomes are common themes in the current literature. When the focus is on inner-city or Medicaid children and their families, African-American children were found to use the emergency department for asthma management more frequently than other groups

(Cohen et al., 2006; Murray et al., 1997; Ortega et al., 2001; Rand et al., 2000). How do ethnic or racial disparities explain asthma prevalence in African-American children? Several studies (Litonjua, Carey, Weiss, & Gold, 1999; Pearlman et al., 2006; Stingone & Claudio, 2006) have consistently found that African-American children, especially those who lived in poor areas, had a higher prevalence of asthma than did other groups of children. Using evidence from the National Health Survey of more than 14,000 African-American children and 49,000 white children having asthma to address racial disparities in childhood asthma, McDaniel et al. (2006) found that African-American children not only had a higher asthma prevalence, but also had low birth weights, had lower family incomes, and were less likely to see a physician regularly. Smith et al. (2005) examined the relationship between race/ethnicity, family income, and childhood asthma prevalence. Using the National Health Survey database of more than 14,000 children, those investigators found that African-American poor children had a considerably higher risk of asthma than did poor white children. The authors made the cogent remark that investigations should move beyond descriptions of ethnicity to explain why these differences occur.

The literature presents an alarming portrait of African-American children with asthma. Because race or ethnicity is a key variable, findings are compared and contrasted among different groups of children with asthma. Although a high prevalence of asthma, possible risk factors, and other specific characteristics among these children and their families are consistently seen, findings are not definitive and even raise more questions. Such findings do not mean that the current portrait is not of value to researchers and clinicians. Nonetheless, the current literature only presents the tip of the iceberg in terms of depth and breadth of social and other issues that these families face daily, affecting their ability to manage their children's health effectively and successfully.

African-American Family Responses to Childhood Asthma

It is important to reiterate that the incidence of asthma among African-American children, particularly for those who live in inner-city areas, is not only significantly higher but also tends to be more severe than that in other groups of children. Additionally, asthma outcomes are poorer in African-American children than in their counterparts. Key to determining the underlying causes of these undesirable findings and the most effective interventions to improve them is the accurate description and understanding of beliefs and practices of African-American caregivers as well as the children with asthma themselves. Therefore one may ask this question: What are the responses of African-American caregivers to childhood asthma?

Although a plethora of multidisciplinary clinical and research literature describes family experiences with childhood asthma, only a modicum of evidence exists about asthma management from African-American family members' viewpoints. In many reports, African-American parents or caregivers represented considerable percentages of study participants. In most published reports, however, at least one other ethnic group (white and/or Latino) is included along with those of African-American caregivers or parents. In most cases the study findings were enmeshed, though participants' ethnicity was often included in demographic data. Several studies (Conn et al., 2005; Koenig, Chesla, & Kennedy, 2003; Lee, Parker, DuBose, Gwinn, & Logan, 2006; Peterson, Sterling, & Stout, 2002; Peterson & Sterling, 2005; Valerio et al., 2006; Yoos & McMullen, 1999) reported perceptions and beliefs about children's asthma and its management. Most of those perspectives came from parents or caregivers who live in urban areas or the inner city and/or are Medicaid recipients.

Demands, Resources, and Asthma Management Strategies

Families and their children with asthma face complex demands associated with the illness. In a study of European-American and African-American parents of school-aged children with asthma, African-American parents, who were about 50% of the study sample, reported that the most time-consuming caregiving demands were simultaneously managing their time at work and the child's school and treatment regimen and that family support was limited (Lee et al., 2006). Sixty-four percent of parents of children with asthma in Valerio et al.'s study (2006) were African-Americans who cited experiencing multiple emotions, including stress and feeling overwhelmed, as they managed their child's asthma. Those parents were knowledgeable about asthma triggers but expressed a need for more asthma education and felt powerless about managing the environment outside their homes.

Use of health services and the services provided by healthcare professionals to manage their children with asthma is a major concern of African-American parents. Parents in one study reported that getting help meant receiving the health care they wanted and found acceptable within the healthcare system. Despite spending time, energy, and family resources, they noted that the results were not always successful (Peterson, Sterling, & Weekes, 1997, p. 139). Peterson-Sweeney, McMullen, Yoos, and Kitzman (2003) reported that the parents (44% African-American) in their study expressed a need for ongoing asthma education, found teaching by primary care providers inadequate, struggled with medication administration, yet wanted their knowledge of and skills in asthma management to be acknowledged and respected. In keeping with this notion, Flores, Abreu, Tomany-Korman, and Meurer (2005), whose sample consisted of 70% African-American parents, found that outpatient and inpatient asthma education was insufficient and exposure to environmental triggers was not sufficiently controlled. Their perspectives formed the basis for determining which factors may contribute to the prevention of hospital admissions of their children because of asthma.

The increasing incidence and prevalence of asthma in children under age 6 warrants a great deal of attention and concern. The qualitative work of Koenig (2006) included African-American parents and their infants and toddlers with asthma. Parents reported feelings of distress and fear of death as they used various strategies to manage these young children. When the child was hospitalized parents reported fear, anger, and helplessness as they witnessed the many procedures and interventions that their infants and toddlers endured (Koenig et al., 2003).

Descriptions of salient characteristics of African-American caregivers provide valuable insights about their asthma management strategies and styles. Sterling and Peterson (2003) reported that the female caregivers of children with asthma in their study managed a family asthma system; were gatekeepers to the child's asthma care; were religious, industrious, and autonomous; had family support; and had significant health problems themselves. In two studies of inner-city parents, depressive symptoms were found in mothers of children with asthma, but those symptoms were not related to the child's asthma morbidity. Nonetheless, mothers with severe depressive symptoms were found to be more likely to take their child to the emergency department (Bartlett et al., 2001, 2004).

Yoos and McMullen (1999) found that African-American parents, who were 46% of the sample, were more accurate in their description of perception, interpretation, and evaluation of asthma symptoms than were white parents. Important to note here, however, is that those in the sample in general did not recognize early symptoms, often leading to the start of interventions late in the child's asthma exacerbation. In a later study, Yoos, Kitzman, McMullne, Sidora-Acoleo, & Anson (2005) found no significant differences between African-American and white parents to call a healthcare provider for their child's asthma symptoms except for "chest tightness" and that African-American children were more likely to report a cough to their parents than other asthma symptoms.

Caregiver Beliefs and Adaptations

Parents expressed specific beliefs that they considered to be barriers to asthma management (Mansour, Lanphear, & DeWitt, 2000). Their most frequent identified barriers, as noted in data from focus groups, included family issues, such as number of caregivers, family conflict issues, associative support, and attitude toward asthma, as well as physical or social environment (allergens, social support, resources), accessibility to a healthcare provider (continuity of care or lack of, relationship with provider), the impact of limiting exercise on their child's quality of life, and the mechanisms of the healthcare system (insurance, accessing healthcare services).

Adherence to asthma treatment regimens is a significant issue and is linked to the extent of the child's morbidity and other positive or negative outcomes. Adherence to prescribed asthma management was often related to medication use, particularly that of controller medications. The literature consistently reports that controller or preventive medication use is less in African-American children than in other groups. More specifically, African-American children use fewer anti-inflammatory asthma medications daily (Flores et al., 2005; Lieu et al., 2002; Walders, Drotar, & Kercsmar, 2000). In Mansour et al.'s (2000) study, parents were also specifically concerned about the use, safety, and long-term complications of asthma medications and modified medication use prescribed by their primary care provider. In a sample consisting of 65% African-American parents of children with asthma,

75% of those parents believed that medications were necessary for their children's health but also had concerns about them. Interestingly, only 22% complied with the prescribed medication regimen (Conn et al., 2005). Other studies found that inhaled corticosteroids were underused (Butz et al., 2006; Rickert et al., 2003) and that parents' fears and diminished treatment expectations were barriers to their use (Yoos, Kitzman, & McMullen, 2003).

Health beliefs, which are often based on cultural values, influenced medication use and, in general, asthma management. Also found was that non-Western approaches to asthma management are also embraced by African-American families. Those approaches included biofeedback, calming measures, breathing exercises, herbal treatment, religious healing, and drinking water or juice (Braganza, Ozuah, & Sharif, 2003; Handelman, Rich, Bridgemohan, & Schneider, 2004; Peterson et al., 2002). The study of Braganza et al. (2003) found that a high proportion of parents perceived complementary alternative medicine to be effective and used it as a first treatment of acute episodes without ever informing their physicians. Not mentioned in the study report, however, is why parents use complementary alternative medicine, what beliefs they have about complementary alternative medicine, and what the cultural implications may be.

Explanatory Models

Explanatory models have been used to study African-American caregivers of children with asthma (Handelman et al., 2004; Peterson & Sterling, 2005; Peterson et al., 2002). An explanatory model depicts how a person responds to a particular illness episode and helps one to understand how he or she makes sense of any illness episode. Explanatory models of asthma influence one's perceptions about the illness and how asthma-related events and situations are communicated (Yoos & McMullen, 1999). In an ethnographic longitudinal study of 20 African-American families living in two cities, Peterson and Sterling (2005) found that families draw on their cultural context to understand asthma, including the cause of the child's condition, triggers, the circumstances necessary for asthma symptoms to appear, and the treatment the child should receive. Another noteworthy theme was "growing out of it" meaning that the trajectory of the child's asthma can range from having asthma, through transitioning, to having grown out of it (Peterson & Sterling, 2005). Although some aspects of African-American caregivers' perceptions of asthma are consistent with healthcare providers, their understanding of the chronic nature of asthma was not shared. In Handelman et al.'s (2004) study of inner-city parents and children with asthma various explanatory models were described, including parental understanding of asthma etiology, pathophysiology, and medications. In both studies (Handelman et al., 2004; Peterson & Sterling, 2005), investigators found that families have their own explanations of asthma with regard to etiology (heredity), symptoms (phlegm, body pains, and wheezing), and chronicity (growing out of it, no asthma when asymptomatic).

What are the responses of African-American caregivers to childhood asthma? The current literature describes caregiver beliefs, psychosocial responses, asthma management strategies, and concerns about healthcare delivery systems/health providers, and explanatory models of asthma. The literature tends to focus on families who live in urban and inner-city areas and/or are Medicaid recipients. African-American caregivers are studied either as a single entity or in combination with other ethnic groups. As a result, specific African-American findings are usually clustered as a single sample response or are embedded within general study results; however, a few studies reported findings based on ethnicity. In any case, discussion of study results within the context of African-American culture is virtually nonexistent.

Issues Pertaining to Study Methods

Because of the increased prevalence of asthma in children and minority children in particular, research on this population has increased, with the goal of improving outcomes for these children. A disproportionately high incidence of asthma among African-American children with asthma is seen not only in epidemiological data but also in the number of African-American children and their caregivers who are study participants. The following overview of studies including African-American participants in the past decade shows various designs and methods, including randomized control, quasi-experimental, descriptive, qualitative, case studies, and focus groups.

The multisite controlled trial, National Cooperative Inner-City Asthma Study, included more than 1,000 children with asthma and their families, of whom more than 70% were African-Americans (Evans, Gergen, Mitchell, et al., 1999). Testing the effectiveness of tailored inventions delivered by case manager social workers, the investigators found the intervention group had significantly better outcomes (hospital and symptom days, unscheduled visits) than the control group. Improved outcomes were sustained by the intervention group during the second year of the study. The investigators noted the importance of recognizing the effects of poverty and challenges of inner-city life when designing interventions geared toward families living in that environment.

A randomized controlled design was used by Levy, Heffner, Stewart, and Beeman (2006) in studying the efficacy of asthma management in medically underserved preponderantly African-American urban schools to reduce school absences and hospitalizations for the treatment of asthma among this population. The intervention group underwent an asthma case management approach, whereas the control group received usual care. Among the difficulties the authors reported were those that related to differences in the educational and medical cultures. They did not mention the possible effect of cultural or ethnic beliefs held by African-Americans and how that might influence asthma management. They did find that best practices for asthma management were not consistently offered in these underserved communities and that nurse case management can result in positive improvements in school-based asthma management.

Klinnert et al. (2005) conducted an environmental, home-based, random-controlled, nurse home visit intervention study. The participants were maternal caregivers and infants 9 to 24 months old in low-income families. Of the 150 participants in the study, 23% of the intervention group and 22% of the control group were African-Americans. The families received nurse home visits for a year aimed at decreasing allergen and environmental tobacco smoke exposure as well as improving symptom perception and management. Although adverse environmental exposure was reduced, no significant difference in respiratory symptoms or medical use was found between intervention and control groups. No discussion was given of the influence of cultural differences within study populations.

Another random-controlled, home-based, nurse intervention study (Brown et al., 2005) of low-income, urban, primarily African-American families of young children found that caregiver education, presence of father or surrogate father in the home, and environmental safety were the family characteristics that significantly affected achieving the learning objectives of the nurse home-visiting educational program. Despite the recognition of family influences, the influence of culture or ethnicity on family behavior was not discussed. Bonner et al. (2002) conducted a study of 100 Latino and African-American families consisting of individualized asthma education interventions. Though the intensive interventions were successful, no mention is given of the difference that ethnicity may have to the study.

An evaluation of an elementary school–based asthma management program in a largely African-American population used a randomized control design (Gerald et al. 2006). Those authors found a significant increase in asthma knowledge among the intervention group but no change in morbidity measurements. They discussed weaknesses with the data used to measure outcomes and indicated that self-report data might be a more reliable and accurate measure. Another problem was the high mobility of the study population, making it difficult to maintain contact. The discussion of the article is thoughtful in stating how asthma school education programs may become successful by closer collaboration with schools and with medical caregivers. Culture and ethnicity are not addressed either as influences on behavior related to asthma management or as values underlying beliefs about chronic illness generally and asthma specifically.

Retention of African-American study participants enrolled in an inner-city community-based asthma intervention study was described by Williams, Wharton, Falter, French, & Redd (2003) using demographic, clinical, residential, and logistical variables. Those authors evaluated data from 489 participants of which 467 (96%) were African-American. Data from the children who remained in the study and those who dropped out were compared. Findings showed that retention was higher for participants enrolled in a second year of the study who lived longer at the same residence. Retention was also higher for those enrolled during a face-to-face follow-up home visit than for those being enrolled at the emergency department. Although the findings are from an African-American population, nothing is stated regarding the influence of race or ethnicity on retention.

Using a quasi-experimental pre- and posttest design, Velsor-Friedrich, Pigott, and Srof (2005) examined the effects of a practitioner-based school asthma program for inner-city African-American children. With Orem's (2001) self-care deficit model used as a framework, the intervention group scored higher than the control group in the self-care abilities (asthma knowledge, asthma self-efficacy, and general and asthma self-care practices). Health outcomes showed no significant difference between the two groups. The model does not address ethnic or cultural factors that are reflected in the findings of this study.

Horner (2004) used a quasi-experimental design to test the effectiveness of group and home-based asthma education for children and parents, respectively. In that pilot study no significant differences were found between groups based on several factors, including ethnicity of the African-American, European-American, and Mexican-American children in the study.

Chan et al. (2005) conducted a cross-sectional survey of 405 white, African-American, and Latino children and adolescents to determine the effects of language on asthma management practices and asthma-related outcomes. The outcomes from 145 African-American children and adolescents were similar to those of the white children, and outcomes for Latinos from English-speaking homes were only slightly worse than for non-Latino white peers.

Lieu et al. (2002) examined racial and ethnic disparities in hospitalization rates for asthma among children in a managed Medicaid program. In that large-scale cross-sectional study, telephone interviews were conducted with parents and existing data were extracted from Medicaid records and the Children's Health Survey for Asthma. The study group found that a black–white disparity existed after adjusting for other sociodemographic variables. Black children had the worse asthma status with the most symptom-days and missed days at school and severity as assessed by parents. This study reported on black children as a subgroup but used racial/ethnicity only as a variable to describe the group. Beliefs and cultural variables that might influence these findings are not discussed. Nonetheless, differences might be attributable to particular healthcare beliefs, and a concept of disease is acknowledged.

In the Harlem Children's Zone Asthma Initiative (Nicholas et al., 2005), a 22-item asthma screening survey was used. Because of the small number of children screened, reporting on subgroups of blacks or Latinos was not possible. The study did confirm the high prevalence and severity of asthma in this target area among school-aged children, boys, Latinos, and children living with smokers, however. The children in that initiative are now receiving an array of services, and the authors are advocating for policies that would cover community-based asthma services. There is no discussion of the cultural implications for such services, although the authors state that to be successful they used an "integrated strategy that built on the existing infrastructure at the involved organizations" (p. 246).

Structured interviews of 60 African-American adolescents and their primary caregivers were used by Walders et al. (2000) to understand the perception of family management of asthma, adherence to treatment plans, and functional morbidity. Those authors found that nonadherence and functional morbidity correlated with caregiver overestimation of adolescent involvement in self-care and that caregiver responsibility declined with increasing adolescent age. The authors noted that the key to understanding study findings is the important issue of African-American family structures and multiple caregivers.

Questionnaires were also used with a convenience sample of 267 primarily African-American parents or primary caregivers of children with asthma aged 18 months to 16 years who participated in a five-session, community-based, asthma educational program (Bryant-Stephens & Li, 2004). The authors found positive results and recommend such programs for inner-city caregivers as part of management of childhood asthma. Mention is given of "complexities of asthma management" but not of the context of the children's family and social life, of which asthma might be only a small part. No mention is made of how culture or ethnicity affects this group of caregivers.

Neighborhood asthma coalitions (NAC) are community-based groups that are being studied as to their efficacy to reduce acute asthma rates in children. Fisher, Strunk, Sussman, Skyes, and Walker (2004) studied 249 low-income African-American patients (100 NAC subjects and 149 control subjects). Data from four NACs were compared with four comparable control neighborhoods. The NACs included educational asthma programs and promotional asthma activities and provided support for caregivers and children with asthma. Data were collected by quarterly telephone interviews from NAC members and from audits of acute care sites. Structural equation modeling showed the NACs were associated with positive change on the Index of Asthma Attitudes scale and lower rates of acute care. Although the reduction in acute care rates was seen among active NAC participants, the social mechanism associated with this finding was not discussed and therefore no basis was provided to build on that finding.

School-based asthma management was studied among 22 inner-city African-American children using a case study approach (McEwen, Johnson, Neatherlin, Millard, & Lawrence, 1998). Both qualitative and quantitative data were collected. Results were reported in terms of peak flow measurements, which significantly decreased bronchodilator use and relieved asthma symptoms, which declined by 75%. No conclusions could be drawn from the school absenteeism data collected, because the cause of absence was not stated and no historical absentee data existed for comparison. Although all participants were African-American, the implications of racial/ethnic influence on the child's asthma management were not discussed.

Focus groups were used in an African-American school (Boyle, Baker, & Kemp, 2004) to elicit specific cultural/ethnic influence of asthma and asthma management. The study involved two focus groups of school children ($n = 19$), one group of parents ($n = 4$), and two of teachers ($n = 18$). Content analysis of data revealed themes about beliefs and behaviors about asthma. The authors found the themes related to culture/ethnicity were "death," "talk about asthma," or the language used to describe symptoms. Those areas warrant further study.

Anderson et al. (2005) conducted a descriptive study that included in-depth interviews of principals and individual surveys of teachers, telephone interviews of parents, and face-to-face interviews of children with asthma in 14 low-income, preponderantly African-American, urban elementary schools. The results show where improvement can occur: clarifying school policies related to severe asthma attacks, correcting inappropriate knowledge of teachers, reducing school absences, overcoming problems with taking medication at school, and correcting children's misconceptions about asthma. The questions used in the interviews and surveys were evidence based, but the beliefs, ethnicity, and culture of the participants were not discussed. One can infer that the parents and children are African-American. Are the teachers also African-American? What beliefs are held by these groups that lead them to give "at least one "inappropriate step" (p. 239) when asked what they would do for a child having a severe asthma attack? This information is important to help in designing interventions that make sense to these groups and will result in improved asthma management for children in these schools.

Kaugars, Klinnert, and Bender (2004) undertook a critical literature review to determine how families affect pediatric asthma. One area they examined was racial or ethnic background, noting that such an undertaking is complex. The most frequent barriers described in their search were patient and family characteristics, environmental factors, health care, and health systems factors. They stated that caregiver beliefs about asthma management need to be understood along with evaluating the cultural competence of the healthcare system practice. Understanding those beliefs and evaluating cultural competence may play a significant role in the outcome of asthma management.

What issues are involved in the methods used for research of African-American families having children with asthma? Many other studies have looked at school-aged, low-income, African-American children in the urban setting (Bartholomew et al., 2006; Cohen et al., 2006; Lee et al., 2006; Flores et al., 2005; Valerio et al., 2006). Although being African-American is a criterion for participation and sometimes a variable, the understanding of beliefs and cultural values of this population are not discussed. As with other cultures, African-Americans are not a homogeneous group and therefore do not all hold the same beliefs (Sterling et al., 1997).

A few of the studies referred to above (Kaugars et al., 2004; Koenig et al., 2003) recognized that family beliefs and concepts about disease influence asthma outcomes and the need for practitioners and the healthcare system to be culturally competent. Most of the reviewed studies, however, did not discuss study findings within the context of sample's culture. One way to address cultural ethnic beliefs is the conduct of qualitative studies or mixed methods. Such studies or methods would facilitate the understanding of underlying beliefs and the "why" of some of the behaviors seen among African-Americans leading to interventions and subsequent research that incorporates this new understanding.

Why Is Culture an Important Issue to Address?

We agree with Galanti (2004) that a "basic working definition of culture is that it encompasses beliefs and behaviors that are learned and shared by members of a group" (p. 2). If one believes, as does Kleinman (1980), that "cultural beliefs and norms channel illness experiences and patient roles" (p. 119), then health research must include the cultural context. As an aside, let us mention that some of the misunderstandings and conflicts in health care come from the difference of values and beliefs held by the healthcare providers and the patient populations for which they care. Kleinman (1980) believes that symptoms are socially constructed, whence the "illness." *Disease* is the term used by healthcare providers. To understand patients, one must understand the illness experience within their cultural construction. Symptoms have a feedback role: If patients perceive a symptom as a serious threat, then treatment might be sought. That feedback loop effectively brings the patient into contact with the healthcare system.

Few of the studies reviewed here take into consideration African-American families' cultures and beliefs in that way via the feedback loop. All studies had a significant number of African-American participants, but few studies incorporated beliefs with behavior and outcomes. Schober and Lacroix (1991) stated that today, lay (here we refer to African-Americans) theories of illness have essentially the same explanatory frameworks of health and illness as they did 300 years ago. Reviewing the literature in 1997, Scharloo and Kaptein found five consistent dimensions that organize illness experiences: identity, cause, consequence, timeline, and controllability. So, the questions of what should be studied and measured and the best method to use are important when studying African-Americans. An analysis of group means may not be the most sensitive or valid way to analyze data; individual or specific family responses or beliefs will be lost. Thus attention given to the design and method section of the study is critical. For example, the high rate of nonadherence was mentioned in several studies discussed here. This nonadherence points to the need to understand the specific beliefs that underlie study participants' behaviors. Marteau and Senior (1997) found that open-ended questions used as part of an unstructured or semistructured interview often elicit comments on causal beliefs of an illness. They are careful to say, however, that other methods, such as rating scales, checklists, and rank ordering, have been used successfully and suggest comparing results using different methods. Peterson et al. (2002) used semistructured open interviews to discover explanatory models and to learn about asthma from African-American caregivers of children with asthma. Their findings show that explanatory models come from the family-lived experience. Marteau and Senior (1997) looked at illness representation and found that the perceptions one has of another person's problem can determine the kind of help offered. That healthcare providers understand patients' culture and beliefs is therefore imperative.

References

Akinbami, L. (2006). *The state of childhood asthma, United States, 1980–2005*. Advance Data from Vital and Health Statistics. U.S. Department of Health and Human Services, Centers for Disease and Prevention, National Center for Health Statistics, Number 381. December 12, 2006, pp. 1–28.

Anderson, E. W., Valerio, M., Liu, M., Benet, D. J., Joseph, C., Brown, R., et al. (2005). Schools' capacity to help low-income, minority children to manage asthma. *Journal of School Nursing, 21*(4), 236–242.

Bartholomew, L. K., Sockrider, M. K., Abramson, S. L., Swank, P. R., Czyzewski, D. I., Tortolero, S. R., et al. (2006). Partners in school asthma management: Education of a self-management program for children with asthma. *Journal of School Health, 76*(6), 283–290.

Bartlett, S., Kolodner, K., Butz, A., Eggleston, P., Malveaux, F., & Rand, C. (2001). Maternal depressive symptoms and emergency department use among inner-city children with asthma. *Archives of Pediatric Adolescent Medicine, 155*, 347–353.

Bartlett, S., Krishnan, J., Riekert, K., Butz, A., Malveaux, F., & Rand, C. (2004). Maternal depressive symptoms and adherence to therapy in inner-city children with asthma. *Pediatrics, 113*(2), 229–237.

Bonner, S., Zimmerman, B. J., Evans, D., Irigoyen, M., Resnick, D., & Mellins, R. (2002). Individualized intervention to improve asthma management among urban Latino and African-American Families. *Journal of Asthma, 39*(2), 167–179.

Boyle, J. S., Baker, R. R., & Kemp, V. H. (2004). School-based asthma: A study in an African American elementary school. *Journal of Transcultural Nursing, 15*(3), 195–206.

Braganza, S., Ozuah, P., & Sharif, I. (2003). The use of complementary therapies in inner-city asthmatic children. *Journal of Asthma, 40*(7), 823–827.

Brooks, A., Byrd, R., Weitzman, M., Auinger, P., & McBride, J. (2001). Impact of low birth weight on early childhood asthma in the United States. *Archives of Pediatrics & Adolescent Medicine, 155*(3), 401–406.

Brown, J. V., Demi, A. S., Celano, M. P., Bakerman, R., Hobrynski, L., & Wilson, S. (2005). A home visiting asthma education program: Challenges to implementation. *Health Education & Behavior, 32*(1), 42–56.

Bryant-Stephens, T., & Li, Y. (2004). Community asthma education program for parents of urban asthmatic children. *Journal of the National Medical Association, 96*(7), 954–960.

Butz, A., Tsoukleris, M., Donithan, M., Van Doren, H., Mudd, K., Zuckerman, I. H., et al. (2006). Patterns of inhaled anti-inflammatory medication use in young underserved children with asthma. *Pediatrics, 118*(6), 2504–2513.

Chan, K., Keeler, E., Schonlau, M., Rosen, M., & Mangione-Smith, R. (2005). How do ethnicity and primary language spoken at home affect management practices and outcomes in children and adolescents with asthma? *Archives of Pediatrics & Adolescent Medicine, 159*(3), 283–289

Cohen, R. T., Celedon, J. C., Hinckson, V. J., Ramsey, C. D., Wakefield, D. B., Weiss, S. T., et al. (2006). Health-care use among Puerto Rican and African-American children with asthma. *Chest, 130*(2), 463–471

Conn, K., Halterman, J., Fisher, F., Yoos, H., Chin, N., & Szilagyi, P. (2005). Parental beliefs about medications and medication adherence among urban children with asthma. *Ambulatory Pediatrics, 5*(5), 306–310.

Evans, R., Gergen, P. J., Mitchell, H., et al. (1999). A randomized clinical trial to reduce asthma morbidity among inner-city children: Results of the National Cooperative Inner-City Asthma Study. *Journal of Pediatrics, 135*, 332–338.

Fisher, E. B., Strunk, R. C., Sussman, L. K., Skyes, R. K., & Walker, M. S. (2004). Community organization to reduce the need for acute care for asthma among African American children in low-income neighborhoods: The neighborhood asthma coalition. *Pediatrics, 114*(1), 116–123.

Flores, G., Abreu, M., Tomany-Korman, S., & Meurer, J. (2005). Keeping children with asthma out of hospitals: Parents' and physicians' perspectives on how pediatric asthma hospitalizations can be prevented. *Pediatrics, 116*(4), 957–965.

Galanti, G. A. (2004). *Caring for patients from different cultures* (3rd ed.). Philadelphia: University of Pennsylvania Press

Gerald, L. B., Redden, D., Wittich, A. R., Hains, C., Turner-Henson, A., Hemstreet, M. P., et al. (2006). Outcomes for a comprehensive school-based asthma management program. *Journal of School Health, 76*(6), 291–296.

Grischkan, J., Storfer-Isser, M., Rosen, C., Larkin, E., Kirchner, H., South, A. et al. (2004). Variation in childhood asthma among former preterm infants. *Journal of Pediatrics, 144*(3), 321–326.

Handelman, L., Rich, M., Bridgemohan, C., & Schneider, L. (2004). Understanding pediatric inner city asthma: An explanatory model approach. *Journal of Asthma, 41*(2), 167–177.

Higgins, P., Wakefield, D., & Cloutier, M. (2005). Risk factors for asthma and asthma severity in nonurban children in Connecticut. *Chest, 128*(6), 3846–3853.

Horner, S. (2004). Effect of education on school-age children's and parents' asthma management. *Journal of the Society of Pediatric Nurses, 9*(3), 95–102.

Joseph, C., Ownby, D., Peterson, E., & Johnson, C. (2002). Does low birth weight help to explain the increased prevalence of asthma among African Americans? *Annals in Allergy Asthma & Immunology, 88*(5), 507–512.

Kaugars, A. S., Klinnert, M. D., & Bender, B. G. (2004). Family influences on pediatric asthma. *Journal of Pediatric Psychology, 29*(7), 475–491.

Kleinman, A. (1980). *Patients and healers in the context of culture.* Berkeley, CA: University of California Press.

Klinnert, M. (1997). Guest editorial. Psychosocial influences on asthma among inner-city children. *Pediatric Pulmonology, 24*, 234–236.

Klinnert, M. D., Liu, A. H., Pearson, M. R., Ellison, M. C., Budhiraja, N., & Robinson, J. L. (2005). Short-term impact of a randomized multifaceted intervention for wheezing infants in low-income families. *Archives of Pediatric Adolescent Medicine, 159*(1), 75–82.

Klinnert, M., Price, M., Lie, A., & Robinson, J. (2002). Unraveling the ecology of risks for early childhood asthma among ethnically diverse families in the southwest. *American Journal of Public Health, 92*(5), 792–798.

Koenig, K. (2006). Families discovering asthma in their high-risk infants and toddlers with severe persistent disease. *Journal of Family Nursing, 12*(1), 56–79.

Koenig, K., Chesla, C., & Kennedy, C. (2003). Parents' perspectives of asthma crisis hospital management in infants and toddlers: An interpretive view through the lens of attachment theory. *Journal of Pediatric Nursing, 18*(4), 233–243.

Koinis, M., & Murdock, K. (2005). Identifying risk and resource factors in children with asthma from urban settings: The context health development model. *Journal of Asthma, 42*(6), 425–436.

Lee, J., Parker, V., DuBose, L., Gwinn, J., & Logan, B. (2006). Demands and resources: Parents of school age children with asthma. *Journal of Pediatric Nursing, 21*(6), 425–433.

Levy, M., Heffner, B., Stewart, T., & Beeman, G. (2006). The efficacy of asthma case management in an urban school district in reducing school absences and hospitalizations for asthma. *Journal of School Health, 76*(6), 320–324

Lieu, T., Lozano, P., Finkelstein, J., Chi, F., Jensvold, N., Capra, A. M., et al. (2002). Racial/ethnic variation in asthma status and management practices among children in managed Medicaid. *Pediatrics, 109*(5), 857–865.

Litonjua, A., Carey, V., Weiss, S., & Gold, D. (1999). Race, socioeconomic factors, and area of residence are associated with asthma prevalence. *Pediatric Pulmonology, 28*(6), 394–401.

Mansour, M., Lanphear, B., & DeWitt, T. (2000). Barriers to asthma care in urban children: Parent perspectives. *Pediatrics, 106*(3), 512–519.

Marteau, T. M., & Senior, V. (1997). Illness representations after the human genome project: The perceived role of the gene in causing illness. In K. J. Petrie & J. A. Weinman (Eds.), *Perceptions of health & illness* (pp. 241–266). Amsterdam: Harwood Academic Publishers.

McDaniel, M., Paxson, C., & Waldfogel, J. (2006). Racial disparities in childhood asthma in the United States: Evidence from the National Health Interview Survey, 1997–2003. *Pediatrics, 117*(5), e868–e877

McEwen, M., Johnson, P., Neatherlin, J., Millard, M. W., & Lawrence, G. (1998). School-based management of chronic asthma among inner-city African-American schoolchildren in Dallas, Texas. *Journal of School Health, 68*(5), 196–201.

Meurer, J., George, V., Subichin, S., Malloy, M., & Gehring, L. (2000). Risk factors for pediatric asthma emergency visits. Milwaukee Childhood Asthma Project Team. *Journal of Asthma, 37*(8), 653–659.

Murray, M., Stang, P., & Tierney, W. (1997). Health care use by inner-city patients with asthma. *Journal of Clinical Epidemiology, 50*(2), 167–174.

Nicholas, S. W., Jean-Louis, B., Ortiz, B., Northridge, M., Shoemaker, K., Vuaghan, R., et al. (2005). Addressing the childhood asthma crisis in Harlem: The Harlem Children's Zone Asthma Initiative. *American Journal of Public Health, 95*(2), 245–249.

Oliveti, J., Kercsmar, C., & Redline, S. (1996). Pre- and perinatal risk factors for asthma to inner-city African American children. *American Journal of Epidemiology, 142*(6), 570–577.

Orem, D. (2001). *Nursing: Concepts of practice* (5th ed.). St. Louis, MO: Mosby.

Ortega, A., Belanger, K., Paltiel, A., Horwitz, S., Bracken, M., & Leaderer, B., (2001). Use of health services by insurance status among children with asthma. *Medical Care, 39*(10), 1065–1074.

Pearlman, D., Zierler, S., Meersman, S., Kim, H., Viner-Brown, S., & Caron, C. (2006). Race disparities in childhood asthma: Does where you live matter? *Journal of the National Medical Association, 98*(2), 239–247.

Peterson, J. W., & Sterling, Y. M. (2005). "Growin' out of it": An explanation of childhood asthma by African American families. In M. de Chesnay (Ed.), *Caring for the vulnerable: Perspectives in nursing theory, practice, and research* (pp. 143–151). Sudbury, MA: Jones and Bartlett.

Peterson, J. W., Sterling, Y. M., & Stout, J. W. (2002). Explanatory models of asthma from African American caregivers of children with asthma. *Journal of Asthma, 39*(7), 577–590.

Peterson, J. W., Sterling, Y. M., & Weekes, D. (1997). Access to health care: Perspectives of African American families with chronically ill children. *Family Community Health, 19*(4), 64–77.

Peterson-Sweeney, K., McMullen, A., Yoos, H. L., & Kitzman, H. (2003). Parental perceptions of their child's asthma: Management and medication use. *Journal of Pediatric Health Care, 17,* 118–125.

Platts-Mills, T. (1997). Editorial. Asthma among inner-city children. *Pediatric Pulmonology, 24,* 231–233.

Quinn, K., Shalowitz, M., Berry, C., Mijanovich, T., & Wolf, R. (2006). Racial and ethnic disparities in diagnosed and possible undiagnosed asthma among public school children in Chicago. *American Journal of Public Health, 96*(9), 1599–1603.

Rand, C., Butz, A., Kolodner, K., Huss, K., Eggleston, P., & Malveaux, F. (2000). Emergency department visits by urban African American children with asthma. *Journal of Allergy Clinical Immunology, 105*(1 Pt 1) 83–90.

Rickert, K., Butz, A., Eggleston, P., Huss, K, Winkelstein, M., & Rand, C. (2003). Caregiver-physician medication concordance and undertreatment of asthma in inner-city children. *Pediatrics, 111*(3), 214–220.

Scharloo, M., & Kaptein, A. (1997). Measurement of illness perceptions in patients with chronic somatic illness: A review. In K. J. Petrie & J. A. Weinman (Eds.), *Perceptions of health & illness* (p. 103). Amsterdam: Harwood Academic Publishers.

Schober, R., & Lacroix, J. M. (1991). Lay illness models in the enlightenment and the 20th century: some historical lessons. In J. A. Skelton & R. T. Croyle (Eds.), *Mental representation in health and illness* (pp. 10–31). New York: Springer-Verlag.

Smith, L., Hatcher-Ross, J., Wertheimer, R., & Kahn, R. (2005). Rethinking race/ethnicity, income, and childhood asthma: Racial/ethnic disparities concentrated among the very poor. *Public Health Reports, 120,* 109–120.

Sterling, Y. M., & El Dahr, J. (2006). Wheezing and asthma in early childhood: An update. *Pediatric Nursing, 32*(1), 27–31

Sterling, Y. M., & Peterson, J. W. (2003). Characteristics of African American caregivers of children with asthma. *American Journal of Maternal Child Nursing, 28*(1), 33–38.

Sterling, Y. M., Peterson, J. W., & Weekes, D. (1997). African American families with chronically ill children: Oversights and insights. *Journal of Pediatric Nursing, 12*(5), 292–300.

Stingone, J., & Claudio, L. (2006). Disparities in the use of urgent care services among asthmatic children. *Annals in Allergy, Asthma & Immunology, 97*(2), 244–250.

Valerio, M., Cabana, M. D., White, D. F., Heidmann, D. M., Brown, R. W., & Bratton, S. L. (2006). Understanding of asthma management: Medicaid parents' perspectives. *Chest, 129*(3), 594–601.

Velsor-Friedrich, B., Pigott, T., & Srof, B. (2005). A practitioner-based asthma intervention program with African American inner-city school children. *Journal of Pediatric Health Care, 19*(3), 163–171.

von Maffei, J., Beckett, W. S., Belanger, K., Triche, E., Zhang, H., Machung, J. F., et al. (2001). Risk factors for asthma prevalence among urban and nonurban African American children. *Journal of Asthma, 38*(7), 555–564.

Walders, N., Drotar, D. & Kercsmar, C. (2000), The allocation of family responsibility for asthma management tasks in African American adolescents. *Journal of Asthma, 37*(1), 89–99.

Williams, S. G., Wharton, A. R., Falter, K. H., French, E., & Redd, S. C. (2003). Retention factors for participants of an inner-city community-based asthma intervention study. *Ethnicity and Disease, 13*(1), 118–125.

Yeats, K., & Shy, C. (2001). Prevalence and consequences of asthma and wheezing in African American and white adolescents. *Journal of Adolescent Health, 29,* 314–319.

Yoos, H. L., Kitzman, H., & McMullen, A. (2003). Barriers to anti-inflammatory medication use in childhood asthma. *Ambulatory Pediatrics, 3*(4), 181–190.

Yoos, H. L., Kitzman, H., McMullen, A., Sidora-Acoleo, K., & Anson, E. (2005). The language of breathlessness: Do families and health care providers speak the same language when describing asthma symptoms? *Journal of Pediatric Health Care, 19*(4), 197–205.

Yoos, H. L., & McMullen, A. (1999). Symptom perception and evaluation in childhood asthma. *Nursing Research, 48*(1), 2–8.

Chapter 17

Life Histories of Successful Survivors of Colostomy Surgery, Multiple Sclerosis, and Bereavement

Mary de Chesnay, Renee Rassilyer-Bomers, Jessica H. Webb, and Rebecca W. Peil

Life histories are often collected during ethnographic research to tell the story of the culture through the eyes of those key informants most representative of the culture. There is a rich tradition of collecting life histories in anthropological research during long periods of fieldwork when the researcher lives within the community and develops relationships over time. However, long periods of fieldwork are not always possible in nursing research, so in this chapter we present an abbreviated way to collect life histories from individuals who have much to teach nurses about living with their health conditions.

Life history differs from autobiography in that the agent of interpretation is the researcher, not the one whose life is being described. The informant tells his or her story to the researcher who then interprets the story in light of the research questions and the cultural context in which the person lives (de Chesnay, 2005). There are many examples of detailed life histories in the anthropological literature (Davison, 1989; Early, 1993; Gmelch, 1986; James, 2000; Levy, 1988; Scheub et al., 1988; Sexton, 1981). Following is a brief description of the methodology with three abbreviated examples of life histories collected by nurses.

Methodology

The methods for these studies were developed by the first author to refine the traditional anthropological techniques for nursing research. The original study is reported in the first edition of this book (de Chesnay, 2005).

A similar method of focusing life history material for briefer reports was developed by Hagemaster (1992), who presented a clear outline for interviews conducted solely as life histories. The usefulness of life narratives was described by Mattingly and Lawlor (2000). Beery, Sommers, and Hall (2002) used an adaptation of Hall's (1996) methodology of focused life stories to explore women's experiences with pacemakers.

In the studies reported in this chapter, the life histories are abbreviated stories told by people who have something to teach others through the recounting of their path to success at overcoming the obstacles associated with their disease or condition. Success for each study was self-defined by the key informant and refers to a sense of prosperity and general satisfaction with accomplishments and success at overcoming obstacles.

It is important to note that the data derived from this study are emic data (from the person's viewpoint) rather than etic (from the researcher's viewpoint). Emic data are more powerful for the purpose of developing culturally appropriate interventions because of the increased likelihood of relevance to the target audience.

There are three methods of data collection in addition to participant observation: a series of semistructured interviews, genograms, and timelines. The research question in all three studies is this: How does one achieve success at overcoming the obstacles associated with the condition (colostomy, multiple sclerosis, bereavement)?

Key informants were recruited purposively. Genograms and specific demographic data about the sample are not presented here to protect participants' privacy. The genogram was developed as a clinical tool in family therapy and is now widely used as an assessment tool in nursing and medicine. The genogram model developed for family therapy (McGoldrick & Gerson, 1986; McGoldrick, Gerson, & Shellenberger, 1999) was adapted by the first author for use in her own clinical practice as a family therapist and as an instrument of research in an earlier study (de Chesnay, Marshall, & Clements, 1988). The purpose of the genogram is to shortcut the analysis of family data.

Genogram questions involved gathering information about the family of origin and successful role models within the family. Interviews included broad questions about the definition of success, facilitators and barriers, and stories from the informants' youth. Generally, three or four interviews lasting about 2 hours were necessary. Interviews were audio-taped for accuracy.

The timeline data collection tool is simply a horizontal line on a blank page with "birth" at the left end and "present age" at the right end. Informants were asked to indicate on the line the critical events in their lives and the ages at which the events occurred. The timeline helped to clarify the sequence of events important to the person. Informants were given copies of the genograms and timelines and were encouraged to change them as needed during the intervals between interview sessions.

After the institutional review board gave approval, the informants were recruited, the consent forms were explained and signed, and the interviews were scheduled, conducted, and analyzed. The first author served as a consultant and resource to the others, but the three studies were conducted autonomously.

"A Second Chance at Life": Life History of a Successful Colostomy Patient (Rassilyer-Bomers)

The key informant selected for this research project was Olivia (her name has been changed to protect her privacy and certain biographical material has been abbreviated to disguise her identity). Referred by her ostomy support group, Olivia demonstrated significant success in her colostomy life-style since surgery 1 year ago. Members of her ostomy group identified her exemplar nature, in her ability to share her colostomy experience with others, and in her active participation in ostomy support groups and education. Olivia is currently constructing a brochure on ostomy care that illuminates tips and suggestions on how to live with an ostomy from her own personal experience. She is a delightful and knowledgeable woman who provided a rich and informative life history with data and concepts that portray the success among colostomy patients.

Olivia is a 54-year-old white woman who grew up in a dual-parent household with two older brothers and one younger sister. Influenced greatly by her father, Olivia learned the significance of hard work, integrity, and morals at a young age. Since her teenage years, Olivia worked numerous jobs to support her college education and well-loved trips to Hawaii. She flourished in school and graduated in the top of her class. Married at a young age of 20, she and her husband have maintained a loving and supportive marriage for the last 34 years. She functioned in numerous capacities as a business manager, wife, and mother to their only son. During his youth, Olivia selected to participate in several of her son's school activities and volunteered for auctions and fundraising. She was noted by others to have coordinated some of the most successful auctions financially for the school. Upon her son's college entrance Olivia returned full time to work in the business realm, until sudden onset of her illness in 1997. Suffering from a gastrointestinal condition that involved fecal incontinence and chronic pain, Olivia remained homebound and ill for approximately 7 years. When the opportunity for surgery approached, Olivia jumped at the chance to get her life back. On February 5, 2004, Olivia underwent a colon resection and colostomy procedure.

Importantly, Olivia has seen herself as a successful person since childhood through adulthood, assisted by the guidance of her father and significant role models in her family. She described herself as a perfectionist, a goal-oriented individual, and a hard worker who strove to complete all that she desired. Ultimately, her strong-willed personality and successful nature culminated in her ability to face the challenges presented by her colostomy surgery.

Olivia's genogram illuminated a family circle consisting of her husband and son. She described her family unit as supportive and close, although her son no longer lives at home. He calls frequently and visits often. Her family of origin comprises her two older brothers, younger sister, and father. Her mother passed away, and her father now lives alone. There are several divorces throughout her generation among her brothers and cousins. Her eldest brother, father, great aunts, and maternal cousins were all noted as successful and supportive individuals.

Olivia was also asked to identify relationships on the genogram that were close versus those that were distant or conflicted. This was important because it reiterates which relationships are sources of support or, conversely, sources of heartache and anxiety. It also provided insight into family dynamics and issues that are currently not resolved.

According to Olivia, she is close to her immediate family of husband and son. She is also close to her father, her maternal aunts, eldest brother, adopted niece of her eldest brother, and eldest nephew of her only sister. These individuals were seen as persons she routinely contacted and had a positive bond to. As for distant relationships, she marked her youngest brother, the rest of her nieces and nephews, and all family members on her mother's side of the family. She considered these relationships distant because of the infrequency of contact, although the relationships are positive.

Finally, the only two relationships that Olivia marked as conflicted were with her mother and her sister. Throughout the interview Olivia referred to her mother as a controlling individual. "She [Olivia's mother] tried to control me. It was okay, especially when I was older, but not when I was growing up." Her mother is now deceased, but when she talks of her past relationship with her she frowns and sounds saddened. This is in large contrast to how she perceives her father, whom elicited a smile and evident pride, when she spoke of him. In regards to her sister, Olivia was not too explicit with why they have a conflicted relationship. She made mention that her sister was selfish at times and not considerate of others. Furthermore, her sister was not a support person during her surgery and recovery, rarely contacting her unless she required something. To recover, Olivia made it clear that she purposely distances herself from her sister and individuals who treat her poorly because of her need to stay positive and heal. She obviously recognizes how healthy and unhealthy relationships in her life impact her overall well-being and has taken steps to surround herself with supportive and caring individuals.

On the timeline, Olivia described numerous events and periods that were significant in her life and influenced her success. In 1961 she suffered from rheumatic fever, which was noted as her first significant experience with illness and recovery. Her first job was as a waitress at a restaurant, which taught her responsibility and independence. In 1968 she was elected corresponding secretary of her high school class, and in 1969 she graduated 16th of 416 students in her high school class and took her first trip to Hawaii. In 1971 she married her husband of 34 years and learned to balance a married life with college and full-time employment. She graduated from a Seattle urban university in 1973 and had her first professional position in 1974. Her advancement to business manager in 1975 gave her greater responsibility and self-confidence. One year later in October 1976 she gave birth to her son and began her role as mother. Olivia noted in 1988 her bout with chickenpox, another unexpected illness. Then in 1997 she began experiencing health problems associated with her gastrointestinal system, thereby leading to the colostomy surgery in February 2004.

Concepts

Knowledgeable

The concept of knowledge was a significant factor in Olivia's colostomy success and was illuminated through her frequent emphasis on the importance of pre- and postsurgical education. Specifically, she gathered knowledge through a personal dedication toward learning, collecting information, and understanding aspects of colostomy life. She clearly mentioned numerous avenues of knowledge retrieval, including doctors, enterostomal nurses, books, Internet sources, and support groups. It was evident that she perceived self-education as significant and that knowledge acquisition was a personal responsibility. She acknowledged her own desire to learn and how she was able to better cope with her ostomy experience using the knowledge she accrued. Examples of statements that portray this concept are as follows:

> I knew that I would have to learn how to take care of it. And so I searched the Internet, that's what I did.
>
> Education is foremost. And you study, and gather as much information as you can. There are some sources out there. . . . UOA, the United Ostomy Association.
>
> I did a personal search, but I did have an incredible doctor. I came in with two and a half pages of questions and he answered them before I even asked them. So he was great, and my ET nurse was great. They were very personable and they had the facts.
>
> The doctors and the ET nurses can provide us teaching, but mostly they don't know what it is like because they don't have one. And that is hard. You need that information, to talk with people who do have it. And it's scary. And it's hard to go to that first support group. Very hard, but it's so worth it.

Confident

Olivia mentioned how important it was to be confident in herself to be successful. She described this in her everyday accomplishments and in the achievements of her colostomy experience. This concept is portrayed as both a trait of her strong-willed nature and in her appreciation for hard work, happiness, and positive attitude. Olivia perceived a sense of humor as a way to develop confidence, along with education and developing a strong knowledge base. Seeking skilled medical staff that she was confident in was essential in her healing process, as well. Olivia also saw support from family members and friends as providing her with the confidence to cope and adjust. These methods enabled her to develop the strength to overcome the hardships involved with colostomy care. She expresses her confidence:

> I would say, [success] is confidence. Confidence . . . postiveness . . . Making goals and reaching them. I think you have to be happy with what you do . . . and reaching your goals is very important.
>
> And then it is important to make little goals. Like don't get upset when you have little explosions and get it all over everything. . . . You have tears the first couple of times, but then you learn to laugh at it now. You laugh and have to have a good sense of humor about it or you won't make it through.
>
> You have to have confidence . . . confidence and trust. And knowing that I was confident in my surgeon, I was not nervous about the surgery itself.
>
> You also have to be comfortable around your stoma. I remember the first time I felt it. I was surprised and fascinated at it. Not many people have the opportunity to see their insides on the outside.

Adaptable

The ability to adapt and adjust to a colostomy life-style was a significant factor as evidenced by her flexibility and how she made life-style changes with ease and acceptance. Her willingness to set goals and follow through in an organized and focused fashion had enabled her to quickly adjust both pre- and postsurgically:

> I had to adjust and focus on healing. Because once you begin to heal, then you can get on with your life.
>
> Well, an ostomy is not a natural thing. But now when I look down at it when I am cleaning and changing, it is no big deal. But when I was even eight to nine months post-op, I used to just stand in the mirror and look and think that was not normal looking, to have a stoma on your stomach. And you just have to get over it and move on, and consider the alternatives of being sick.
>
> But no matter how long you have the ostomy, it does hit you sometimes. And you learn to turn it into positives. It's an ongoing process.

Discussion

The concepts of knowledge, confidence, and adaptation portrayed through this research are supported in the literature, although further research is necessary to validate and apply these findings. Although the review of literature identified a gap in research regarding colostomy success, numerous articles identified these concepts in relation to colostomy care.

In a literature review completed by Black (2004), stoma patients were examined in regards to the psychological, sexual, and cultural issues that presented when faced with a change in body image. She defined successful adaptation as a return to everyday activities and relationships. Factors that influenced this adaptation included the disease process, diagnosis, treatment, and nursing care both in the hospital and in the community. Furthermore, those patients who had strong feelings of personal competence demonstrated fewer psychosocial problems (Black, 2004). Education and willingness to learn about the stoma also presented with less psychological and sexual issues. Similarly, the results of this study illustrated Olivia's need to change her life-style so she could return to her normal endeavors and activities. She educated herself so she could feel competent and comfortable with her stoma and had significant support from her doctor and ostomy nurse before and after her surgical procedure.

Bekkers et al. (1995) examined self-efficacy in regards to the psychosocial adaptation of patients to stoma surgery. It more clearly identified the role of self-efficacy and confidence as the direct link with positive postoperative adjustment and accelerated adaptation. The concept of confidence in this research study was thus validated as an important source of success for colostomy patients. Olivia required support, guidance, and strong feelings of self-worth and competence to be successful, which are components of psychosocial adaptation illuminated in the literature (Bekkers et al., 1995).

"I'll Show You": Life History of a Successful Multiple Sclerosis Patient (Webb)

Florence (pseudonym) is a 46-year-old white woman who has worked in the healthcare field for 12 years. She was diagnosed with multiple sclerosis at the age of 30. Shortly before her diagnosis she began to struggle with severe fatigue and cognitive difficulties. She remembers being "lucky if I could get the bed made and dinner done all in the same day," which was in stark contrast to her usual productivity. These struggles continued throughout the early years of living with her multiple sclerosis (MS) until she decided to take matters into her own hands.

Florence has created a unique intervention for people with MS who have fatigue. To protect her identity, no specifics are given regarding this intervention. She uses the intervention on a regular basis, and it "has turned my life around." In addition to helping her deal with her own fatigue, her intervention has helped thousands of others who deal with the challenges presented by MS-related fatigue. She feels compelled to continue improving her intervention and therein helping more people with MS. She believes that success happens in steps and "there is no end," so when she reaches one step of success she has to keep on moving. This idea, which she truly appears to live by, is illustrated when she comments, "you've always got to be challenging, progressing, moving."

Florence has been married to the same man for 16 years. Together they have a 15-year-old son and a 19-year-old daughter. She acknowledges that her husband has contributed to her success, describing him as "probably the one who believed in me the most." She believes his encouragement throughout the years has enabled her to reach many of her goals.

Her genogram showed a family of origin that was intact and nuclear for two generations. Divorce is present among her siblings, however; her husband's family is intact and nuclear with no divorce. She has one surviving parent, and all her siblings are still living. Florence is the only one who lives outside of the state where her family originated. Her genogram also reveals no other family members with MS.

On the timeline she indicated the following ages at which significant events occurred: age 30, when she was diagnosed with MS; age 31, when she moved; age 31, when she began working for a local veterinarian; age 32, when she discovered a precursor to her intervention; age 35, when she finished her education; age 40, when she developed her intervention; and age 42, when she received confirmation that her intervention was beneficial. It should be noted that throughout Florence's life she was motivated by many people telling her she "couldn't do" something or doubting her ability. These occurrences are not documented on the timeline due to her vague recollection of specific occasions; however, she believes these were significant because they were constant motivators to prove them wrong.

Concepts

Motivational Styles

Throughout Florence's life she had been motivated by many people, including her parents, siblings, employers, husband, and colleagues. The means by which she was motivated were varied. Some people motivated her through encouragement and support, some through doubting her ability to accomplish certain goals, and others by withholding affection and praise unless she performed well. She acknowledges that all these methods ultimately worked to motivate her to perform her best; however, she admits that the people who doubted her, were skeptical of her, and challenged her where the most influential. As she reflected through her past accomplishments, she saw that the most significant successes throughout her life were all motivated by someone doubting her ability:

> And, you know, I've always been like that . . . you tell me I can't do something, I'm going to do it. I mean, you just lit a fire under me.

MS-Related Fatigue

MS-related fatigue affected her life in a variety of significant ways. She found she was unable to fulfill her daily activities, she struggled with the tasks necessary to keep her home, and was unable to continue her education program because of the way the fatigue affected her cognition. She felt as though the fatigue ruled her entire life, and finding a means by which to alleviate the fatigue was the only way she was able to function. Throughout the duration of her disease, desperation prompted her to try a variety of treatments for her fatigue. She strongly believed that without a solution to MS-related fatigue she never would have accomplished the goals she set and, hence, never achieved her success:

> The fatigue fed everything. It was just that horrendous fatigue, just horrendous, which really bothered me because it would take me 3 hours to make a bed.
>
> There were times when I'd try and mow the lawn and I'd go about 25 feet and I'd have to stop and go lie down. That's one thing with an MS patient with fatigue, they've got to lie down and now I know why. So I'd have to lie down and then I'd mow another 25 feet. . . . and that's how I mowed my yard. It would take me all day.

Coping

Dealing with a chronic disease forced Florence to find ways to cope with many ongoing challenges. She also found that in spite of the fact that her disease was chronic, new obstacles unearthed themselves to confront her. This reflects one of the characteristics of MS: its tendency to exacerbate and cause new symptoms to appear or cause current symptoms to worsen, or both. Both the anticipated challenges and the novel limitations required that she use a variety of coping mechanisms to overcome them:

> You know the biggest piece of advice I would give, and one that I've lived by too, is you've got to stay positive.
>
> I think that the period of time where I didn't feel well, I started to realize that if the house wasn't dusted, it wasn't the end. If everything wasn't perfect, it wasn't the end. Or for dinners, I just started thinking, okay we'll have sandwiches tonight, we don't need to have a big, nice dinner.

Self-Worth from Productivity

Throughout the interviews it became very clear that Florence derived her sense of self-worth from being able to accomplish tasks. She believes this started in childhood and was reinforced by the way her mother raised her. She struggled greatly with her drive to be productive during the times her MS symptoms limited her ability to work. Her MS limited her abilities in many ways: fatigue, weakness, inability to use her extremities, parasethias, and cognitive dysfunction. The transcripts were reviewed very closely and the sense of self-worth was never discussed without being associated with productivity:

> My worth is what I can get done and what I can accomplish.
>
> No one was going to know . . . to me to be disabled was oh, you can no longer be productive, that's the way I looked at it.
>
> My family was good about that. They didn't . . . oh, here, let me do that . . . because some days I would have welcomed that, you know. But I would have gotten accustomed to that, too. And, you know what, that's not good. Everybody needs to feel worth. You know that they're contributing something.

Discussion

Florence used the skepticism of others to motivate her to achieve her goals time and time again. For her, it was the most powerful source of motivation. She was able to take the negativity of others and turn it into fuel for her endeavors. Although this type of motivation may not be the most appropriate method for a healthcare provider in all cases because it could have a poor outcome for some, it sheds some light on the potential variety of motivators. These findings show that some patients may respond to being challenged.

The current available literature is aimed in two primary areas: school achievement for children and adolescents and advancement in the workplace. The paucity of available data in this area and the repeated implication that specific motivational styles significantly affected the participant's success suggest a need for further research.

The data revealed in this study appear to support the altered quality of life caused by MS-related fatigue that has been reported in MS literature (Merkelbach, Sittinger, & Koenig, 2002). The study participant described the overwhelming effects both physically and cognitively that fatigue had on nearly every aspect of her life. In fact, it was her own horrible experience with fatigue that inspired her to create her unique intervention for fatigue. Finding relief for MS-related fatigue opened doors for the participant that would have otherwise stayed closed. The data collected in this study seem to suggest that finding ways to ameliorate fatigue in persons with MS may act as a precursor for success. The treatment of Florence's fatigue provided her with the energy and cognitive clarity she needed to create and refine her own intervention for fatigue. The data of this study did not seem to support the findings of Parmenter, Denney, and Lynch (2003), which suggest no differences in cognitive function related to fatigue severity. Florence described increased cognitive difficulties during times of increased fatigue.

The concept of coping in persons with MS is present in the literature (Aikens, Fischer, Namey, & Rudick, 1997; Jean, Paul, & Beatty, 1999; Mills & Allen, 2000). The data in this study suggest it was essential for the participant to find ways of coping to adjust to her disease. In fact, she found many different ways of coping with her disease and the circumstances it presented. Through denial, acceptance, redefining what was important, and focusing on the positive aspects of life Florence was able to find peace with her illness and limitations. This idea is consistent with research that points to people with MS utilizing a variety of different coping mechanisms.

Currently, there is a lack of research data associating self-worth and productivity. The findings of this study suggest that productivity, or the amount one accomplishes, can greatly affect how one feels about themselves. Such findings have practical implications for allied healthcare fields such as vocational rehabilitation, occupational therapy, physical therapy, and recreational therapy. Staying productive and accomplishing self-defined goals is an essential piece of healthy living for MS patients and can often be accomplished with the help of allied health services. As discussed earlier, the study participant never spoke of self-worth except within the context of her accomplishments. This indicates how critical productivity can be to one's life. The deficiency of data in this area in conjunction with the participant's powerful message regarding the impact of productivity on her self-worth illustrates a need for further investigation on the topic.

"Making Sense out of the Madness": A Life History of Successfully Overcoming Grief (Peil)

This informant was known to the investigator as someone who experienced the loss of her husband approximately 15 years previously, when he died in his early thirties after a short illness. At the time, Kate (a pseudonym) lived with her husband and their two small children in a West Coast suburban area. The couple shared a career in the social services, working primarily with developmentally disabled adults. Together, they also founded a summer camp that mixed children from poor and well-to-do backgrounds, and eventually they integrated developmentally disabled children into this camp as well. Kate and her husband shared dreams that they made into a reality of service to others. Shortly after his death, Kate changed direction and began to do grief work, first in a hospital working with children and later in a school. A couple of years after his death, Kate moved to the Pacific Northwest and created a practice to counsel other widowed persons. Her current urban practice includes private counseling, support groups, retreats, and children's support after the death of a parent. It is expanding to incorporate other holistic elements, such as homeopathy and massage.

Kate defines her success at overcoming grief as, "the ability to move through the intense part of the pain . . . coping with the situation until the point at which . . . I reinvested in life. . . ." She continues, "Success would mean living a full life again, or having a life that felt . . . full and whole. I'm not living in the pain anymore, I'm happy in my life,

I'm fulfilled." Her definition corresponds well with the following previously published definition: "to adapt successfully despite the presence of significant adversity." Now, more than a decade after the loss of her husband, Kate considers herself healed.

Concepts

Expressing Grief

Kate's mother died when she was 20, and at that time no one around her expressed any outward emotion. "My dad couldn't even mention her name . . . could barely look at me 'cause I looked just like her. I mean everything about the grief experience was kinda sick." Kate learned from this experience. "When [my husband] died, I knew how I *wasn't* going to do it. And that was by pretending everything was okay." In fact, when asked what, if anything, was easy after the loss of her husband, Kate says, "Well, I didn't have a hard time grieving. That was easy. Some people do; they can't cry."

During the interviews Kate discussed the importance of letting emotion out through various media, including meditation, yoga, journaling, and even swimming. This is in addition to expressing grief verbally with friends, family, counselors, and a support group. It is important "to express your grief in healthy ways and get it out, not just let it simmer . . . you know, not being in a vacuum and just keeping it all inside." She also mentions the importance of humor during such a hard time: "I could *never* have gotten through without my sense of humor." Whereas stifling grief leads to poor outcomes, expression of grief through as many avenues as possible allows the griever to let it out and begin to work through the long process.

Seeking Social Support

When Kate's mother died, "I got *no* support. *Nobody* knew how to help me. I mean it was gross." When her husband died, Kate took an active role and reached out to find help. Kate credits a wide variety of people and other supports for helping her overcome her grief. "I feel like my therapist saved my life . . . I mean, of course, I would've but I didn't— I *feel* like I couldn't have." In addition to individual therapy, Kate participated in a group for those recently widowed. "I can't even imagine doing it without a support group."

Not surprisingly, Kate developed a new network of widowed friends from her support groups, and for awhile after her husband's death she felt more comfortable associating with her newly widowed friends than with her close-knit group of established friends. "I mean, I kind of didn't want to be with our [common] friends very much initially after he died, just because it was too painful. . . . I got really involved with some other widows that were in my group . . . and they were probably the people I wanted to be with the most during that time. . . . I didn't have to be mad at my widow friends 'cause they were in the same boat as me."

Though she lived in the southwestern United States when her husband passed away, Kate had a close friend in the Pacific Northwest who, at the time, was in graduate school and still single. Because this friend had a close-knit group of friends of her own, Kate "escaped" to visit them often and ended up moving to the Northwest 2 years after her husband died. "[My friends in the Northwest] weren't married yet, you know, [they] were single, so I fit better with them—even though I was a bit older—than I fit with my old friends."

In addition to the above factors, Kate says she "couldn't have gotten through it without [my husband's] family. . . ." She states the importance of having an established group of friends before being widowed. "You're not always beautiful in grief . . . so if you have some—a good track record before, usually your friends can kinda hang in." More than simply expressing grief individually, it is crucial to seek the support of others in similar situations as well as those who know how to help guide through the grief experience.

Spirituality

At least as important as the support of other people, Kate emphasizes spirituality, in a broad sense, as among the most important of factors that help widows overcome the death of a spouse. She views spirituality as the belief that, "There's something more than just chaos . . . something greater than just us as individuals. You can see that something greater if two people come together . . . caring about each other or extend[ing] love." Her idea of spirituality ascribes meaning to an event that may not have made any sense before.

"'Spiritual' sounds religious to people and I don't mean religion; I mean . . . spirit, but some people aren't comfortable with that concept. But, it exists for everyone whether it's called that or not. . . . I talk with people about . . . you know your spiritual hammock—that there's something that kind of holds you in the universe or something. And so being in touch with that—not necessarily defining it, but having a sense that you're not just in this . . . world that has no, that it's just this chaotic thing." Kate never explicitly mentions God. Instead, she emphasizes spirituality as something that helps one ascribe meaning to an experience that at first makes no sense.

In the process of making sense of something so chaotic, Kate also discusses the importance of "going deeper." "What I try to do with people is help them get a sense that grief is something that you move through, and that as you move through it, you go deeper, and what I mean by deeper is spiritually deeper. I may not use that word with people but that is what happens is spiritually you're going deeper so you're connecting to something more." Spirituality, that is, "going deeper" to find meaning in the grief experience, is crucial to its positive outcome.

Helping Others

Several times Kate mentions the fact that her husband was also a helper, not only in his career but in helping neighbors with gardening projects. In addition to working together in special education, he and Kate also founded "a camp for kids, mixing inner-city kids with rich kids, and . . . trying to kind of have positive things come from that mix. And we ended up also adding developmentally disabled adults and kids."

> I remember right after he died, I started thinking . . . about doing something around intensive care units and how I wanted to make some changes in the hospital situation to support the families and patients, and then it kind of shifted to wanting to

have this center. That was . . . practically from the moment of [my husband's] death that I really started kind of thinking about, okay, what would it be and. . . ? And mostly it was because I needed *so* much and my kids needed *so* much. . . . I went back [to the hospital] a few months after he died and spoke about what was horrible and what was good . . . they need more training on grief.

Around the same time she began volunteering at the hospital where her husband died. "I started volunteering there in the bone marrow transplant unit with kids, thinking . . . I don't know, I just knew I needed to do that. I can't believe I would. I *hate* hospitals. I hate— I mean I can't believe that I went back into that hospital day after day."

It was very painful for Kate to continue working in the same job after her husband died, and after a few months she moved on to other work.

I felt as passionate about special ed when I was in my special ed life as I do about this I think . . . I was *definitely* passionate about that and I thought, 'I will never do anything else in my whole life. I love this work.' And then, you know, this big thing happened and I completely went off on a whole different path.

However, she never stopped serving others who were vulnerable. She worked for the school system and another hospital before moving to the Northwest and founding the center where she works now.

I've always been in the social service field. . . . I mean I don't feel like the work I do now is so different from the work I used to do. It's just a different group of people.

Almost from the moment of his death, Kate had plans to create a multifaceted center for others who had experienced the loss of a partner at a young age as well as for their children.

So I started thinking, what I really would love to have is this retreat place . . . that would be kind of set apart from the real world or something, where we would have this place where people could come, with their kids . . . there would be massage and a hot tub and . . . just this warmth and nurturing and support. And people could come and do a retreat, and just kind of get support, they would get support, and they'd just be able to kind of rejuvenate, and then go back and kind of suffer through the week. . . . So anyway, I started talking with friends about [this dream] and we'd make jokes about it . . . it was just kind of this huge part of my life was this dream of having this someday . . . we just talked about it a lot, and for me it was a thing that helped me live . . . made some sense out of the madness. . . . sustained me in some really deep way. I remember thinking . . . am I just dreaming about this because I need something to hold onto while I get through this? And I thought, well it doesn't really matter.

When she decided to found the center where she works now, it seemed to come naturally. "So that was really helpful. . . . I mean I had experience in some of that kind of stuff, and in community too. . . . Everything kind of came together from the different parts of my life in a good way." "It's so weird how when somebody dies, how your life just, like, goes this totally different way . . . but [this is] partly why I love working with people so much because I can see how huge it is, you know, when somebody dies. And, it's like, I *really* get it." Transforming grief into something to help others through similar processes benefits both the helper and the more newly bereaved.

Discussion

The key informant of this study reiterated time and again the importance of getting grief out and not keeping it stifled, which is supported by Erich Lindeman, who observed that avoidance of intense pain and expression led to less effective grieving (Schwartz-Borden,1992). Kate's strategies of expression through talking, reading, writing, and swimming concur with the literature that emotional expression is very important in the resolution of grief (Maercker, Bonanno, Znoj, & Horowitz, 1998).

Many others have cited the support factors of family and friends in particular in aiding effective grief (Clauss-Ehlers & Levi, 2002; Greeff & Human, 2004; Kaunonen, Tarkka, Paunonen, & Laippala, 1999; Larson & Dearmont, 2002; Walters & Simoni, 2002). Like much of the research, Kate reported the importance of social support, particularly through friends (new recently widowed friends as well as established friends) and her husband's family.

Hutch (2000) believes that that essence of a "spiritual life" is converting loss into gain, regardless of a person's religious beliefs. In fact, this very accurately describes what Kate did through her grief. Her definition of spirituality— "making some sense out of the madness"—closely matches Hutch's description. Quite interestingly, the fact that Kate moved through her grief to help others through theirs shows how she turned loss into gain not only spiritually, but in a very tangible way as well. On the other hand, Kate never explicitly mentions the idea that her personal losses could have been much worse in spite of the heartache they cause, as Hutch also suggests is the essence of human spirituality (2000).

Kaunonen et al. (1999) discussed the helpfulness to the bereaved of not only accepting support, but of reaching out to other grieving family members. Kate took this a step further and now not only works on behalf of helping her own family, but of helping widowed persons in her greater metropolitan area. Her personality has clearly been a helping one through her whole life, but being widowed herself shifted her focus to helping others in similar situations.

Conclusion

Life history is a methodology that offers insight into the factors that key informants perceive as contributory to their success. Examining the life histories of an MS patient, colostomy patient, and individual grieving for a lost spouse, one can gain perspective on the similarities inherent in the success of persons facing chronic illness and loss. Although these studies examine stories that are vastly different in origin and only investigate one key informant from that culture, the universal concepts that surface are helpful in illuminating possible future research topics for development of interventions to assist these groups of patients. The three commonalities that emerge from the exploration of these life histories include coping, support, and desire to help others.

Coping

Coping with chronic illness and loss was foundational for all three life histories. With regard to Olivia, the colostomy patient, her ability to cope was intertwined with her pursuit of information regarding her condition. She sought out educational resources from books, online resources, and informed individuals so that she had better understanding of her life-changing body-altering surgery. Learning about the diet regime and ostomy equipment also enabled her become proactive in her health care and gave her insight into some of the complications that occur with poor diet and equipment failure. Furthermore, knowledge gave her confidence to examine the commonalities of successes and challenges others with ostomies faced, thereby appreciating her own experience and allowing her to cope.

Likewise, Florence, the MS patient, learned to cope both with her chronic illness and with the subsequent complications that emerged from this disease process. She remained positive and began developing more realistic goals and expectations for herself, which took into consideration her fatigue. Florence began to realize that everything did not have to be perfect and that it was okay to forgo some of the small tasks that she always tried to complete before her diagnosis. Developing her intervention for MS-related fatigue also was a mechanism allowing her to cope. She believed that by combating her fatigue, she was better able to meet her goals and activities of daily living.

When Kate lost her husband, she began coping by expressing her grief. She knew that internalizing grief and allowing it to simmer was unhealthy. Kate cried and verbalized her grief to family, friends, and counselors. Furthermore, she talked of the importance of spirituality in understanding the death experience. Delving into spirituality gave her peace and the ability to cope with the devastating loss of her husband.

Support

Support was especially important to Olivia, who sought the help and presence of positive family members and friends. She needed acceptance because of body image changes and the taboo of colostomy surgery. Family and friends who were willing to discuss her surgery and condition demonstrated abiding support and acceptance of her. Her husband was also seen as a special support person because of his continual assistance caring her for postoperatively. More importantly, though, he demonstrated the same love and intimacy has always displayed, despite the ostomy and her change of appearance. It was with the support of others that allowed Olivia the confidence to successfully adapt and come to peace with her chronic illness.

Florence describes her support differently. Unlike Olivia, she surrounded herself with individuals who both supported her and doubted her abilities. The negative and skeptical people in her life motivated her to succeed and to prove them wrong. In this way, lack of support offered her a means of support. However, Florence also regards her family as very supportive by providing her with reassurance and by sustaining her self-worth.

When Kate described the first experience she had with death, she noted that she received no support when her mother passed on. Therefore when her husband died she sought others that would give her the support she needed. Kate saw a counselor and also participated in a widow's group. She saw the support of others who had similar experiences with losing a spouse as essential to help move through the grieving process. In fact, she moved to the Pacific Northwest to be close to friends that she felt comfortable with and supported by.

Helping Others

Olivia made it clear that helping others was part of her success and recovery. She became well-informed about colostomies via research and personal experience. Olivia felt obligated and proud to share this information with others facing similar situations. Her participation in her local United Ostomy Association chapter allowed her the chance to talk with others about their current experiences and to discuss with potential patients needing surgery for their chronic illnesses. Furthermore, she is creating a brochure that offers tips and suggestions to make ostomy life a little easier. Development of educational materials that are surprisingly lacking for ostomy patients is her contribution and legacy.

Florence developed an intervention to help combat MS-related fatigue. Her own struggle with fatigue was encompassing all aspect of her life and limiting her ability to meet her goals. Although this intervention was developed for her own use, she shares it with other MS patients battling this relentless exhaustion. She has helped others live a more normal life, despite this chronic illness.

Kate's work helping others precedes her husband's death by working in social services with disabled and impoverished youth. However, after her husband's passing she knew she needed to help others, especially those grieving for loved ones who have died. Initially, Kate volunteered with children in a bone marrow transplant unit, despite her dislike for hospitals. When she moved to the Northwest, she then founded a center for individuals who lost a partner and their children. She has helped others face the death of someone close and develop healthy coping skills to successfully grieve.

These resilient women transcended their own distress and not only survived successfully but also found unique ways to help others who experience similar suffering. Their stories serve as powerful reminder to nurses of the healing power of making the decision to succeed.

Acknowledgment

We are grateful to Dr. Kathleen Martín, Professor, Department of Anthropology, Florida International University, for her early guidance and support in learning the life history approach.

References

Aikens, J. E., Fischer, J. S., Namey, M., & Rudick, R. A. (1997). A replicated prospective investigation of life stress, coping, and depressive symptoms in multiple sclerosis. *Journal of Behavioral Medicine, 20*, 433–445.

Beery, T., Sommers, M., & Hall, J. (2002). Focused life stories of women with cardiac pacemakers. *Western Journal of Nursing Research, 24*(1), 7–27.

Bekkers, M. J., Van Knippenberg, F. C., Van Den Borne, H. W., Poen, H., Bergsma, J., & Van Berge Henegouwen, G. P. (1995). Psychosocial adaptation to stoma surgery: A review. *Journal of Behavioral Medicine, 18,* 1–31.

Black, P. (2004). Psychological, sexual, and cultural issues for patients with a stoma. *British Journal of Nursing, 13,* 692–697.

Clauss-Ehlers, C. S., & Levi, L. L. (2002). Violence and community, terms in conflict: An ecological approach to resilience. *Journal of Social Distress and the Homeless, 11,* 265–278.

Davison, J. (1989). *Voices from Mutira: Change in the lives of rural Gikuyu women.* Boulder, CO: Lynne Reinner.

de Chesnay, M. (2005). "Can't keep me down": Life histories of successful African Americans. In M. de Chesnay (Ed.), *Caring for the vulnerable: Perspectives in nursing theory, practice, and research* (pp. 221–231). Sudbury, MA: Jones and Bartlett.

de Chesnay, M., Marshall, E., & Clements, C. (1988). Family structure, marital power, maternal distance, and paternal alcohol consumption in father-daughter incest. *Family Systems Medicine, 6*(4), 453–462.

Early, E. (1993). *Baladi women: Playing with an egg and a stone.* Boulder, CO: Lynne Reinner.

Gmelch, S. (1986). *Nan: The life of an Irish traveling woman.* Prospect Heights, IL: Waveland.

Greeff, A. P., & Human, B. (2004). Resilience in families in which a parent has died. *American Journal of Family Therapy, 32,* 27–42.

Hagemaster, J. (1992). Life history: A qualitative method of research. *Journal of Advanced Nursing, 17,* 1122–1128.

Hall, J. (1996). Geography of childhood sexual abuse: Women's narratives of their childhood environment. *Advances in Nursing Science, 18*(4), 29–47.

Hutch, R. A. (2000). Mortal losses, vital gains: The role of spirituality. *Journal of Religion and Health, 39,* 329–337.

James, D. (2000). *Doña María's story.* Durham, NC: Duke University.

Jean, V. M., Paul, R. H., & Beatty, W. W. (1999). Psychological and neurological predictors of coping patterns by patients with multiple sclerosis. *Journal of Clinical Psychology, 55,* 21–26

Kaunonen, M., Tarkka, M.-T., Paunonen, M., & Laippala, P. (1999). Grief and social support after the death of a spouse. *Journal of Advanced Nursing, 30,* 1304–1311.

Larson, N. C., & Dearmont, M. (2002). Strengths of farming communities in fostering resilience in children. *Child Welfare, 81,* 821–835.

Levy, M. (1988). *Each in her own way: Five women leaders of the developing world.* Boulder, CO: Lynne Reinner.

Maercker, A., Bonanno, G. A., Znoj, H., & Horowitz, M. J. (1998). Prediction of complicated grief by positive and negative themes in narratives. *Journal of Clinical Psychology, 54,* 1117–1136.

Mattingly, C., & Lawlor, M. (2000). Learning from stories: Narrative interviewing in cross-cultural research. *Scandinavian Journal of Occupational Therapy, 7,* 4–14.

McGoldrick, M., & Gerson, R. (1986). *Genograms in family assessment.* New York: W. W. Norton.

McGoldrick, M., Gerson, R., & Shellenberger, S. (1999). *Genograms: Assessment and intervention.* New York: W. W. Norton.

Merkelbach, S., Sittinger, H., & Koenig, J. (2002). Is there a differential impact of fatigue and physical disability on quality of life in multiple sclerosis? *The Journal of Nervous and Mental Disease, 190,* 388–393.

Mills, N., & Allen, J. (2000). Mindfulness of movement as a coping strategy in multiple sclerosis: A pilot study. *General Hospital Psychiatry, 22*, 425–431.

Parmenter, B. A., Denney, D. R., & Lynch, S. G. (2003). The cognitive performance of patients with multiple sclerosis during periods of high and low fatigue [Electronic version]. *Multiple Sclerosis, 9,* 111–118.

Scheub, H., Mack, B., Schildkrout, E., Obbo, C., Wilks, I., Romero, P., et al. (1988). *Life histories of African women.* London: Ashfield.

Schwartz-Borden, G. (1992). Metaphor—visual aid in grief work. *Omega: Journal of Death & Dying, 25,* 239–248.

Sexton, J. D. (1981). *Son of Tecún Umán: A Maya Indian tells his life story.* Prospect Heights, IL: Waveland.

Walters, K. L., & Simoni, J. M. (2002). Reconceptualizing Native women's health: An "indigenist" stress-coping model. *American Journal of Public Health, 92,* 520–524.

"Staying with HIV/AIDS": A Compressed Ethnography of Zambian Women

Terra Grandmason

As the leading cause of death in sub-Saharan Africa, HIV/AIDS results in severe physical, economic, and social disturbances. Women represent 57% of HIV infections in Africa, with Zambian women 1.4 times more likely to be infected than men (United Nations General Assembly Special Session on HIV/AIDS, 2005). This study explores the experiences of women in Zambia who face unique socioeconomic and sociocultural challenges while bearing the greatest disease burden.

This ethnography sought to increase understanding of how Zambian women living with HIV/AIDS subsist in an environment where supports may be nonexistent or strained to the breaking point. The focal question asked was in what form and to what extent is support present in the women's lives. The answer emerged as a detailed account of enduring and overcoming uncertainty and loss, drawing a picture of how nine impoverished Zambian women are "staying with HIV," the local syntax used to describe their HIV-positive status, denoting a life permanently impacted by an incurable, impairing, and fatal virus. The research question was in what form and to what extent is support present in the lives of HIV-positive low-income Zambian women?

Literature Review

In addition to social and emotional needs, support needs among women living with HIV in sub-Saharan Africa may include food, money, medicine, physical assistance, future orphan care, and health teaching (Harding, Stewart, Marconi, O'Neill, & Higginson, 2003; Plattner & Meiring, 2006). Meeting these needs are complicated amid deteriorating resources due to prolonged poverty, urbanization, and the impact of HIV/AIDS on local and national economies (Dyson, 2003; UNAIDS, 2004; World Bank, 2005). In South Africa and Zambia, monthly incomes fell 66–80% in households affected by AIDS (Barnett & Whiteside, 2002; Steinberg et al., 2002).

Because men were disproportionately affected early in the HIV/AIDS epidemic, single-parent households are now largely female headed (Moore & Vaughan, 1994; Niehaus,

1994; UNAIDS/UNFPA/UNIFEM, 2004; World Bank, 2005). Marital rates in the region are decreasing, and widows may be unable to find new partners to help provide for them (Hunter, 2007; World Bank, 2005). Limited employment opportunities may be further hindered by HIV-related pain or fatigue, forcing women to rely on such uncertain work as selling produce or transactional sex (Hunter, 2007; Keogh, Allen, Almedal, & Temahagili, 1994).

Widespread stigma associated with HIV/AIDS is another obstacle to support. The risk of eviction, rejection, or shame from social networks and potential discrimination in accessing financial, educational, and occupational resources often result in women hiding their HIV status (MANET, 2003; Plattner & Meiring, 2006). This increases isolation and decreases the likelihood of women accessing available supports (Ciambrone, 2002). Women often face blame, condemnation, and accusations of promiscuous sexual behavior if their HIV status is discovered (Panos Institute, UNICEF, 2001). Negative social consequences may also emerge from life-style alterations such as choosing not to breast-feed or not to have more children (Lawson, 1999).

Psychosocial support is important for dealing with the struggles of real and feared discrimination, unmet needs, and the difficult act of disclosing one's status (Ciambrone, 2002; Chaava, 1990; Kayawe, Kelly, & Baggaley, 1998; Uys, 2003). It also improves retention of HIV-related information, overall well-being, and performance of daily duties despite insomnia, pain, or fatigue (Eisenberg, Kemeny, & Wyatt, 2003; Hughes, Jelsma, Maclean, Darder, & Tinise, 2004; Keogh et al., 1994; UNFPA, 2006). This is important because depression and suicidal ideation often occur after discovery of HIV status (Keogh et al., 1994; Plattner & Meiring, 2006; Swindells et al., 1999). However, acceptance of one's own HIV-positive status and the establishment of a closer relationship with a higher power were found to contribute to well-being and a sense that there must be a purpose for one's HIV infection (Plattner & Meiring, 2006).

As well as facing a unique set of obstacles due to a disadvantaged social and economic position, women also share the wider African experience of lacking desperately needed resources and services. Women carry a greater burden of stigma surrounding HIV/AIDS, which limits their willingness to access supports. Despite general acknowledgment that support is beneficial, it is unclear to what extent different supports are present or impact the lives of women. In sub-Saharan Africa where a variety of factors impact the existence and access to support, few studies explore the experience of support among HIV-positive women. For the purposes of this study, no published literature was found that focused on support among HIV-positive Zambian women.

Methodology

This research was conducted using a compressed ethnographic research design to accommodate a shortened research time frame (LeCompte & Schensul, 1999).

TABLE 18-1. **Participant Demographics**

Marriage status	Widowed 78%	Married 11%	Unknown 11%
Work status	Unable 44%	Sporadic 33%	Stable job 22%
Had children	Yes 100%	No 0%	Unknown 0%
Experienced death of at least one child	Yes 56%	No 0%	Unknown 44%
Caring for orphans	Yes 33%	No 22%	Unknown 44%
Participate in community outreach	Yes 78%	No 11%	Unknown 11%
Taking anti-retro-virals (ARVs)	Yes 56%	No 22%	Unknown 11%
Disclosed status to > 1 important friend or family member	Yes 78%	No 22%	Unknown 0%
Belong to HIV/AIDS support group	Yes 78%	No 22%	Unknown 0%

Sample

A purposive sample of nine women was obtained. Women ranged in age from 38 to 48 years, with education levels ranging from grades 7 to 12. All participants were accessing outpatient services at the hospice. Further demographics are shown in Table 18-1. The women's experiences and perspectives of support were explored during the interview, and their stories were analyzed for this study. Interviews with local nongovernmental organization heads and HIV/AIDS service providers were also conducted to verify data interpretation and to provide a broader perspective of support available to the sample population.

Setting

One of the poorest nations in the world, Zambia has an AIDS rate of 16.5% among 15- to 49-year-olds (UNDP, 2005; UNAIDS, 2004). Median age is 16 years, and life expectancy is 37.5 years, which has fallen 14 years over the past two decades. In 2003 Zambia instituted free HIV treatment. The semiurban AIDS hospice in Lusaka Province, where this study was conducted, is one of many locations providing this free HIV treatment. Participants in this study resided in surrounding densely populated compounds, which are illegally created shantytowns now largely considered legal residences and house the majority of Zambians (Kunda, 2004).

Data Collection and Analysis

Data were collected over 4.5 weeks through participant observation and open-ended interviews, allowing research to be guided by cultural concepts. Follow-up interviews were not conducted because of time constraints. Cultural informants and AIDS-based organizations and agencies provided feedback and assistance to ensure accurate data interpretation. Participant observations and informal discussions were recorded by note-taking in a daily diary.

Interviews

A semistructured questionnaire consisting of nine broad open-ended questions guided interviews. Key cultural informants provided feedback on interview approach, question design, and English syntax used in questions. Three pilot interviews were conducted in Nyanja with translation assistance before deciding to conduct interviews one-on-one in English to increase privacy and confidentiality and to control how questions were asked and interpreted. It is critical to note that the interview guide in ethnographic research is almost never final, and each key informant was approached as an individual within her own immediate context. All interviews were conducted in a safe and private location and tape-recorded as per consent.

Participants considering participation were provided the equivalent of US $2, the cost of two local meals. This was approved by cultural informants as an appropriate sum that was not so great that women would feel coerced to participate. It was clarified with women that compensation for considering the interview was theirs to keep, and they were not obliged to consent to or participate in the research.

Participant Observation

The researcher lived primarily with a local Zambian female-headed household, the residents of which were key cultural informants. She also resided part time on hospice grounds, with patients and staff acting as key cultural informants. Participant observation occurred in both locations. At the hospice this occurred during volunteer work, support group meetings, home-care visits, discussions, and interactions with patients and staff. Away from the hospice this was conducted at social gatherings, meals, meetings with organizations, and walking or traveling daily on local buses.

Limitations

Without being conducted in local languages, the depth and comprehensiveness of the data may be constrained. To maximize the ability of the researcher to conduct her own interviews, cultural informants and research participants were selected with relatively high English proficiency, which resulted in a higher than average education level among participants. Also, the time allocated for data collection was sufficient to complete the research but prevented follow-up interviews with the nine interviewees.

Data Analysis

Nine participant interviews were analyzed, at which point data saturation was reached. Using de Chesnay's (2005) qualitative data analysis format, transcripts and notes were confidentially coded for emerging categories, themes, and concepts. Coded and interpreted data were shared with cultural informants for further analysis and feedback. These data were not shared with participants because of the short time frame and challenges contacting and locating participants before the study ended. Triangulation through interviews, observations, and feedback from key informants helped ensure accuracy of procedures and findings. Careful field notes were kept and reviewed regularly.

Findings

Four major concepts emerged from interviews with the nine participants on the topic of support: uncertainty, encouragement, staying with HIV, and free mind.

Uncertainty

Uncertainty emerged as an ever-present threat and source of hope for women both before and after knowing their HIV status. Uncertainty was the constant awareness that one's situation could change rapidly and unexpectedly at any moment. Uncertainty complicated the struggle to secure food, housing, medical care, income, children's education, and children's futures. Women described uncertainty in their ability to control interactions with men, including husbands, and in predicting reactions to their HIV status. Institutional uncertainty was acknowledged in the form of corruption and unreliable service sectors. Although uncertainty appeared to afford hope that a situation could improve unexpectedly, it was most often described as contributing to loss, fear, and grief.

Loss was a significant component of uncertainty, including lost husbands, children, siblings, relationships, jobs, health and physical abilities, normalcy, and the will to live. The desire to prevent more loss was expressed by many, and past losses were described as painful reminders of needs no longer met. One woman described losing family members, and a critical support source, due to HIV:

> There are a number lost. All my elder brothers, they are all gone. Then my immediate brothers, they are all gone. . . . I'm missing my sisters. . . . The one who was so close to me, she was fond of me. When I saw her sick, I didn't want her to be sick. Even when she died, even now, because she used to go to South Africa, most of the time when I see these trucks I think—maybe she's coming. And I forget that she's dead, she's gone for good. So now I'm lonely, she used to encourage me. We used to play together most of the time. Whatever we used to do, she was there next to me.

Encouragement

Encouragement was described as an expression of concern, providing assurance that women's lives were valued and worth living. It was seen as an expression of faith that women could and should continue forward. Encouragement was derived from the physical presence of others, physical acts of support such as assistance during illness, supportive words, or material and financial gifts and loans. Self-encouragement was derived from personal resolve, prayer, faith, a connection with God, and a sense of purpose. Encouragement assisted women to seek their HIV status and reinforced their ability to stay with HIV.

To Seek Status

Encouragement to go for HIV testing was reported to be an influencing factor in the decision to get tested. This occurred through education about HIV symptoms and risk factors and assurance that women would be supported or have a future if found to be HIV positive. Despite numerous factors influencing the decision to test, most women ultimately credited the encouragement of healthcare providers who had informed them about symptoms and risks. Assurances were provided through free anti-retro-virals (ARVs), an expanding service sector assisting those with HIV/AIDS, and a perceived decrease in stigma. One woman shared her perception on the evolving social and medical context surrounding HIV/AIDS:

> That time when you used to hear about HIV/AIDS, [people] used to fear. We had that fear. You say "hah! I have to die" and you have to keep it to yourself. It's not like the way it is now . . . now it's open, a number of people, they want to help . . . Now I say, I do think if this drug, free drugs were there that time when my brothers and sisters were sick, I think this time, they were going to be well . . . they were going to be there, they were going to be helped.

To Stay with HIV

Encouragement was reported to contribute to self-acceptance of HIV status while assisting women to continue "staying with HIV" amid uncertainty, illness, pain, depression, and other daily struggles. Encouragement by family members was provided through physical, emotional, material, and financial support. Encouragement was also gained through faith, personal beliefs, supportive gestures, organizations, and supportive policies assisting women to seek testing, access treatment, learn about HIV, accept their status, implement self-care behaviors, and maintain hope and belief in their future. Support groups were highly valued sources of encouragement, teaching women how to live with HIV while providing a forum to share experiences and escape feelings of isolation or loneliness, as one woman stated:

> When I joined the support group, life for me changed because I also receive encouragement from my fellow friends. When we meet together, you can see that

we are not the only one going through it, this HIV virus, there are many. So, we encourage each other.

Women valued the encouragement during illness, particularly not being left alone with their thoughts and being assisted to eat, walk, take medications, and maintain hygiene. Encouragement was also important to continue accessing health care and treatment despite ongoing challenges such as affording transportation and enduring physical pain or side effects. One woman described the encouragement her father provided:

> My father encouraged me, in fact . . . when I started taking my drugs, I informed dad about it. . . . Then he said "ok, its ok, look, continue. Maybe you, your life will be prolonged. It's not you alone, there are a number of people . . . no, as long as you are well, it's ok. Because you'll continue doing things on your own. . . . If you get better, its better you do things, what you can manage you'll be able to do . . . you'll be helping your children also. You'll raise up those children, you'll see that to the time when they grow up, and then when they will be married also."

Staying with HIV

"Staying with HIV" is the central concept emerging from this study. This term was used by participants to describe the process of living with HIV, with the understanding that the virus had moved permanently into their lives. This process began after women accepted their status and involved piecing together support, normalizing life with HIV, and finding purpose.

Piecing Together Support

This process of seeking and accessing various resources promoted daily survival and helped prevent or manage HIV-related complications. This occurred through the piecing together of financial, nutritional, shelter, physical, medical, educational, decisional, social, emotional, and spiritual/religious support. Women highlighted the necessity of being "open" to receiving support, expressing both gratitude for support received and frustration over the ongoing struggle and inability to provide for themselves. Many felt resented, and alluded to guilt or shame, for having to ask for help. Although anyone could be a potential support, identified sources are shown in Table 18-2. These were mentioned during the open interview process and were not derived from comprehensive surveying of support sources.

Short-term or temporary support came in the form of monetary or nutritional gifts and loans from family, friends, and churches and in the form of physical support during acute illness from family and healthcare providers and from "piece work," such as a one-day or week-long job. Long-term or ongoing support came from educational resources improving understanding of HIV, consequently informing women's decisions and actions. Support groups, counselors, friends, and healthcare providers were identified as education sources:

> I get advice from the doctors, they teach us to look after ourselves carefully, to maintain good diet. It's something which was difficult to know, to really know that a good diet would be helping someone [with HIV] be strong. We always said, "since I get a low salary, I just buy whatever I buy, as long as the days are going." But this time I've learned that even some other foods do help . . . even keeping the home clean, even if that means [spending] money.

Family members were identified as sources of ongoing support, providing shared housing, transportation, money for medicines, food, and emotional comfort. Because of the financial struggle faced by families, their support was often described as erratic. As one woman shared, "I've got a sister who I stay with. When they told me to buy medicine, she

TABLE 18-2. Identified Sources of Support

Support Sources (number of categories identified as support for)	Educational/ Information	Emotional	Decisional	Social	Physical	Medical	Nutritional	Financial	Spiritual/ Religious	Shelter
Family (9)	X	X	X	X	X	X	X	X		X
Church/ congregation (7)		X		X	X		X	X	X	X
Friends (7)	X	X	X	X	X		X	X		
Spouse (7)	X		X	X		X	X	X		X
Support groups (6)	X	X	X	X			X		X	
Counselors (5)	X	X	X			X			X	
God/prayer (5)		X	X		X	X			X	
Income generation (5)				X		X	X	X		X
Healing/recovery (4)	X	X	X						X	
Healthcare providers (4)	X		X		X	X				
Others with HIV (4)	X	X	X	X						
Children (3)		X			X	X				
ARVs/medicine (2)					X	X				
Media (1)	X									

buys medicine. Sometimes she can manage, sometimes she cannot . . . when she don't have money I don't buy the medicine."

Dependence on others was reported to be necessary because of the difficulty securing employment, attributed to HIV-related physical limitations, gender, or a lack of opportunity. All women pieced together informal work, although many were currently unable due to physical limitations. "Piece work" was heavily relied on and described as often physically demanding activities such as cleaning and selling vegetables, fish, beer, or transactional sex. One woman offered a reflection on trying to make ends meet:

> You wake up around 4 [am] and you know that the following day you don't have anything [food] to give the children. You just start thinking—what am I going to do? Sometimes poverty, it can lead you in something bad. You plan of something which is not good, at the end of the day, you regret . . . for example, just a man. Yeah a man asks you maybe to sleep with him, because like here, women they know that automatically if you sleep with a man, at the end of it, they will give you something . . . and that something is not that you are going to please yourself. Maybe you've got a family, you've got the children, you're a single parent. When you get that little money you can buy something for the children at home.

There was consensus that the process of piecing together support was ongoing and always difficult. One woman stated, "It's a strange type of life. It's hard, but we have to continue in it, there's nothing else we can do." The mental and emotional strength to continue was attributed to prayer, social interactions, and support groups. Each woman identified God as a major source of support, providing them with hope and working through others to help them. Reflecting on it all, one woman stated, "I can say, we're just, sometimes we're just surviving by God's grace."

Normalizing Life with HIV

Despite an ongoing struggle to survive and awareness that their life was now different from others' lives, women described a process of normalizing life with HIV. This reportedly began after acceptance of their HIV status and occurred through connections with other HIV-positive persons.

Women described support groups as a setting where they shared the experiences and hardships of living with HIV, asked questions, and gained reassurance that they did not face HIV alone. While talking about her HIV support group, one woman stated, "It's a life that I've found to say, it's something normal. Even though you are HIV positive, you are just like any other person, it's only that you are having the virus in your body."

Disclosure was also identified as an indirect component of normalizing life with HIV, because isolation and loneliness were reportedly exacerbated by hiding HIV status. Eight of the nine women interviewed eventually chose to disclose their status to important people in their lives, some disclosing the same day they received test results and others waiting 2 to 3 years. One woman was still unable to tell family, despite the fact they were not identified as a source of support, for fear of being poisoned or otherwise harmed. Overall, disclosure was a positive experience resulting in increased support and understanding:

> I felt isolated by then. It was like I was living in another world. You know when you are keeping something from people, it's like you're in another world. Of which, people don't really know who you are. But as for now, I don't really feel that way because I told them the secret that I have. You know when you are keeping something it's like carrying a burden of which you don't even want anyone to know. But since now everyone knows, even when I get sick they know "oh, it's this [HIV]."

Finding Purpose

This was expressed as a process of finding purpose and meaning in life with HIV. Purpose was derived from the desire to stay alive to ensure the future of children. It was also derived by contributing in some way to the well-being of others. Most women reported that HIV/AIDS outreach work provided purpose and meaning, as one woman stated:

> In my life I really wanted to help people who are sick . . . that's the kind of life I really like to lead. So as for me to find myself here at the hospice, it's really a pleasure. I visit the people that are sick. I help them in any way they want me to help. So I think I'm trying to fulfill what I wanted.

Many of the women whose physical deterioration had reversed after treatment viewed themselves as proof to others that there is life after an HIV diagnosis. Community members reached out to them as HIV experts who could assist others potentially suffering from HIV. A number of the women also believed that HIV had taught them and their families a great deal, as one woman stated:

> I think it was for a purpose that I had to be HIV positive. So that I should know what other people are really going through. So ever since I knew that, I've come to learn a lot . . . it also helped my family to really know what's happening to some people, to really understand some diseases. That's a very good experience.

Finally, most women were assured through their belief in God that there was purpose in their disease status. One woman reflected, "I'm still around, maybe for a purpose. God he reserved my life because, so that I can teach others also."

Free Mind

A free mind was desired by all women and broadly defined as freedom from worry and protection from uncertainty. Worry was attributed to lack of security and uncertainty over food and nutrition, finances, the future of their children, stable shelter, health, and life expectancy. A free mind was achieved in the short term through discovering HIV status, understanding the ongoing illnesses suffered, having food for tomorrow, not being left alone during illness, getting treatment, or engaging in prayer. In the long term a free mind was thought to be acquired through stability (stable finances, nutrition, shelter, and physical health), self-sufficiency (freedom from dependency through employment and physical health), and the knowledge that children's futures were secure (through a designated care provider to prevent orphanhood and complete their education).

Stability

Stability was described as the acquisition of financial security, food security, permanent housing, and the knowledge that a woman could manage her health to remain functional and productive. Stability was also identified as the ability to go to sleep at night without worrying about tomorrow, such as whether she could pay school fees or feed her children.

Self-Sufficiency

Although not necessary to achieve stability, which could be provided by others, self-sufficiency was viewed as financial independence, resulting in overall empowerment and freedom from dependency on others. Despite being in a stable relationship one woman stated, "All I want is a job, so that I should take 100% responsibility for myself." Acquired and maintained through income-generating activities that allowed them to single-handedly maintain stability and secure the future of their children, women largely envisioned opening their own businesses. One woman stated, "If I could create something, I can do business. Here if I can have a shop, I can do business." Each woman reported that getting a business started required upfront resources she could not secure.

Securing a Future for One's Children

The ability to secure their children's future was a long-term goal for the eight women who had living children. Although stability and self-sufficiency enabled women to create a stable future for children, if the women were to die before seeing children into adulthood, this responsibility was seen to fall to others.

All women believed that a permanent house to leave to children would protect them, particularly from a future on the street. Only one woman had a secure house, which was left by her deceased husband. All women believed their children were too young to be on their own and care for each other (children ranged from ages 2 to 19 years), but they agreed that if necessary the children could manage if they had secure housing. One woman stated the following:

> I must have a house. But whatever comes, if it's my death, those children must stay good, they should not suffer, they must be in one place. . . . I'm staying with my mother, and that house of my mother is for my family. So, if I die, those children, they'll never keep them.

All women with living children also valued the education of their children, citing constant concern over the struggle to pay school fees or ensuring future caregivers would continue to educate orphaned children. Education was described by many as a way to ensure their children had a successful future, especially female children.

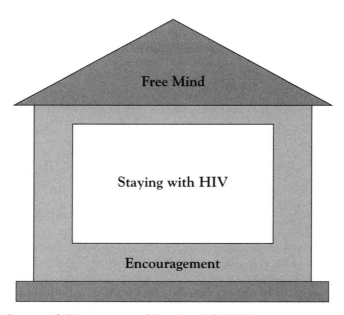

Figure 18-1 Structural Components of Staying with HIV

Discussion

Among the four emergent concepts (uncertainty, encouragement, staying with HIV, and free mind), the concept of staying with HIV was central to the findings and imbued in each of the other concepts: It must proceed on a base of uncertainty, it is strengthened and fostered by encouragement, and it allows the pursuit of a free mind. The interrelationship of these concepts is displayed in Figure 18-1.

Staying with HIV assumes the central position in the model. This concept represents the point at which women acknowledged and accepted that HIV had moved permanently into their lives (as represented in Figure 18-1 by a house or hut). For the women interviewed this consisted of piecing together supports, normalizing life with HIV, and finding purpose in their illness. Consistent with Plattner and Meiring (2006), this study found acceptance of HIV status to be a contributing factor to overall well-being, as was the ability to find meaning in one's illness. It is important to note that the ability of women to stay with HIV was not realized in social isolation but was greatly bolstered through internal and external encouragement.

Encouragement is an umbrella term used by women to describe the many internal and external supports that were both provided to and accessed by them. It contributed to the discovery and acceptance of one's own status and reinforced the process of staying with

HIV and maintaining hope and a vision for the future. Whether attained actively or passively, encouragement appeared to be critical to fostering resiliency and resourcefulness, strengthening the willpower of women to continue staying with HIV despite uncertainty and sometimes intense emotional and physical suffering.

Although a free mind is desirable to most of humanity, the free mind described and sought by participants was not excessive in expectation but challenging in the face of widespread poverty, gender inequality, and limited national or community infrastructure to aid in its realization. In a climate of uncertainty there is wisdom in the desire to achieve self-sufficiency. Yet vehicles must be identified or expanded to boost women's abilities to become self-sufficient.

Conclusion

This study looked at the role and experience of support among HIV-positive Zambian women. It discovered an array of support needs and a complicated interrelationship between support, culture, and poverty among women living with HIV. This study found that among the women interviewed, "staying with HIV" was a dynamic process that was key to survival, personal knowledge, gaining a sense of normalcy, and deriving meaning from life with HIV. To promote and strengthen the process of staying with HIV, the following conclusions are offered:

1. *The most acutely needed form of support is assistance to achieve self-sufficiency.* Women were hard-pressed to meet daily needs and were unable to plan ahead for future needs. They lacked control over the timing, type, quantity, and quality of support provided from any given source. Despite the high value placed on any existing support, they were limited in their reliability and capacity to assist. Economic empowerment leading to self-sufficiency has been found to be a crucial component empowering women to meet subsistence needs, provide for families, and acquire greater control over their lives and bodies (MANET, 2003; Pronyk et al., 2005; Sachs, 2005; SEF/RADAR, 2005).

2. *Encouragement can help promote earlier utilization of free testing services and ultimately decrease morbidity and mortality.* It is not news that barriers to testing still exist despite national policy supporting free testing and treatment. Women choosing to know their HIV status must still reside in an environment perceived to be saturated with fear and stigma surrounding HIV (Guay et al., 1999; Maman, Mbwambo, Hogan, Kilonzo, & Sweat, 2001).

In this study most women attributed their decision to test to encouragement and teachings received from healthcare providers. Most women did not discuss HIV or their plan to test with family or friends before diagnosis, and most did not receive their encouragement to seek testing. Because of the importance of emotional and decisional support from partners, family, and friends, their encouragement directing women to seek testing is critical and must be promoted (Guay et al., 1999; Thabo, 2006).

Most participants waited to test until experiencing the death of a husband or multiple acute or chronic illnesses. Encouragement to seek earlier testing can help decrease the suffering and financial toll inflicted by HIV-related illnesses, possibly prompting life-saving testing of partners or children or preventing mother-to-child transmission.

3. *Fostering a sense of normalcy among HIV-positive women is necessary for well-being.* Most women interviewed highlighted stories about experiencing a sense of normalcy, times they did not feel alone in their struggle with HIV, or where they did not feel "different" from others. This was attributed to the creation and maintenance of relationships with other HIV-positive individuals, particularly within support groups providing ongoing support and counseling (Ciambrone, 2002; Krabbendam, Kuijper, Wolffers, & Drew, 1998).

4. *Finding purpose in life with HIV contributes significantly to meaning and self-worth.* Women appeared to derive significant purpose and meaning from their illness, which was attributed to a deepened understanding of suffering and the realization that they could help to prevent HIV or minimize suffering in others. Women participated in community outreach and education on HIV prevention, education, and promotion of voluntary counseling and testing (VCT). Many women also volunteered to assist others during illnesses or death. The role most of the women played in their own communities as HIV outreach workers was crucial for their own sense of purpose and fulfillment and had the added benefit of addressing stigma and increasing awareness within families and communities.

This study supported the findings of Plattner and Meiring (2006), who found that belief in something greater than oneself contributed to hope and meaning, ultimately assisting those living with HIV to continue forward in life with both purpose and a vision of the future.

The recommendations for healthcare and service providers are as follows:

1. *Strengthen support groups.* Support groups are a critical source of support that must be bolstered with greater informational, material, and financial resources to teach women about HIV and how to live successfully with the virus while providing a supportive setting to create a sense of normalcy. Support groups also have the potential to assist women in accessing other resources, finding purpose in their illness through organized outreach work, and potentially contributing to self-sufficiency by serving as a vehicle for microcredit, cooperative, or reimbursement ventures.

2. *Increase encouragement from healthcare providers.* Encouragement from healthcare providers was effective when women were educated about HIV, symptoms, risks, treatment options, self-care, and medications. All women should be informed

about the benefit of seeking early versus late testing, and those who are HIV positive should be continually educated about HIV and areas where they may be able to self-advocate (e.g., requesting pain medications, company during illness, educating care providers or families, instituting behavior changes). Although women may not immediately seek VCT, encouragement empowers them with the knowledge necessary to recognize and act on symptoms and risks.

3. *Promote and provide incentive for HIV-positive women to engage in community outreach work.* Community outreach by HIV-positive women provided a sense of purpose and was often viewed as a personal or religious calling. By using their lives as an example for others, they increased community understanding of HIV, the needs of those infected, and the prolonged and productive life possible with testing and treatment sought in a timely manner. Incentives to engage in this work could foster the continuation of valuable outreach work increasing community awareness of HIV while also contributing to individual self-sufficiency. Incentives could include financial, nutritional, or material reimbursement. Support groups offer a structure that can and are being used to provide such incentives.

This study serves as an initial investigation using a compressed ethnographic design. Further research is necessary to deeply examine the role of support among women living with HIV/AIDS in Zambia from a variety of angles. This study cannot be considered representative because all participants were accessing medical services and 78% belonged to a support group. The median education level of 10 years was higher than the national average of 6.6 years. These were likely the result of recruiting women conversationally fluent in English who were accessing hospice services. Also, the median age of 41.3 years was higher than statistics noting Zambian women most affected by HIV/AIDS are between the ages of 30 and 34 years (United Nations General Assembly Special Session on HIV/AIDS, 2005). This study should be conducted with HIV-positive women from various educational levels and age ranges. It would be ideal to repeat this study in a rural and an urban locale.

Acknowledgments

Gratitude and deep appreciation are extended to the hospice counselor and the nine women who participated in this study. Special thanks must be given to Dr. Mary de Chesnay, an inspiring professor and exceptional research chair, and Dr. Barbara Anderson, the research committee member whose reviews and edits were invaluable in writing this study. A deeply personal thank-you must also be expressed for the support and mentorship of Dr. Peter Kareiva and the support and encouragement of Carol and Katy Mumba, Auntie Lillian, Michele Brommelsiek, Linda Lovick, Juan Sheenan, Leonard Haamunga, Sr. Stanislawa, Ida Mukuka, Malele Dodia, Thomas Kapakala, Beene, Karolina Sczpakowska, Mulenga Muleba, and Janelle Tuttle.

References

Barnett, T., & Whiteside, A. (2002). *AIDS in the twenty-first century: Disease and globalization*. New York: Palgrave Macmillan.

Chaava T. (1990). Approaches to HIV counseling in a Zambian rural community. *AIDS Care, 2*(1), 81–87.

Ciambrone, D. (2002). Informal networks among women with HIV/AIDS: Present support and future prospects. *Qualitative Health Research, 12*(7), 876–896.

de Chesnay, M. (2005). "Can't keep me down": Life histories of successful African Americans. In M. de Chesnay (Ed.), *Caring for the vulnerable: Perspectives in nursing theory, practice, and research* (pp. 221–231). Sudbury, MA: Jones and Bartlett.

Dyson, T. (2003). HIV/AIDS and urbanization. *Population & Development Review, 29*(3), 427–442.

Eisenberg, N. I., Kemeny, M. E., & Wyatt, G. E. (2003). Psychological inhibition and CD4 T-cell levels in HIV-seropositive women. *Journal of Psychosomatic Research, 54*(3), 213–224.

Guay, L., Musoke, P., Fleming, T., Bagenda, D., Allen, M., Nakabiito, C., et al. (1999). Intrapartum and neonatal single dose nevirapine compared with zidouvodin for prevention of mother-to-child transmission of HIV-1 in Kampala Uganda: HIVNET 012 randomized trial. *Lancet, 354*, 795–802.

Harding, R., Stewart, K., Marconi, K., O'Neill, J. F., & Higginson, I. J. (2003). Current HIV/AIDS end-of-life care in sub-Saharan Africa: a survey of models, services, challenges, and priorities. *BMC Public Health, 3*(33), 1–6.

Hughes, J., Jelsma, J., Maclean, E., Darder, M., & Tinise, X. (2004). The health-related quality of life of people living with HIV/AIDS. *Disability and Rehabilitation, 26*(6), 371–376.

Hunter, M. (2007). The changing political economy of sex in South Africa: The significance of unemployment and inequalities to the scale of the AIDS pandemic. *Social Science & Medicine, 64*, 689–700.

Kayawe, I., Kelly, M., & Baggaley, R. (1998). HIV counseling and testing. *World Health, 51*(6), 12–13.

Keogh, P., Allen, S., Almedal, C., & Temahagili, B. (1994). The social impact of HIV infection on women in Kigali, Rwanda: A prospective study. *Social Science & Medicine, 38*(8), 1047–1053.

Krabbendam, A., Kuijper, B., Wolffers, I., & Drew, R. (1998). The impact of counseling on HIV-positive women in Zimbabwe. *AIDS Care, 10*(suppl. 1), S25–S37.

Kunda, M. (2004). Illegal compounds difficult to provide services-council. *The LRF News*, 48. Retrieved January 9, 2007, from http://www.lrf.org.zm/Newsletter/january2004/features.html

Lawson, A. L. (1999). Women and AIDS in Africa: Sociocultural dimensions of the HIV/AIDS epidemic. *International Social Science Journal, 51*(3), 391–400.

LeCompte, M. D., & Schensul, J. J. (1999). *Designing & conducting ethnographic research. Ethnographer's toolkit, v.1*. Walnut Creek, CA: AltaMira Press.

Maman, S., Mbwambo, J., Hogan, N. M., Kilonzo, G. P., & Sweat, M. (2001). Women's barriers to HIV-1 testing and disclosure: Challenges for HIV-1 voluntary counseling and testing. *AIDS Care, 13*(5), 595–603.

MANET. (2003). *Voices for equality and dignity: Qualitative research on stigma and discrimination issues as they affect PLWHA in Malawi*. Lilongwe, Malawi: Author.

Moore, H., & Vaughan, M. (1994). *Cutting down trees: Gender, nutrition, and agricultural change in the northern province of Zambia, 1890–1990*. Portsmouth, NH: Heinemann.

Niehaus, I. (1994). Disharmonious spouses and harmonious siblings: Conceptualising household formation among urban residents in QwaQwa. *African Studies, 53*(1), 115–135.

Panos Institute, UNICEF. (2001). *Stigma, HIV/AIDS and prevention of mother-to-child transmission: A pilot study in Zambia, India, Ukraine and Burkina Faso.* New York: UNICEF.

Plattner, I. E., & Meiring, N. (2006) Living with HIV: The psychological relevance of meaning making. *AIDS Care, 18*(3), 241–245.

Pronyk, P., Kim, J., Hargreaves, M., Makhubele, M., Morison, L., Watts, C., et al. (2005). Microfinance and HIV prevention: Emerging lessons from rural South Africa. *Small Enterprise Development, 16*(3), 26–38.

Sachs, J. (2005). *The end of poverty: How we can make it happen in our lifetime.* London: Penguin.

SEF/RADAR. (2005). *The IMAGE Intervention.* Retrieved February 15, 2007, from http://www .lshtm.ac.uk/genderviolence/reports/imagebrochforweb.pdf

Southern African Regional Poverty Network (SARPN) (2005). *Zambia poverty and vulnerability assessment* (Rep. No. 32573). Human Development Division, Africa Region. Hatfield, South Africa: World Bank.

Steinberg, M., Johnson, S., Schierhout, G., Ndegwa, D., Hall, K., Russell, B., et al. (2002). *Hitting home: How households cope with the impact of the HIV/AIDS epidemic. A survey of households affected by HIV/AIDS in South Africa.* Report compiled for the Henry J. Kaiser Family Foundation and the Health Systems Trust. Retrieved August 13, 2007, from www.hst.org.za/uploads/files/hittinghome.pdf

Swindells, S., Mohr, J., Justis, J. C., Berman, S., Squier, C., Wagener, M. M., et al. (1999). Quality of life in patients with human immunodeficiency virus infection: Impact of social support, coping style and hopelessness. *International Journal of STD and AIDS, 10*(6), 383–391.

Thabo, T. F. (2006) Social and psychological factors associated with willingness to test for HIV infection among young people in Botswana. *AIDS Care, 18*(3), 201–207.

UNAIDS. (2004). *2004 Report on the global AIDS epidemic.* Geneva: UNAIDS.

UNAIDS/UNFPA/UNIFEM. (2004). *Women and HIV/AIDS: Confronting the crisis.* Geneva: UNAIDS.

UNDP. (2005). *Human Development Report 2005.* New York: UNDP.

UNFPA. (2006). *Sexual and reproductive health needs of women and adolescent girls living with HIV: Research report on qualitative findings from Brazil, Ethiopia, and the Ukraine.* New York: United Nations Population Fund.

United Nations General Assembly Special Session on HIV/AIDS. (2005). *Follow-up to the Declaration of Commitment on HIV/AIDS. 2005 Zambia Country Report.* United Nations General Assembly Special Session on HIV/AIDS.New York: United Nations.

Uys, L. R. (2003). Aspects of the care of people with HIV/AIDS in South Africa. *Public Health Nursing, 20*(4):271–280.

Gender Differences in Barriers to Adolescent Honesty with Advanced Practice Nurses

Andrew R. Kruse

The purpose of this study was to examine gender differences in adolescents' perceived barriers to honesty with advanced practice nurse. Although adolescents' use of primary care is the lowest in the United States (Clowers, 2002; Klein, McNulty, & Flatau, 1998; Lindberg, Lewis-Spruill, & Crownover, 2006), research indicates that adolescents are not always honest with providers during healthcare visits (Breslin, 1998; Diaz et al., 2004; Farrant & Watson, 2004; Ginsburg & Menapace, 1997). Withholding or fabricating information during healthcare visits greatly influences the quality of care provided and can have significant consequences. Adolescents are vulnerable as a result of the major physical and emotional changes they are experiencing and the many life-style choices they are making. A primary care provider may be the only person an adolescent can turn to for treatment, help, guidance, or truth regarding risky behaviors (Summers et al., 2006). It is imperative that providers are aware of the perceived barriers adolescents have toward achieving this relationship so that each barrier can be addressed individually to improve the quality of health care provided.

Many studies have examined the qualities in a provider that are important to adolescents (Clowers, 2002; Klostermann, Slap, Nebrig, Tivorsak, & Britto, 2005; Rutishauser, Esslinger, Bond, & Sennhauser, 2003). Results have consistently shown that adolescents want a provider who is respectful, competent, honest, trustworthy, and provides confidential health care (Ginsburg & Menapace, 1997; Klostermann et al., 2005).

Extensive research has also explored adolescents' interpretations and understanding of confidentiality (Atkinson, Schattner, & Margolis, 2003; Breslin, 1998; Donovan, Mellanby, Jacobson, Taylor, & Tripp, 1997; Farrant & Watson, 2004; Ford, Thomsen, & Compton, 2001; Klein et al., 1998; Klostermann et al., 2005; Lindberg et al., 2006; McPherson, 2003; Rutishauser et al., 2003). Confidentiality is seen as a major barrier to health care for adolescents, significantly affecting their ability to trust. A perceived lack of confidentiality has been found to deter adolescents from accessing health care while also causing them to be dishonest with their provider (Breslin, 1998; Diaz et al., 2004; Farrant & Watson, 2004; Ginsburg & Menapace, 1997).

Considering the wealth of information surrounding adolescents and confidentiality, it is startling that no research has been performed on barriers to honesty in the patient–provider relationship. Patient honesty is imperative in providing quality health care, yet no research exists examining other deterrents to adolescent honesty. Possible reasons adolescents may withhold information could include a fear of parental punishment, judgment from the provider, embarrassment, a lack of trust, or the inability of the provider to help them. This study attempts to examine some of the possible reasons that adolescents may be dishonest with providers.

Methodology

Design

This is a preliminary psychometric study, so a mixed design was chosen to provide basic descriptive data and to examine relationships. A comparative design was used because research indicates that adolescents have different beliefs toward healthcare issues based on their gender (Atkinson et al., 2003; Farrant & Watson, 2004). Participants were asked to fill out questionnaires containing eight vignettes. Once completed, participants were asked to meet in a focus group to discuss their perspectives on barriers to adolescent honesty. A female observer was present to help record the discussions and to increase the comfort level of females. Focus groups were audio-taped.

Sample and Setting

Permission was granted to distribute a self-administered questionnaire during an introductory psychology class. All 17 students present willingly participated, although three surveys were excluded because of missing data. The sample consisted of six men and eight women who ranged in age from 18 to 25 years. The mean age for men was 19.6 years, with an age range of 18 to 22. The mean age for women was 20.1 years, with an age range of 18 to 25. Most participants were sophomores (66%), with freshmen and juniors each comprising 16% of the male participants. Half of the female participants were sophomores (50%), whereas 38% were freshman and 12% were juniors at the university. After completing the questionnaire in class, only one male participant chose to attend the focus group.

The study was conducted in a small private conference room on the university campus. Pizza and various snacks were provided to participants as a form of incentive.

Instruments

Once consent forms were signed, the participants were asked to complete a basic demographic survey. A self-administered questionnaire containing eight vignettes was developed for this study, similar to de Chesnay's (1982) methodology. Each vignette depicts a unique situation in which an adolescent is not telling the truth to the advanced practice nurse. Participants are given nine possible reasons that the patient did not tell the truth and asked to rank all reasons the adolescent is being dishonest by marking the best explanation of why the patient lied with a "1," the second best reason the patient lied with a "2," the third best reason the patient withheld the truth with a "3," and so on.

Vignettes were chosen to provide baseline descriptive data and as a way to provide a segue into the focus group discussions. If asked to report personal experience, the sample would have been limited to those who have withheld information from a provider in the past. By using fictional situations instead of personal experience, it was anticipated that the subjects would be more likely to be candid.

Data Analysis

Once coded as nominal data, the questionnaire results were analyzed using an ungrouped frequency distribution. The results were then compared and plotted on a histogram. The data were analyzed according to vignette, barriers, and gender of subject. Qualitative data were analyzed using content analysis. The vignettes were first analyzed by examining participant responses to each vignette (1–8). This revealed the most likely and least likely barriers to adolescent honesty according to each scenario. This approach allowed a direct comparison of answers between males and females for each vignette as well as a way to analyze the influences a particular situation may have on responses.

The data were also analyzed according to barriers, or reasons that the adolescent was dishonest, by adding the points (1–9) that participants assigned to each response in every vignette. The total was then divided by the number of responses to arrive at the average number of points given to each response. Therefore the lower the number, the more often participants chose that response as the reason that an adolescent was dishonest with the provider. This approach revealed what participants believed were the most significant and least significant barriers to adolescent honesty with a provider while allowing clear gender comparison.

Validity and Reliability

Face validity was attained by reviewing the vignettes with adolescents. Content validity was determined by a panel of three experts who had experience with adolescents. The questionnaire and its administration were standardized to increase reliability. Results were coded as nominal data, and all tests were administered by one person.

Content analysis provided guidelines for reliability of qualitative data. Systematic checks of accuracy of coding were performed throughout data analysis (Downe-Wamboldt, 1992). The interview data were reviewed with a methods expert.

Limitations

This study has several limitations, including a small convenience sample that limited data analysis to a simple frequency distribution. The qualitative data were generated not by a group but by the only person who came to the focus group. Adequate time to complete the questionnaire may not have been provided for participants with learning disabilities or those who speak English as a second language. Because of the age of participants the data collected may not be representative of younger adolescents. The data may not be generalizable to all adolescents, because the sample only includes college students from a private Jesuit University.

Results

Areas of Agreement

Analysis of the vignettes primarily revealed agreement between male and female responses (Table 19-1). Both male and female participants believed "embarrassment" and a "fear of telling parents" were the most likely barriers to cause dishonesty. Male participants chose "embarrassment" or "fear of telling parents" as the most significant barrier in all scenarios, whereas females chose one of these two barriers for seven of eight scenarios. The barriers "not nurse practitioner's business" and "the issue is not a big deal" were chosen by both male and female participants as the least likely barriers to cause dishonesty.

TABLE 19-1.   Analysis of Vignettes: Most Significant and Least Significant Barriers According to Vignette*

Topic of Question	Male Participants			Female Participants		
	Significant Barrier	Possible Barrier	Not a Barrier	Significant Barrier	Possible Barrier	Not a Barrier
Vignette 1: Sexually transmitted disease	A, B	F	G	B, A	E, D	I, G
Vignette 2: Smoking	B	A, D	G, F	B, F	H, A, D	G
Vignette 3: Drinking	B	I, D	E	B	I, H	A
Vignette 4: Pregnancy	B	F, D, A	I, G	A, B	F, D	I, H, G
Vignette 5: Depression/ suicide	B	C, F	E, D	B	C, E, G, A	I, H
Vignette 6: Sex	B,	B, C, F	I	A	E, F	I, G, H, A, C
Vignette 7: Marijuana	B	F, A	E, H	F	I, B, H	G
Vignette 8: Drinking/ rape	A	B, D	I, G	A	B, D, F	I, C

* Letters in the table refer to the responses to each item in the vignettes. See Table 19-2 for the exact responses that correspond to each letter.

TABLE 19-2. Analysis of Barriers: Average Score for Each Barrier in Order of Significance

Male Participants		Female Participants	
Barriers	**Score**	**Barriers**	**Score**
B) Going to tell parents	2.69	B) Going to tell parents	3.25
A) Embarrassed	3.02	A) Embarrassed	3.94
D) Lack of confidentiality	4.25	F) Negative reaction/judgment	4.09
F) Negative reaction/judgment	4.48	E) Lack of trust	4.81
C) NP won't understand	5.48	D) Lack of confidentiality	4.95
H) Not NP's business	5.52	H) Not NP's business	5.45
I) Issue is not a big deal	6.48	C) NP won't understand	6.09
G) NP is unable to help	6.72	G) NP is unable to help	6.09
E) Lack of trust	6.96	I) Issue is not a big deal	6.94

NP, nurse practitioner

Analysis of the barriers revealed that both female and male participants scored the barrier "fear of telling parents" as the most likely reason that the adolescent in the scenarios was dishonest (Table 19-2). On the 1–9 scale male participants gave an average score of 2.69, whereas female participants rated this response as 3.25. Men and women were also in agreement in the second most significant barrier, "embarrassment," with men giving an average score of 3.02 and women giving an average score of 3.94. Receiving a negative reaction from the provider was also fairly influential, being rated as a 4.48 by men and a 4.09 by women.

Agreement was also found in some of the least likely reasons for dishonesty (Table 19-2). Feelings that "the issue was not a big deal" was rated as not influential, 6.48 by males and 6.94 by females. An "inability of the provider to help" was also seen as an unlikely reason to be dishonest, 6.72 by males and 6.09 by females.

Areas of Difference

Data analysis of the vignettes revealed several differences between male and female participants (Table 19-1). Female participants, more than male, believed that a very significant barrier to honesty was a "negative reaction or judgment" from the provider. The data also revealed that female participants were more likely to believe that "lack of trust" and "none of the nurse practitioner's business" were barriers. Data analysis of the barriers revealed several major differences between male and female participants (Table 19-2). It was found that "lack of trust," rated 6.96 by the men, was rated 4.81 by the women.

Many participants wrote in their own barriers as a response to the vignettes. There were nine possible barriers, with a 10th option to write in any response that participants believed were missing. All 17 questionnaires were used in the analysis of the added barriers because survey completion was not necessary. Of the 14 added barriers, 6 were similar to existing barriers, such as "none of the nurse practitioner's business," "lack of confidentiality," "feeling judged," and "embarrassment," and they were coded as such.

Two unique barriers were mentioned by several people as the number one reason the adolescent was dishonest. Two participants expressed that the difficulty and anxiety of admitting a problem to someone is significant and can cause dishonesty. In addition, three participants mentioned that dishonesty could occur if the adolescent is still unsure of what to do about an issue. Furthermore, single participants mentioned that an adolescent is likely to be dishonest because "marijuana use is not legal," a misunderstanding that "provider's only deal with physical problems," and that an adolescent may have a "different interpretation of sexually active."

Incomplete Questionnaires

Three of the 17 questionnaires were only partially completed. Two of those questionnaires were filled out by ranking only the top three barriers to each vignette. What the participants completed seems congruent with the data from the rest of the participants. The third questionnaire was filled out sporadically, with some vignettes being filled out completely but most only partially completed. This participant wrote in answers to four of the eight vignettes, and the responses completed seemed to differ from the rest of the data.

The Interview

One participant, a 19-year-old male sophomore, attended the focus group; however, he was very talkative and provided quality data through his many opinions and insight. The interview lasted approximately 75 minutes. Discussion with the participant revealed that his age was ideal for this research. He was young enough to provide recent experiences as an adolescent but mature enough to accurately analyze and articulate those experiences to provide relevant data.

The interview revealed that the questionnaire depicted an accurate representation of adolescent experiences with providers. The participant expressed that the questionnaire seemed both relevant and valid. The directions were described as clear, and the survey itself was seen as straightforward. The participant believed that similar answers were given for most scenarios but answered honestly throughout.

The barriers were all seen as legitimate and likely reasons that an adolescent may be dishonest with a provider. The barrier that he believed was least likely to cause dishonesty was that a "nurse practitioner is unable to help." He believed that nurse practitioners can always provide some sort of help. The participant wrote in one barrier on two different vignettes as the most significant barrier to honesty. He believed that the anxiety of admitting a problem may prevent an adolescent from being honest, because it is often easier to avoid an issue than to confront it.

The participant did not recognize gender as affecting his responses to the questionnaire. Upon further discussion it was revealed that the participant believed it is easier for males to discuss personal and more embarrassing issues, such as sex, with a provider of the same gender. It should be noted that there was no female input regarding this information, and therefore it may not apply to female adolescents.

The participant believed that dishonesty is largely dependent on the situation. He believed that there are primarily two types of situations in which adolescents are dishonest. When adolescents are dishonest regarding personal or sexual issues, such as sexual experience, sexually transmitted diseases, and pregnancy, it is primarily due to feelings of embarrassment, shame, or fear of judgment. The other situation involved illegal use of substances, such as drug, alcohol, or tobacco use. This dishonesty revolves around a fear of punishment and a lack of confidentiality, a fear of telling parents, or fear of judgment.

When asked why adolescents may not be completely honest, the participant had many responses, though the most important was clearly the idea of a lack of "situational trust." This was defined by the participant as a feeling of trust toward the provider at a specific moment, independent of past history and all other factors. When asking a question it is the responsibility of the provider to make the situation trustworthy.

The participant's personal experience provided insight to this term. When asked if he was using illegal substances at an initial visit with an ophthalmologist, he honestly replied "no." Situational trust was provided by the ophthalmologist through the privacy he offered, the "chill" attitude he portrayed, the way he talked to the patient as a friend, and by explaining why he was asking such a personal question. When asked if he was sexually active by his family provider of 15 years, of whom he trusted completely, the participant was dishonest. This was because the question was asked abruptly, causing him to feel shocked and embarrassed, reacting quickly, in an attempt to avoid the situation.

When asked how providers can promote situational trust with an adolescent patient, many suggestions were offered. The provider should promote a relaxed yet professional environment, using "loose" dialogue, and approaching personal questions casually. Privacy should be provided to the adolescent and confidentiality should be explained. A provider should lead up to personal questions gently, while explaining the importance of the questions being asked.

The participant discussed that some adolescents may not initiate a conversation about a personal issue because of the anxiety they experience. When asked of ways in which a provider can improve openness in these situations, it was suggested to start vague, by asking if the patient has anything they would like to discuss. Reinforce confidentiality, and explain that the provider is open and available to answer any questions. Become more specific, asking "do you have any questions about sex, smoking, drugs, etc." The participant believed that most adolescents have something they are curious about but are afraid to ask. Gently easing into the questions provides "situational trust," whereas specifically asking about sensitive issues eases the difficulty of bringing up a difficult topic.

The participant also proposed the use of posters and brochures to increase the awareness of adolescents. The participant stated that while in the waiting room he reads any available material offered by the office. He suggested that this would serve as a nonconfrontational means to prepare adolescents for personal questions while also increasing adolescent awareness.

Discussion

Several conclusions were drawn from the data:

1. Adolescents are not always honest with providers.
2. The two most significant barriers to adolescent honesty are embarrassment and fear that the provider will tell their parents.
3. Barriers to honesty are often scenario specific.
4. Situational trust promotes honesty.
5. Males and females have different barriers.
6. Male participants are in more agreement than female participants regarding barriers to honesty.

Adolescent dishonesty with providers was a premise on which the questionnaire was based and therefore is not able to be supported by the quantitative data. In agreement with Breslin (1998), Ginsburg and Menapace (1997), Diaz et al. (2004), and Farrant and Watson (2004), the focused interview revealed that adolescents are not always honest with their provider. This was revealed through the participant's personal experience of dishonesty with a provider. In addition, the participant made many references to adolescent dishonesty and provided insight into ways to promote honesty with adolescent patients.

Surprisingly, limited research has examined the impact that the fear of parents finding out has on an adolescent. Although "confidentiality" was seen as a significant barrier to honesty for both male and female participants in this study, in contrast to past research (Atkinson et al., 2003; Breslin, 1998; Klostermann et al., 2005; Rodriguez, Sheldon, Bauer, & Perez-Stable, 2001; Sankar & Jones, 2005) "confidentiality" did not have the impact on honesty that it has had in other studies. The most significant barrier unanimously became a "fear that the provider will tell their parents." This result, also seen by Donovan et al. (1997), may indicate that in regards to adolescents the primary concern is not confidentiality but the portion of confidentiality involving telling their parents.

"Embarrassment" was also revealed as a primary barrier to honesty, in agreement with past research (Cunningham, Tschann, Gurvey, Fortenberry, & Ellen, 2002; Lindberg et al., 2006; Sankar & Jones, 2005). Some research does not support "embarrassment" as a barrier to honesty (Rodriguez et al., 2001), though this may be attributed to the idea that embarrassment could be a much more significant barrier to honesty for adolescents. Adolescents may be more likely than adults to be embarrassed, due to peer pressure, limited experience, or a fear of being abnormal.

The interview participant believed that dishonesty largely depended on the situation. He expressed that when dealing with issues of sexuality, barriers to honesty primarily involved feelings of embarrassment or a fear of judgment. Barriers to honesty regarding the illegal use of tobacco, alcohol, or drugs involved a fear of judgment, punishment, or parental discovery.

The data analysis of the vignettes confirmed the ideas stated in the interview. When the vignettes were separated according to topic, very different responses were elicited from participants. Vignettes involving illegal activity, such as drinking, smoking, or marijuana use, revealed that "embarrassment" was not consistently seen as a barrier but that a "fear of telling parents" was a significant barrier (Table 19-1). In addition, a feeling that "the issue is not a big deal" was seen as a possible or significant barrier.

When analyzing vignettes concerning sexual involvement, it was found that reasons for dishonesty were somewhat different. The most likely reason for dishonesty, for both male and female participants, was "embarrassment," followed by "a fear of telling parents." "Judgment" by the provider was found to be a more significant barrier to honesty than with illicit substance use. In contrast, feelings that the issue was "not a big deal" and an "inability of the provider to help" were the least likely to cause dishonesty, according to both male and female participants.

The interviewee revealed that adolescents may be more likely to be embarrassed or fearful of judgment about sexual questions because sex is seen as a taboo topic by society. Adolescents using substances illegally may believe that substance use is a part of adolescence and that there is nothing wrong with it; hence, they are not embarrassed. The interview participant believed that many adolescents are aware of the repercussions of illicit substance use and are therefore afraid to be punished by their parents.

Though the quantitative data cannot support situational trust, the idea was brought up numerous times in the focused interview. This term, described by the participant as a feeling of trust toward a provider at a specific moment, includes many of the barriers that were examined in the quantitative portion of the research. The idea of situational trust encompasses embarrassment, confidentiality, a fear of telling their parents, a lack of trust, and fear of judgment. These are all identified barriers to honesty that would be relieved by providing situational trust.

Situational trust has significant implications for practice by putting the responsibility of adolescent honesty back on the provider. Situational trust is not necessarily dependent on trust, a relationship, or a history but on creating an environment that encourages honesty and provides support, while taking the time to work with the adolescent. Therefore a provider can no longer look at adolescent dishonesty as an absolute and must see it as something that they can affect.

Although most of the data are very similar for both male and female participants, there are some significant differences. The data analysis of the vignettes revealed several differences between male and female participants when organized according to topic (Table 19-1). Regarding tobacco, alcohol, and marijuana use, female participants believed that a very significant cause of dishonesty was a "negative reaction or judgment" from the provider. This response was not consistently seen by the male participants. Female participants also tended to believe that dishonesty was often caused by feelings that it is "none of the provider's business," whereas male participants did not reflect this in their answers. In contrast, male participants expressed "embarrassment" as a significant reason for dishonesty when discussing illegal substance use, whereas female participants believed "embarrassment" was one of the least likely reasons an adolescent would be dishonest. When discussing sexual situations female participants, more than male, found that a "lack of trust" would be more likely to contribute to dishonesty.

The most noteworthy difference is that, according to the analysis of the barriers (Table 19-2), the male participants believed that a "lack of trust" of the provider was the least likely reason an adolescent would be dishonest (average score, 6.96), whereas the female participants believed that it was a fairly significant cause of dishonesty (average score, 4.81).

Analysis of the vignettes (Table 19-1) revealed that although male participants believed that a "lack of trust" was a neutral barrier in regards to most situations, it was not seen as a barrier to honesty in the vignettes involving alcohol and marijuana use. In contrast, female participants believed a "lack of trust" was a possible barrier in sexual situations.

Klostermann et al. (2005) explained that to adolescents trust is influenced by confidentiality, competence, honesty, and respect and is a core attribute adolescents seek in a provider. This implies that trust can be interpreted by the participant in several different ways. It is possible that "lack of trust" is not considered a significant barrier to the participants, because some of the attributes that make up the idea of trust are included as individual barriers in the questionnaire, so it no longer has the level of impact it did when it involved confidentiality. In addition, although it may be an important quality of a provider, it may not be a barrier to honesty.

Analysis of the barriers revealed that the average score given to each barrier was more extreme for the male than for the female participants. As seen in Table 19-2, the range of average scores for all nine barriers is 2.69–6.96 for male participants and 3.25–6.94 for female participants. The less extreme averages are a result of the difference in range of scores attributed to each response by individual participants (for all eight vignettes). Male participants had a smaller range of scores for six of the eight barriers, causing their averages for each barrier to be more extreme and indicating more agreement about the significance of barriers among the male participants. Although this does not confound the data, the implications for practice are slightly more difficult to discern among female participants, because the results are less clear.

These results could be an inaccurate side effect of an uneven sample size. As the sample grows, variability is expected. Though the sample size for this research was nearly even, six males and eight females, it is likely that two more male participants would increase the range of scores, resulting in a similar effect as the female participants. In addition, these data could be skewed by one participant who has very different views from the rest of the participants. This would cause extreme ranges, with altered average scores.

Implications for Practice

This study generated several implications for practice, and these are presented as suggestions for how providers might interact with adolescents to encourage their candor. First, utilize situational trust to provide an environment conducive to honesty. During the interview the participant expressed that situational trust is a significant element to promoting honesty, for which the provider is directly responsible. Providing situational trust encourages honesty through a nonthreatening atmosphere, which reassures the patient of the provider's motives. When asked how to promote situational trust with an adolescent patient, the participant had several suggestions. A relaxed yet professional attitude was expressed as especially important. This is obtained by being both respectful and respectable while using a "loose" dialogue without medical jargon on the same level as the patient. Doing this provides a casual and comfortable atmosphere for the adolescent while showing them that you are a friend who wants to help, as opposed to an adult who wants to punish.

Privacy should be provided to the patient, without parents present and with the door closed. The participant also explained that it is important to lead up to personal questions gently. This limits the amount of shock that an adolescent may experience when abruptly raising sensitive topics, ideally preventing reactive responses that are often dishonest in an attempt to avoid the issue. It is also important to show the adolescent patient that it is acceptable to be honest.

Adults, such as parents, teachers, and coaches, are often seen as authority figures to adolescent patients. Consequently, their personal lives are often withheld from adults. To promote honesty and disclosure, confidentiality should be explained because it is imperative that providers are not seen as authority figures. Furthermore, before asking personal questions of an adolescent patient, an explanation should provide the importance of the questions asked. The participant's personal experience revealed that many adolescents do not think about why personal questions are asked and do not realize that dishonesty could have repercussions. Finally, the participant believed it was important that personal questions are asked casually, like all other questions, without being intense or drawing any extra attention.

By providing situational trust a provider addresses many of the issues that arose in this research. Although the most significant barriers to honesty were seen as "embarrassment" and a "fear of telling parents," situational trust addresses those barriers while also lessening the effects of other barriers, such as "confidentiality" and "lack of trust." The most significant difference between male and female participants was that female participants, more than male, believed a "lack of trust" was a significant barrier to honesty. Situational trust addresses this issue by increasing the level of trust with a provider. Furthermore, although this study found that barriers to honesty are scenario specific, providing situational trust addresses this issue as well. During a routine visit providers are often unaware of whether an adolescent's issue of concern involves sexual issues or illicit substances. Therefore it would be wise to provide situational trust in an attempt to lessen the effects of all barriers to honesty, as opposed to only those barriers relevant for the scenario.

Second, if dishonesty is suspected, provide as much situational trust as possible and gently approach the question again. According to the participant in the interview, he was not offended when his provider asked him if he used illicit drugs a second time. This was because the provider explained the importance of the question, provided privacy, and casually ensured confidentiality. This does not imply that all adolescents who deny use of illicit substances should be asked a second time or that those who seem to be dishonest should be asked more than twice. Adolescents may respond poorly, feeling that you do not trust them, but by being clear and honest, by providing situational trust, they may come to understand the importance of the question and respond candidly to the question. Third, be specific when asking if patients have anything they would like to discuss.

The interview revealed that many patients have personal issues they would like to discuss but because of anxiety they do not initiate a conversation. Though situational trust should still improve honesty, anxiety is a unique barrier because the adolescent may want to discuss the issue. The participant in the interview suggests approaching sensitive issues slowly, from a broad perspective. Preface the question with an explanation of confidentiality and ask "is there anything else you would like to discuss with me?" This is a non-threatening question that prepares the adolescent for more sensitive questions. Unfortunately, the participant pointed out that many providers do not follow up this question, and many patients do not bring up their issues. The participant suggested following up the vague question with more specific questions, such as "If you have any questions about sex, drugs, depression, alcohol, etc., I am open to all of them, and this is completely confidential. There is no such thing as a bad question." This may help reassure them that their question is valid or that this is an appropriate situation to ask.

A fourth suggestion is to know the state laws regarding adolescents because it is important for providers to be honest with their patients, particularly when they are looking for honesty in return. Specifically, providers need to be clear about confidentiality laws regarding drug treatment, sexually transmitted disease testing, mental health treatment, abortion, contraception, and pregnancy.

Fifth, provide material for adolescent patients to read while waiting. In accordance with McPherson (2005), the participant from the interview recommended utilizing the waiting room and exam room to provide information for the patient to read. This material could include confidentiality laws, services provided, common questions that adolescents can ask about, or personal questions that the provider may ask. This material provides a nonconfrontational approach to sensitive topics, allowing the patient to recognize the provider as a resource. It also provides the patient time to prepare for sensitive questions and evaluate any issues they may want to address. This material can be provided in a variety of ways, such as posters or brochures. McPherson (2005) suggests free posters and booklets regarding sexual health advice from Brook (www.brook.org.uk).

Finally, the provider should provide adolescent patients with a nonconfrontational way to address their concerns. For example, the interview participant mentioned that most adolescents have sensitive issues they would like to discuss but experience too much anxiety to initiate a conversation about it. To ease an adolescent's anxiety of bringing up an issue, an additional form could be provided with the initial paperwork. This form could list several sensitive issues, such as sexual history and drug or alcohol use. The adolescent can check the boxes of the issues they would like to discuss, and the provider can then initiate a conversation about the issues. This provides a nonconfrontational means to initiate a conversation with a provider.

Conclusion

This study, although preliminary, indicated that adolescents do edit what they tell providers and may not be candid in busy healthcare settings if providers do not take the time to establish rapport and trust with the patient. Anything the provider can do to make it safe for the patient to be candid will have a positive effect on both the relationship and healthcare outcomes.

References

Atkinson, K., Schattner, P., & Margolis, S. (2003). Rural secondary school students living in a small community: Their attitudes, beliefs and perceptions towards general practice. *Australian Journal of Rural Health,* 11, 73–80.

Breslin, M. (1998). When physicians assure confidentiality, teenagers are willing to talk openly. *Family Planning Perspectives,* 30, 52.

Clowers, M. (2002). Young women describe the ideal physician. *Adolescence, 37*(148), 695–705.

Cunningham, S. D., Tschann, J., Gurvey, J. E., Fortenberry, J. D., & Ellen, J. M. (2002). Attitudes about sexual disclosure and perceptions of stigma and shame. *Sexually transmitted infections, 78*(5), 334–338.

de Chesnay, M. (1982). *Problem framing and change strategies: A survey of Georgia registered nurses.* Unpublished doctoral dissertation, University of Alabama, Birmingham.

Diaz, A., Neal, W. P., Nucci, A. T., Ludmer, P., Bitterman, J., & Edwards, S. (2004). Legal and ethical issues facing adolescent health care professionals. *The Mount Sinai Journal of Medicine, 71*(3), 181–185.

Donovan, C., Mellanby, A. R., Jacobson, L. D., Taylor, B., & Tripp, J. H. (1997). Teenagers' views on the general practice consultation and provision of contraception. *British Journal of General Practice, 47,* 715–718.

Downe-Wamboldt, B. (1992). Content analysis: Method, applications and issues. *Health Care for Women International, 13*(3), 313–321.

Farrant, B., & Watson, P.D. (2004). Health care delivery: Perspectives of young people with chronic illness and their parents. *Journal of Paediatrics and Child Health, 40,* 175–179.

Ford, C. A., Thomsen, S. L., & Compton, B. (2001). Adolescents' interpretations of conditional confidentiality assurances. *Journal of Adolescent Health, 29,* 156–159.

Ginsburg, K. R., & Menapace, A. S. (1997). Factors affecting the decision to seek health care: The voice of adolescents. *Pediatrics, 100*(6), 922–931.

Klein, J. D., McNulty, M., & Flatau, C.N. (1998). Adolescents' access to care: Teenager's self-reported use of services and perceived access to confidential care. *Archives of Pediatrics & Adolescent Medicine, 152,* 676–682.

Klostermann, B. K., Slap, G. B., Nebrig, D. M., Tivorsak, T. L., & Britto, M. T. (August 2005). Earning trust and losing it: Adolescents' views on trusting physicians. *The Journal of Family Practice, 54.* Retrieved October 3, 2005, from http://wwwjfponline.com

Lindberg, C., Lewis-Spruill, C., & Crownover, R. (2006). Barriers to sexual and reproductive health care: Urban male adolescents speak out. *Issues in Comprehensive Pediatric Nursing, 29,* 73–88.

McPherson, A. (2005). ABC of adolescence: Adolescents in primary care. *British Medical Journal, 330,* 465–467.

Rodriguez, M. A., Sheldon, W. R., Bauer, H. M., & Perez-Stable, E. J. (2001). The factors associated with disclosure of intimate partner abuse to clinicians. *The Journal of Family Practice, 50*(4), 338–344.

Rutishauser, C., Esslinger, A., Bond, L., & Sennhauser, F. H. (2003). Consultations with adolescents: The gap between their expectations and their experiences. *Acta Paediatrica, 92,* 1322–1326.

Sankar, P., & Jones, N. L. (2005). To tell or not to tell: Primary care patients' disclosure deliberations. *Archives of Internal Medicine, 165,* 2378–2383.

Summers, D., Alpert, I., Rousseau-Pierre, D., Minguez, M., Manigault, S., Edwards, S., et al. (2006). An exploration of the ethical, legal and developmental issues in the care of an adolescent patient. *The Mount Sinai Journal of Medicine, 73*(3), 592–595.

Experiencing Homelessness: A Grounded Theory Study of Formerly Homeless Mothers

Pamela M. H. Cone

America
It is cold at night
But worst at dawn
That dawn's early light
When the flag is
Still there
Waving in the faces of Americans
Sleeping
In the streets
Cold
Hungry
Forgotten by their government
Ignored by mankind
But living
In
America the beautiful

—*By G. C. Plebe, homeless in San Francisco (1998)*

Homelessness adversely affects the spirit, mind, and body (Golden, 1992; Seltser & Miller, 1993), causing increased vulnerability, especially among homeless women with children (Averitt, 2003). A widespread and growing problem, homelessness continues to stretch the already limited resources of shelters and service-providing agencies in the United States. Single female-headed households are the fastest growing segment of the homeless population (Netburn, 2005), but relatively little is known about this subgroup of the homeless (National Coalition for the Homeless, 2006).

Homelessness and motherhood seem contradictory; motherhood implies protectiveness and nurturance, whereas homelessness implies extreme vulnerability (Banyard & Graham-Berman, 1998). This vulnerability includes both individual and group susceptibility to health problems (de Chesnay, 2005), impacting both the mother and groups of single-female–headed households living on the streets. People living in poverty, people of color, and people who are marginalized because of race, age, gender, ethnicity, immigrant status, or sexual preference are among the most vulnerable people groups (Flaskerud, 1999). Being homeless places women with children in several of these categories; mothers and their families are extremely vulnerable and at high risk for multiple health problems, a serious concern for society because women are usually responsible for the social fabric of the family and community (Munhall, 1994; Seltser & Miller, 1993). This chapter focuses on the problem of homeless mothering.

Statement of the Problem

Oer the last 20 years there has been a sharp rise in interest regarding homelessness; indeed, there are numerous research studies among the homeless, yet little is known about the needs and experiences of homeless single women with children and the strategies necessary to survive and to reintegrate into mainstream society. Many factors contribute to homelessness, including poverty, unemployment and underemployment, family crises, sociopolitical factors such as affordable housing, family disintegration, domestic and neighborhood violence, mental illness and substance abuse, and catastrophes (Blair, Jacobs, & Quiram, 1999). America's current socioeconomic and sociopolitical climate has negatively impacted the family, resulting in a nationwide rise in family homelessness (Whitehead, 2002). In Los Angeles County the homeless family is the most rapidly increasing group among the homeless population, with homeless single mothers being the fastest growing segment (Netburn, 2005; State of the County, 2003). Homeless families, in particular homeless single mothers, have complex needs involving multiple dimensions: physical, social, emotional, psychological, and spiritual. Unfortunately, the growing numbers of homeless families give clear evidence that current programs of assistance are not meeting their needs.

Definition of Homelessness

The Stewart B. McKinney Homeless Assistance Act of 1987, Public Law 100-77, describes a homeless person as someone "who lacks a fixed, regular, and adequate night-time residence or a person who resides in a shelter, welfare hotel, transitional program or place not ordinarily used as regular sleeping accommodations, such as streets, cars, movie theatres, abandoned buildings, etc." (Weingart Center #1, 2000, p. 1). Not readily evident in this definition of homelessness is the temporary stay with friends or family. This type of transitional residence for the homeless is often overlooked in work among the homeless (Averitt, 2003). Homeless women with children often access these types of transitory living situations as they attempt to meet the needs of their children without actually living on the streets.

Although homelessness is reported worldwide, the United States has a significant and growing problem with homelessness (Blair et al., 1999). It is a widespread problem that affects most large cities, particularly the larger metropolitan areas, such as Los Angeles and New York (Institute for Children and Poverty, 1998; Netburn, 2005; U.S. Conference of Mayors, 2001). At the turn of this century the number of homeless was estimated at 3.5 million, or 1% of the U.S. population (Urban Institute, 2000). A June 16, 2005, press release from the Los Angeles Homeless Services Authority revealed that every night there are about 91,000 homeless individuals in Los Angeles County alone (Netburn, 2005). This is the largest homeless population in any major city in the United States.

Many sociopolitical and socioeconomic factors influence the changing profile of the homeless. Although white males, veterans, the mentally ill, and substance abusers continue to number significantly among the homeless population, family homelessness is on the rise. Twenty years ago families with children represented a relatively small percentage of the homeless who accessed emergency shelters. Currently, their numbers have increased 10-fold (Institute for Children and Poverty, 1998). This alarming new trend is demonstrated in a recent survey revealing that women and girls comprise almost one-third of the homeless population in Los Angeles County (Netburn, 2005). Homeless women, especially those with children, are increasing in numbers each year. Between 1970 and 1990 there was a 46% increase in the number of poor families headed by a single female (U.S. Bureau of Census, 1998). At the turn of the century families made up 40% of the U.S. homeless population; in 84% of these homeless families a mother with 2.2 minor children under 6 years of age heads a typical family unit (Weingart Center #1, 2000). The increasing percentage of homeless children younger than age 5 years raises a number of issues related to the long-term effects of homelessness, such as health deficits, developmental delays, and learning problems (Choi & Snyder, 1998; Drake, 1992; Oliviera, 2002).

Homeless mothers comprise the fastest growing segment of the homeless population, but qualitative research from their own perspective is limited. It is this literature gap that was the motivation for this grounded theory study of formerly homeless mothers, who are often marginalized and disenfranchised because of their homeless status.

Methodology

The purpose of this grounded theory study was to explore and understand the homeless experience from the perspective of women with children who lived the phenomenon. The research question for the pilot study was as follows: How did formerly homeless mothers experience and survive homelessness?

This study used a qualitative mode of inquiry with a grounded theory design (Glaser & Strauss, 1967) and a feminist theory focus on the exploration of women's issues from the perspective of women who had experienced the phenomenon (Lorber, 1998). The grounded theory approach helps the researcher to explore, understand, and explain a social process and generate new theory regarding the phenomenon (Audiss & Roth, 1999).

The researcher immerses in the data to identify concepts and their meanings, to define and explain relationships and patterns, and to develop theory that emerges from the data What emerges is a new way of explaining the phenomenon, one that has "grab" and makes sense to those experiencing it (Artinian in Chenitz & Swanson, 1986). This understanding of emergence from versus forcing of data is consistent with Artinian's explanation that the discovery mode breaks through the analysis and allows the researcher to "identify the core variable or the process that describes the characteristics of a particular social world" (1986, p. 17), namely the world of the formerly homeless mother.

Vulnerable populations, such as the homeless, are often difficult to access for research (Chiang, Keatinge, & Williams, 2001). This is particularly true of homeless mothers, with their concern over society's negative view on homeless mothering (Page & Nooe, 2002; Russell, 1991). Data gathering occurred in a variety of settings, primarily among formerly homeless mothers in the Greater Los Angeles area. On receiving approval from the institutional review board of the University of California, San Francisco, participants were sought through multiple methods. Advertisements were placed in local papers, and flyers were placed in homeless shelters to access shelter workers who may have been previously homeless as well as in areas frequented by homeless and formerly homeless people. Gatekeepers in various organizations working with the homeless helped facilitate entrée to formerly homeless mothers via a support letter. In addition, recruitment fliers and invitation letters were provided to the gatekeepers for distribution to the target population. As only those who contacted the researcher were asked to participate, there is no record of formerly homeless mothers who refused to participate.

Purposive and theoretical sampling strategies were used to select participants and to determine saturation or clarification of theoretical categories during the data collection and analysis phases, which occur simultaneously in a grounded theory study (Egan, 2002). Glaser (1978) advocates continuing data collection until saturation occurs, a process that requires trusting the data and the emergent categories rather than preconceived notions. Theoretical saturation was achieved with 12 participants, although 30 were included in the entire study. Data collection and analysis was done over three waves of participant interviews: seven in the first wave, three in the second wave, and eight in the third wave. In addition to the sample of participants who were interviewed, first-hand stories of homeless mothers were selected from a review of the literature. All met the inclusion criteria of the interview sample.

Participant inclusion criteria were formulated with concerns for vulnerable populations in mind (Flaskerud, 1999). These criteria included women at least 18 years old who spoke and understood English, were mothers at the time of their homelessness, and identified themselves as formerly homeless (i.e., homeless for at least 3 weeks and off the streets for more than 6 weeks). These durations are based on the literature review. Having their children with them on the streets was not a requirement.

Each interview was conducted in an open-ended fashion and began with a grand tour question (Glaser & Strauss, 1967), giving each participant the opportunity to articulate her story of homelessness. Participants were encouraged to describe their perceptions and experiences related to homelessness in as full detail as possible. Spending time listening to the women's stories in the way that they wanted to tell them was an essential strategy to begin building rapport and trust in this vulnerable group (Ensign & Panke, 2002). A set of more detailed questions was then asked: How do women with children experience becoming homeless? What are the believed needs of homeless mothers? How did they prioritize these needs? What strategies did they use to meet these needs? How did the process change over the course of the homeless experience? How did they manage to get off the streets? Who or what helped them to get into stable housing? What made them feel no longer homeless? At various times during the interview, the researcher refocused the discussion and pinpointed and validated salient issues. No difficulties were encountered, and none of the participants became upset during the interview. The interview ended with a summary and a "you told me . . . " sentence. Participants were allowed to validate or correct the researcher's understanding of her experiences. Although no financial reward can adequately compensate for the open sharing of painful stories, the participants agreed to accept $20 in remuneration for participating in the study.

With 18 verbatim-transcribed participant interviews and 12 literature-based stories, 30 cases were available for data analysis. The grounded theory analytical approach uses the constant comparative method of data analysis. Data analysis began with open coding of the first interview and continued until themes emerged, and categories were identified and saturated. As data were analyzed the researcher asked the data topical questions regarding homelessness. What do homeless mothers identify as primary needs or concerns when homeless? What structures are there for meeting needs? How does the process of perceiving and meeting needs unfold? What key structures or persons assisted them in overcoming homelessness? These questions were particularly helpful when analyzing the first-hand accounts from the literature. They also provided the researcher with evidence of fit with the emerging theory.

Findings

Grounded theory analysis of the stories of formerly homeless mothers revealed the multiplicity and complexity of the needs that they faced during their entire homeless experience. Initially, the process of experiencing homelessness was found to encompass three stages with several themes in each. This process changed over time. In addition, three stages to the process of experiencing homelessness were discovered: (1) becoming homeless (disconnection), (2) navigating homelessness (survival), and (3) overcoming homelessness (reconnection; Table 20-1). All three stages were seen in both the stories of study participants and of the cases extracted from the literature, though the course through the processes proceeded at a different pace for each mother. The themes are losing financial resources, experiencing a crisis, losing social supports, searching for food and safe shelter, facing hardships, learning coping and survival strategies, connecting with someone, revaluing of self, figuring out solutions, and reintegrating into society.

TABLE 20-1. Process of Experiencing Homelessness from Disconnecting to Reconnecting

Disconnecting: Becoming Homeless →	Surviving: Navigating Homelessness →	Reconnecting: Overcoming Homelessness
• Losing financial stability • Experiencing a crisis • Losing social supports	• Searching for food and safe shelter • Facing hardships • Learning coping and survival strategies	• Connecting with someone • Revaluing of self • Mutually finding solutions • Reintegrating into society
Context: Homeless motherhood Conditions: Living on the streets or in other temporary situations		Context: Formerly homeless motherhood Conditions: No longer living on the streets or in other temporary situations

Becoming Homeless

The process of becoming disconnected and homeless is complex and involves multiple factors, including poverty and financial instability, a crisis of some sort, and a fragile social network that failed to help when a crisis occurred. Poverty has been identified as a predisposing factor to homelessness (Timmer, Eitzen, & Talley, 1994). One mother reported, "I was out here by myself for a while, I worked two jobs. I tried to pay the rent. It didn't work. . . . I was literally, nothing in my pocket. I have no education. I had no job. I had nowhere else to go, no family, no friends." Another woman told her story:

> I'm estranged from my family, there's a lot of bad blood between us you would say. . . . I was uh, living in an apartment that was practically three quarters of my income. I was never able to buy clothes or uh, let's say dish liquid and toilet paper, stuff that, the necessity thing, that you need when you in an apartment. And this actually been goin' on for 18 months and then finally I just got tired of not, of goin' without these things, so I decided to stop payin' my rent. And then I lost my place.

Eviction from home or losing one's home for any reason was a crisis that could potentially precipitate homelessness, especially for those who were already financially unstable and without adequate social networks. All participants reported that they became disconnected from family and other social supports before becoming homeless. One said, "I got no family, nobody helped me an' my baby. . . . I ended up livin' with people. You know, stayin' here, tryin' to stay there. It got to be inconvenienced, so I had to get out." Pre-homeless disconnection appears to be a predisposing factor to becoming homeless. When social networks failed, other coping strategies became strained and eventually gave out as well, leaving the mother homeless.

Navigating Homelessness

The second stage included themes about feeling devalued and marginalized, learning strategies to ensure safety and to find food and shelter, and enduring multiple types of hardships. Jack London (1903, 1998), in his anthropology of the East End of London entitled, *The People of the Abyss*, wrote that everywhere he turned disenfranchised and hopeless people teetered on the edge of the abyss, where suffering was a constant bedfellow and death a friend. Survival depended on motivation and the energy to discover new coping strategies. Benchmarks of this stage included a sense of aloneness and the need to meet the basic needs of survival. Mothers had a motivational factor of caring for their children, which drove their activities of survival, but they often lacked the energy to find new ways to cope (Munhall, 1994). Some strategies were unusual, as evidenced by one mother who said, "I had my son with me and we didn't have nowhere to go. So I went in Sears and put on some clothes and was gonna walk out and the security camera got me and I had to go to jail . . . my son was put into foster care . . . "

One participant, who called herself Diva, explained, "You know, it's a hard life out there. I never ate out the trash can. I never got that far, but I did sleepin' out the sidewalk; and that's something I always said, I'll never do that. I mean it. You wouldn't get through out there. You find yourself doin' things you said you'd never do."

Navigating homelessness as a survival strategy that is both instinctive and learned emerged as the participants discussed the pitfalls and shoals of homelessness as they tried to survive in "the jungle" of homelessness. Unfortunately, the very strategies that enable the homeless to survive are those that are countercultural, leading to marginalization of those most in need of assistance (Banyard, 1995; Lindsey, 1998; Miller & Keys, 2001). Although some mothers had histories of substance abuse, others began to use alcohol after becoming homeless, finding that the physical and emotional pain of homelessness was dulled by its use (Brehm, 2005; Choi & Snyder, 1998). In addition, the assistance programs available for the homeless often have structural and procedural guidelines that make it difficult for women with children to access the services that they and their children need (Banyard & Graham-Berman, 1998). Some of the mothers were fleeing domestic violence, and they had access to special shelters; however, these were often filled and had long waiting lists (Bassuk, 2001; Belcher, Green, McAlpine, & Ball, 2001).

One woman, called Precious, reported, "I didn't have a place to live. So I went to a shelter. Because I was homeless and staying in shelters, I didn't have a stable environment for my daughter and she was removed on her first birthday. And that really became, no more shelters for me, no more nothing, I just I took to the streets."

Overcoming Homelessness

The final stage was the process of getting off the streets and into stable life-styles. Connecting with someone, revaluing self, mutually finding solutions, and reintegrating into society were the themes of this stage. Reconnection began with a one-on-one contact with a caring individual who reached out and kept on reaching out until the mother responded and established a long-term connection. This began the process of revaluing of self, a significant step toward overcoming homelessness as these women who had been disenfranchised and marginalized began to see themselves as individuals who mattered to someone. "I was on probation," said one mother, "and they helped me move to a place . . . which is a recovery program for men and women. And they accepted me and I was pregnant, and they accepted me." Feeling revalued and affirmed as a person enabled most of the mothers to be ready to work out solutions to their problems, a process they wanted to do with the care providers rather than have done for them (Toohey, Shinn, & Weitzman, 2004). Mutuality was an important part of the entire overcoming process, and the women believed they needed to take ownership of their process of getting out of homelessness.

This theme was expressed by Diva, who said, "The support group, the [Sober Living] program, they helped a lot. Only, the, the main issue is, YOU HAVE TO WANT TO DO IT [capitals added by author to denote vocal emphasis]. You have to want to do it FOR YOU [vocal emphasis]. You know you can pray, and that's good and ask God to help you. But you have to want to do it. Can't nobody else do it for you!"

Through mutual problem solving, the practical assistance these women with children received was thus tailored to their needs as well as their skills and abilities. One mother put it this way:

> The most helpful was the social worker there. She helped me quite a bit. She sent me on a . . . to participate on a . . . like a day program. I went there for support and then she made referrals to places like this. . . . This is how I got here to this building. She sent my name here. And put me on a waiting list here. And that was very motivating. After being in a place like that for a while, that really inspired me. It made me feel really good.

Becoming reintegrated into mainstream society was the final phase of the last stage of experiencing homelessness. This included finding jobs and homes and settling into lifestyles that were supported by a social network providing a measure of interdependence. Many mothers were involved with church groups that provided this support, whereas others became part of various organizations that assisted the homeless. These women believed they needed to give back in some way to the society that had assisted them in overcoming homelessness.

Implications

Analysis of data revealed a number of initial themes in this study among formerly homeless mothers. These themes included losing financial resources and stability, experiencing a crisis event, and losing family and social support; followed by searching for food and safe shelter, making choices to survive, and feeling marginalized; and, finally, connecting with someone, feeling affirmed and valued as a person, finding practical solutions, finding a place to live, and becoming financially stable to get out of homelessness. As various themes were analyzed and compared, it became evident that there was a basic social process, experiencing homelessness, similar to the findings of some other researchers. A comparison of the early findings of this study to the model of homelessness by Grigsby and Bauman (1990) revealed that the loss of personal support from family, social support from friends, and community support from organizations found in that study parallel those experienced by homeless mothers. For example, the fragmentation of social supports precipitated the mother with a disabled daughter into homelessness. Literature on social support abounds, and it is clearly a relevant issue in this study (Toohey et al., 2004). The experience before homelessness is a key factor. Interestingly enough, loss of family support seems to precede loss of other social support. Grigsby, Bauman, and Gregorich (1990) in their work, *Disaffiliation to Entrenchment: A Model for Understanding Homelessness,* developed a model of becoming homeless that closely parallels what this researcher found with these homeless women and their children.

In addition, the second stage, navigating or surviving homelessness, had similar findings to those of several other research studies among the homeless (Golden, 1992; Meadows-Oliver, 2003; Menke & Wagner, 1997). The deep impact of the homeless state on the sense of self among these mothers is seen more clearly in light of social interactions and interpersonal connections defined by symbolic interactionism (Blumer, 1969), which addresses the social structures that are in place and assists in understanding the social norms of today. Homeless mothers must negotiate the social structures that are in place and the meanings that are attached.

Philosopher and phenomenologist Martin Heidegger (1962) sees this socially constructed self as being time and place oriented, a critical concept when dealing with homeless mothers. Even the language related to the homeless situation has an impact on how the woman with children who has no home views herself. Philosopher Charles Taylor (1997) writes that "our identity is partly shaped by recognition or its absence" (p. 225). The failure of society to see and understand the individual identity of a homeless person can cause real harm to homeless people, diminishing their already low self-esteem and increasing their suffering. Indeed, Taylor believes that when we as a society mirror a negative or distorted image of someone or a group of people, we are actually misrecognizing them. This misrecognition can be very destructive and can result in the depreciation, oppression, stigmatization, and marginalization of homeless people (Miller & Keys, 2001; National Coalition for the Homeless, 2006). When working with homeless mothers, the restoration of self is a big step in the process of overcoming difficult life situations (Kozol, 1988).

Those who overcome homelessness indicate that social support is critical to their success and to their ability to take their place in the social world as a mother. "What is particularly crucial here is the social dimension of this need to see ourselves as worthy and responsible human beings" (Seltser & Miller, 1993, p.106). The overcoming stage had some similarities with the findings of Kennard (2002), whose dissertation study explored spiritual strategies that resulted in a renewal of spirit that involved a revaluing and strengthening of the inner person. The part that was missing from anything found in an extensive review of the literature was the reconnection piece. The one-on-one connection with a single individual who genuinely cared was the key to overcoming homelessness. This leads the researcher to hypothesize that building social networks on a personal basis must be included in any plan for overcoming homelessness.

Limitations of the Study

Qualitative research methods such as grounded theory rely on the researcher's perspective and ways of thinking and understanding throughout data analysis. This means that there is a subjective element inherent in the analysis. However, such subjectivity is acceptable when rigor has been maintained throughout the study. Although there is evidence in the literature of many gerund grounded theories reported as basic social processes, not every grounded theory study results in one. This study resulted in the discovery of a basic social process, but according to Glaser (1996), a basic social process is only one of many theoretical codes. Another limitation of the study is the gender issue, because only women were interviewed. On the other hand, it is the perspective of the homeless mother that is of interest to the researcher, so that limitation is a necessary one.

Every research study has advantages and disadvantages to the method chosen. Grounded theory has the advantage of having theory development as its focus (Glaser, 2001); a disadvantage to this method is that not every grounded theory study results in theory development. This can be frustrating for the researcher. Often, it is difficult to determine significance and generalizability, as one can with quantitative studies. On the other hand, it is rewarding to discover a process that truly explains a particular phenomenon.

Homeless women with children have many complex challenges as they navigate their life situation and try to overcome it. Grounded theory offers a means of understanding how homeless mothers experience and overcome their homelessness.

Conclusion

According to Glaser (2001), the grounded theory perspective is particularly suited to understanding a process that occurs over time. With a vulnerable population, gaining entrée and enrolling enough participants is often a serious challenge, and there can be limitations relating to participants. Fortunately, this researcher was able to build rapport with a number of gatekeepers over time spent working in homeless shelters and clinics. Some of the women had histories of substance abuse or domestic violence, or some had diagnoses of mental illness and needed a specialized program before they could go into transitional housing. These women have actually received more attention in the research arena than those whose homeless experience was precipitated by poverty, job loss, or a crisis event such as illness or death of a spouse. This last group "fell through the cracks" as one formerly homeless mother put it.

Analysis of formerly homeless mothers' stories reveals the multiplicity of needs that homeless mothers face during homelessness and the emergence of the process of experiencing homelessness. It is a process that occurs over time, moving from disconnection to reconnection. The establishment of long-term connections and reliable social networks is crucial to helping these families to get off and stay off the streets. This is a major breakthrough when considering program planning and development for homeless single-female-headed families.

Strategies that have proved to be successful include such programs as "Homes for the Homeless" in New York City (DaCosta Nunez, 1996) and PATH (2002) in Los Angeles. What these programs have in common is their focus on a broad range of services and extended support through the time these families self-identify as ready to be independent. Programs for homeless families need to be flexible and multifaceted. In addition, they need to encourage establishment of mutual support networks that mend the torn fabric of societal connections for these families. Providing food and shelter helps keep them alive, but personal caring contacts with homeless mothers gives them encouragement, raises their self-esteem, and helps motivate them to change.

Family homelessness can be overcome, as these formerly homeless mothers have demonstrated. Leaders in society, such as healthcare providers, need to work with homeless families to help them reintegrate into mainstream society and avoid becoming another homeless statistic.

Acknowledgments

This chapter is based on the author's dissertation study among formerly homeless mothers. Dr. Catherine Waters, dissertation chair and professor at University of California San Francisco, and Dr. Barbara Artinian, grounded theory methodologist, professor emeritus at Azusa Pacific University, gave invaluable assistance throughout the course of the project. In addition, some financial support for data collection and analysis was provided by the Iota Sigma Chapter of Sigma Theta Tau International. Findings were presented at local (LA Urban Health Conference), national (National Council for Family Relations), and international (Bergen University Grounded Theory Workshop) conferences.

References

Artinian, B. M. (1986). The research process in grounded theory. In W. C. Chenitz & J. M. Swanson (Eds.), *From practice to grounded theory: Qualitative research in nursing.* Menlo Park, CA: Addison-Wesley.

Audiss, D., & Roth, T. (1999). Application of grounded theory to content definition: A case study. *Top Health Information Management, 19*(3), 47–51.

Averitt, S. S. (2003). "Homelessness is not a choice!" The plight of homeless women with preschool children living in temporary shelters. *Journal of Family Nursing, 9*(1), 79–100.

Banyard, V. L. (1995). "Taking another route": Daily survival narratives from mothers who are homeless. *American Journal of Community Psychology, 23*(6), 871–891.

Banyard, V. L., & Graham-Berman, S. A. (1998). Surviving poverty: Stress and coping in the lives of housed and homeless mothers. *American Journal of Orthopsychiatry, 68*(3), 479–489.

Bassuk, E. L. (2001). *Multiply homeless families: The insidious impact of violence.* Unpublished paper presented for the Housing Policy Debate, PAIS International database.

Belcher, J. R., Green, J. A., McAlpine, C., & Ball, K. (2001). Considering pathways into homelessness: Mothers, addictions, and trauma. *Journal of Addictions Nursing, 13*(3/4), 199–208.

Blair, C., Jacobs, N. R., & Quiram, J. (1999). *Homelessness in America: How could it happen here?* Wylie, TX: Information Plus.

Blumer, H. (1969). *Symbolic interactionism: Perspective and method.* Englewood Cliffs, NJ: Prentice-Hall.

Chenitz, W. C., & Swanson, J. M. (1986). *From practice to grounded theory: Qualitative research in nursing.* Menlo Park, CA: Addison-Wesley.

Chiang, V. C., Keatinge, D., & Williams, A. K. (2001). Challenges of recruiting avulnerable population in a grounded theory. *Nursing and Health Sciences, 3,* 205–211.

Choi, N. G., & Snyder, L. (1998). Voices of homeless parents: The pain of homelessness & shelter life. *Journal of Human Behavior in the Social Environment, 2*(3), 55–77.

Da Costa Nunez, R. (1996). *The new poverty: Homeless families in America.* New York: Insight Books/Plenum Press.

De Chesnay, M. (Ed.). (2005). *Caring for the vulnerable: Perspectives in nursing theory, practice, and research* (2nd ed.). Sudbury, MA: Jones and Bartlett.

Drake, M. (1992). The nutritional status and dietary adequacy of single women and their children in shelters. *Public Health Report, 107,* 312–319.

Egan, T. M. (2002). Grounded theory research and theory building. *Advances in Developing Human Resources, 4*(3), 277–295.

Ensign, J., & Panke, A. (2002). Barriers and bridges to care: Voices of homeless female adolescent youth in Seattle, Washington. *Journal of Advanced Nursing, 37*(2), 166–172.

Flaskerud, J. H. (Ed.) (1999). Emerging nursing care of vulnerable populations. *Nursing Clinics of North America, 34*(2), 261–539.

Glaser, B. G. (1978). *Theoretical sensitivity: Advances in the methodology of grounded theory.* Mill Valley, CA: Sociology Press.

Glaser, B. (1996). *Gerund grounded theory: The basic social process dissertation.* Edited with assistance of W. D. Kaplan. Mill Valley, CA: Sociology Press.

Glaser B. (2001). *The grounded theory perspective: Conceptualization contrasted with description.* Mill Valley, CA: Sociology Press.

Glaser, B. G., & Strauss, A. L. (1967). *The discovery of grounded theory: Strategies for qualitative research.* Chicago: Aldine.

Golden, S. (1992). *The women outside: Meanings and myths of homelessness.* Berkeley, CA: University of California Press.

Grigsby, C., Baumann, D., & Gregorich, S. E. (1990). Disaffiliation to entrenchment: A model for understanding homelessness. *Journal of Social Issues, 46*(4), 141–156.

Heidegger, M. (1962). *Being in time.* Translated from German by J. Macquarrie & E. Robinson. New York: Harper.

Institute for Children and Poverty. (1998). *Ten cities, 1997–1998: A snapshot of family homelessness across America.* New York: Institute for Children and Poverty.

Kennard, K. A. (2002). Renewal of the spirit: Exploring the religious and spiritual coping strategies of the homeless. Unpublished dissertation from City University of New York. *Dissertation Abstracts International, 62,* no. 12A.

Kozol, J. (1988). *Rachel and her children: Homeless families in America.* New York: Fawcett Columbine.

Lindsey, E. W. (1998). The impact of homelessness and shelter life on family relationships. *Family Relations, 47*(3), 243–252.

London, J. (1903, 1998). *The people of the abyss.* London: Pluto Press.

Lorber, J. (1998). *Gender inequality: Feminist theories and politics.* Los Angeles: Roxbury.

Meadows-Oliver, M. (2003). Mothering in public: A meta-synthesis of homeless women with children living in shelters. *Journal for Specialists in Pediatric Nursing, 8*(4), 130–136.

Menke, E. M., & Wagner, J. D. (1997). The experience of homeless female-headed families. *Issues in Mental Health Nursing, 18*(4), 315–330.

Miller, A. B., & Keys, C. B. (2001). Understanding dignity in the lives of homeless persons. *American Journal of Community Psychology, 29*(2), 331–334.

Munhall, P. L. (Ed.). (1994). *In women's experience.* New York: National League for Nursing.

National Coalition for the Homeless. (2001). *Homeless families with children. NCH Fact Sheet #7.* Washington, DC: Author.

National Coalition for the Homeless. (2006). *Who is homeless? NCH Fact Sheet #3.* Washington, DC: National Coalition for the Homeless. Retrieved August 17, 2007, from http://www.nationalhomeless.org/publications/facts/Whois.pdf

Netburn, M. (2005). *The Los Angeles homeless services authority releases key data from its first homeless count.* Retrieved August 21, 2007, from http://www.lahsa.org/pdfs/Current/Press%20Release%20Final.pdf

Oliviera, N. L. (2002). The nutrition status of women and children who are homeless. *Nutrition Today, 37*(2), 70–77.

Page, T., & Nooe, R. M. (2002). Life experiences and vulnerabilities of homeless women: A comparison of women unaccompanied versus accompanied by minor children, and correlates with children's emotional distress. *Journal of Social Distress and the Homeless, 11*(3), 215–231.

PATH. (2002). *Issue brief.* Washington, DC: Projects for Assistance in the Transition from Homelessness, a branch of the Department of Mental Health Services.

Plebe, G. C. (1998). *Poetry from the Street Sheet, a publication of the Coalition on Homelessness.* San Francisco: Coalition on Homelessness.

Russell, B. G. (1991). *Silent sisters.* Baltimore: Hemisphere Publishing Corporation.

Seltser, B. J., & Miller, D. E. (1993). *Homeless families: The struggle for dignity.* Chicago: University of Illinois Press.

State of the County. (2003). *State of the County Report: Los Angeles 2000–2002.* Los Angeles: United Way.

Taylor, C. (1997). *Philosophical arguments.* Cambridge, MA: Harvard University Press.

Timmer, D. A., Eitzen, D. S., & Talley, K. D. (1994). *Paths to homelessness: Extreme poverty and the urban housing crisis.* Boulder, CO: Westview Press.

Toohey, S. M., Shinn, M., & Weitzman, B. C. (2004). Social networks and homelessness among women heads of household. *American Journal of Community Psychology, 33*(1–2), 7–20.

Urban Institute. (2000). *A new look at homelessness in America.* Retrieved August 21, 2007, from http://www.urban.org/publications/900366.html

U.S. Bureau of Census. (1998). *Poverty in the United States: 1997.* Washington, DC: Author.

U.S. Conference of Mayors. (2001). *A status report on hunger and homelessness in America's cities: 2001.* Washington, DC: Author.

Weingart Center #1. (June 2000). *Who is homeless in Los Angeles? Just the Facts.* Los Angeles: Institute for the Study of Homelessness and Poverty.

Whitehead, D. (2002). *Statistics on homelessness.* Washington, DC: National Coalition for the Homeless.

Chapter 21

The Use of Community-Based Participatory Research to Understand and Work with Vulnerable Populations

Ellen Olshansky

Health disparities and lack of access to health care among some disadvantaged populations have received increasing attention and concern among healthcare providers and health policymakers (Minkler, Blackwell, Thompson, & Tamier, 2003; U.S. Department of Health and Human Services, 2000). As healthcare providers and policymakers have become more concerned about the health of vulnerable populations, more research has been developed to better understand their plight. The goal of these research studies is to develop effective interventions. These studies, however, often fail to present the perspective of those who are vulnerable, resulting in less than optimal interventions. The purpose of this chapter is to present an overview of community-based participatory research (CBPR) as an approach to learning about and working effectively with vulnerable populations.

Vulnerable populations encompass those groups with decreased access to care and increased risk for illness and accidents. In trying to intervene with various vulnerable populations, it is imperative that healthcare providers understand their perspectives rather than imposing on them what we believe to be their experiences. Without such understanding we may unwittingly exacerbate problems, and community members who are vulnerable may believe they are being given edicts, are disempowered, and have no voice in the solution to their problems. An example is the exclusion of women from clinical trials with the disastrous results that findings related to men were simply applied to women without scientific evidence for the clinical significance of these findings. Women as a population became vulnerable by virtue of being excluded from research. At this point the National Institutes of Health mandates the inclusion of women unless there is obvious rationale for excluding them. Such inclusion, however, does not guarantee that the perspectives and voices of women are included in the research. The issue of appropriate recognition of women's issues continues to be argued and debated (Parascandola, 2006).

Many researchers use open-ended approaches to understanding the experiences of others, including asking open-ended questions without imposing variables a priori. This approach yields important data that would not otherwise be generated. However, this research is done "on" the participants. CBPR takes a different approach. It actively involves the participants as coresearchers. Clark and colleagues (2003) addressed the need for community members themselves to contribute to identifying the needs within their communities. This chapter presents an overview of this method and then describes why it is appropriate for working with vulnerable populations.

Overview of Community-Based Participatory Research

CBPR is an action-oriented research method that involves a team approach inclusive of all participants. "All" participants refers to the researchers and the "researched" as equal members of the research team, all with an important voice in the research. Rather than referring to the process of doing research "on" people, this approach refers to doing research "with" people. The "people" are those members of a community of interest, those who are most directly affected by the phenomenon being studied. The members of a community also work in tandem with the researchers, leading to a collegial research effort within an environment of collaboration rather than the traditional hierarchical environment. One important goal of CBPR is to empower those who have not been empowered (e.g., those who are vulnerable) by helping to eliminate oppressive situations and/or conditions contributing to marginalization and vulnerability.

CBPR engages community members as active participants in the research. An important aim of this research is to generate an understanding of the community members' perspectives and needs so as to develop interventions that meet the needs of the community members. The concept of action is integral to CBPR (in fact, some refer to this kind of research as "participatory action research" or "action research") because the overt goal of this research is to take constructive action. CBPR is most appropriate for addressing the needs of vulnerable populations because it encourages the direct and active involvement of the members of those populations. Such an approach seeks to mitigate inequalities and oppression among vulnerable groups.

In recent years CBPR has received increasing attention. Seymour-Rolls and Hughes (2000), Minkler et al. (2003), and Israel, Schulz, Parker, and Becker (1998) addressed the importance of this approach to research in better understanding the nuances and complexities in communities of interest. Olshansky and colleagues (2005) described how CBPR can be used to understand and alleviate health disparities. At the Eastern Nursing Research Society a research interest group was recently formed with a specific focus on CBPR, reflecting the increasing interest in this approach to research.

Israel and colleagues (1998) aptly described eight key principles of CBPR:

1. Recognizing that the community is the unit of study

2. Building on the strengths already present in the community

3. Continually facilitating collaboration and partnership in each phase of the research

4. Integrating knowledge and action (e.g., knowledge alone is not enough; it must be coupled with action for social change)

5. Promoting the alleviation of social inequality by colearning

6. Using an iterative process

7. Focusing on wellness and an ecological perspective of health

8. Partnering in the dissemination of research findings

This chapter uses the framework presented by Israel and colleagues. The next section presents an in-depth look at each of these principles, followed by a focus on the applicability of each to working with vulnerable populations.

Principles of CBPR: Applicability to Vulnerable Populations

1. *Recognizing that the community is the unit of study.* This principle addresses the central focus of CBPR: the community and the factors that influence the community must be understood and addressed to understand the issues of the individual within the community. The concept is consistent with the ecological framework that addresses social, political, economic, environmental, and sociological factors as part of the community context and contributing to the experience of individuals within the community. Although the experiences of each individual are important and each individual is unique, the focus is on the community in which the individual experiences situations and problems. Individual differences within communities are taken into account to develop a comprehensive understanding of the complexities within communities.

2. *Building on the strengths already present in the community.* This principle embraces the attitude that those within the community already have strengths despite the fact that they are vulnerable by virtue of unequal access to care and perhaps oppression by other dominant groups. In the spirit of empowerment it is important to learn from them how they view their strengths, how they would like to use their strengths to tackle the problems identified, and how they can improve on present strengths. It is imperative that the community members articulate these strengths and why they view them as strengths. Reciprocally, it is imperative that the members of the research team truly listen to and hear the community members' descriptions of how they cope with situations, how they have managed in the past, and what their views are in regard to how to continue to manage and move forward despite the vulnerabilities that they experience on a daily basis.

   Focusing on strengths encourages empowerment among the members of the community. They believe they have something to offer rather than being told what they should do by the researchers or health professionals. In addition, the researchers can learn from the community participants. Rather than, as is traditionally done, imposing their views on the community participants, the researchers can begin to understand what works best for the community participants.

3. *Continually facilitating collaboration and partnership in each phase of the research.* Collaboration and partnership are signature aspects of CBPR. To develop a collaborative partnership with the members of a vulnerable community requires much planning (Kelly, 2005). It takes time to develop a true partnership with members of the community, particularly when there has been a lack of trust of researchers from an academic or other institution among vulnerable community members. Taking the time initially to develop trust, enabling the entrée of the traditional researcher into the community, is crucial to the success of the research. Strategies for achieving this trusting relationship include going into the community and conducting focus groups on site (as opposed to having the community members travel to the location of the researcher).

It is important that the researchers venture out of the "ivory tower." Community members, likewise, need to know that they have an open invitation to the researcher's location, but of overriding importance is for the researchers to enter the context of the community members. By doing so they strive to understand the context and to reverse the often stereotypical view of the ivory towers of academia. Gaining entrée into the community and developing trust among the community members is only the beginning of this collaboration and partnership. Community members are considered equal partners in the research. They have an active voice in determining the research question, in designing the research method, in contributing to the data collection and analysis, and in disseminating the research results. They work in partnership as equal members of the research team.

It is important to recognize the unique skills and contributions made by each member of the research team. The community members are the experts in the actual phenomenon under study. The traditional researchers are the experts in research methodology, including collection and analysis of data, and writing up or presenting research results. Therefore each member of the research team contributes based on his or her area of expertise, but all members of the research team are involved in all the steps of the research process to greater or lesser degrees.

Focus groups are commonly used in CBPR as a way to involve all members of the research team and to elicit perspectives from the various members of the research team. Focus groups are a way of facilitating discussion within an atmosphere of openness, where the goal is to hear the various perspectives and views of community members and the traditional research members. The focus group serves several purposes. It helps each member of the team to get to know one another and to hear each person's perspectives and description of their experiences. It also helps the members to come together in a collaborative manner as they begin to understand each person's experiences, focusing on the differences among them while also looking for and eventually being able to define commonalities. The focus group allows the members to more clearly define the research problem, the focus of the research, and to identify the goals and outcomes of the research.

4. *Integrating knowledge and action.* A crucial component of CBPR is action, in the form of developing and implementing interventions within the community that will help to alleviate the problems identified. CBPR is a form of research with the overt purpose of making social change to alleviate disparities, oppression, and other factors that lead to vulnerability. CBPR is true "translation research" because the translation into practice occurs in an immediate and ongoing fashion from the moment the research commences and throughout the entire process. By working closely and collaboratively with community members who desire constructive social change, the emphasis on action to achieve this constructive change is paramount in CBPR. This approach is germane to nursing education as nursing students are a strong voice for social change necessary to improve health disparities among vulnerable populations (Reimer-Kirkham, Van Hofwegen, & Hoe-Harwood, 2005).

5. *Promoting the alleviation of social inequality by colearning.* The principles discussed above contribute to alleviating social inequality. This principle is directly related to the principle of integrating knowledge and action. To alleviate social inequality it is imperative that constructive social change leads to social emancipation and alleviation of oppression. Such social change is truly constructive only if those less fortunate (those who are vulnerable) are empowered. Integrating this principle into CBPR reflects the complexity of this research approach. This research process includes developing collaborative partnerships, involving all members of the community actively in the research project, overtly seeking to make social change in a constructive manner, and doing all of this while empowering those less fortunate. In fact, without such empowerment the other aspects of the research will not be achieved. Lofman, Pelkonen, and Pietila (2004) aptly described the importance of the involvement of the community members to address unequal power relationships.

6. *Using an iterative process.* An iterative process is one in which each of the phases of a study are conducted in a circular, as opposed to a linear, fashion. Each phase is not a discrete part of the process. Each phase informs the next phase, and subsequent phases may lead to returning to previous phases to make changes based on continuous learning throughout the CBPR process. This iterative process is central to all qualitative research. CBPR uses qualitative research methods through focus groups, eliciting perspectives of informants in their own words, and approaching data in an interpretive manner. The research begins in an inductive manner as the research question is open ended, and the goal is to learn the perspectives of the members of the community without imposing preconceived variables. As the research continues certain variables that are generated through the research process receive greater focus based on continuing data to support these variables. In qualitative terms this is referred to as saturation of data (Strauss & Corbin, 1998). At this point data collection becomes more deductive, focused on

looking for further evidence of predetermined and emerging variables. Previous data are then reanalyzed with the explicit purpose of looking for data or evidence to support the existence of these variables. This iterative process involves going back and forth with data collection that influences data analysis, which then furthers data collection.

7. *Focusing on wellness and an ecological perspective of health.* CBPR proposes multiple and interacting factors within ones' social context that influence and are influenced by health. This ecological perspective embraces the notion that context is a key factor in understanding how to promote wellness. The context includes biological, psychological, environmental, social, and interpersonal factors. Health and wellness occur within this context. Using CBPR, the research team seeks to understand the factors in this ecological perspective. These factors are uncovered by open-ended questions and participant observation.

8. *Partnering in the dissemination of research findings.* As noted earlier, in CBPR all members of the research team are involved in all aspects of the research process, including the dissemination of research findings. Traditionally, the dissemination of research has consisted of researchers writing for publication or presenting at conferences. These publications and conferences have been refereed (i.e., reviewed by a panel of experts who are also researchers and scholarly peers). In CBPR those peer reviews continue, but research findings are also disseminated in magazines and meetings of the lay public. Those publications that are sent to peer-reviewed journals will, ideally, include the lay community members as coauthors. The research data and findings are "owned," in a sense, by all members of the research team, a key aspect of CBPR.

CBPR and Vulnerable Populations

Vulnerable populations often lack a voice in regard to what they need and to how these needs could best be met. It is more common for presumed "experts" from health care and other arenas to dictate solutions to vulnerable populations. This dominant attitude, although perhaps well meaning, is usually counterproductive. It keeps vulnerable populations in vulnerable positions. They continue to lack a voice. A CBPR approach seeks to address these limitations of the traditional approach to assisting vulnerable populations. CBPR aims to assist the vulnerable in attaining and maintaining a voice, to recognize those who are vulnerable as the true "experts" about the issues they are experiencing, and to ultimately assist them toward partnership in social change.

Implementing a CBPR Approach with Vulnerable Populations

Even after establishing the critical need for CBPR in alleviating inequalities and oppressions suffered by vulnerable groups, it remains difficult to implement such an approach. Many barriers exist, but one goal of nurses and other healthcare providers and researchers is to work actively to overcome those barriers. This section presents strategies for implementing CBPR in research and healthcare settings.

In academic research settings there needs to be support for such an approach. The National Institutes of Health recognizes the need for CBPR, reflected in a recent call for research proposals incorporating CBPR. In educational settings, this approach should be included in research courses in undergraduate and graduate programs.

Academic researchers and healthcare clinicians should partner with one another to develop research programs that include community members. An ideal CBPR project would include academic researchers, clinicians, and community members. In addition, health policy experts and members of health insurance companies could also be included in such research. All these participants in the research process can contribute important perspectives. The research team is expanded to include the voices of the community members. The community members then have the opportunity to voice their concerns to these various members of the healthcare team.

References

Clark, M. J., Cary, S., Diemont, G., Ceballos, R., Sifuentes, M., Atteberry, I., et al. (2003). Involving communities in community assessment. *Public Health Nursing Journal, 20*, 456–463.

Israel, B. A., Schulz, A. J., Parker, E. A., & Becker, A. B. (1998). Review of community-based research: Assessing partnership approaches to improve public health. *Annual Review of Public Health, 19*, 173–202.

Kelly, P. J. (2005). Practical suggestions for community interventions using participatory action research. *Public Health Nursing, 22*(1), 65–73.

Lofman, P., Pelkonen, M., & Pietila, A.M. (2004). Ethical issues in participatory action research. *Scandinavian Journal of Caring Science, 18*, 333–340.

Minkler, M., Blackwell, A. G., Thompson, M., & Tamier, H. (2003). Community-based participatory research: Implications for public health funding. *American Journal of Public Health, 93*, 1210–1213.

Olshansky, E., Sacco, D., Braxter, B., Dodge, P., Hughes, E., Ondeck, M., et al. (2005). Participatory action research to understand and reduce health disparities. *Nursing Outlook, 53*, 121–126.

Parascandola, M. (2006). From exclusion to inclusion: Women and minorities in clinical trials. *Research Practitioner, 7*(2), 52–64.

Reimer-Kirkham, S., Van Hofwegen, L., & Hoe-Harwood, C. (2005). Narratives of social justice: Learning in innovative clinical settings. *International Journal of Nursing Education Scholarship, 2*(1), Article 28.

Seymour-Rolls, K., & Hughes, I. (2000). *Participatory action research: Getting the job done.* Action Research E-Reports, 4. Retrieved August 13, 2007, from http://www.fhs.usyd.edu.au/arow/arer/004.htm

Strauss, A., & Corbin, J. (1998). Basics of qualitative research: Techniques and procedures for developing grounded theory. Thousand Oaks, CA: Sage.

U.S. Department of Health and Human Services. (2000). *Healthy people 2010: Understanding and improving health.* Washington, DC: Office of Disease Prevention and Health Promotion.

Immigrant Vulnerability: Does Capitalism in the United States Matter?

Jenny Hsin-Chun Tsai

International migration (or immigration) is an ancient phenomenon. With globalization this old phenomenon is happening faster and becoming more diversified than ever before. In 1997 in the United States alone 25.8 million persons, or 9.7% of the total U.S. population, were immigrants (Schmidley & Gibson, 1999). In 2000 immigrants increased to 28.4 million, representing 10.4% of the nation's total population (Lollock, 2001). Schmidley and Gibson's (1999) projection indicates that from 1995 to 2050, 40% of the total immigrant population will be Hispanic, 30% will be from Asia and the Pacific Islands, 20% will be non-Hispanic whites, and 10% will be African-American. As a result, demand for culturally competent care is knocking on the doors of clinicians, educators, researchers, and healthcare administrators harder than ever before.

Scientists believe that as a result of the extensive changes involved in immigration, the health of immigrants is threatened and their risk for poor health is increased after resettlement. In other words, changes experienced during transition add to the vulnerability of immigrants (Meleis, 1996). With regard to mental health many works show various kinds and degrees of adverse mental health consequences for immigrants and refugees: Ödegaard's (1932) investigation in the United States regarding mental illness in adult immigrants; Rutter et al.'s (1974) survey of children in the United Kingdom; Munroe-Blum, Boyle, Offord, and Kates' (1989) study of children in Canada; Baider, Ever-Hadani, and DeNour's (1996) work with Russian immigrants in Israel; Barnes' (2001) screening of recent refugees in the United States; Griffin and Soskolne's (2003) cross-sectional study of Thai migrant agricultural workers' psychosocial distress in Israel; and Sundaram, Oin, and Zøllner's (2006) investigation of suicide risks among foreign-born individuals in Denmark, to name a few.

Studies from other scholars further show factors that are associated with the health status and vulnerability of immigrants. For example, Anderson's study (1985) with Indo-Canadian and Greek women in Canada found that the women's help-seeking experiences were affected by their own perceptions of health, inability on the part of health professionals to grasp the circumstances of their lives, and their experiences of discrimination.

Studies with Polish immigrants (Aroian, 1990), Iranian immigrants (Lipson, 1992), and Korean immigrants (Nah, 1993) in the United States showed that language and occupational accommodation were two key factors for successful resettlement. The existence of ethnocultural communities in the area where immigrants move was also found to be important for immigrants' psychosocial adaptation and health (Baker, Arseneault, & Gallant, 1994; Tsai, 2006). Weitzman and Berry's work with poor immigrant women in New York (1992) indicated that being poor and being an immigrant contributed to these women's limited use of U.S. medical care and poor health status. These women faced even greater barriers to health care than did poor and uninsured Americans.

Transition during immigration and resettlement adds to the vulnerability of immigrants. Nevertheless, this vulnerability is not a static self-contained entity. Immigrant vulnerability is produced in ongoing interaction with social, economic, political, and cultural structures of the receiving country. Chopoorian (1986) reminded the nursing profession that a lack of consciousness about social, political, economic, and cultural factors prevents nursing from arriving at a comprehensive view of human health. Such a lack of consciousness about these issues keeps the profession in a peripheral role in the larger arena of social, economic, and political affairs of the United States. To promote the health of immigrants, as Anderson (1991) suggested, health professionals need to "acquire, through their education, a theoretical base that allows them to analyze the socioeconomic and political factors that influence health care delivery" (p. 716) and other aspects of everyday life.

Partial findings of a critical ethnographic study (Tsai, 2001) are presented in this chapter to show the effects that the receiving country's economic structure has on the vulnerability of immigrants. This is illustrated through events of their daily lives, their psychosocial reactions, and the adaptive strategies they used during resettlement in the receiving country. Implications for U.S. health professionals are discussed thereafter.

Description of the Study

This critical ethnographic study took place in a metropolitan area in the northwest region of the United States between 1998 and 2000. The study was designed to explore how immigrant families' lives are shaped by the larger societal context of the receiving country. Data were collected from nine Taiwanese immigrant families recruited through community snowball referrals. Participants were protected through compliance with the university-approved procedures for human subjects.

Sample

A total of 29 participants, representing these nine families, contributed to the overall data. Of the 29 participants, 16 were parents with a mean age of 45.3 years (standard deviation [SD] ± 2.4). Nine completed college (16 years) in Taiwan, and four had advanced education (three master's degrees and one doctorate) in North America. As for the 13 children, they were between 8 and 21 years of age, with a mean of 16.1 years (SD ± 3.7). Their education ranged from second grade to first year of college. These families arrived in the United States as immigrants between January 1989 and August 1998 through three mechanisms: own employment (*n* = 3), sponsored by siblings who were naturalized U.S. citizens (*n* = 4), and returning to the United States (*n* = 2) (in which case, one of the key family members already had permanent resident status or citizenship in the United States). Most families (*n* = 8) lived in middle-class areas.

Data Generation

Participants were interviewed one to three times, alone or with other family members. All interviews were semistructured and were conducted primarily in Chinese. English was occasionally used with children who were limited in Chinese proficiency or to convey certain ideas. All interviews were conducted at home, with the exception of one participant who chose to meet at a restaurant because his parents and sibling did not participate. The length of visit for each interview ranged from 1.5 to 10 hours. Interviews were recorded on audiotape with the consent of the participants. During the interview visits, observations were undertaken to learn about family dynamics, family structure, family affect, daily family activities, the physical home environment, network contacts, and opinions about extrafamilial environments.

In addition to interviews and observations, each participant completed a demographic and immigration questionnaire at the end of the first interview. The children's version had 21 items and collected each child's demographic information. The adult version had 41 items that gathered each adult participant's individual information and his or her family information. Both Chinese and English versions were available. Assistance was available at the scene to help them complete the questionnaires.

Data Analysis and Scientific Rigor

Descriptive statistics (frequency, mean, and SD) were used to analyze the questionnaire data. Narrative analytical technique (Riessman, 1993) guided the analysis of the interview data. In the first step interviews were transcribed from audiotapes to paper (in Chinese). Both verbal and nonverbal communications were preserved in the Chinese transcripts. After close examination of the Chinese transcripts, portions of the Chinese language transcripts (i.e., narrative segments) were selected, translated, and preserved in the English language transcripts for in-depth analysis.

Substantive and methodological codes were written next to the highlighted narrative segments. Other analytical notes were also written next to the related narrative segments. Ongoing comparisons of stories across different family members in the same family and across families were made during the analysis process. Ongoing consultation with senior researchers and colleagues with diverse backgrounds, as well as confirmation with participants, refined the analysis. Fewer and fewer new codes were generated with each newly analyzed interview after half of the interviews were analyzed. Codes gradually merged and became more abstract and analytical. HyperRESEARCH (1999), a computer-assisted qualitative software, was used to manage the data and emerging codes.

Findings

The in-depth analysis revealed that four aspects of U.S. societal context shaped the everyday lives of immigrants. One of these was economic: the norms, values, and practices defined by U.S. capitalism. (The others were immigration policy, Western imperialism, and social class.) Marketing culture, insurance, and credit were the three themes of the economic context identified in the data related to U.S. capitalism.

Marketing Culture

Marketing culture refers to "the degree with which the norms and practices of business for selling products and making profits for business owners influence immigrants" (Tsai, 2001, p. 168). Similar to what occurs in the rest of the U.S. population, families in this study received multiple phone calls, mailings, or in-person visits for various product sales and donations. Taiwan is a capitalist country, yet the economic structure and culture differ from those of the United States. The United States emphasizes individualism and the free market. Taiwan emphasizes collectivism and tighter government control.

Participant families had different cultural knowledge about and conceptions of telecommunications and product sales. Many of them complained about their contacts with sales representatives in the United States. "Ordering magazines is the same [problem]. They knock on your door all the time. Ask you to order, ask you for donation. Many of this type of problem," said one family (Tsai, 2001, pp. 168–169). They were distressed, bothered, and frustrated by these practices and the hassles derived from these practices. As one participant said, "We only called Taiwan for a few minutes. Why it cost so much?! We later knew the reason [because we did not sign up for any long-distance promotion plan]. There is only one phone company in Taiwan. You just need a phone and then you have everything" (mother of two, living in the United States for 18 months at the time of the interview) (Tsai, 2001, p. 168).

Some families were concerned and worried about being cheated or having financial or even legal complications because "there are charges against some wrongdoing all the time in America. Lawsuits are everywhere" (Tsai, 2001, p. 169). The levels of frustration and worry were found to be higher in the participant families who were less proficient in English or who did not have friends or relatives in the area to which they moved.

Families usually thought of strategic solutions to decrease their stress level and protect themselves after a few bad experiences with sales people. For instance, some families chose to say no to everything and stick with whatever (telephone company, magazine subscription) they had at the time. After learning from friends or relatives with knowledge about the U.S. marketing culture, another strategy was sometimes adopted by the immigrants: speaking with a strange foreign accent or improper grammar in hopes that this would stop salespersons from further explaining their products. Some families adapted to the U.S. marketing culture by adjusting their personal perceptions. They treated the money lost to purchasing products they regretted as the "tuition" they had to spend as part of their immigration journey. "Be careful" was the phrase used by some participants throughout the interviews.

Insurance

Insurance is "the types and amounts of insurance necessary to adequately protect the families" (Tsai, 2001, p. 171). Health and life insurance were exported from the United States to Taiwan decades ago. Thus Taiwanese are familiar with the concepts of health and life insurance. Because of the increasing use of cars in Taiwan, car insurance was adopted in Taiwan in the mid-1990s. After participant families immigrated, they began to realize that there are many more types of insurance in the United States and, as one participant said, "everything needs to be insured." The expense of insurance was much higher than they had expected.

The participant families' greatest concern was the cost of health insurance. Taiwan has a universal healthcare system. Having to purchase one's own health insurance when not employed was a new concept to families who were new to the United States. For one family that emigrated as an investment, they did not know that they needed to purchase individual health insurance until they were involved in the local Taiwanese community. Families felt helpless with the high cost of health insurance; at the same time they could not go without insurance. Unfortunately, the road to finding a health insurance plan was not straightforward either. There are many insurance plans offered by different companies. Before participant families could even make a decision, they had to learn about copayments, deductibles, preferred doctors, prevention, and so forth. For participant families who spoke limited English, choosing an insurance plan was challenging. They had to rely on relatives or friends in the area (more so than did those who were comfortable with English) to resolve the insurance issues.

To overcome the problems with insurance, the first step was staying as healthy as possible to avoid healthcare expenses while the family was looking for jobs that offered benefits. One family said, "When we just got here, we had no insurance. Could not get sick! We bore with it for half a year. Took some over-the-counter drugs [when we're sick]" (Tsai, 2001, p. 173). Some families flew back to Taiwan for their healthcare needs, usually the nonemergency kind, because as one participant said, "add a round trip ticket on top of [the treatment cost], I still have plenty left. It's still cost-effective" (Tsai, 2001, p. 172). A few families would just pay for the insurance regardless of the cost because they knew the importance of having insurance in the United States.

Credit

Credit refers to "the degree of which the value of credit affects immigrant families in the U.S." (Tsai, 2001, p. 174). In capitalism credit means money and profits (Weber, 1992). Credit history, a widely used concept in the United States, is used to assess a prospective customer's potential for profit making for the business owner. A good credit history means a potential for making profits from this prospective customer. However, credit history is not a concept that exists in Taiwan. Thus families living in the United States for the first time were surprised and confused when apartment managers asked about credit history and requested investigation fees. Although families in the study were lucky enough to have the investigation waived, some of them had friends who could not even rent a place because they had no credit history at the time. One family said that a friend had to pay 6 months rent in advance in cash to secure the place.

The lack of credit history not only presented problems for immigrants' access to housing, it also hampered their ability to get loans and credit cards and, ironically, chances to build up their credit history. In the area of loan and credit card applications, no family was lucky with these services. As one unhappy family described their experience, "American banks were not willing to loan to us because he wants you to use credit as deposit, right? Chinese use properties as deposit for loans. That's the difference" (Tsai, 2001, p. 128). Families eventually turned to Chinese-owned banks for help. Regardless of the fact that the process with Chinese-owned banks was not completely smooth, families at least got the loan or credit card from the bank as a start.

Discussion

Decades of studies of immigrant experiences have informed us of the resettlement experience and the threats to immigrant health in countries such as Canada, the United Kingdom, and the United States. Analysis of the stories of nine Taiwanese immigrant families reveals that immigrants' everyday life is inseparable from the economic structure of the receiving country. Three capitalist practices—the marketing culture, insurance, and credit—create a living context that increases immigrants' vulnerability in the United States.

The financial burden, potential legal ramifications, and limited access to housing, loans, and health care are not the kinds of experiences that immigrants to the United States anticipate before their immigration. Literature has shown that when people move into a new country they have to adapt, to varying extents, with regard to the language used by the receiving country, the physical environment, the culture, the systems, the loss of social support, and economic survival (Aroian, 1990; Baker et al., 1994; Lipson, 1992; Sam & Berry, 1995; Tsai, 2001). The adaptive processes can last from years to a lifetime. These unexpected experiences are additional stressors that place immigrants in the United States at risk while they are attempting to manage the other demands they must face as immigrants. Moreover, as part of the capitalist environment or economic structure, people in the United States are always bombarded with sales promotions for new products, business changes, new insurance coverage, and increases in healthcare costs. Even Americans who were born and raised in the United States struggle to understand the changes and choices available to them and to deal with these economic practices.

Immigrants, particularly new immigrants, easily get lost in the massive amount of information thrown at them. Making an informed decision is a much more challenging and stressful process for new immigrants than for native-born Americans and established early-wave immigrants. In other words, immigrants' vulnerability exists on a continuum. The degree of the vulnerability increases when the receiving country's economic structure intersects with immigrants' language challenges, unfamiliarity with the systems, and/or limited access to local social networks for support. In this study the participant families (who had been in the United States no more than 10 years) discussed their self-doubt about the decisions they made; they revealed their worries and frustration about the financial and legal consequences of their decisions. Unlike those citizens born in the United States, immigrants can face deportation for numerous legal issues (e.g., not reporting an address change to the immigration authority, speeding tickets, credit problems, or crime). Thus not only are immigrants concerned about the same financial and legal consequences as the people of the receiving country, but they also need to worry about the legal consequences specifically tied to their immigration status.

Navarro (1993, 2003) argued that the problems of the U.S. healthcare system can not be understood without including capitalism—the moving force behind the financing and delivery of health services in the United States—in the discussion. Health insurance companies are controlled by corporate owners and have a tremendous power over how services are provided by healthcare providers. Profit and efficiency are the bases for their decision. Insurance premiums are raised to cover growing medical costs and ensure profits. As a result, employers shift the cost of insurance premiums to their employees and/or provide limited choices of insurance plans or no insurance at all. More people become uninsured and face greater barriers to access health care for treatment and illness prevention (Asplin et al., 2005; Himmelstein, Woolhandler, & Hellander, 2001; Kleinke, 2001; Taylor, Larson, & Correa-de-Araujo, 2006). Because capitalism in the United States has such an intimate relationship with immigrants' everyday experience, I would further argue that this economic framework has not only shaped the nation's healthcare system, it also has driven the production of goods and marketing, the creation of insurance policies, and access to those things that fill basic needs. To decrease immigrants' vulnerability and promote their health, it is absolutely essential to include capitalism in the discussion.

Implications for Health Professionals

Health professionals have ample opportunities to work with immigrants: in acute care settings, primary care settings, long-term care facilities, community clinics, workplaces, home settings, and schools. In fact, health professionals are in a valuable position to ensure health equity for immigrants. Presented here are some ways for health professionals to be true health advocates.

As a microlevel approach, during visits health professionals should include questions that can help them better understand the effects of the U.S. capitalist economic structure and practices on the stress levels and well-being of immigrant clients. Because immigrant clients are already using their individual resources (e.g., personal intelligence and knowledge, social networks) to develop sufficient strategies to overcome those stressors, health professionals can (should) serve as another resource for these clients. If immigrant clients do not have enough individual resources to develop effective adaptive strategies, health professionals should then initiate the discussion and collaborate with the clients to formulate some potentially practical and successful strategies.

In addition to changing their own practices, health professionals have to share their knowledge with their colleagues and policymakers to heighten their awareness of the effects of the receiving country's economic structure on immigrants' vulnerability and health status. Thus fewer health professionals and policymakers will use culture or language barrier as a catch-all category to explain all immigrant experiences (McGrath, 1998; Tsai, 2003). Instead, they will have a more comprehensive understanding of immigrants' experiences and healthcare needs. As a result, more health professionals and policymakers will provide relevant interventions for the immigrant population and engage in the reconstruction of social and health policies that are driven by U.S. capitalism—a system that goes beyond immigrants' control yet has a tremendous effect on their everyday life.

Conclusion

Immigrants are at a higher risk for poor health. Nevertheless, their risk is not solely a result of language skills, education, levels of assimilation to the receiving country, or knowledge about the systems of the receiving country. The historical, sociocultural, economic, and political structures play significant roles in shaping immigrants' everyday experiences and health status. This chapter provides some preliminary insights into the effects of the U.S. economic structure on immigrant vulnerability. To provide culturally competent care to the immigrant population, further investigation into each of these structural effects and their interactions with immigrants' vulnerability is crucial. Cross-national comparison is needed as well. Of course, it is also necessary to have more health professionals and policymakers who can recognize that the health experiences and stresses immigrants identify are indeed products of complex social processes. Immigrants then will not be blamed for their problems while the "causes" of the problems lie in the larger societal context.

Acknowledgments

This chapter is based on the author's dissertation study. The study was supported in part by the American Nurses Foundation, the Psi-Chapter-at-Large of the Sigma Theta Tau International, the Robert Gilbert Foundation of the Association of Child and Adolescent Psychiatric Nurses, and the Hester McLaws Nursing Scholarship Fund of the University of Washington School of Nursing. An earlier version of this chapter was presented at the 2nd State of Science Congress in Washington, DC, in September 2002.

References

Anderson, J. M. (1985). Perspectives on the health of immigrant women: A feminist analysis. *Advances in Nursing Science, 8*(1), 61–76.

Anderson, J. M. (1991). Immigrant women speak of chronic illness: The social construction of the devalued self. *Journal of Advanced Nursing, 16*, 710–717.

Aroian, K. J. (1990). A model of psychological adaptation to migration and resettlement. *Nursing Research, 39*(1), 5–10.

Asplin, B. R., Rhodes, K. V., Levy, H., Lurie, N., Crain, A. L., Carlin, B. P., et al. (2005). Insurance status and access to urgent ambulatory care follow-up appointments. *Journal of the American Medical Association, 294*, 1248–1254.

Baider, L., Ever-Hadani, P., & DeNour A. K. (1996). Crossing new bridges: The process of adaptation and psychosocial distress of Russian immigrants in Israel. *Psychiatry, 59*, 175–183.

Baker, C., Arseneault, A. M., & Gallant, G. (1994). Resettlement without the support of an ethno-cultural community. *Journal of Advanced Nursing, 20*(6), 1064–1072.

Barnes, D. M. (2001). Mental health screening in a refugee population: A program report. *Journal of Immigrant Health, 3*(3), 141–149.

Chopoorian, T. J. (1986). Reconceptualization of the environment. In P. Moccia (Ed.), *New approaches to theory development* (pp. 39–54). New York: National League for Nursing.

Griffin, J., & Soskolne, V. (2003). Psychosocial distress among Thai migrant workers in Israel. *Social Science and Medicine, 57*, 769–774.

Himmelstein, D., Woolhandler, S., & Hellander, I. (2001). *Bleeding the patient: The consequences of corporate health care.* Monroe, ME: Common Courage.

HyperRESEARCH (Version 2.03). (1999). Thousand Oaks, CA: ResearchWare.

Kleinke, J. D. (2001). *Oxymorons: The myth of a US health care system.* San Francisco, CA: Jossey-Bass.

Lipson, J. G. (1992). The health and adjustment of Iranian immigrants. *Western Journal of Nursing Research, 14*(1), 10–29.

Lollock, L. (2001). *The foreign-born population in the United States: March 2000, current population reports.* U.S. Census Bureau, Current Population Reports P20-534. Washington, DC: U.S. Census Bureau.

McGrath, B. B. (1998). Illness as a problem of meaning: Moving culture from the classroom to the clinic. *Advances in Nursing Science, 21*(2), 17–29.

Meleis, A. I. (1996). Culturally competent scholarship: Substance and rigor. *Advances in Nursing Science, 19*(2), 1–16.

Munroe-Blum, H., Boyle, M. H., Offord, D. R., & Kates, N. (1989). Immigrant children: Psychiatric disorder, school performance, and service utilization. *American Journal of Orthopsychiatry, 59*(4), 510–519.

Nah, K. (1993). Perceived problems and service delivery for Korean immigrants. *Social Work, 38*(3), 289–296.

Navarro, V. (1993). *Dangerous to your health: Capitalism in health care.* New York: Monthly Review Press.

Navarro, V. (2003). Policy without politics: The limits of social engineering. *American Journal of Public Health, 93*, 64–67.

Ödegaard, O. (1932). Emigration and insanity. *Acta Psychiatrica et Neurologia,* (suppl. 4), 11–206.

Riessman, C. K. (1993). *Narrative analysis* (Vol. 30). Newbury Park, CA: Sage.

Rutter, M., Yule, W., Berger, M., Yule, B., Morton, J., & Bagley, C. (1974). Children of West Indian immigrants. I. Rates of behavioral deviance and of psychiatric disorder. *Journal of Child Psychology and Psychiatry, 15*, 241–262.

Sam, D. L., & Berry, J. W. (1995). Acculturative stress among young immigrants in Norway. *Scandinavian Journal of Psychology, 36*(1), 10–24.

Schmidley, A. D., & Gibson, C. (1999). *Profile of the foreign-born population in the United States: 1997.* U.S. Census Bureau, Current Population Reports P23-195. Washington, DC: U.S. Government Printing Office.

Sundaram, V., Oin, P., & Zøllner, L. (2006). Suicide risk among persons with foreign background in Denmark. *Suicide & Life-Threatening Behavior, 36*(4), 481–489.

Taylor, A. K., Larson, S, & Correa-de-Araujo, R. (2006). Women's health care utilization and expenditures. *Women's Health Issues, 16,* 66–79.

Tsai, J. H. C. (2001). *One story, two interpretations: The lived experiences of Taiwanese immigrant families in the United States.* Unpublished doctoral dissertation, University of Washington, Seattle.

Tsai, J. H. C. (2003). Contextualizing immigrants' lived experience: Story of Taiwanese immigrants in the United States. *Journal of Cultural Diversity, 10,* 76–83.

Tsai, J. H.-C. (2006). Xenophobia, ethnic community, and immigrant youths' friendship network formation. *Adolescence, 41*(162), 285–298.

Weber, M. (1930/1992). *The protestant ethic and the spirit of capitalism* (A. Giddens, Trans.). London, UK: Routeledge.

Weitzman, B. C., & Berry, C. A. (1992). Health status and health care utilization among New York City home attendants: An illustration of the needs of working poor, immigrant women. *Women and Health, 19*(2/3), 87–105.

Unit Four

"The world is a dangerous place, not because of people who are evil, but because of people who don't do anything about it."

■ ■ ■

Albert Einstein

PRACTICE

Predisposition to Non–Insulin-Dependent Diabetes Mellitus among Immigrants from the Former Soviet Union

Nataly Pasumansky

Scientific articles and media report a worldwide epidemic of diabetes. Surveys about prevalence of diabetes in the United States report that diabetes has increased 33% between 1990 and 1998 and is steadily increasing (Levetan, 2001). According to a report from the Centers for Disease Control and Prevention (CDC), diabetes is currently the sixth leading cause of death in the United States. Prevention and treatment of diabetes is a difficult task and needs both a cultural and an individual approach. The National Diabetes Information Clearinghouse emphasized that certain ethnic groups have an increased percentage of diabetes among adults 20 years old and older. Many cultural groups, new immigrants among them, are known to have an increased incidence of diabetes. With the stress of immigration and change of life-style and diet, new immigrants are more prone to diabetes. One such group, immigrants from the former Soviet Union, needs special attention because of its many elderly and chronically ill persons.

Immigrants from the former Soviet Union often have poor dietary habits and sedentary life-styles that put them at risk of developing obesity, a major risk factor for diabetes. With the collapse of the former Soviet Union, many people there became poor and resorted to a diet they could afford, which is usually high in calories and carbohydrates with few fresh fruits and vegetables. In addition, with little emphasis on prevention, former Soviet Union immigrants have little awareness of healthy diet and life-style options; therefore diabetes is often diagnosed late while the disease is already in progress. After immigration persons with diabetes and pre-diabetes have a difficult time learning a new language and finding a job, causing them to pay less attention to their health. In addition, these immigrants often are poor and have no access to basic health care.

Healthcare access for immigrants from the former Soviet Union is also complicated because of their diversity. They come to the United States from different republics of the former Soviet Union. Most of them come from Russia and the Ukraine. Most of them know the Russian language; however, some immigrants that come from other places, such as Latvia or Uzbekistan, do not know or are not fluent in Russian. In addition, they have different customs and religions. Even though interpreter services may be helpful, it is still not easy to accommodate the diverse cultural groups in this vulnerable population.

Nurse practitioners who manage former Soviet Union immigrants require understanding of specific cultural behavior and dietary habits. Advanced practice nurses may be particularly appropriate to care for Russian-speaking immigrants because they usually spend more time with patients than the physician. In addition, advanced practice nurses provide individualized treatment plans that are cost-effective. Nurse practitioners may have more expertise at gaining patients' trust because of the additional time with the patient and their traditional education to treat, including life-style modifications. With an increased knowledge of health practices and the historical background of immigrants, nurse practitioners may have higher compliance rates among their patients.

A culturally sensitive approach in diabetes education and treatment was suggested in many publications (London, 2002; Public Health, 2001). Diabetes treatment depends on factors such as stress, diet, and healthy life-style; therefore cultural aspects and trends are building blocks for understanding how to treat diabetes in Russian-speaking immigrants. However, little is known about Russian-speaking immigrants and diabetes. Nurse practitioners need to assess risk factors and develop plans for prevention of diabetes and diabetic complications in the immigrant population of the former Soviet Union.

Literature Review

A cultural approach in diabetes treatment and prevention is important for nurse practitioners and other healthcare providers. Literature currently addresses diabetes in different ethnic groups, such as the Chinese, Vietnamese, Cambodians, and Latinos (Adams, 2003; Mull, Nguyen, & Dennis, 2001; Rankin, Galbraith, & Huang, 1997). The increased mortality rate of Russian immigrants from chronic diseases including diabetes was a major concern for Israel and has been studied from a variety of perspectives (Ben-Noun, 1994; Rennet, Luz, Tamir, & Petersburg, 2002). Chronic diseases are reported as significantly higher in Russian Jewish immigrants than in Israeli veterans (Brodov, Mandelzweig, Boyco, & Behar, 2002; Rennet et al., 2002). This problem of chronic diseases among Russian immigrants significantly influenced Israeli mortality statistics and required a change in the Israeli medical system. However, little is known about diabetes among the community of immigrants from the former Soviet Union in the United States.

Preventative Care Practices among Immigrants from the Former Soviet Union

The literature indicates that in Russia health promotion is poor and people usually went to their provider only if they had health problems, especially among the middle aged. Female Russian immigrants tend to not use health-screening resources such as blood pressure, cholesterol screening, Pap smear, mammography, and breast self-examination. According to Ivanov and Buck (2002) immigrants from the former Soviet Union do not believe in health prevention and usually would not visit a clinic for screening examinations. In addition, women did not receive information about the need for such screening measurements. (Ivanov & Buck, 2002). Heavy cigarette smoking, high alcohol consumption, poor dietary intake, and little attention to physical fitness have contributed to chronic health problems in the Russian population (Duncan & Simmons, 1996). A major identified problem was the absence of basic health screening measurements such as cholesterol testing, high blood pressure screening, Pap smear, and mammogram (Duncan and Simmons, 1996). Authors did not mention, however, the importance of glucose screening for this population with multiple risk factors.

Russian articles about diabetes report that people are aware of healthy life-style, healthy diet, and health promotion, but they pay more attention to those things when they have a health problem. According to Russian Federation Ministry of Health, there was no appropriate preventative care for diabetes. In 2003 when the Ministry of Health did an investigation in Tumen (a medium-sized city in Russia), millions of patients were diagnosed with diabetes. Those patients already had serious cardiac problems as a result of hidden diabetes (Ministry of Health, Russian Federation, 2003). In one article Manvelov (1999), a Russian physician, wrote that 50% of patients who suffered a cerebrovascular accident may have had diabetes as a risk factor before the cerebrovascular accident occurred. He also stated that the diabetes rate in Russia is about 4–5%, but in some populations it may be as high as 20%. This high prevalence of diabetes among Russians discloses as well the genetic component of diabetes, making it a unique problem for Russian immigrants in the United States or elsewhere in the world.

The adverse effects of diabetes, similar to other chronic conditions (e.g., cardiovascular diseases), may be minimized with appropriate nonmedication care. "Medical nutritional therapy, exercises and diabetes education" can treat diabetes and prevent complications (Levetan, 2001). In addition, social support is a most important factor for prevention of diabetes complications. Russian families can be very supportive, but they may not understand the importance of prevention or early treatment of diabetes. Even though immigrants from the former Soviet Union are usually highly educated, they have little disease prevention knowledge. The CDC Task Force recommended diabetes education information in the community (CDC, 2005). However, because of the language and cultural barriers, Russian-speaking immigrants do not attend community education meetings. Education one-on-one by a nurse practitioner may be more beneficial for them.

Diet and Obesity among Russian-Speaking Immigrants

Dietary habits vary within different cultural groups. Russian-speaking immigrants are a diverse group and have different eating patterns. However, knowing the most common Russian diet pattern is important for nurse practitioners to discuss dietary changes if needed. Brown (2003) emphasized that more studies are needed to examine nutritional habits among ethnic groups and how important it is for healthcare providers to understand patients' specific cultural diet and to help them adjust to a healthier life-style.

Diet habits depend on cultural differences and vary from country to country within the former Soviet Union. Dietary habits in Russia are typically high in carbohydrates and fat and low in vegetables. Oystragh (1980), a Russian-speaking physician in Australia, conducted a study on Russian Jewish immigrants in Australia. In his practice he performed routine urine and serum glucose tests on new patients and found 15 diabetic patients among 158 patients (9.49%). This was compared with the average Australian incidence of 3.0%. He attributed the increased diabetes rate to two main factors: the high-stress period of immigration and a diet "extremely high in starches, where potatoes, bread, cakes, biscuits are eaten in almost every meal" (Oystragh, 1980, p. 270). The author observed only a small group of immigrants, but he believed this small group provided an accurate picture of the dietary habits of many Russian immigrants.

Obesity as a result of poor dietary habits is a major risk factor for developing non–insulin-dependent diabetes mellitus (NIDDM). Nikitin (1989) found that people who migrate to the eastern region, Siberia, increased their risk of developing diabetes. He found obesity to be an important risk factor. More than half of women who migrate to Siberia experienced a rapid weight gain during the first years of migration (Nikitin, 1989). One recent study of 644 Russian immigrants in New York found an increased risk in these immigrants to developing diabetes. Immigrants from the former Soviet Union are "invisible minorities" with high diabetes risk, and the main predisposition factor among them is obesity (Hosler, 2003).

Popkin (1998) collected data from a Russian longitudinal monitoring survey and found a consistent increase in adult, particularly elderly, obesity. Popkin (1998) found the overall increase in total obesity was more than 5 percentage points per 10-year period in Russia. Popkin (1998) also emphasized that NIDDM and many cardiovascular conditions related to NIDDM, such as hypertension, dyslipidemia, and atherosclerosis, are increasing rapidly in poor countries.

Zabina et al. (2001), conducting a study in Russia, found that, as in the United States, the cause of chronic diseases is typically related to life-style risk factors such as poor diet and inadequate physical activity. According to their survey of 542 men and 1,151 women living in Moscow, more than half of the men were currently smoking and more than half of the men and women had a body mass index of more than 25, signifying an obesity problem (Zabina et al., 2001). This study is consistent with the findings of Duncan and Simmons (1996) in which physical assessment data of 30 Russian immigrants showed that 65% of participants were overweight but only 14% of them were advised to lose weight. Duncan and Simmons (1996) questioned whether immigrants from the former Soviet Union are aware of obesity as a health problem.

To the contrary, studies by the Russian Federation Ministry of Health showed that Russian immigrants who have been diagnosed with diabetes are aware of the importance of diet in the treatment of diabetes, because many studies published in Russian are about a healthy diet in diabetes (Sharafertdinov, Mesheryakoba, & Plotnikova, 1997). However, a review of the Russian-language literature did not show any encouraging information about diabetes prevention and suggestions for diet change before disease onset.

Medication versus Natural Remedies

In the former Soviet Union, as in other countries and in the United States, there is a variety of medication treatments for diabetes. However, the use of natural remedies in Russian cultures remains open to discussion. In a dated article by Wheat, Brownstein, and Kvitash (1983), former Soviet Jewish patients were found to consider all drugs as poison and believed more in natural remedies. Today, the use of natural remedies for diabetes treatment in the Russian community is relatively unknown. As in many other countries, urban and highly educated people may not even be aware of treatment with natural remedies, but the rural population may believe in natural remedies as a best choice of treatment. Nurse practitioners as primary care providers need to know the risks and benefits associated with these natural remedies.

Multiple studies in Russia about the use of natural remedies have shown an increased interest in them. A study on green coffee was conducted at the Moscow Center for Modern Medicine, Russian Ministry of National Defense. Green coffee contains 55% chlorogenic acid, which is an antioxidant. Volunteers for the study received 90 mg/d chlorogenic acid or placebo. Results showed that blood glucose levels dropped 15–20% in those who received chlorogenic acid but not in the placebo group. The researchers concluded that chlorogenic acid has a potential role in the management of diabetes (Fields, 2003).

Another study used tea made from blueberry leaves (known as *chai cherniki* in Russian) for gastric colic and diabetes. Blueberry leaf extract contains caffeoylquinic acid and hydroxicinnamic acid (Jimenez del Rio, 2003). The study, also conducted at the Moscow Center for Modern Medicine, showed that blueberry leaf extract "possesses physiologically significant glucose-reducing potencies" (Jimenez del Rio, 2003).

It is not known from the literature review if those remedies are used often by Russian-speaking patients in the former Soviet Union or by immigrants. More studies are needed in the United States for detecting risks and benefits of those natural remedies because they are not widely used in the United States.

Stress and NIDDM

Immigrants from the former Soviet Union, like other immigrants, experience high psychological stress. Smith (1996) noted that Russian immigrants leave to escape very poor living conditions and joblessness but often face the same problems after entering the United States. They tend to end up in inner-city apartments with crime problems, low status, and low paying jobs. With the stress of adapting to these multiple factors, Russian immigrants pay little attention to their health. Brodov et al. (2002) studied 13,742 patients of two cohorts (Soviet Union and Israeli born) and found the statistically significant difference in mortality between the two groups (14.7 and 18.5, $p < 0.001$, respectively). The main causes of mortality rates in this study were many chronic diseases, especially coronary artery disease. However, the authors suggested that the reason for those chronic diseases was psychological stress. Stress has an adverse effect on many chronic diseases, NIDDM among them.

Many Russian-speaking immigrants may consider stress as a major risk factor of NIDDM onset (Meyerovich, 2003; Sidorov, Novikova, & Solov'ev, 2001). Multiple studies show how stress affects glycemic control negatively in clients that already have type 1 or type 2 diabetes. Conversely, little research evaluated stress and diabetes onset. Peyrot, McMurray, and Kruger (1999) found that stress affected glycemic control mostly because stress causes poor regimen compliance. These authors also suggested a connection between stress and diabetes onset.

Fukunishi, Akimoto, Horikawa, Shirasaka, and Yamazaki (1998), with a sample of 600 people, suggested that poor utilization of social support was associated with the onset of glucose tolerance abnormality. These authors suggested that lack of social support from family, relatives, and friends as well as other stress-related factors were negatively correlated with glucose tolerance tests in persons not known to have diabetes. Despite those findings, stress is not discussed as a risk factor for diabetes onset during healthcare visits. However, with Russian-speaking immigrants who might believe in the relationship between diabetes and stress, stress should be discussed by nurse practitioners during office visits.

Case Studies

The case studies below illustrate the problems in caring for immigrants from the former Soviet Union with diabetes. These case studies were recorded after telephone interviews with chosen participants. The names and some minor details were altered to protect the privacy of the participants.

Case Study 1

Boris S., a 75-year-old male refugee, emigrated with his family from Sverdlovsk, a large city in Russia, to the United States 8 years ago. Before emigrating, Boris worked as an engineer in a factory where he sat most of the day. He had almost no physical activity after work. He was overweight, liked to eat foods high in simple sugars, and had no family history of diabetes. Boris was diagnosed with diabetes in Russia 10 years ago. After noticing he was thirsty all the time, he went to a local endocrinologist who did a blood sugar examination. The endocrinologist sent Boris home, stating that Boris had no problem with his sugar. However, Boris continued to suffer from excessive thirst, and people around him noticed he was drinking water all the time. Boris went to an endocrinologist again, and the endocrinologist sent him for a glucose tolerance test. "They let me drink sugar and then tested my blood every hour," stated Boris. After this test the physician diagnosed him with type 2 diabetes. The endocrinologist told Boris that the first time he visited he had pre-diabetes, but now his diagnosis was diabetes. The endocrinologist said his diabetes was caused by working in the stressful environment at the factory, but he didn't mention that Boris was overweight.

The endocrinologist gave Boris some diabetic Polish medication for 1 month. Boris did not receive any specific education regarding his diabetes and was sent home without a glucometer. Every month he came to the endocrinologist to check his blood sugar and to receive his diabetic medications. Boris was also aware that he should avoid simple carbohydrates in his diet, but it was difficult for him. Every once in a while Boris would eat food not recommended in his diabetic diet.

After Boris came to the United States, he was diagnosed with hypertension and coronary artery disease requiring open heart bypass surgery. In addition, he had spinal stenosis, making it difficult for him to do any exercises because of the back pain. "Physicians here recommend physical activity such as walking and bicycling, but I can't do anything because shooting pain in my spine and legs and in addition I walk like on pillows and cannot feel my legs well because of my diabetes neuropathy, so I continue to be overweight. When my son came to visit me I noticed that he is getting big and I suggested him immediately start to lose weight," stated Boris.

Boris now visits his primary care provider every 3 months. He checks his blood glucose at home. Boris does not believe in natural remedies. His main diet now consists of vegetables, some fruits, oatmeal, buckwheat, and all kind of meats. His primary care provider instructs him on leading a diabetic life-style, and he tries very hard to follow those instructions.

Case Study 2

Marina P., 67 years old, emigrated as a refugee from Ukraine, Kiev. She was diagnosed with diabetes 14 years ago in the Ukraine. Before emigrating she worked as an accountant in a sewing factory. At work she sat most of the time and did not have time for physical activity. As a result she became overweight, but she did not believe it was a health problem. For 2 years before she was diagnosed with diabetes mellitus, she was thirsty all the time and had urinary urgency. Despite her symptoms she did not seek medical help and continued to live with this "discomfort." Marina's friend, who was a physician, noticed that Marina frequently went to the restroom and suggested she have her blood sugar checked.

When Marina went to the clinic to have her blood and urine checked, she already had diabetes. The physician suggested that there was something wrong with Marina's pancreas but did not mention her weight and her life-style. Initially, her physician suggested keeping a low carbohydrate diet and prescribed medications. However, Marina saw no improvement, so she began taking a Hungarian medication for diabetes. She did not have a glucometer at home; instead, she checked her blood sugar once a month in a local clinic.

At the time of her immigration to the United States 9 years ago Marina had very high blood glucose, kidney problems, arthritis, neuropathy, and poor vision. It was suggested that she take insulin, but she insisted on taking oral medications. As a first step Marina was referred to dietitian and her daughter helped her with translation. She received prescriptions for three different types of diabetic medications and now her blood sugars are stable and within normal limits.

Marina received education from her primary care provider and dietitian and decided not to go to diabetes educator or support groups. For now, her diet consists mostly of vegetables, buckwheat, and meat. She likes potatoes and used to eat them in every dish, but the dietitian asked her to reduce the amount of potatoes she consumed to preserve a healthy diet. She still needs to reduce her weight but finds it difficult because of severe arthritis and diabetic neuropathy. "Diabetes is distorting everything," said Marina.

Case Study 3

Tatyana, 52 years old, emigrated from Yarkutsk, a city in the north of Russia. The patient was diagnosed with diabetes in Russia about 15 years ago. Tatyana was diagnosed shortly after she moved to Novosibirsk, in the southern part of Russia. She related how in the North she stopped eating fresh fruits and vegetables because they were not available; she ate them only during the summer because she grew them in her backyard. She also gained weight at that time. After the diagnosis she did not take medication but checked her blood sugar every month in a local clinic. At that time Tatyana did not received any education or information about diabetes, but she read literature on her own to learn more about the disease.

In the 5 years after the initial diagnosis, Tatyana moved to the United States and her diabetes was not under control. Tatyana also discovered that she had hyperlipidemia and hypertension and her multiple aches in her legs and arms actually were signs of diabetic neuropathy. Tatyana also easily contracted ear and other bacterial infections, which she learned may be because of her diabetes and not from a weak immune system, as she was told in Russia.

In the United States Tatyana started to take new medications for diabetes, hypertension, and hyperlipidemia and was referred for diabetic education. Tatyana refused to go to the diabetic education program and started to read a lot of books and articles about diabetes. Tatyana believes in natural remedies and uses them too for her condition.

Recently, Tatyana was informed that her diabetes was not under control and she needed to start insulin injections. Tatyana refused to start the insulin treatment. She said that she had been under a lot of stress and that is why her diabetes was not under control. She was sure that stress was a main factor in diabetes control. Tatyana read about a new injectable medication, which she requested instead of insulin. Now Tatyana's blood sugars are under better control, and she now feels better and even has less body aches. However, she refuses to accept that she may need insulin injections in the future.

Case Study 4

Svetlana, 70 years old, emigrated from Novosibirsk, Russia. She was diagnosed with diabetes 15 years ago in Russia. Her mother was also diabetic and died from diabetes complications. Svetlana was very anxious to discover she has diabetes. In Russia Svetlana was told to change her diet by not eating any sweets, but she hasn't had any specific treatment for diabetes. Once a month she went to a local clinic to check her blood sugar.

When Svetlana moved to the United States she already had hypertension, coronary artery disease, and hyperlipidemia. Svetlana started a complex medication treatment and went with an interpreter to a diabetes education program. Svetlana learned a lot about life-style modifications and healthy diet and tried to lose weight. Svetlana started to eat a lot of vegetables and healthy grains that she used to eat in Russia and a limited amount of potatoes, white bread, and sweets.

Now, despite all attempts to keep Svetlana's blood sugar under control, her diabetes was still not controlled and she started to develop neuropathic pain in her legs. Svetlana was told that she needed to initiate insulin treatment. She was very reluctant and didn't want to use insulin like her mother for the rest of her life. With proper explanation that included cultural awareness of her concerns, Svetlana finally agreed to start insulin treatment and went to a diabetic education center to learn how to start insulin initiation.

Case Study 5

Oleg, 44 years old, emigrated from a small city in Ukraine 10 years ago. Oleg is a truck driver, and on his annual physical examination it was discovered that he had diabetes with Hgb A1C-12. Blood tests showed that he also had hyperlipidemia. Oleg was invited for a follow-up and diabetes treatment initiation. Oleg was overweight but had no symptoms of polyuria, polydipsia, or polyphagia. Oleg's diet consisted of a lot of white bread, potatoes, and other starch. As a truck driver Oleg sat a lot during his work and did not have time for physical activity after work.

Oleg was shocked when he was told he had diabetes. He said he had been under a lot of stress lately at his work and that was the reason for his diabetes diagnosis. He agreed to start medication treatment for his diabetes but wanted natural remedies because he didn't want to take "all those chemicals that are harmful for his body." He also was sure he could be cured with medications, life-style and dietary changes, and reduced stress. Oleg refused to go to a diabetes education program and asked a Russian-speaking provider to educate him one on one.

Case Study 6

Anna, 56 years old, emigrated to the United States from Kharkov, a large town in Ukraine. She was diagnosed with NIDDM soon after emigrating. Anna does not believe in any medications; therefore, she started to increase her physical activity and to follow a strict diet after diagnosis. Her diet consisted mostly of vegetables and some meat. Anna stated that she ate a lot of cabbage. In addition, she started to take natural remedies that were sent to her from Ukraine, and later she found some natural remedies, similar to Ukrainian, in the United States. Her blood sugars still were not under control, and she was also diagnosed with hyperlipidemia. Anna tried medication for her cholesterol, but the medication "destroyed her liver" and she stopped taking it.

Anna is not overweight, but her blood sugars are not under control. Despite all attempts from several physicians, she refuses to take any prescription medications for diabetes and hyperlipidemia and takes only natural remedies. Anna also refused to go to a diabetes education center, saying she knows everything about diabetes. Recently, her electrocardiogram showed some changes, and she was referred to cardiologist.

Discussion

These case studies are examples of urban educated immigrants diagnosed with diabetes before or after immigration to the United States, except case studies 5 and 6. In case studies 5 and 6, they were diagnosed with diabetes in the United States, but they were included in the case studies because after immigration they continued to have similar diets and life-styles as before immigration. Because of their diabetes these people have multiple complications, and in the United States they continue complex treatment including blood glucose control and prevention of further complications of diabetes. Despite the fact that these people are from different cities and countries of the former Soviet Union, Russia, and Ukraine, they have similar stories.

These case studies show the poor awareness of diabetes along with the absence of preventive measures after diagnosis of diabetes. Most of the case study participants believed that natural remedies were the first line of treatment for diabetes and all "chemicals" were harmful for them, but some of them had no awareness of natural remedies. All case study participants believed they had diabetes because of stress or that stress has a significant impact on developing diabetes. Most of the case study participants were reluctant to attend group education at diabetic education centers and preferred education one on one with the healthcare provider. These case studies show that before diabetes education by the healthcare provider, they paid less attention to diabetes risk factors such as poor diet and sedimentary life-style. With proper education after diagnosis all case study participants changed their life-style but continued to include in their diet healthy products that they were familiar with before immigration. In the United States case study participants became more aware of their condition and achieved better glycemic control, but sometimes it was too late to prevent many of their diabetic complications.

Consistent with the case studies, Sharafertdinov et al. (1997) showed the typical diet for many former Soviet Union diabetic patients. These Russian-speaking immigrants with diabetes prefer dishes with cereals, such as buckwheat and grains (e.g., rye wheat), or whole wheat bread as a main dish. Nurse practitioners need to be aware that Russian-speaking immigrants may prefer a specific type of diet and help them to find healthy alternatives that meet their ethnic preference; for example, they could encourage in addition to healthy grains a diet with more vegetables and other healthy products that are available at the market. In addition, nurse practitioners should inform these clients that although American restaurants, including fast food restaurants, may have healthy meals, they often offer portions that are too large for people who are trying to reduce their weight. Referral to a dietitian who is knowledgeable about this group may be very helpful for Russian immigrants.

These aforementioned case studies give a general picture of immigrants from the former Soviet Union with diabetes, but this picture is limited to these several cases only. The diversity of Russian-speaking immigrants is a very important aspect and needs to be taken into consideration in any study about this cultural group.

Implications for Practice

As the worldwide incidence of diabetes increases, multiple studies are conducted about diabetes. Prevention and treatment of diabetes should involve a cultural approach because diet and life-style, major risk factors in diabetes, have strong cultural components. Studies conducted in the United States and other countries receiving Russian-speaking immigrants show an increased risk of type 2 diabetes in this population. However, with proper diabetic education, diabetic complications may be prevented. Prevention of diabetes and diabetic complications is essential for new immigrants who are poor and have limited access to health care. Nurses need to emphasize the importance of diabetes prevention and educate patients about issues such as stress, diet, life-style, pre-diabetes, metabolic syndrome, and other risk factors for diabetes and about the complications related to late diagnosis of existing problems.

From this literature review of Russian clients and diabetes, two specific cultural variables were identified: use of natural remedies and stress. A nurse practitioner might be surprised that a Russian patient would refuse to accept the standard treatment for diabetes and instead prefer to take natural remedies. However, with appropriate cultural understandings and knowledge about those natural remedies, the nurse practitioner is better able to explain how natural remedies may be more helpful when combined with other treatment plans.

Stress in Russian culture is considered to be a main risk factor for diabetes onset. Nurse practitioners may forget to discuss stress as a risk factor for diabetes onset because they are more concerned about obesity and sedentary life-style factors that seem more important in preventing or treating diabetes. In this group of patients, however, a discussion with a nurse practitioner about stress-related risk factors is important. It is reasonable to discuss stress because these immigrants, having moved to another country to begin a new life and often having to learn a new language, experience tremendous stress.

Smith (1996) mentioned another important point for nurses. She explained that Russian immigrants often ask to see only physicians and not nurses or nurse practitioners. They even may become angry about seeing a nurse instead of a physician. This reaction is understandable because in the former Soviet Union the role of the nurse is mainly to obey the commands of physicians, and the nurses in those countries are usually not allowed to make decisions regarding patient care. In addition, Russian immigrants may not know the role of nurse practitioners because, simply, in their former countries this specialty does not exist. Nurse practitioners may need to first discuss with patients the role of nurses and nurse practitioners.

The literature review and case studies discussed in this chapter aim to help nurse practitioners understand why Russian-speaking patients need unique approaches to care. It may be very useful for the prevention of diabetes or diabetic complications if Russian-speaking immigrants seeking care for any health problems also receive education or screening for diabetes. In addition, nurse practitioners educating about healthy life-style habits, including a healthy diet, provide the client with the opportunity to be part of the care management team in health promotion and maintenance.

Reviewing the literature about Russian-speaking immigrants and diabetes showed that little is known about diabetes prevention among the Russian-speaking ethnic group, who clearly have a predisposition for diabetes. Case studies were used to illustrate some of the problems that Russian-speaking immigrants with diabetes face. More studies are needed about diabetes rates among Russian immigrants, their diet patterns, and the effect of specific diets on the development of diabetes.

References

Adams, C. R. (2003) Lessons learned from urban Latinas with type II diabetes mellitus. *Journal of Transcultural Nursing, 14,* 255–265.

Ben-Noun, L. (1994) Shchihutmahalot chroniot vemaafyanim sociodemografiim ecel olim hadashim mihever haamim beshana harishona. [Chronic diseases in immigrants from Russia (CIS) at a primary care clinic and their socio-demographic characteristics.] *Harefuah, 127,* 441–445.

Brodov, Y., Mandelzweig, L., Boyko, V., & Behar, S. (2002). Is immigration associated with an increase in risk factors and mortality among coronary artery disease pat? A cohort study of 13,742 patients. *Israel Medical Association Journal, 4,* 326–329

Brown, D. (2003) More studies need to examine habits within ethic groups. *Journal of the American Dietetic Association, 103,* 706.

Centers for Disease Control and Prevention. (2005). *Diabetes projects: Guide to community preventive services.* Retrieved October 17, 2007, from http://www.cdc.gov/diabetes/projects/community.htm

Duncan, L., & Simmons, M. (1996). Health practices among Russian and Ukrainian immigrants. *Journal of Community Health Nursing, 13,* 129–137.

Fields, C. (2003). *Applied food sciences announces weight loss benefits to its green coffee antioxidant extract.* Retrieved October 17, 2007, from http://www.npicenter.com/index.asp?action=NBViewDoc&DocumentID=4388

Fukunishi, I., Akimoto, M., Horikawa, N., Shirasaka, K., & Yamazaki, T. (1998). Stress coping and social support in glucose tolerance abnormality. *Journal of Psychosomatic Research, 45,* 361–369.

Hosler, A. (2003) *Diabetes among immigrants from former Soviet Union. International diets.* Retrieved June 5, 2003, from http://www.dietconsultants.com/russian-diet.html

Ivanov, L. L., & Buck, K. (2002). Health care utilization patterns or Russian-speaking immigrant women across age groups. *Journal of Immigrant Health, 4,* 17–27.

Jimenez del Rio, M. (2003). *Blueberry leaves extract: Diabetes & more.* Retrieved October 17, 2007, from http://www.annieappleseedproject.org/bluebleavexm.html

Levetan, C. (2001). Diabetes prevention. How about now? *Clinical Diabetes, 19,* 34–38.

London, F. (2002). Improving compliance. What we can do. In *2002 PDR diabetes disease management guide* (2nd ed., pp. 501–505). Montvale, NJ: Thomson PDR.

Manvelov, L. C. (1999) Saharnyi diabet kak factor riska celebrovaskulyarnyh zabolevanii. [Diabetes as a risk actor for cerebrovascular accidents.] *Lechashii vrach, 9,* 1–9. Retrieved October 17, 2007, from http://www.osp.ru/doctore/1999/09/09.htm

Meyerovich, M. (2003). Somatic symptoms among recent Russian immigrants. *American Medical Association.* Retrieved July, 7, 2003, from http://www.ama-assn.org/ama/pub/article/8401-1959.html

Ministry of Health, Russian Federation. (2003). *Phederal'naya celevaya programa—saharnyi diabet.* Retrieved July, 17, 2003, from http://www.minzdrav-rf.ru/in.htm?rubr=130

Mull, D. S., Nguyen, N., & Dennis, J. M. (2001). Vietnamese diabetic patients and their physicians: What ethnography can teach us? *Western Journal of Medicine, 175,* 307–311.

Nikitin, Y. P. (1989) Problemasaharnogo diabeta v regionah Sibiri. [The problem of diabetes mellitus in the Siberian regions.] *Vestnik Akademii Meditsinskikh Nauk, 5,* 35–39.

Oystragh, P. (1980) Diabetes mellitus in Russian Jewish immigrants. *Australian Family Physician, 9,* 269–270.

Public Health Seattle and King County. (October, 19, 2001). *New community-based diabetes activities will help bridge the health gap for minority communities.* Retrieved October 17, 2007, from http://www.metrokc.gov/health/news/01101801.htm

Peyrot, M., McMurry, J. F. Jr., & Kruger, D. F. (1999). A biopsychosocial model of glycemic control in diabetes: Stress, coping and regimen adherence. *Journal of Health and Social Behavior, 40,* 141–158.

Popkin, B. M. (1998). The nutrition transition and its health implications in lower-income countries. *Public Health Nutrition, 11,* 5–21.

Rankin, S. H., Galbraith., M. E., & Huang, P. (1997). Quality of life and social environment as reported by Chinese immigrants with non-insulin-dependent diabetes mellitus. *The Diabetes Educator, 23,* 171–176.

Rennet, G., Luz, N., Tamir, A., & Peterburg, Y.(2002). Chronic disease prevalence in immigrants to Israel from the former USSR. *Journal of Immigrant Health, 10,* 29–33.

Sharafertdinov, K. H., Mesheryakoba, V. A., & Plotnikova, O. A. (1997). Izmenenie poslepishevoi glikemii pod vliyaniem nekotoryh uglevodosoderzhashih produktov u bol'nyh saharnym diabetom. [Change of postprandial glycaemia under effect of some carbohydrate containing food in patients with type II diabetes.] *Lechebnoe Pitanie, 1,* 27–30.

Sidorov, P. I., Novikova, I. A., & Solov'ev, A.G. (2001). Rol' negativnyh social'nyh i psichologicheskih factorov na poyavlenie i kurs lechenia saharnogo diabeta. [The role of unfavorable social and psychological factors in the onset and course of diabetes mellitus.] *Terapevticheskii Archiv, 73,* 68–70.

Smith, L. (1996). New Russian immigrants: Health problem, practices, and values. *Journal of Cultural Diversity, 3,* 68–73.

Wheat, M. E., Brownstein, H., & Kvitash, V. (1983) Aspects of medical care of Soviet Jewish émigrés. *The Western Journal of Medicine, 139,* 900–904.

Zabina, H., Schmid, T. L., Glasunov, I., Potemkina, R., Kamardina, T., Deev, A., et al. (2001). Monitoring behavioral risk factors for cardiovascular disease in Russia. *American Journal of Public Health, 91,* 1613–1614.

Barriers to Healthcare Access for Latino Service Workers in a Resort Community

Caroline Cogen

The purpose of this chapter is to identify the barriers and propose strategies to improve access to health care by Latino service workers in an affluent resort community in the western United States. Many traditionally underserved populations in rural communities have difficulty accessing health care because of the lack of medical facilities. Access is especially problematic in affluent resort communities in which there is great disparity between the "haves" and "have-nots." During the winter the area discussed in this chapter is a major ski resort. In summer hikers and others interested in the great outdoors enjoy the peace and splendor of the mountains.

The healthcare resources are examined in the community for the Latinos who provide a major role in the service industry. These people work in low-paying jobs that are critical to the smooth operation of a resort area, yet those who function as housecleaners, maids in hotels, restaurant workers, and so on are often "invisible" in the sense that, if they do their jobs well, they are not really noticed by the wealthy individuals they serve. The project was inspired by the author's commitment to the community as a part-time resident and an advanced practice nurse with a strong sense of social justice regarding the poor and underserved.

Little research has been conducted in resort communities. Barriers exist that are sometimes politically determined. For example, one cannot open a healthcare clinic in this resort area and receive federal funding based on the physician-to-population ratio because the ratios do not accurately reflect the physicians available to provide health care for this population. Based on the U.S. Census Report (USCR, 1990–2004) there are 21,000 residents in this resort community and 71 physicians. However, these numbers do not represent physicians actually providing care in the community. For example, the only local community hospital has just 31 physicians on the medical staff. According to the Wood River Medical Society approximately half of the physicians work part-time and are therefore not available to assume a full patient load (Smith, personal communication).

The resort area of interest has a population of 21,000 residents, most of whom are part-time residents. According to local officials there are 2,400 housing units in the primary resort area and 1,600 of theses homes are second homes, reflecting the affluence of the community (Foley, 2004). An overwhelming financial disparity exists between the permanent residents, who range from minimum-wage workers to the wealthy elite. Like most famous tourist destinations, the resort is known for plush golf courses and snow-covered mountains. But because of the remote geographical area, the businesses rely on local residents to work in the service industry. The harsh winters and treacherous mountain terrain make long-distance commuting from outlying towns difficult. Most of those who work in the service sector earn minimum wage or less and commute from outlying cities 40 miles away.

The first section of the chapter consists of a literature review on access issues in the United States. The second part is a description of a ski resort in the western United States that struggles to serve the healthcare needs of the underserved residents of the community.

Literature Review

Barriers to Health Care

Barriers to healthcare access were a major theme in many articles reviewed for this chapter (Anderson, 1995; Probst, Moore, Glover, & Samuels, 2004; U.S. Department of Health and Human Services, 2002). Individual barriers particularly relevant to Latino service workers include economic issues, immigration status, transportation, and language. Individual barriers are distinct from cultural barriers, which include beliefs, norms, customs, and rituals that prevent particular groups from seeking health care (Hunter, Gaylord, Britnell, & Ashford-Works, 1998).

Economic Issues
The cost of healthcare services is a major barrier. Latinos often forego treatment because they do not have the money to pay for services and are unable to obtain health insurance. This is especially problematic for immigrants who do not have legal status (Anderson, 1995). Johnson (2001) stated that vulnerable people cannot afford the cost of health care. The lack of financial resources was cited throughout the research literature as the number one reason for not accessing health care. Even those individuals who have insurance do not have enough money for the copayments or deductibles even with the reduced rate some clinics offer. A related barrier is the lack of medical clinics and providers who accept Medicaid or who offer a sliding fee scale to care for the large number of uninsured and indigent people (Kaiser, 2003). Failure to be flexible on payments leads to longer appointment times, waiting room delays, and excess usage of emergency departments by individuals who do not want to wait for appointments.

The median income for the vulnerable group examined in this chapter is less than $44,000 annually (Kaiser, 2003). This rural town's service-worker population does not have the disposable income to pay for insurance premiums or healthcare cost. Low-income wage earners do not earn enough money to purchase health insurance and cover the cost of basic needs. These workers see the importance of health insurance but choose to pay bills, obtain food, and cover rent rather than purchase insurance. They have little, if any, discretionary income. Some fear that if they already owed previous bills they could not receive additional medical assistance. If the medical bills remain unpaid, many fear retribution by authorities, particularly immigration officials.

Immigration Status
Although the issue of undocumented Mexican-Americans is particularly timely given the attention currently being paid to the U.S. border problems, it is unclear how many of these people have found their way to the community of interest. It is likely that the workers who are employed by the major facilities are legal, but there are many landscapers and construction workers who come and go and might not be legal immigrants. One model program was created for newly legalized immigrants in Chicago (McElmurray, Park, & Busch, 2003).

Transportation
Barriers such as transportation and language also are a common theme. Transportation was an issue because many immigrants do not have drivers' licenses or even know how to drive. Rural areas do not have public transportation. The service workers rely on friends who have cars, but the friends who have cars are more likely to work during clinic times and are not available to drive them to appointments. Additionally, because of the enormous costs of housing, local service workers are forced to live 25–40 miles out of town and carpool or shuttle into work each day. Scheduling a medical appointment requires them to take a day off from work to see a primary care provider in another town.

Language
Because Spanish is the primary language among Latino service workers and most Anglos do not speak Spanish, it is difficult to communicate with each other. In the resort area 90% of the population is white and English speaking, with 10% Spanish speaking or another language as their first language (USCR, 1990–2004). The Latinos in the resort area find it difficult to make a doctor's appointment, let alone understand all that was said to them during their appointments. The language barrier for Latinos who are not fluent in English if the providers do not speak Spanish is enormous (Johnson, 2001).

Cultural Values

For some of the Latino service workers, who are mainly from Mexico, a strong cultural value is to be tough and not need health care. Perceived illness in the Latino population is a weakness (Anderson, 1995). The practice of waiting until the health problem has reached a crisis point appears to contribute to the difficulty Latinos face when accessing health care. It is important to note that though the Latino adults may wait and postpone their own health care, they do not have the same expectation of toughness from their children. Parents put the needs of their children before themselves at any financial cost.

Another cultural barrier is that some Latinos rely on *curanderos* (traditional healers) or friends for advice. *Curanderos* treat with home remedies, herbs, and over-the-counter medications (Doty & Ives, 2002). Sometimes the advice of *curanderos* and friends or family members conflicts with that given by the healthcare establishment. Denial also plays a role in access in that young people might see themselves as invincible and believe that nothing bad can happen to them. Like youth in many cultures, they might minimize their injuries or symptoms. Denial might happen on two levels in that they might not attend to dangerous or unhealthy practices or they might "tough it out." This reaction is consistent with Anderson's (1995) work on the cultural value of being tough and traditional notions about machismo (Galanti, 2003).

Healthcare Literacy

Additional healthcare barriers found in the literature (Vezeau, 2005) include the complexity of the healthcare forms, leading to two major problems. The first problem is the inability to complete medical forms, leading to frustration and avoidance of medical services (Anderson, 1995). The second problem is that individuals with little or no recorded health history are the ones least able to provide accurate medical information in times of crisis (Mercer, 2001).

Another problem identified in the literature was the lack of clinics with a Spanish translator. In a study by the Association of Community Organization for Reform (2004), hospitals were contacted to determine whether a Spanish-speaking interpreter was available. The law requires that all hospitals provide an interpreter upon request, yet over 50% did not offer this assistance (Association of Community Organization for Reform, 2004). The problems associated with incomplete or inaccurate communication about health history and status are obvious and critical.

Demographic Trends

The United States is experiencing a shift in demographic trends, including an increase in cultural diversity. Demographers predict that the next two decades will bring racial and ethnic minority populations to a numerical majority in the United States (Sue & Sue, 1999). The reality is that African-Americans, Native American, Alaska Natives, Asian-Americans, Pacific Islanders, and Latinos accounted for 30% of the population in 2000 (U.S. Department of Health and Human Services, 2001). These population groups are projected to increase to 40% of the population by 2025 (U.S. Department of Health and Human Services, 2001). In response to these demographic changes, social workers and medical professionals have attempted to prepare for these population shifts by creating initiatives and standards related to cultural diversity and practice. The professional responses have yielded mixed successes.

The Latino population in the United States is characterized by its rapid growth, with a projected increase to 97 million by 2050, representing one-fourth of the U.S. population. Mexican-Americans comprise almost two-thirds of Latino-Americans with the remainder of Puerto Rican, Cuban, South American, and Central American, Dominican, and Spanish origins. Latinos are highly concentrated in the southwest United States, with 60% living in California, Arizona, New Mexico, Colorado, and Texas. However, other states have also seen increases in Latinos. From 1990 to 2000 the number of Latinos more than doubled in Arkansas (170%), North Carolina (129%), Georgia (120%), Nebraska (108%), and Tennessee (105%) (USCR, 1990–2004).

Many of North Carolina's county departments of health, social services, and other community service agencies are experiencing a steady rise in the number of Latino families they serve, and with good reason. North Carolina has the fastest growing Latino population in the United States.

It is a mistake to assume that Latinos are a homogeneous culture. In fact, Latinos are an extremely diverse group. They include individuals with a wide range of characteristics from many different countries, regions, socioeconomic backgrounds, cultures, and races. For example, Spanish language nuances can dramatically affect interpretation from country to country.

Cultural Competence

Nurse practitioners continue to strive toward cultural competence. McPhatter (1997) viewed cultural competence in terms of transforming knowledge and awareness of culture into interventions that support and sustain healthy functioning within the appropriate cultural contest. More recently, de Chesnay, Wharton, and Pamp (2005) described cultural competence in terms of acting in a way that is respectful of the values and traditions of the patient while performing nursing actions.

Sociopolitical Environment and Unresponsive Professions

The broader sociopolitical environment affects the practitioner's work with culturally diverse groups. Sue and Sue (1999) pointed out that traditional medicine might serve to oppress multiethnic groups. The ethnocentric bias of the medical establishment values compliance or adherence with its own regimens and protocols. If patients do not comply or adhere, they risk punitive messages by their healthcare providers.

Sue and Sue (1999) speculated that the underutilization of health and mental health services is related to the cultural insensitivity and inappropriateness of formalized services for culturally diverse groups. Findings from the Commonwealth Fund Minority Health Survey (LaVeist, Diala, & Jerrett, 2000) support this speculation. Data from this survey revealed that 43% of African-Americans and 28% of Latinos, in comparison with 5% of whites, believed that because of their cultural background, a healthcare provider treated them poorly. The lack of professionals' ability to practice in a culturally competent way further oppresses their patients who face biased behavior within the larger society.

High-Needs Populations

Latinos are relatively underrepresented among people who are homeless or have children in foster care. However, they are present in high numbers in several other vulnerable populations who experience health disparities. For example, Latino-Americans are 9% more likely to be incarcerated, compared with 3% of non–Latino-Americans. Latino men are nearly four times as likely as white men to be imprisoned at some point during their lifetime (Weich & Angulo, 2000).

Latinos who served in Vietnam were at higher risk for war-related posttraumatic stress disorder than were black and non-Latino white veterans. Many suggest refugees from Central America experienced considerable civil war–related trauma in their homelands. Studies have found rates of posttraumatic stress disorder among Central American refugee patients ranging from 33% to 60% (Weich & Angulo, 2000).

In general, Latino-Americans have rates of alcohol use similar to non-Latinos. However, Latinas usually have lower rates of alcohol and drug use than their male counterparts. Rates of substance abuse are higher among U.S.-born Mexican-Americans compared with Mexican-born immigrants. Specifically, substance abuse rates are twice as high for U.S.-born Mexican-American men than for Mexican-born men but are surprisingly seven times higher for U.S.-born Mexican-American women than for Mexican-born women (Weich & Angulo, 2000).

Latinos with diabetes are at higher risk of heart disease, but they can reduce that risk, according to a new national health awareness campaign unveiled recently by the National Diabetes Education Program during the National Council of La Raza's annual conference. By controlling blood sugar, blood pressure, and cholesterol, people with diabetes can live longer healthier lives (U.S. Department of Health and Human Services, 2002). U.S. Department of Health and Human Services Secretary Thompson announced the campaign, *Si Tiene Diabetes, Cuide Su Corazon*, aimed at helping Latino-Americans better understand the need to control all aspects of their diabetes (U.S. Department of Health and Human Services, 2004).

Availability of Mental Health Services

In 1990 about 40% of Latinos either did not speak English at all or did not speak it well. Although the percentage of Spanish-speaking mental health professionals is not known, only 1% of licensed psychologists who are also members of the American Psychological Association identify themselves as Latino. Moreover, there are only 29 compared with 173 non-Latino white providers per 100,000 (LaVeist et al., 2000). If these proportions of Spanish speaking to non–Spanish speaking hold true for other healthcare professionals, then the problems of communication become enormous.

Access to Mental Health Services

Nationally, 37% of Latinos are uninsured, compared with 16% of all Americans. This high number is driven mostly by Latinos' lack of employer-based coverage—only 43% compared with 73% for non-Latino whites (LaVeist et al., 2000). Although Latino service workers in the community of interest might value insurance, they view it as discretionary and have no room in their meager budgets for spending on luxuries such as health insurance.

Appropriateness and Outcomes of Mental Health Services

Few studies on the mental health resources of Latinos are available. One randomized study found that members of low-income Spanish-speaking families were more likely to suffer a significant exacerbation of symptoms of schizophrenia in highly structured family therapy than in less structured case management. Several studies have found that bilingual patients are evaluated differently when interviewed in English as opposed to Spanish, thereby influencing outcomes (Johnson, 2001).

One national study found that only 24% of Latinos with depression and anxiety receive appropriate care, compared with 34% of whites. Another study found that Latinos who visited a general medical doctor were less than half as likely as whites to receive either a diagnosis of depression or antidepressant medicine (LaVeist et al., 2000). The extent to which Latinos attempt to access mental health services is unclear, but these services might be considered a luxury for people who are not well educated.

Need for Mental Health Care

There was no difference in the frequency of mental disorders among Latino-Americans living in the resort community to that of non-Latino white Americans (Kaiser, 2003). Adult Mexican immigrants have lower rates of mental disorders than Mexican-Americans born in the United States, and adult Puerto Ricans tend to have lower rates of depression living on the mainland (U.S. Department of Health and Human Services, 2001). It is not clear that methods of measurement are standardized, so the existing studies have limited applicability.

Some researchers have found that Latino youth experience proportionally more anxiety and delinquency behaviors, depression, and drug use than do non-Latino white youth. Among older Latinos, one study found that over 26% of the sample was depressed. When depression was related to physical health, only 5.5% of those without physical health problems were depressed (U.S. Department of Health and Human Services, 2001).

Culture-bound syndromes seen in Latino-Americans include *susto* (fright), *nervios* (nerves), *mal de ojo* (evil eye), and *ataque,* which may include screaming uncontrollably, crying, trembling, verbal or physical aggression, dissociate experiences, seizure-like or fainting episodes, and suicidal gestures (U.S. Department of Health and Human Services, 2001).

In 1997 Latinos had a suicide rate of about 6% compared with 13% for non-Latino whites. However, in a national survey of high school students, Latino adolescents reported more suicidal ideation and attempts proportionally than nonwhites and blacks (U.S. Department of Health and Human Services, 2001).

State of the Art of the Literature Regarding Access to Health Care

Areas of Agreement

The major area of agreement in the research literature was that the Latino population is in crisis when trying to access health care. The Latinos state that there are language difficulties when trying to make appointments because the clinic personnel did not speak Spanish (Mercer, 2001). If they are able to explain that they need an appointment, they still have difficulty expressing their symptoms and the nature of the medical problem. The Latinos state that sometimes when trying to access healthcare clinics they are confronted with humiliation and embarrassment at not being able to speak English and are treated disrespectfully. This makes it difficult and anxiety-producing to try to access health care.

The literature documented a critical need for federal and state policymakers to acknowledge Latino health disparities and lead the way to better health and quality of life for this population. For example, research with significant funding conducted under the auspices of federal agencies is lacking. Although there are strong disparities among income levels, rates of uninsured individuals, and the low education level of this population, only recently have federal agencies begun to take notice. For example, the resort community of interest in this chapter recently received a large amount of funding from the Department of Health and Welfare to help meet the community needs (Mason, 2005).

The articles reviewed seem to show consensus that Latino individuals face many unique challenges when trying to access health care. The challenges include cost of services, inability to access services, and cultural and language barriers. Johnson (2001) also pointed out other issues repeatedly mentioned in the literature, including long waits, clinic times, and disrespectful treatment from healthcare providers. Hunter et al. (1998) urged providers to remember not to generalize rural communities but to embrace the differences of the communities and ethnic populations. This idea is particularly relevant to policymakers.

Areas of Disagreement

There is disagreement as to whether individual resort communities or large suburban areas should be studied in future research when addressing the healthcare needs of Latinos and the underinsured. Mercer (2001) pointed out that the population is diverse and varies greatly from county to county across the United States. Therefore studying the needs of larger populations does not address the needs of Latinos from specific rural resort areas. Other studies do not mention this and imply that individual communities are not different enough to warrant studying each for culturally based solutions. Both arguments have some value. If the statement by Mercer were true that the diversity between counties is great, then it would be prudent to do further research within subgroups to develop health guidelines for each country of origin.

Another area of disagreement in the literature is concerned with the relative importance of different types of barriers to health care. Johnson (2001) found that the number of clinics was a larger barrier to accessing health care than a language barrier between provider and patients (Carson, Jenssen, & Synder, 2004). However, most of the studies reported language as the number one barrier.

A final area of inconsistency is related to the effect of long wait times in clinics. Johnson (2001) stated that although it is necessary to do further research, a standardized method for retrieving data is necessary before further research should be conducted. The lack of standardized methods of collecting data is a source of confusion in the literature and makes interpretation difficult and generalizability limited.

Gaps

A major gap in the literature is the lack of information on barriers to health care for Latinos in affluent communities. This chapter is an attempt to address this problem by focusing on a specific rural community and the needs of that population. However, the nature of resort communities might indicate that the problems faced by Latinos in the ski resort described here might be similar to those issues in other types of resorts with affluent and disadvantaged groups.

Overall, the published research on the healthcare barriers facing Latino populations in the United States, particularly in rural areas, is lacking or suspect. Some of the workers do not have immigration papers and so avoid contact with government agencies and remain unaccounted for (Carson et al., 2004).

The Latino population continues to grow and is the largest minority group in the United States, and it is becoming more difficult for the healthcare system to ignore the needs of this population. There is an abundance of reports and articles based on observation and trends relating to the healthcare needs of Latinos, but there is a limited amount of actual research conducted. Most publications seem anecdotal or theoretical. On the positive side, the amount of research in this field is likely to increase because of the rapid growth and critical needs of this population. In Idaho alone, 50% of the Latinos are uninsured, according to the Idaho Department of Health (2004). The sheer numbers of people who are uninsured will create the demand for more research and new models.

Community Description: The Resort Community

An attempt to create a new model was inspired by the author's involvement in the community of a ski resort in a western state. This rural area has many Latino service workers who hold menial jobs and yet are critical to the local economy. The community of interest is a summer and winter resort area located in the western United States. This resort is considered by many to be one of the most desirable and exclusive vacation destinations in the United States and attracts people of means and influence. The mountain community has a beautiful setting located at 6,000 ft. elevation in the Pioneer Range of the Rocky Mountains and is home to many famous people. It is not uncommon to shop at local supermarkets and stand beside celebrities who are also shopping for groceries.

The area was first developed as a mining town in the 1800s, and its successes and failures were dependent on the productivity of the mines, true for many similar towns of this region. In 1936 Averill Harriman chose this specific area as the location of the first ski resort in the United States. The Union Pacific Train Line was extended to the region, and the main lodge was built in 1936. Since that time the area has flourished with the rapid expansion of the ski industry and other sports activities. Summer recreation, such as golfing, tennis, hiking, and bicycling, has become extremely popular and attracted even more tourists than the winter sports.

There is a stable but small population of people living year-round in the vicinity who support the local economy. Full-time residents include wealthy retirees, professionals such as attorneys and real estate developers, and small business owners as well as low-wage service workers. The average income for this county is $44,000 exceeding the per capita income for the United States, which was $14,000 in 2001 (Rogers, 2006). This resort community has a per capita income of $31,000 in the county with 8% of the population living below poverty (USCR, 1990–2004). The county has the highest cost of living compared with the surrounding communities. The high cost of living makes it difficult for service workers to afford housing in the town itself, so they live outside and commute to work.

The service workers in particular are extremely important to the economy of the resort area. They are the principal labor force for the businesses that flourish here. However, there is great disparity between the income of the tourists and part-time residents in comparison with full-time workers, even professionals. For example, registered nurses have a starting wage of $19.00 per hour compared with Washington State at $24.00 per hour (USCR, 1990–2004). The salaries of nannies, restaurant workers, construction workers, and other service workers vary depending on their employers. Though the salaries or hourly wages might be slightly better than in a middle-class urban neighborhood, the cost of living is so much higher that proportionately workers do not keep as much of their wages.

Statistics show that since 2000 this resort community had one of the largest population increases in this region, with expected growth to continue (USCR, 1990–2004). Ownership of a vacation home is a growing trend in ski resorts. The second-home debate centers around whether the part-time residents contribute to the community's wealth or burden it. In this community 36% of the residents are part-time residents. Amazingly, approximately 70% of the jobs in this resort community are in the heart of the local ski resort, though half of the service workers live elsewhere (USCR, 1990–2004).

The argument that vacation home owners in resort communities consume the local economy is that these part-time residents displace full-time residents on fixed incomes, consume unnecessarily large quantities of resources, drive up real estate prices, and do not contribute to local business (Foley, 2004). Herein lies one of the complex issues when trying to create free clinics to support the total community. The affluence of the residents skews the basis on which federal funds are allocated. The mean income appears much higher than usual due to the extreme wealth of the few versus the low income of the many permanent residents. This resort community ranks 44 on the list of the 50 counties in the state of study in 2005 to receive federal monies and currently receives $205 tax dollars for every man, woman, and child residing in this community compared with the statewide average of $839 per capita (Mason, 2005). These statistics are staggering and explain the vast disparity in income and resources in this area.

As a long-term visitor to the region, the author has become concerned about the healthcare options available to the large segment of the population who are either uninsured or underinsured. There are many physicians and other healthcare providers and a new modern hospital. However, these professionals appear to primarily serve the more affluent members of the community. Through discussions with community members it was mentioned that although there was access to health care through the local emergency department, the fee schedule was not adjusted for the poorer patients. An unplanned trip to the emergency department for something as minor as a sinus infection becomes a financial burden and a deterrent to most of the Latino service workers.

This area is not unlike many successful resorts in that the popularity and success of the resort area cannot continue to grow unless the needs of the large working population are met. The local political leaders in the area are cognizant of this looming problem but have thus far not been successful in developing affordable and easily attainable health care for all.

It is quite apparent that there are gaps about what is known concerning access to health care for Latino service workers in resort communities. There is great diversity among the resort communities as well as the Latinos who work in them. Therefore it is imperative to examine a specific community in depth, because the research indicated that each community is so diverse that generalizing the implementation plan is impossible (Association of Community Organization for Reform, 2004). Each community needs to develop its own plan for providing access to service workers, but monies are not allocated to make it possible.

The Ski Resort

It is clear that community leaders recognize a problem with access to care for the Latino service workers. For example, a prominent figure of the local hospital stated that he recognized the extent of the problem but offered no solutions. In fact, he mentioned that the hospital is not interested in developing a free or low-cost clinic for this segment of the population. He stated that the emergency room and clinics were available to all of the community but admitted that there were substantial costs involved.

Members of the major medical group in the community were contacted and also had no interest in developing more facilities for this population of patients. The hospital has recently closed its medical staffing. This means that a new physician moving into the area cannot obtain hospital privileges until a current member of the medical staff retires, dies, or moves. This decision was made to protect the income of the current physicians practicing in the area and to prevent physician turnover. This creates a successful medical practice but deters new physicians from moving to the area, physicians who may be willing to see more low-income and underinsured patients.

The ski resort community likewise does not meet the requirements of a medically underserved area. The resort had 74 physicians in 2002, compared with 54 in 1996. This computes to 3.6 physicians per 1,000 patients for this community (American Medical Association, 1996–2002). Based on these data, one might believe there is no need for more physicians to support the population. However, the report does not detail which of the 74 physicians work part-time, seasonally, accept charity cases, or use a sliding scale. Though these data make the physician coverage seem adequate, there are large gaps in the medical care delivered to this community. For example, the new local hospital and various clinics do not offer sliding scale fees for underinsured patients.

Random phone calls were made to the hospital emergency department and several independent clinics to inquire about the availability of services to those without insurance. The clinics contacted stated that if patients are willing to accept a lengthy wait and make regular monthly payments at the standard fee, they would be able to see the patient.

The demographic data are alarming for this resort community. Although there appears to be an adequate number of physicians to serve the population, this is not so because most physicians will not see uninsured or underinsured patients, and there is not an adequate medical center to serve this portion of the population. Thus these people are forced to leave the community to obtain basic health care. However, because they live far away from the community, they would not be able to work on the days they need to see a provider.

This community is not designated a medically underserved area because of the physicians-to-population ratio, so the area would not qualify for federal funds. As stated previously, the number of physicians available is quite misleading because many physicians work part-time and are completely unavailable to the service workers and indigents. Although it may still be possible to qualify for some federal funding, the process could be quite lengthy with no guarantees for success. This situation is a catch-22 for the service workers who must choose between accessing care in their home towns or working.

Other Resorts

Like the ski resort just described, other recreation resort areas experience similar situations when trying to deliver health care to underserved or underinsured members of their community. Though not rural in the same sense as the ski resort, the resort community of Hilton Head Island, South Carolina, experienced the same healthcare disparities as the ski resort, but one local physician found an answer. Dr. Jack McConnell, a retired physician on Hilton Head Island, observed the disparity of health care for the service workers of Hilton Head. Committed to making a change, Dr. McConnell met with a group of local retired physicians to share his vision of opening a free clinic and 13 of the 29 physicians agreed to join forces and help. At the time, although all the physicians agreed with the concept, many were very skeptical that such a clinic could open (Graves, 1996).

McConnell convinced the state that this clinic would be supported entirely by donated funds. High malpractice insurance and medical license renewal fees were a deterrent for many retired physicians. After convincing the state legislators for a special exception from state requirements, he purchased malpractice insurance at a reduced fee. Likewise, South Carolina allowed an exemption of medical license fees, which allowed the retired physicians to practice medicine at this free clinic. In July 1994 the doors opened to this healthcare clinic for the needy. Named "Volunteers in Medicine Clinic," the clinic now has more than 35 doctors, 50 nurses, and over 200 lay people who donate their time each week (Graves, 1996). The Hilton Head clinic is a model of how a community that does not meet the state and federal requirements of a medically underserved area can support the underserved population with volunteers who offer a wealth of experience in health care.

Aspen, Colorado, is another wealthy ski resort claimed by many to be the fourth richest town in the United States with demographics similar to the community of interest in this chapter, Aspen has a population of 14,000 people. Of those, 90.5% are considered white and 6.5% are Latino. Service workers maintain the viability of this ski resort. Without these people the economy of Aspen would be severely compromised. Aspen experiences a continued loss of revenue as mentioned in the Aspen Retail Analysis Report of 2003 (BBC Research & Consulting, 2003).

Aspen and other ski resorts such as Vail and Breckenridge have continued to face a decline in retail consumerism according to the Aspen Retail Study (BBC Research & Consulting, 2003). The population of Aspen has decreased by 1.2% since 2004 (USCR, 1990–2004). With one local hospital willing to see the indigent population and additional hospitals 30 miles away, healthcare access again becomes a factor in providing for the community. Aspen is feeling a loss in revenue for 3 consecutive years. An extensive report by the city's planning committee does not mention other possibilities for this loss, such as lack of service workers to provide for the seasonal influx of tourists. Without support systems to provide for the working population, people are choosing to move to areas where housing and services are affordable.

Discussion

Two issues stand out as particularly significant in the literature: access to healthcare facilities and inadequate numbers of healthcare facilities available to the most vulnerable members of the population. These must be addressed if the needs of the working poor are to be served. The community residents were not aware that the hospital functions as a closed medical unit. This concept of staffing is of particular interest when discussing issues of healthcare access. Although a closed medical unit does not discourage physicians to independently practice in the community, only a designated number of physicians are given privileges to the hospital. Therefore highly qualified physicians are not able to open practices in this town because of their inability to gain admitting privileges.

The vulnerable population of interest in this chapter is Latino service workers: residents who commute in from outlying towns to work in service-oriented jobs in the ski resort. In this resort community 10.7% of the population is Latino. The average household income for a Latino family in the community is $44,000 (U.S. Department of Health and Human Services, 2004). The community is 90% white and 10.7% Latino, with an average age between 25 and 44 years of age, including a 4% unemployment rate that fluctuates during seasonal activities (U.S. Department of Health and Human Services, 2004). The community draws from this particular population to maintain the businesses' operating status. Without this population, many of the businesses would not be able to function, particularly during the high season.

The services offered to the community focus on serving the elite tourist population, leaving few services for the Latino population. For example, there is one local hospital that serves the resort community, allowing access to health care by all individuals, but the fee for service does not vary depending on income. There are no discount stores to purchase low-cost basic needs such as undergarments. To purchase these items one would have to travel 25–40 miles out of the resort community. This is a huge burden in the winter season when it is not uncommon to have 2–3 feet of snow fall in one night and 12-foot drifts, making the roads impassible even if one had a car.

The term *rural* has no single accepted definition. For the purpose of this chapter, the following are commonly viewed as rural indicators: low population size and density, distance from urban areas, low degree of urbanization, and types of economic activity (U.S. Department of Health and Human Services, 2004). One of the difficulties in receiving federal monies is the inability to measure this community as medically underserved. Because of the number of wealthy residents full and part time the statistical numbers do not show a need for designation as underserved. The economic separation of this town is significant, from the wealthy elite to the working poor with a relatively small middle class. The working poor are defined here as individuals who spent at least 27 weeks in the labor force but whose income fell below the official poverty line, which for this community is $31,000 annual income or less (U.S. Department of Health and Human Services, 2004).

The economic disparity in this population leads to one of the major problems for the Latinos: lack of accessible health care. In a community with a population of 21,000, 8% were earning below the federal poverty level, earning less than the per capita annual salary of $31,000 (USCR, 1990–2004). This is an important problem on many levels, not only from an economic standpoint, but also in terms of the resources related to the ability to purchase health insurance. Addressing the problem of health care for the vulnerable population of Latino service workers in this rural town is critical for the growth of the community. The amount of residents earning below the federal poverty level may not be significance in itself, but when one considers that this community has the highest cost of living than any other local region, the number of poor people becomes highly relevant.

With the lack of healthcare facilities or existing resources in the community, many of the underserved workers relocate, leaving the resort community without support workers. Each year there are more unopened businesses and longer wait times at the local restaurants and lodging cafeteria due to lack of workers. In December 2006 the local ski mountain did not open at the desired time due to lack of employees.

There are many good reasons to do future studies to help determine and understand the reasons for the current decline in the number of available workers. If specific causes were isolated for the loss of low-income support workers, the community could focus on solutions to ensure that the populations of this community received adequate care from local resources. In addition, and more importantly, restructuring the community services would help the entire community by reducing the crime rate and providing a better society in which to live, significantly improving the economy.

Conclusion

Preliminary results of this community examination indicated a need for affordable and convenient healthcare services for Latino service workers. Solutions for addressing the lack of facilities include reallocating existing services, adding needed services, analyzing the success of similar resorts, and developing a new model for this community. The disparity between the income and financial status of the two major groups is profound and will not change. Ultimately, the success of the community depends on the availability of low-income workers, so a solution must be found to accommodate their needs. Expecting them to travel back to the outlying towns in which they live is neither fair nor economically practical.

A more reasonable approach to this problem is to develop a private clinic staffed by a physician and two or three nurse practitioners. Much of the clinic's funding could be obtained from fees generated from patients on a sliding scale. Public awareness would be increased and contributions could be obtained. The local hospital raises approximately $1 million per year in donated funds from this small but affluent community. Public funding from the city council and county health department may also be available. For as little as $250,000 for the first year, a model program could be opened and expanded with donated services, sliding scale fee-for-service, and grant funding.

This chapter was an attempt to raise questions about how a resort community can support Latino service workers' needs for affordable health care. The literature review revealed that specific types of barriers exist for this population in accessing health care. Once healthcare barriers are understood, appropriate solutions may be considered. Solutions may include the creation of a free clinic with both public and private funding and volunteer services from retired physicians and nurse practitioners. In lieu of this, expanding existing facilities with improved transportation, communication, and access may be possible. Either alternative will provide much-improved health care for this underserved community.

As the diversity of these small rural resort towns increases, so will the need for highly specialized physicians and nurse practitioners. Communities such as this resort will need to restructure services or risk losing workers due to decreased productivity related to illness. A plan to eliminate health disparities among Latinos and underserved populations requires a comprehensive and coordinated approach by health and human service organizations, commitment from different levels of government, and full participation of the private sector.

References

American Medical Association. (1996–2002). *Physician characteristics and distribution in the U.S.* Retrieved October 17, 2007, from http://www.ama-assn.org

Anderson, R. M. (1995). Revising behavior model of access to medical care. *Journal of Health and Social Behavior, 36,* 1–10.

Association of Community Organization for Reform. (2004). *Speaking the language of care: Language barriers to hospital access in American cities.* Retrieved August 21, 2007, from http://acorn.org/fileadmin/Additional_Accomplishments/National_report.pdf

BBC Research & Consulting. (2003). *The Aspen retail study.* Retrieved May 12, 2006, from www.aspenpitkin.com

Carson, K. L., Jenssen, L., & Synder, A. (2004). *The health and nutrition of Hispanic migrant and seasonal farm workers.* Harrisburg, PA: The Center for Rural Pennsylvania, Pennsylvania State University.

De Chesnay, M., Wharton, R., & Pamp, C. (2005). Cultural competence, resilience and advocacy. In M. de Chesnay (Ed.), *Caring for the vulnerable: Perspective in nursing theory, practice, and research* (pp. 31–42). Sudbury, MA: Jones and Bartlett Publishers.

Doty, M. M., & Ives, B. L. (2002). *Quality of health care for Latino population, finding from the commonwealth fund 2001 health care quality survey.* Washington, DC: The Commonwealth Fund, Families USA.

Foley, G. (2004). *Can our valley find a balance?* Retrieved August 21, 2007, from http://www.mtexpress.com/index2.php?ID=10048

Galanti, G. (2003). The Hispanic family and male-female relationships: An overview. *Journal of Transcultural Nursing, 14*(3), 180–185.

Graves, T. (1996). Open arms healing hands. *UT Medicine Magazine,* Spring.

Hunter, R., Gaylord, S., Britnell, M., & Ashford-Works, C., (1998). *Making a difference in rural communities: A guide for trainees in the health professions.* Chapel Hill, NC: Carolina Geriatric Education Center, University of North Carolina.

Johnson, M. D. (2001). Meeting the health care needs of a vulnerable population: Perceived barriers. *Journal of Community Health Nursing, 18,* 24–28.

Kaiser, H. J. (2003). State the facts on-line, Idaho minority health median family income by race/ethnicity. Retrieved April 18, 2005, from http://www.statehealthfacts.kkf.org

LaVeist, T. A., Diala, C., & Jerrett, N. C. (2000). *Minority health in America.* Baltimore: Johns Hopkins University Press.

Mason, R. (2005). *Blaine county benefits from $4.3 million dollar investment from the Department of Health & Welfare.* Retrieved May 12, 2006, from http://www.healthandwelfaredept.org

McElmurry, B. J., Park, C. G., & Busch, A. G. (March 6, 2003). The nurse-community health advocate team for urban immigrant primary health care. *Journal of Nursing Scholarship, 35*(3), 275–281.

McPhatter, A. R. (1997). Cultural competence in child welfare: What is it? How do we achieve it? What happens without it? *Child Welfare, 76,* 225–278.

Mercer, M. M. (2001). *Initiatives to improve access to rural health care services a briefing paper.* Phoenix, AZ: Arizona Health Care Cost Containment System, William M. Mercer, Incorporated.

Probst, J., Moore, C., Glover, S., & Samuels, M. (2004). Person and place: The compounding effects of race/ethnicity on rurality and health. *American Journal of Public Health, 94*(10), 1695–1703.

Rogers, G. (January 2006). *Blaine county profile.* Retrieved May 11, 2006, from www.cl.idaho.gov

Sue, D., & Sue, D. (1999). *Counseling the culturally different.* New York: John Wiley & Sons.

U.S. Census Report (1990–2004). *U.S. Census report Blaine County Idaho.* Retrieved January 26, 2006, from www.quickfacts.census.gov

U.S. Department of Health and Human Services. (2001). *Mental health: Culture, race, and ethnicity. A supplement to mental health: A report of the Surgeon General.* Rockville, MD: Author.

U.S. Department of Health and Human Services. (2002). *Healthy people 2010.* Washington, DC: National Academies Press.

U.S. Department of Health and Human Services. (2004). *The 2004 HHS poverty guidelines.* Retrieved April 16, 2006, from http://aspe.hhs.gov/poveryt/04.shtml

Vezeau, T. (2005). Literacy and vulnerability. In M. de Chesnay (Ed.), *Caring for the vulnerable: Perspective in nursing theory, practice, and research* (pp. 407–418). Sudbury, MA: Jones and Bartlett Publishers.

Weich, R., & Angulo, C. (2000). *Justice on trial: Racial disparities in American criminal justice system.* Retrieved April 16, 2006, from www.HRW.org/backgrounder/usa/race

Barriers to Tuberculosis Screening among Filipino Immigrants to the United States

Gloria Q. Natividad

The purposes of this chapter are to identify the barriers to tuberculosis (TB) screening among Filipino immigrants and to suggest strategies for healthcare providers to implement in caring for this population in the community. Identification of these barriers will enable providers to create interventions to prevent the spread of the disease in the community. Although the focus of this chapter is on Filipino immigrants to the United States, the concepts are universal and might be extended to Filipino immigrants in a variety of countries.

Tuberculosis

TB was the leading cause of morbidity and mortality worldwide until the middle of the 20th century. By the late 1970s the disease had been almost eradicated; however, because of the spread of HIV, TB made an alarming resurgence in the urban areas of the United States. In addition, there was a widespread epidemic of HIV and TB in other parts of the world such as Asia, Africa, and South America, mostly because of inadequate health care delivery due to poverty. Drug-resistant TB also emerged because of poor treatment and management of the disease. Today, TB is a threatening global problem.

Even with an overall decrease in the number of TB cases in the United States over the last few years, the number of cases among people born outside the United States has increased. For example, in 2003 in Washington State in the western United States, TB affected the minority population as follows: Asians had the highest incidence rate (28.5%), followed by African-Americans (16.8%), Native Americans (16.6%), and Hispanics (8%) (Washington Department of Health, 2004). According to the World Health Organization (WHO) the Philippines ranks fourth in the world for the number of cases of TB. Because there is a substantial Filipino immigrant population in the United States, this statistic is significant for physicians and nurse practitioners who serve this population.

Screening is a critical part of knowing whom to treat. It is inherently difficult to screen for TB for a variety of reasons, which include the large pool of infected persons and reactivation rates of person with past episodes of the disease, sometimes from decades past (Matsunaga, Yamada, & Macabeo, 1998). If high-risk persons are given preventive therapy, new cases can be reduced. However, identifying those with a high risk is a major challenge, particularly if they report feeling well and do not view themselves as having any disease. Additionally, distinguishing TB infection from TB disease is often difficult, even for the TB worker. Knowing the barriers to screening TB enables providers to screen and treat infected patients to reduce the incidence of this communicable disease among Filipinos and other members of the larger community who associate with them.

Infection

The American Lung Association defines TB as an airborne infection caused by the bacterium *Mycobacterium tuberculosis*. Although TB primarily affects the lungs, other organs and tissues may be affected as well. There is a difference between being infected with TB and having TB disease. An individual with TB infection has TB bacteria present in the body but the body's immune system is preventing the disease from becoming active. Someone who has TB is sick and can spread the disease if not properly treated. Several symptoms indicate active TB, such as prolonged coughing (including hemoptysis), repeated night sweats, unexplained weight loss, anorexia, fever, chills, and general lethargy. TB is a communicable disease and can be spread by an airborne pathogen through coughing, sneezing, laughing, talking, and singing. Repeated and lengthy exposure is usually necessary to contract the disease. TB infection cannot be spread by touch or by sharing utensils with the infected person.

Latent TB infection is a condition in which living tubercle bacilli are present in an individual without producing the clinically active disease. The infected individual usually has a positive tuberculin skin test but does not have symptoms related to the infection. The person has a normal chest x-ray, does not have positive bacteriological examinations (smear and culture), is not infectious, and is not considered a case of TB. However, the infected individual remains at lifelong risk of developing the disease.

Multidrug-resistant TB is a state wherein a person has drug resistance to isoniazid and rifampin, the first-line drug treatment for TB. This condition can usually be prevented by initial treatment of TB patients with four drugs and ensuring adherence to the regimen by administering TB medications under directly observed therapy. Clinicians who are not familiar with the treatment of this condition should consult a specialist.

Prevention of TB Infection

Avoiding contact with the person carrying the TB bacteria is the preferable method of avoiding TB infection. However, because the disease carrier frequently does not know that she or he is carrying it, controlling the spread of the disease can be quite difficult. The bacillus Calmette-Guérin (BCG) vaccine is the only vaccine available against tuberculosis. Intracutaneous inoculation with BCG is currently used in many parts of the world, especially in young children, to prevent tuberculosis even though its protection does not extend into their adult years. At the present time health authorities do not recommend the use of the BCG vaccine in the United States except in two situations. First, BCG is recommended for infants and children with negative tuberculin tests who are at high risk of intimate and prolonged exposure to persistently untreated or ineffectively treated patients with infectious TB. Second, it is also recommended to tuberculin-negative infants and children in groups where the rate of new infection exceeds 1% per year and for whom the usual surveillance and treatment has been attempted but are not operationally feasible. These groups include persons without regular access to health care or groups who have demonstrated inability to effectively use existing accessible care.

In the Philippines the primary means of preventing TB infection is the BCG vaccine. According to a survey done in 1997, BCG coverage has improved. However, the prevalence of TB infection and annual risk of TB infection has remained essentially unchanged since the 1981–1983 nationwide TB prevalence survey, largely due to the inadequacies of the national TB control program (Tupasi, Radhakrishna, & Quelapio, 2000a; Tupasi et al., 2000b).

To protect healthcare workers against nosocomial spread of the disease, the following steps should be followed. For someone who has a negative skin test, annual or periodic skin testing continues. If a healthcare worker has a positive skin test, then a chest x-ray is recommended. If the chest x-ray is negative, an explanation of the signs and symptoms of active TB follows with instructions for the healthcare worker to contact Occupational Health as soon as the signs and symptoms of active TB appear. If the chest x-ray is positive, treatment is recommended with referral to an infectious disease specialist. Healthcare workers caring for TB patients (in a negative pressure room) must wear appropriate respirators and follow the structural safety precautions of the workplace.

Screening and Diagnosis

The tuberculin skin test, purified protein derivative (PPD), is used to screen patients who did not receive the BCG vaccine in childhood. However, it is a poor diagnostic tool because although a TB-infected person will test positive if he or she is in an active stage of TB, so will someone without TB in reaction to the test. The booster effect suggests that the patient retains the memory of delayed type hypersensitivity at *M. tuberculosis*. The Centers for Disease Control and Prevention (CDC) suggest that a second test that is also positive be followed up with a chest x-ray to rule out active TB. It takes 6 to 12 weeks after exposure to TB for a successful exposure that develops into an infection.

Treatment of TB

The overall goals for the treatment of TB are to cure the individual patient, to minimize death and disability from TB, and to interrupt the transmission of *M. tuberculosis* to other persons. TB treatment regimens must include multiple drugs to which the organisms are susceptible. Treatment with a single drug can lead to the development of a bacterial pop-ulation resistant to that drug. Likewise, the addition of a single drug to a failing anti-TB regimen can lead to resistance to that drug. In the United States the Food and Drug Administration has approved two fixed combination drugs: Rifamate, which contains iso-niazid and rifampin, and Rifater, which contains isoniazid, rifampin, and pyrazinamide.

Directly observed therapy is an anti-TB program managed by the Health Department wherein a community volunteer is assigned to a patient to ensure the patient takes the daily drug treatment over the required period. In the Philippines local remedies (39%) and herbal products (38.6%) were identified as main treatment for TB. Families with an income below 2,000 pesos ($40.00/month) were most likely to use local remedies. They were also most likely to believe that TB is not a curable disease (Portero-Navio, Rubio-Yeste, & Pasicatan, 2002).

TB and Filipinos

In 2003 persons born outside the United States accounted for more than 53% of all new TB cases. Sixty-four percent of all TB cases in Washington State were from Asia and Southeast Asia (53%), followed by Central and South America (20%) and Africa (12%). The highest case numbers came from Mexico (27%), the Philippines (23%), Vietnam (18%), and India (13%) (Washington Department of Health, 2004).

Economic Factors

According to a WHO report (Wise, 1998), more than one-third of all Filipinos live below the poverty line, and the problem of TB is particularly acute in poor areas. Cramped and overcrowded housing, poor ventilation, low immunity due to malnutrition, delayed diag-nosis, and overpriced drugs all contribute to the escalating incidence of TB (Wallerstein, 1999). According to Wallerstein, 1 in 10 of those infected go on to develop the disease and infect up to 15 other persons per year.

Directly observed therapy has shown encouraging results in pilot areas. It was imple-mented nationwide in the Philippines in 2001, but the budget of the Philippine govern-ment is inadequate and doctors can only provide free drugs to 30% of patients, compared with Vietnam and Cambodia (90%) and China (50%). Many TB patients in the Philippines must buy drugs from a pharmaceutical company, where they pay a high price. Most of the patients use the drug only until symptoms disappear, which contributes to the develop-ment of drug-resistant strains of TB (Wallerstein, 1999).

Cultural Factors

According to the president of the TB clinic in the Philippines, patients with TB-like symptoms do not seek treatment due to the stigma attached to the illness because TB is perceived as a shameful and unclean disease (Easton, 1998). To remedy this misconception about the disease, the Philippine Coalition against TB was established in 1994.

Yamada, Caballero, Matsunaga, Agustin, and Magana (1999) conducted focus group research regarding attitudes toward TB in immigrants from the Philippines to the United States. Comments and beliefs from the focus group participants shared several themes: causation and mechanism of TB, social and psychological implications of TB, and treatment of TB (Yamada et al., 1999). According to the study, in Filipino culture TB is perceived to be caused by several different factors. Respondents viewed TB as a highly contagious disease and commonly believed that one could contact TB by passing a sufferer on the street, engaging in casual conversation, or sharing eating utensils, telephones, or beds. To prevent spread it was believed that the clothes of a sufferer had to be boiled. Some respondents believed that even the smell from the open coffin of a victim of TB could produce the illness.

With respect to mechanism of the disease, those surveyed believed that cough, bloody cough, weight loss, and fatigue were all symptoms of TB. In addition, they believed that the body becomes dry when someone has TB and that this dryness makes if difficult to produce phlegm, so blood is coughed out as a result. Some believed that in severe TB, the lungs are filled with water. Others believed that the body actually shrinks, so the shoulders appear high as a result. Many also saw the disturbance of sleep by cough as a prominent feature, and they also thought that TB worsened with alcohol abuse. Finally, most indicated that death was the worst consequence of TB.

Participants in the Philippine immigrant focus groups considered the victims of TB to be infectious and therefore requiring isolation. The general attitude toward the victim of TB was stigmatization. The infected individual was thought to be dirty and was considered an outcast and shunned by society. Members of the focus group expressed the following (Yamada et al., 1999):

> They don't see you as a person when you have TB. The family members do not come to you because they feel you are dirty, and they are afraid that they will get the disease. They do not want to talk to you because they do not want to inhale the air that you breathe . . . especially the children since their resistance to infection is still low.

There are also psychological implications to having TB. The life of the victim of TB is characterized by suffering. Victims focus on their disease and impending death to the exclusion of all else, losing interest in work and other aspects of life. The stigmatization of TB leads to feelings of shame, isolation, and loneliness. Consequently, some sufferers avoid medical attention; they would rather not know the diagnosis. Some sufferers may become mentally incapacitated. The consequence of social stigmatization appears to include features that border on clinical depression.

Portero-Navio et al. (2002) interviewed Filipinos in Manila and suburbs regarding their knowledge and attitudes about TB. Only 24% of those interviewed knew that TB is due to germs (bacteria or microbes). Most linked TB with poor living conditions (86.2%) and air pollution (75.3%). More than half (63.8%) blamed smoking as a clear cause of the disease, and nearly one-third (31.2%) believed that it was an inherited pathology.

Educational Factors

Portero-Navio et al. (2002) also found that knowledge of how TB is transmitted correlates significantly with level of education. Respondents with a college education were more likely to know that a bacterium causes TB, whereas those with little or no formal education believed it was inherited. Interviewed subjects indicated normal breathing as the main mode of transmission of TB (55%), although only 21% indicated dissemination by droplet during coughing as the disease vehicle (Portero-Navio et al., 2002).

Family Relations

Auer, Sarol, Tanner, and Weiss (2000) studied how TB patients seek health assessment in Manila. They found that the family plays an important role. This is not unexpected in the Philippines, where the family remains an important source of support throughout adulthood. Therefore health communication to promote health and prevent illness should be conveyed to more than one member of the family. Underscoring the importance of this, the findings showed that 28% of respondents reported someone else with TB in their household when they themselves came for a medical check. The conclusion is that family-based health communication can be strengthened by encouraging those seeking care to always be accompanied by a family member and enabling community health workers to adequately convey health communication messages to the families in their houses.

Another significant social consequence of TB is that many Filipinos believe that someone with TB is prohibited from immigrating to the United States and thus unable to join family members who reside there. In fact, the infected person can receive treatment and then emigrate when no longer contagious.

Filipino Providers

Studies of the health-seeking behavior of TB patients in India, Pakistan, the Philippines, and Vietnam showed that more than half of these patients had consulted a private physician at some point. Moreover, use of private healthcare providers was not clearly related to socioeconomic status and extended to all social strata. However, in the Philippines in particular, the study showed that many cases of drug-resistant TB resulted from inadequate administration by the physician.

Manalo, Pineda, and Montoya (1998) investigated health care providers' knowledge, attitudes, and practices for TB. Findings of the study were as follows: (1) there are many misunderstandings about how TB is transmitted, (2) there is a need for wider acceptance of tuberculin testing and isoniazid chemoprophylaxis, and (3) there is considerable neglect of sputum examinations for diagnosis and treatment monitoring. Treatment was generally consistent with the recommendations of the national TB program: 42% were giving triple regimens and 29% were giving quadruple therapy. However, there were serious shortcomings in the management of retreatment cases with only 1% of respondents correctly identifying the algorithm proposed by the council of TB.

The need to update the skills and practices of private practitioners and health center staff is indicated by both overuse and inappropriate use of x-rays and the failure to examine sputum in accordance with current policy. There was also a conflict in the area of disclosure: The survey revealed that more than half of the physicians objected to the mandatory reporting of new TB cases. The providers based their success in attracting TB patients to their offices on confidentiality and on flexibility and kind treatment by providers (Auer et al., 2000).

U.S. Immigration and TB

In 1990 many Filipino veterans of World War II entered the country without medical screening or restrictions after being granted citizenship by the Immigration Act of 1990. By 1993 according to the TB Control Division of San Francisco Department of Public Health, the number of Filipino cases of TB had increased. This group of Filipino national veterans is an exception to the medical screening requirements of the Immigration Act: All other applicants for immigration visas are required to receive medical screening that includes examination for TB (CDC, 1990).

There is a reporting or notification program to identify immigrants at high risk for TB in the Philippines. This overseas screening process is intended to prevent infectious persons from entering the United States and to ensure that new arrivals who are at high risk for TB or have active TB receive medical services. Visa applicants 15 years or older must have a chest x-ray performed before they enter the United States. If the x-ray is suggestive of TB, acid-fast bacilli smears must be obtained, and applicants may not enter the United States until they have started on anti-TB therapy and their smears are negative. In addition, they must apply for a waiver signed by the local health department in their intended U.S. destination and complete therapy overseas before they are permitted to enter the United States (Washington Department of Health, 2004).

Solutions

Cultural Solutions

There are barriers to overcome in gaining patient participation: (1) culturally derived health beliefs that differ from those of Western medicine, (2) inability to communicate with medical providers in the patients' primary language, (3) inability to afford cost of medical evaluation and treatment, and (4) lack of familiarity with the access points to medical care. Of these, communication is the most obvious challenge. To facilitate communication, educational materials written in the patient's own language should be gathered from the CDC and other similar sources. The use of bilingual healthcare providers would also give support to U.S. immigrants. These bilingual staff members could translate appointment letters, reminder cards, and other information used for screening. Considerable time should be spent with each person screened to explain in detail the definition of TB, the procedure of placing tuberculin skin test, and the implications of the test.

Especially where cultural and language differences exist, it is necessary to explain the distinction between infection and disease and to provide assurances to clients with positive reactions. The disease process must be explained particularly because many who might know about the disease are unfamiliar with the idea of taking medication for a latent infection. Teaching materials should be developed to assist in providing a sufficiently detailed explanation. In addition, having the patient repeat explanations in their own words will help avoid polite "yes" responses to an oversimplified "do you understand?" query.

Assurance should be given at the outset that follow-up tests and preventive treatment would be at no cost and safe from report to Immigration and Naturalization Service agents. To ensure accuracy and standardization of information given to clients, a detailed algorithm should be developed in collaboration with providers, agency partners, and bilingual health education experts. History questions and key informational phrases should be translated into simple language that is understandable at various educational levels (D'Lugoff, 2002).

A patient-centered viewpoint should be emphasized, with particular emphasis on cultural and social influences on patients' beliefs and practices. A culturally competent approach is one in which providers seek to educate themselves about such influences. Practitioners must question individual patients about their personal beliefs, but prior knowledge of such perspectives will foster successful clinical partnership. As Yamada et al. (1999) emphasizes, practitioners who care for the Filipino patient with TB should focus patient education around the degree of its transmissibility and the manner in which it may be reduced.

In addition, community-based educational interventions among Filipino immigrants about the true degree of transmissibility of TB may lead to less stigmatization and, consequently, to less hiding of illness. If TB service providers are not required to inquire about immigration status and can ensure members of the community that legal immigrants are not deported if they develop active TB, it may increase cooperation and adherence to therapy. Such efforts may foster community-wide TB control. Two kinds of educational materials may help in this regard: culturally sensitive materials that the health worker can give to the patients and materials for the health workers themselves.

Economic Solutions

Health communications alone are insufficient for adequate control of TB. They cannot reduce a delay to treatment unless health services are available, affordable, and acceptable. There is no substitute for competent, efficient, and patient-oriented personnel who effectively engage patients in a productive treatment alliance, but medicines must be readily available. Efforts to promote a directly observed therapy strategy must account for the human aspect of clinical interactions. The technical and organizational aspects of TB control should not detract from appreciation of the human aspect of treatment and control strategies.

To stop the worldwide transmission of TB, adequate sources of funding must be identified to ensure that every TB patient has access to effective diagnosis and treatment. The social and economic inequities surrounding TB must be reduced. New preventive, diagnostic, and therapeutic tools and strategies must be developed and implemented to eliminate the disease.

Provider Solutions

As medical providers, physicians and advanced practice registered nurses (APRNs) should provide leadership in public health advocacy for TB prevention and control. Among other things, they could develop community partnerships and strengthen community involvement in TB control, educate the public and train healthcare providers to maintain excellence in TB services, and develop and implement a program of research into the behavioral factors related to TB treatment and prevention and rapidly transfer findings from research studies into practice (D'Lugoff, 2002).

D'Lugoff (2002) also urged providers to increase the capacity of TB control programs to implement targeted testing and treatment programs for high-risk persons and provide technical, programmatic, and research support aimed at reducing the incidence of TB as an opportunistic disease in countries with high HIV burdens. In addition, they could ensure appropriate care for patients with multidrug-resistant TB and monitor their response to treatment and treatment outcomes and support the development of the state- or area-specific TB elimination plans that contain communications activities to build support for TB elimination. An example of an excellent provider is described by Tracy Kidder (2003) in his book, *Mountains Beyond Mountains*. The book profiles Paul Farmer, a Harvard Medical School alumnus who had a passion for medicine and a particular interest in caring for TB and HIV patients. He established health clinics in Haiti and Peru, where he dedicated his time to finding treatment and funding for the poorest of the poor who cannot afford health care. His quest is to solve the challenge of giving treatment to multidrug-resistant TB.

Agency Solutions

One of the best ways to overcome agency barriers to effective treatment of TB is through use of the Internet. The CDC (2004) published an interactive core curriculum that can be accessed online; it provides detailed guidance in curing and treating a TB patient. As Internet access becomes more widely available, providers around the world can view this updated information and apply the guidelines for treating TB disease to their own practice.

The American Thoracic Society and CDC published new guidelines for TB control efforts. These guidelines are for targeted tuberculin skin testing of populations at high risk of infection and the treatment of latent infections for all these found to be infected (Geiter, 2000).

In the Philippines there are government or independent agencies who can help decrease poverty and thus decrease the barriers to effective TB treatment. For example, a Catholic organization, Couples for Christ, has been doing an excellent job working with the government to help rebuild the nation. Couples for Christ founded the Gawad Kalinga Foundation, which builds houses for the poor with donated building materials and volunteer labor. They have built entire villages for the poor and plan to build 700,000 homes in 700 villages in 7 years. This will alleviate some of the overcrowding in the squatter areas of the Philippines and therefore lessen the risk of spreading communicable diseases such as TB.

State of the Art of Literature

Areas of Disagreement in the Literature

Matsunaga et al. (1998) stated that screening is a difficult and overwhelming task because of the challenge of determining whether the patient has TB disease or TB infection. However, many believe that screening is a lower priority activity than either case finding, completion of therapy, or contact follow-up. Screening should be undertaken only after consideration of overall costs and benefits to TB prevention and control programs.

Another area of disagreement is the BCG vaccine. The CDC core curriculum for TB disease states that BCG vaccination is not generally recommended in the United States. Reasons for their recommendation include the low risk of infection with *M. tuberculosis*, the variable effectiveness of the BCG vaccine against pulmonary TB, and the vaccine's interference with the ability to determine tuberculin reactivity. However, the University of Texas states that the BCG vaccine is recommended for infants and children with negative tuberculin tests. In addition, if they are at high risk of intimate and prolonged exposure to persistently untreated or ineffectively treated patients with infectious TB, then they will be exposed and contract the disease. Tuberculin-negative infants and children in groups where the rate of new infection exceeds 1% per year and for whom the usual surveillance and treatment has been attempted but are not operationally feasible must get or obtain the vaccine because they are high risk (Nash, 1995).

Areas of Agreement in the Literature

Many agree that TB has become a threat to world health with regard to morbidity and mortality. However, with proper investigation, screening, and treatment the disease can be controlled and eradicated. As far as Filipinos are concerned, they have a higher risk of contracting TB because their country is a developing nation.

Gaps

Many articles have been written regarding TB and Filipino culture and their knowledge of the disease, but few address the barriers to treatment and how to remove them to decrease the incidence of TB in this country. However, some studies address the same issues in other ethnic groups with needs that are similar to those of the Filipino people. Adopting some of these same solutions can help solve the problems surrounding the screening and treatment of TB among the Filipino people.

Case Studies

In this section two brief fictional case studies are presented to illustrate how some of the solutions discussed in this chapter might be applied in real-life situations.

Case Study 1

Pilar is a 55-year-old woman who was living in Manila and then came to the United States to join her daughter. When she petitioned to enter the United States she was very excited to join her daughter. However, Pilar had to go through a series of screenings, such as a physical examination, chest x-ray, and interview. She was concerned that she would not pass the immigration health screening for TB because she had heard of stories of people who were denied of coming to this country due to TB infection. Fortunately, because her x-ray showed no cavitations suggestive of TB, she was able to come to the United States to join her daughter and her grandchild.

Pilar's daughter Nena had come to the United States 5 years previously as a mail-order bride who met her husband through pen-pal letters. Pilar's family was poor in the Philippines, but her daughter now has a better economic situation because of her marriage. Nena has a young daughter and strongly desires her mother to take care of her child because in Filipino culture, it is more desirable for family members to take care of children than outsiders.

When Nena's child started school, Pilar grew lonesome staying at home while everyone in the household was away during the day, so she decided to apply at a local hospital in the nursing home department as a housekeeper. As a preemployment requirement she had a skin test for TB, which turned out to be positive. Her PPD test had 12-mm induration. She did not know what it meant so she asked her friends if she could still work for the company. She decided to go to the International District walk-in for consultation, and she was diagnosed with latent TB. She spoke very little English so she was referred to one of the Filipino providers practicing in the clinic. Because she was afraid she would not get the job, she decided to go to this clinic for a second opinion.

Because Pilar had latent TB, not active TB, she got the job as a housekeeper. The employee health nurse advised her to make sure she completed the routine checks every year to monitor signs of TB disease for someone who has TB infection. The nurse also taught her to watch for signs and symptoms such as night sweats, fatigue, loss of appetite, and weight loss and that these should be reported to the employee health nurse or her primary care provider.

Case Study 2

Juan came to the United States as a veteran of World War II and qualified to come to the United States without previous health screening. It was difficult for him to get a job because he was in his sixties. His business in the Philippines was farming. Hoping to establish his own business, he went to eastern Washington. He heard about an opportunity to work as a fruit picker in the Yakima Valley area, so he decided to go to work for a company there and learn the business. He had been having night sweats, but he thought it was just because of the hot weather. He also had lost weight, but he was attributing this to his poor appetite because he was a little depressed about being away from his family.

He finally went to a local provider when he started coughing. Because this was the first encounter with the provider, he had to give his work history and profile. After taking Juan's history, the provider realized that Juan had been with migrant workers and decided to do a PPD test because he had been in contact with a high-risk group for contracting TB.

The PPD skin test result was positive, and an x-ray revealed cavitations. He was admitted to the local veterans hospital where he was in isolation for 3 days to collect 3 days worth of specimens for acid-fast bacilli and cultures to determine the sensitivity of the organism to medications. He was started on the recommended treatment, and his case had to be reported to the Department of Health. Because he did not have a family member in the United States, he was assigned a health worker for directly observed therapy treatment upon discharge. The provider had limited knowledge of the treatment so he consulted the infectious disease reference and recommended a liver function test before instituting the four-drug regimen recommended by the CDC. Because his liver function tests were within normal limits, Juan was able to receive the first line of treatment. He was given instructions to watch for persistent symptoms and let the provider know if his current medication was not making him feel better while waiting for the sensitivity result of the acid-fast bacilli culture. He was also told that if there was no improvement he would have to be treated with a different regimen. However, a few days later the cultures grew *M. tuberculosis,* which was sensitive to all four drugs. He was able to remain on the medications he was already taking. His treatment regimen lasted 9 months and he recovered well.

Conclusion

The review of literature reveals the difficulty of performing effective TB screening. Effective screening involves identifying persons who have been in contact with infectious TB, screening contacts to determine whether they have TB infection or disease, and providing appropriate therapy when indicated. Providers must screen persons in high-risk populations and subgroups within the community, identifying those infected with TB and providing treatment for latent TB infection as indicated. It is therefore the job of the provider to ensure appropriate therapy is initiated and completed. As Matsunaga et al. (1998) stated, "identifying persons who have TB disease is a daunting and difficult task." Screening is particularly difficult and poses a great challenge among Filipinos, whose knowledge of the disease is skewed by their belief and culture and influenced by their economic and educational status.

Knowing the background of Filipinos and their cultural viewpoints would help to identify their needs and enable effective screening and treatment, especially in those areas that contribute significantly to the U.S. TB burden. A collaboration between WHO and the National Health Agency of the Philippines can improve TB control in the Philippines so there will be less risk of infection when Filipinos emigrate to the United States. In the United States government agencies and private practitioners can help communities foster nontraditional and public–private partnerships to improve the effectiveness of their communication activities, with particular attention to culturally appropriate materials. All organizations must coordinate their efforts to control and eradicate the disease.

References

Auer, C., Sarol J. Jr., Tanner, M., & Weiss, M. (2000). Health seeking and perceived causes of tuberculosis among patients in Manila, Philippines. *Tropical Medicine and International Health, 5*(9), 648–656.

CDC. (1990). *Tuberculosis in Philippine national World War II veterans immigrating to Hawaii.* Retrieved August, 16, 2007, from http://www.cdc/gov/mmwr/preview/mmwrhtml/00021462

CDC. (2000). *Core curriculum on tuberculosis.* Retrieved on August 16, 2007, from http://www.cdc.gov/tb/pubs/corecurr/default.htm

D'Lugoff, M. L. (2002). Tuberculosis screening in an at-risk immigrant Hispanic population in Baltimore City: An academic health center/local health department partnership. *Journal of Cultural Diversity, 9*(3), 79–85.

Easton, A. (1998). Tuberculosis controls in Philippines have failed so far. *British Medical Journal, 117*(7158), 557.

Geiter, L. (2000). *Ending neglect: The elimination of tuberculosis in the US.* Washington DC: National Academy Press.

Kidder, T. (2003). *Mountains beyond mountains.* New York: Random House.

Manalo, M. F., Pineda, A. Jr., & Montoya, J. C. (1998). Knowledge, attitudes and practices for tuberculosis among Filipino family physicians: A comparative analysis by practice setting and location. *Philippine Journal of Microbial Infectious Diseases, 27*(1), 6–12.

Matsunaga, D. S., Yamada, S., & Macabeo, A. (1998). *Cross-cultural tuberculosis manual: Cultural influences on TB-related beliefs and practices of Filipinos, Vietnamese, Chinese and Koreans.* Retrieved April 25, 2007, from http://www.ethnomed.org

Nash, D. R. (January 1995). *Center for pulmonary infectious disease control, brief consults, tuberculosis II.* Tyler, TX: University of Texas Health Center.

Portero-Navio., J. L., Rubio-Yuste, M., & Pasicatan, M. (2002). Socio-economic determinants of knowledge and attitudes about tuberculosis among the general population of Metro Manila, Philippines. *The International Journal of Tuberculosis and Lung Disease, 6*(4), 301–306.

Tupasi, T. E., Radhakrishna, S., & Quelapio, M. I. (2000a). Tuberculosis in the urban poor settlements in the Philippines. *International Journal of Tuberculosis Lung Disease, 4,* 4–11.

Tupasi, T., Radhakrishna, S., Pascual, M., Quelapio, M., Villa, M., Co, V., et al. (2000b). BCG coverage and annual risk of tuberculosis infection over 14-year period in the Philippines assessed from the Nationwide Prevalence surveys. *International Journal of Tuberculosis Lung Disease, 4*(3), 216–222.

Wallerstein, C. (1999) Tuberculosis ravages Philippine slums. *British Medical Journal, 319*(7207), 402.

Washington Department of Health. (2004). *Washington State guidelines for prevention, treatment and control of tuberculosis.* Olympia, WA: Washington Department of Health.

Wise, J. (1998). WHO identifies 16 countries struggling to control tuberculosis. *British Medical Journal, 316,* 11–13.

Yamada, S., Caballero, J., Matsunaga, D. S., Agustin, G., & Magana, M. (1999). Attitudes regarding tuberculosis in immigrants from the Philippines to the US. *Family Medicine, 31*(7), 477–482.

Effective Treatment Plans for Female Veterans with Posttraumatic Stress Disorder

Patricia M. Jergens

The purpose of this chapter is to provide information regarding posttraumatic stress disorder (PTSD) and to suggest treatment plans to assist female veterans experiencing the disorder. Implications for advanced practice nurses (APNs) include how to establish whether single or combination treatment plans are more beneficial for the population and the supporting evidence for each of the therapeutic treatment plans available. In addition, gaps in the research literature are identified to suggest where future research may be directed to promote a better understanding of the disorder.

PTSD is one of the most common mental health problems associated with the experience of traumatic events. After the American Civil War PTSD was known as the Da Costa Syndrome ("soldier's heart") in which cardiac symptoms associated with increased irritability and arousal were experienced after a traumatic event (Grinage, 2003). However, until PTSD was recognized as a psychiatric disorder in 1980, it was characterized as "shell shock," "battle fatigue," or the "post-Vietnam syndrome." PTSD is a complex psychiatric disorder that involves the dysregulation of biological, behavioral, cognitive, and interpersonal systems after a traumatic event (Liebschutz, Frayne, & Saxe, 2003). Individuals who have experienced events such as a threat of death to themselves or someone else, either through an act of violence, accident, war, disaster, or chance encounter of a corpse or body parts, may experience long-term mental distress (Schurr & Friedman, 2001).

Extensive studies conducted on PTSD show that symptoms associated with PTSD are linked to combat stressors and also to various traumatic events that may be experienced by anyone in the course of a lifetime. In particular, the events of September 11, 2001, raised the need to study PTSD in the general population. The focus of this chapter, however, is female veterans.

Overview of PTSD

Diagnosis

To make the diagnosis of PTSD a precipitating traumatic event is necessary, though not sufficient, because many people survive traumatic events that lead to PTSD. The symptoms must last for 1 month and must disrupt one's normal activities before the diagnosis of PTSD can be made. To make the diagnosis more difficult to ascertain, often the symptoms may occur months or years after the traumatic event and can persist for years. Symptoms may last for a short period of time only to recur years later, triggered by an event that may or may not be related to the original incident.

Baxter (2004) identified a cluster of symptoms that have been consolidated into the following three groups that characterize the emotional and physical symptoms seen with PTSD:

- Reexperiencing the trauma, which may include distressing and intrusive recollections of an event, distressing dreams related to an event, hallucinations or flashback episodes that give an impression that the event is happening again, and intense psychological distress (e.g., passing the site of the traumatic event or symbolic association of an event with the traumatic event)

- Marked avoidance of usual activities such as a deliberate effort by the survivor to avoid conversations, thoughts, or feelings related to the trauma; avoidance of people, places, and objects related to the trauma; difficulty in recalling important aspects of the trauma; withdrawal from significant activities; and feelings of isolation

- Increased symptoms of arousal such as sleep alterations, outbursts of anger, difficulty in concentrating, constant vigilance, and an increased startle response

Before a patient can be diagnosed with PTSD, the symptoms must disrupt the patient's normal activities for at least 1 month. To make diagnosis even more complicated, approximately 80% of patients have been reported to have at least one comorbid psychiatric disorder, which may include depression, alcohol or drug abuse, and other anxiety disorders (Bradley, 2003). Foa, Davidson, and Frances (1999) outline the following common problems seen with PTSD:

- Panic attacks: Individuals who have experienced a trauma may have a panic attack when exposed to something that reminds them of the trauma. A panic attack involves intense feelings of fear or discomfort that are accompanied by physical or psychological symptoms (racing heart, sweating, shortness of breath, chest pain, and dizziness).

- Depression: Individuals may become depressed after experiencing a trauma and may no longer take interest or pleasure in things they once did.

- Suicidal thoughts and feelings: This may be seen when the depression becomes so severe the individual may believe life is no longer worth living.

- Substance abuse: Individuals may turn to use of alcohol, prescribed medications, or illicit drugs for a means to deaden the pain they are experiencing.

- Feelings of alienation and isolation: Individuals with PTSD have an increased need for social support. They often feel alone or isolated after experiencing a traumatic event and find it difficult to reach out or enlist the help of others.

- Feelings of mistrust and betrayal: Individuals who have experienced a trauma may feel betrayed and let down by the world, by fate, or by God.

- Anger and irritability: These are common reactions for individuals who have experienced a traumatic event. However, this response may interfere with their treatment and recovery.

It is important to realize that many of the associated problems and symptoms may improve when the PTSD symptoms are successfully treated. However, often symptoms are only alleviated temporarily and may recur.

Diagnosis of PTSD can be further described as an acute attack or chronic episode. An acute episode of PTSD lasts longer than 1 month but less than 3 months, and the symptoms seriously interfere with the person's ability to function. If these symptoms extend past 3 months, the individual should receive recommendations to seek professional help. A chronic episode exists when an episode lasts longer than 3 months, and once a chronic episode is established resolution often is not possible without treatment (Kubany, Leisen, Kaplan, & Kelly, 2000).

There can be many difficulties diagnosing PTSD. Sometimes the female veteran may be reluctant to disclose the traumatic event. This may be due to depression, feelings of guilt, substance abuse or other comorbidities on the part of the patient. It can be beneficial for the practitioner to use direct or nonjudgmental questions such as "Have you ever been attacked or threatened?" or, "Have you ever been in a severe accident or natural disaster?" to elicit the possible diagnosis of PTSD (McPherson, 2003).

At the same time, a healthcare provider can ask questions that establish a link between a traumatic event experienced by a patient and the symptoms. According to Breslau, Peterson, Kessler, and Schultz (1999), screening questionnaires for PTSD show a sensitivity of 80% and specificity of 97% for the diagnosis of PTSD. Questions such as "Do you have diminished interests in activities?" "Do you have problems sleeping?" and "Do you find it hard to feel or show affection for others?" assist the practitioner in the diagnosis of PTSD in female veterans.

Epidemiology

It is estimated that there is an 8–9% prevalence rate of PTSD in the United States, with the condition being twice as common in women. The epidemiology of PTSD has been directly linked to the likelihood of PTSD severity. Duration has been linked to the severity and duration of the trauma, with the most recognizable population being that of the combat veteran. It is further suggested that 25–30% of individuals experiencing a traumatic event will in all likelihood develop symptoms associated with PTSD, although the response to the trauma is directly related to how the individual reacts to stressors in normal everyday life (Grinage, 2003).

Though PTSD can occur from many avenues, the most commonly seen stressors include: motor vehicle accidents in which crash victims have been seen to develop PTSD as early as one week after an accident; natural or man-made disasters, such as those seen in the events of September 11, 2001; physical and psychological torture, seen with the systematic destruction of personality, family, formal and informal institutions, and community; and childhood sexual abuse. Comorbid substance abuse is also often seen with PTSD, with women being diagnosed significantly less often with the disease process than men (Schumann & Miller, 2000).

Pathophysiology

Although the exact cause of PTSD is unknown, it is known that the central nervous system normally responds to overwhelming threats with a fight or flight response, yet with PTSD the body fails to return to its pretraumatic state. In a normal fear response there is the activation of the fight or flight reaction that increases catecholamines and cortisol in response to the severity of a stressor (Grinage, 2003). This acute stressor activates several physiological responses, including activation of the hypothalamic–pituitary–adrenal (HPA) axis with release of adrenocorticotropic hormone, epinephrine, norepinephrine, glucagons, and cortisol. In turn, the release of catecholamines induces anxiety, tachycardia, shortness of breath, and diaphoresis (Schumann & Miller, 2000). In the normal fight or flight response the release of cortisol stimulated by the corticotropin-releasing factor via the HPA axis acts as a negative feedback loop to suppress sympathetic activation and release of additional cortisol (Grinage, 2003).

In individuals with PTSD cortisol levels are subnormal, which causes a state of chronic adrenal exhaustion from inhibition of the HPA axis by persistent severe anxiety The HPA axis and the sympathetic nervous system become disassociated and cause uncontrolled release of catecholamines, affecting memories of the trauma and exacerbating the symptoms when the individual is exposed to cues associated with the trauma (Grinage, 2003).

PTSD among Female Veterans

It has been shown that 43–63% of female veterans enlisted in the military experience high rates of sexual harassment, sexual assault, and physical violence during their military careers. Also, 90% of female veterans being treated at Veterans Affairs facilities have reported experiencing frequent harassment, and 37% have reported being raped during their tours of duty (David, Cotton, Simpson, & Weitlauf, 2004). In the National Vietnam

Veterans Readjustment study, researchers found that 27% of female veterans suffered from PTSD at some point during their postwar lives. However, it was also noted that female veterans participating in this study reported they were less likely to have recurrent symptoms of PTSD if they had family and community support to turn to in times of need (Taft, Stern, King, & King, 1999).

Frayne et al. (2004) studied 30,865 female veterans and found that even though depression was linked to poor physical health, women with PTSD are even more likely to have medical conditions such as hypertension, obesity, emphysema, low back pain, and cancer. PTSD is associated with a greater burden of medical illness than seen with depression. Approximately 4,348 female veterans from the above sample reported that they were diagnosed with PTSD, 7,580 with depression, and 18,937 never diagnosed with either condition. Nearly 90% of the women who reported to have been diagnosed with PTSD complained about having at least one medical condition associated with their symptoms, including arthritis, chronic lower back pain, obesity, or hypertension (Bender, 1999).

The Women Veterans Working Group (1995) identified the following major stressors in female veterans suffering from PTSD who served as doctors, nurses, and aviation staff or volunteers in different wars:

- Witnessing greater number of deaths (of youth, friends, and relations)
- Determining the severity of casualties and making painful decisions, such as who should die and who should get medical care
- Male chauvinism
- Overwork (15–20 hours per day) in a stressful environment
- Sexual harassment, which included minor incidents such as stealing of undergarments to major incidents such as torture and rape (Sometimes the soldiers used rank and authority to influence female soldiers. The results reflected in a negative fashion if a woman refused to comply with the request.)
- Working in unhygienic conditions (sharing of bathrooms, dressing rooms, and bedrooms)
- Problems with professional relationships
- Lack of preparation for an upcoming situation
- Fear of biochemical attack (wearing masks to protect themselves and their future children from disabilities)
- Isolation

It is not known exactly why some individuals have minor symptoms after a trauma and others suffer more and for longer periods. Women who have been victims of some kind of traumatic experience often have more symptoms than men. It would appear that women are more sensitive to stimuli related to trauma, and if a woman experiences trauma directly, the median duration of her illness increases to 5 years as compared with 2 years with men (Breslau et al, 1999). It has been shown that the following factors increase the likelihood that an individual will develop PTSD (Foa et al., 1999):

- The more severe the trauma
- The longer the trauma lasted
- The closer the person was to the trauma
- The more the times the person has been traumatized
- If the trauma was inflicted by another (i.e., rape)
- If the individual experiences negative reactions from friends and relatives

Coronary heart disease and myocardial infarction are known to have higher occurrence rates with female veterans as compared with male veterans, with the contributory factor in this case being a higher level of hostility associated or expressed by women. It was shown that anger and hostility is higher in traumatized women, is positively related to the development of PTSD, and can have a negative impact on the response to treatment (Butterfield, Forneris, Feldman, & Beckham, 2000).

Most women who experience trauma have short-term symptoms. These short-term symptoms may be considered a normal response to a stressful event, especially if symptoms disappear in a few months. However, those symptoms that persist, worsen, or extend past 3 months should be considered serious and these women strongly advised to seek professional help (Feeny, Zoellner, & Foa, 2000).

Women vastly underreport sexual assaults. Only one-third to one-half of the women take the initiative to disclose the event to a friend or family member. Often, women are not diagnosed with PTSD, because they do not feel confident to disclose the rape to a practitioner unless directly asked. This is a common problem found among female veterans who do not relate their symptoms to their experience of war (Feeny et al., 2000). Women often do not recognize that they are experiencing symptoms of PTSD and so reinforce their fears by avoiding memories associated with the traumatic event. Hence, expressing ones feelings, talking, or writing about an event can help a patient in the recovery process.

It is estimated that the fiscal and human cost of PTSD is showing a 60% increase in medical costs over those patients without PTSD (Baxter, 2004). The end cost may be difficult to measure, but it can be very costly to maintain quality of life for patients with PTSD. When added to the cost of war, the prevalence of PTSD becomes even more alarming.

Essential Aspects in the Treatment of PTSD

The U.S. Department of Veterans Affairs has provided detailed information on the treatment of PTSD. A stepwise approach to the understanding of PTSD is essential, beginning with a detailed evaluation of the patient's situation and the development of an effective treatment plan that is comprehensive. The first step of the treatment begins with the safe removal of the patient from a crisis situation. The patient's problems such as exposure to trauma (ongoing domestic or community violence, sexual abuse, or homelessness), depression, suicidal attempts, disorganized thinking, and drug or alcohol addiction must be attended on an urgent basis. The following are essential components, besides pharmacotherapy, in the treatment of PTSD (Paul, 1985):

- Education: Female veterans and their families should be informed about the nature of the PTSD, its causes, and how it can affect perfectly normal people and their families. The complete understanding of the short- and long-term effects of the disorder and other problems associated with it must be brought to light. In essence, treatments must be clearly identified.

- Exposure: The female veteran can be exposed to the traumatic event through imaging that allows her to recapture the event in a safe controlled environment. At the same time it allows the individual to understand her reactions to the event and precipitating causes.

- Understanding: The female veteran must be allowed to understand and examine her feelings such as anger, shame, or guilt.

- Building confidence: Building confidence in female veterans with PTSD is another contributing factor in their treatment. They should be made to feel proud to have served their country. Moreover, their services and decisions during the traumatic event should be appreciated. They should be made to realize their valuable contribution. Such strategies help a patient regain her lost confidence.

Pharmacotherapy

Several forms of therapy have been applied to the treatment of PTSD. Drug therapies include tricyclic antidepressants (amitriptyline, imipramine), agents with anticonvulsant and mood-stabilizing properties (carbamazepine, Depakote), benzodiazepines, monoamine oxidase inhibitors, and selective serotonin reuptake inhibitors (SSRIs) (sertraline, paroxetine, fluoxetine, nefazodone). These medications are used singly, in combination with other medications, or in combination with other therapies to receive the most effective outcome possible. Drug therapies are used based on the previously stated hypothesis that a traumatic experience has interrupted the normal function of the neurochemicals of the brain, causing aberrant symptoms associated with PTSD (i.e., hypervigilance, depression, and anxiety) when exposed to cues associated with the trauma.

Tricyclic antidepressants and monoamine oxidase inhibitors were the first antidepressants to be used in the treatment of PTSD, with a special emphasis on their antipanic effect. Tricyclic antidepressants (amitriptyline, imipramine, and desipramine) have all been studied for their effects on PTSD symptoms and were not found to be effective in alleviating symptoms of avoidance or numbing. Tricyclics are not used primarily because of their adverse side effects and potential for toxicity (Schoenfeld, Marmar, & Neylan, 2004).

Monoamine oxidase inhibitors also were used for their antipanic effects and have been effective in treating some aspects of anxiety and depression. However, because of their potentially harmful adverse side effects in conjunction with many other medications and risk for hypertensive crisis, they too are used only as second- or third-line usage for the treatment of PTSD (Schoenfeld et al., 2004).

SSRIs have been shown to help modulate excessive external stimuli and reduce feelings of fear and helplessness (Schoenfeld et al, 2004). SSRIs, such as sertraline, paroxetine, and fluoxetine, have demonstrated efficacy across the range of PTSD symptoms and therefore have become the first-line treatment for the disorder (McRae et al., 2004). The use of benzodiazepines for treatment of PTSD reportedly does not support efficacy, have been noted to have adverse consequences in their use, and currently are not recommended by the International Society for Traumatic Stress Studies (Mellman, Clark, & Peacock, 2003).

McRae et al. (2004) compared the effectiveness, safety, and tolerability of nefazodone and sertraline for the treatment of PTSD. Participants for this study were men and women between the ages of 18 and 65 years, met the criteria for PTSD as directed by the *Diagnostic and Statistical Manual of Mental Disorders* (DSM-IV), and did not fall into the wide range of exclusion criteria. After a 1-week, single-blind, placebo, wash-out period, participants were assigned to 12 weeks of double-blind treatments with nefazodone or sertraline. Treatment was initiated at 25 mg twice daily for sertraline and 50 mg twice daily for nefazodone, with dosage changes made at no less than weekly intervals. Stable dosing of medication was made by the 4th week of the study, and after the treatment participants were referred for continued treatment. Twenty-three of the original 36 participants completed the 12-week trial and were shown to stabilize on an average daily dose of 463 mg nefazodone and a daily dose of 153 mg for sertraline. The effectiveness of the study indicated improvement of PTSD symptoms to include depression, sleep disturbances, anxiety, and quality of life over time using both medications (McRae et al., 2004).

SSRIs have proven to be effective in treating panic attacks, which makes them more attractive in the treatment of PTSD. Open-label and double-blind trials of sertraline, paroxetine, fluoxetine, fluvoxamine, and citalopram have established that SSRIs are the pharmacological treatment of choice for PTSD (Schoenfeld et al., 2004).

Treatment Modalities for PTSD

Several treatment modalities have been suggested to be successful in the treatment of PTSD, and though these therapies have shown promise in the relief of certain characteristics associated with PTSD, it is important to determine which therapy best suits the individual in need. Exposure therapy, also known as flooding, requires the female veteran to focus on and describe details of a traumatic experience in a therapeutic manner. It allows her to repeatedly confront these feared memories or situations to which at some point these memories become less frightening and dangerous (Rothbaum & Schwartz, 2002).

Marks, Lovell, Noshirvani, Livanou, and Thrasher (1998) addressed the efficacy of exposure therapy either alone or in combination with cognitive restructuring therapy and relaxation without exposure therapy or cognitive restructuring in the treatment of PTSD. This study consisted of 87 participants who were randomized to have 10 weekly sessions of one to four treatments, with follow-ups at weeks 11, 15, 24, and 36. Inclusion criteria for this study included individuals with PTSD for 6 months or more, ages 16–35 years, and absence of melancholia or suicidal intent, organic brain disease, past or present psychosis, and antidepressant use unless the participant had been receiving it for more than 3 months.

Those who were involved in the exposure therapy group were asked to talk in the present tense about what they had undergone, their response, its meaning, and what they smelled, heard, saw, felt, and tasted. They were to describe the critical aspects of the trauma repeatedly until the distress of the situation diminished. In the cognitive restructuring group, participants were taught to spot dysfunctional thoughts and elicit rational alternative thoughts and reappraise believes about themselves, the trauma, and the world. The combination of exposure and cognitive restructuring group was subjected to alternating sessions of each and was given homework assignments that consisted of exposure and cognitive tasks from the previous session. The individuals participating in the relaxation group were given one of three relaxation tapes that they listened to in their session and each night at home for 1 hour. They were then to write down any feelings of anxiety in a daily diary.

At the end of the session and at a 6-month follow-up, individuals participating in the exposure group and the cognitive restructuring group were noted to have a decrease in symptoms associated with PTSD (anger, guilt), and although the combination therapy also showed some improvement similar to that of the individual groups, the relaxation group only showed moderate improvement in PTSD symptoms (Marks et al., 1998).

Cognitive behavioral therapy is another well-known treatment for those suffering from PTSD. This type of therapy uses a combination of exposure therapy, contingency management, behavioral activation, modeling, and biofeedback to help in the reduction or elimination of unwanted reactions to external situations, one's thoughts and feelings, and bodily sensation or functions. Therapists believe that this technique is successful in teaching patients how to replace undesirable responses (Department of Veterans Affairs, 2005).

Zayfert and DeViva (2004) addressed cognitive behavioral therapy for treatment of PTSD and hypothesized that individuals would have residual insomnia posttherapy in the absence of continuing nightmares and hypervigilance. This study consisted of 27 participants seen in a rural tertiary medical center in which 100% were white, 89% female, 59% married or cohabitating, and 70% employed with a mean average age of 37.2 years. Individuals participating in this study reported their trauma experience was childhood sexual or physical abuse, adult sexual or physical abuse, accidents, witnessing violence/death, or other traumas. Participants received 16 individual sessions, which included image exposure, cognitive restructuring, problem solving, and activity scheduling. Cognitive behavioral therapy for insomnia was not included in this study.

Pretreatment results of this study showed that of 25 participants, 22 reported insomnia and 16 reported severe insomnia, with insomnia rating more severely than any other symptom associated with PTSD. At posttreatment 13 of 27 patients reported insomnia, 7 of whom had reported insomnia at pretreatment. The study found that even though all patients who reported nightmares and hypervigilance at posttreatment also reported insomnia, their frequencies were too low to analyze and were not reported by 77% of those with posttreatment insomnia. Twelve patients who reported experiencing trauma in bed, the bedroom, or in darkness reported insomnia at posttreatment, compared with 4 of 15 who were not traumatized in a sleep-related context. Six participants reported taking sleep medication pretreatment and five continued posttreatment (Zayfert & DeViva, 2004).

Although study results supported the hypothesis that insomnia would persist in the absence of continuing nightmares and hypervigilance, the researchers noted that other symptoms of PTSD did improve. It is necessary to note several limitations in this study. First, the sample size of 27 patients is small, consisting of only white women. Second, treatment was tailored to individual needs and treatment termination was based on resolution of symptoms, so patients who received significant amounts of treatment without resolution of symptoms dropped out of the study. Replication of this study with a larger population and stricter guidelines may prove to be more beneficial.

Trauma-focused group therapy was developed for patients who might not tolerate individual exposure therapy. This treatment involves exposure in a group context that includes psychoeducation, cognitive restructuring, relapse prevention, and coping skills training.

Schurr et al. (2003) in cooperation with the Department of Veterans Affairs assessed the effect of trauma-focused group therapy on PTSD. This study obtained the participation of 360 veterans randomly assigned to receive trauma-focused group therapy or a present-centered treatment that involved the same characteristics seen in the trauma-focused group yet avoided the trauma focus. Weekly treatment was provided to groups of six members for 30 weeks, followed by five monthly sessions, with assessment of the severity of PTSD as the primary outcome. Measurements were taken at the end of the initial session and at 18 and 24 months and included psychiatric symptoms, functional status, quality of life, physical health, and service utilization.

The aim of the study was to determine whether the widespread use of trauma-focused group therapy would be beneficial for veterans who use the Veterans Affairs medical system; however, the results of this study showed this not to be true. Though the posttreatment assessments of PTSD severity improved dramatically from baseline, the intention-to-treat analysis showed no difference between therapy groups. It is also important to note that the dropout rate for trauma-focused group therapy was higher than that seen with present-centered therapy. It is also suggested that the study did not find a treatment effect for trauma-focused group therapy, yet placed value on enhancing the delivery of cognitive behavioral treatments in the clinical practice setting.

Finally, prevention intervention refers to a general group of approaches that offer education to recently traumatized individuals about the nature of the response to trauma and encourages and facilitates disclosure of the traumatic events and the immediate emotional responses to the trauma. It is believed that such processes serve to modify the initial perception of cognitive processing of the event or the biological cascade that may be triggered by the trauma and as such assist the individual in forming realistic perceptions and mitigate against the development of a chronic and maladaptive adjustment (McFarlane & Yehuda, 2000).

State of the Art of Literature

Areas of Agreement

Research has shown agreement in the pathophysiology of PTSD in that it involves the dysregulation of the HPA axis with dissociation of the central nervous system, and the complexity of this dysregulation reflects the difficulty in treating the disorder. Furthermore, antidepressants, particularly SSRIs, have shown efficacy in all symptom clusters associated with PTSD and should be used as a first-line treatment for the disorder. There is also general agreement that patients who do not respond to one agent initially may respond to another agent and that response to pharmacotherapy is relatively slow.

Areas of Disagreement

Disagreements seen in many of the studies related to the treatment of PTSD are associated with the longevity and order of treatment. Some studies suggested that treatment longevity should range from 6 months to 1 year depending on the severity of the disorder, whereas other research found a beneficial treatment range of 2 years or more. Also, some studies suggest the use of pharmacological measures alone to relieve the symptoms experienced by female veterans with PTSD, whereas other research suggests that pharmacological measures in combination with therapeutic measures are the best means of eliminating the symptoms associated with the disorder.

The number of different treatment modalities also proves interesting when comparing the different avenues that can be taken. Multiple studies with respect to the different treatment modalities have suggested that one outweighs the other. As stated previously in this chapter, treatment modalities include exposure therapy, cognitive restructuring therapy, cognitive behavioral therapy, trauma-focused group therapy, and prevention intervention. Each study for this literature review compared and contrasted different treatment modalities, yet many agreed on different treatment modalities as being the most effective. Hence, the disagreement stands on which treatment modality is better for the treatment of PTSD.

Gaps in Literature

The major gap in the literature is related to effective treatment plans for women suffering from PTSD. A significant number of studies address PTSD, but these studies are generally related to the treatment of men suffering from the disorder and suggest that these are just as effective for treating women suffering from the same disorder. Additionally, gaps are seen in the recognition of the disorder. This is especially noted when a female patient presents to the primary care clinic with somatic complaints or intermittent complaints of anger, sadness, depression, or anxiety. Studies have not shown how to expand the knowledge base of the APN, which would allow them to recognize and clearly diagnose the symptoms of PTSD and diagnose it as such.

Nursing Implications

APNs are essential in the diagnosis and treatment of women suffering from PTSD. The primary care APN is often the first medical provider a patient may see, and yet the patient may not address or even acknowledge they are showing or having symptoms associated with PTSD. It is essential for the APN to recognize that a patient is in need and initiate a conversation with the patient in a manner that can address her possible needs. It is further essential that the APN and the patient collaborate on the need for medication, education, support, anxiety management, and life-style modification to prevent needless emotional pain and suffering. Additionally, it is essential that the patient be aware of the necessity of compliance to the treatment so that a successful treatment can be obtained.

APNs assume a critical role in facilitating a team and/or organizational approach in the diagnosis and treatment of PTSD. Therefore it is vital that these women are greeted in a manner that allows them to be separate from men, because women often associate men with a threat and the internal feelings being harbored by them may be enhanced and may deter them from seeking the help they desperately need. The APN, team, and/or organization should be able to provide them with a means to obtain support in a safe environment, help them to develop skills for managing their overwhelming emotions, and help them to develop the means to take control of their perceived threats and empower themselves.

Case Study

Captain C.F., RN, BSN, is a 43-year-old woman who was the charge nurse in a small combat support hospital located in Kuwait during Operation Desert Storm. She worked 12-hour shifts, 7 days a week, and was often the only nurse assigned to the night shift, accompanied by one corpsman. She was responsible for single-handedly covering a small six-bed intensive care unit, 12-bed medical unit, and the emergency department, which included the responsibility of stabilizing and maintaining patients while waiting for air evacuation. In addition, she was an integral part of the triage team that was implemented when wounded soldiers arrived at the unit.

The triage system in combat is one that is not very palatable. C.F. had to think of herself as a soldier first, nurse second, and a woman last. She had to get past the nurturing, loving, and mothering aspect of being a woman and nurse, where it is ingrained that one does the best they can for all, to being a soldier and having to preserve the fighting force first. She would have to triage the patients into categories of immediate, delayed, minimal, or expectant. Patients who were categorized as immediate may need surgery to save a life or limb, required minimal operating time, and had an expected good quality survival. Those in the delayed category may require a time-consuming surgery, but delaying care would not jeopardize the life, and stabilization would minimize the effects of the delay. Those in the minimal category had minimal or minor injuries and could be treated by support staff and sent back to the front. Individuals placed in the expectant category were those who had serious or multiple injuries that were too complex and time consuming and would require considerable personnel and resources, which were often not available. These individuals would often be medicated for comfort and set aside to die.

Each night C.F. feared that she would receive a call with inbound trauma victims. She often would not know the extent of the injuries until they arrived and before their arrival would worry about whether she would have a surgeon or specialist available to help care for the injured. On any given night she would dwell upon availability of ventilators of which there were only three, wondering how she would be able to choose which patient would be lucky enough to get what was available. To make things worse, she would worry about the availability of sufficient oxygen to support the respiratory needs of her patients. Oxygen was a prime necessity in the care of her patients and was one she often didn't have enough of. The insufficient supply of oxygen occurred frequently because oxygen trucks were often delayed due to the inability to get through bombed out roads, ongoing road clearing of burnt-out vehicles due to roadside bombing, and frequent bombing of medical supply vehicles.

Captain C.F. treated many severely injured and mutilated military men and heard these men screaming in pain and asking to die just to alleviate the extreme pain they were enduring. One of her biggest stressors was treating the enemy, the same men who caused the mutilation and devastation of her countrymen she saw and treated each day. During many of her tours of duty there would be SCUD missile alerts, and not knowing whether it was real or not, she would have to dawn her chemical gear. This made her work even more difficult because these suits accentuated the already smoldering heat (often 112 degrees or higher) in which she worked.

Just days before the end of C.F.'s tour of duty, she attempted suicide by overdosing on medication she was given for depression and intermittent anxiety episodes. She voiced her reasoning for wanting to end her life as she felt dead inside already, and each time she watched one of her countrymen die a piece of her died as well. She feared that she would not be able to return to the States to her previous nursing job after experiencing all the horrific things she did while in Kuwait. She didn't believe she could stand the mundane complaints of everyday life, the complaints of fellow nurses who had to work extra hours to cover a shift, or listening to honking motorists because they were impatient and in a hurry to get home. She believed that these inconsequential complaints were illegitimate when compared with the few if any complaints voiced by the injured countrymen she cared for each day.

C.F. is home now and works at a Veterans Affairs hospital caring for some of the same men and women she treated while in Kuwait. She attends frequent support groups with other nurses who experienced some of the same traumas and has very supportive family and friends. However, C.F. continues to find it difficult to put her past behind her because the war in Iraq is still ongoing, and she has constant reminders, either on the television or in the newspaper, of what continues in Iraq and to her fellow countrymen.

Conclusion

It is clear that future developments in the treatment of female veterans suffering from PTSD depends on a healthy understanding of the components of the disorder that can be attained through further research directly related to these specific individuals. Having a thorough understanding and more precise characterization of the nature and range of the stress responses in female trauma victims has the potential to lead to significant improvements in the effectiveness of the treatment of victims of trauma. Having a broad understanding of the disorder allows the APN to help empower the female victim and move her from being the victim to becoming the survivor living in the present.

PTSD is exceedingly complex and requires an interdisciplinary multidimensional approach in the management of the disorder. The complexity of PTSD symptom clusters combined with comorbidities suggests that the APN needs to recognize and understand when to refer individuals for further psychiatric evaluation and treatment. Finally, APNs who provide primary care have a unique opportunity to assist the female veteran to organize their internal or external resources, allowing the individual to achieve the most beneficial treatment possible.

References

Baxter, A. (2004). Posttraumatic stress disorder and the intensive care unit patient: Implications for staff and advanced practice critical care nurses. *Dimensions of Critical Care Nursing, 23*(4), 145–150.

Bender, E., (1999). Chronic health problems often accompany PTSD in women. *Clinical and Research News, 23*(17), 36.

Bradley, D. (2003). Diagnosis and management of post-traumatic stress disorder. *Journal of American Family Physicians, 68*(12), 2401–2409.

Breslau, N., Peterson, E., Kessler, R., & Schultz, L. (1999). Short screening scale for DSM-IV, Post traumatic stress disorder. *American Journal of Psychiatry, 156*, 908–911.

Butterfield, M., Forneris, C., Feldman, M., & Beckham, J. (2000). Hostility and functional health status in women veterans with and without posttraumatic stress disorder: A preliminary report. *Journal of Traumatic Stress, 13*(4), 735–741.

David, W., Cotton, A., Simpson, T., & Weitlauf, J. (2004). Making a case for personal safety: Perceptions of vulnerability and desire for self-defense training among female veterans. *Journal of Traumatic Stress, 19* (9), 991–1001.

Department of Veterans Affairs. (2005). *Cautions regarding cognitive behavioral interventions provided within a month of trauma.* Retrieved June, 18, 2005, from http://www.ncptsd.org

Feeney, N., Zoellner, L., & Foa, E. (2000). Anger, dissociation, and posttraumatic stress disorder among female assault victims. *Journal of Traumatic Stress, 13,* 89–100.

Foa, E., Davidson, J., & Frances, A. (1999). The expert consensus guideline series: Treatment of posttraumatic stress disorder. *Journal of Clinical Psychiatry, 60*(16), 14–76.

Frayne, S., Seaver, M., Loveland, S., Christiansen, C., Spiro, A., Parker, V., et al. (2004). Burden of medical illness in women with depression and posttraumatic stress disorder. *Archives of Internal Medicine, 164*(12), 1306–1312.

Grinage, B. (2003). Diagnosis and management of post-traumatic stress disorder. *American Family Physician, 68*(12), 2401–2408.

Kubany, E., Leisen, M., Kaplan, A., & Kelly, M., (2000). Validation of a brief measure of posttraumatic stress disorder: The distressing event questionnaire (DEQ). *The American Psychological Association, 12*(2), 197–209.

Liebschutz, J., Frayne, S., & Saxe, G. (2003). *Practical guidelines for handling abuse issues in clinical settings.* Philadelphia: American College of Physicians.

Marks, I., Lovell, K., Noshirvani, H., Livanou, M., & Thrasher, S. (1998). Treatment of posttraumatic stress disorder by exposure and/or cognitive restructuring. *General Psychiatry, 55,* 317–325.

McFarlane, A., & Yehuda, R. (2000). Clinical treatment of posttraumatic stress disorder: Conceptual challenges raised by recent research. *Australian and New Zealand Journal of Psychiatry, 34,* 940–953.

McPherson, D. (2003). Anxiety disorders. In *Family medicine: Principles and practice* (6th ed., pp. 285–288). New York: Springer.

McRae, A., Brady, K., Mellman, T., Sonne, S., Kileen, T., Timmerman, M., et al. (2004). Comparison of nefazodone and sertraline for the treatment of posttraumatic stress disorder. *Depression and Anxiety, 19,* 190–196.

Mellman, T., Clark, R., & Peacock, W. (2003). Prescribing patterns for patients with posttraumatic stress disorder. *Psychiatric Services, 54*(12), 1618–1621.

Paul, E. (1985) Wounded healers: A summary of the Vietnam nurse veteran project. *Military Medicine, 150*(11), 571–576.

Rothbaum, B., & Schwartz, A. (2002). Exposure therapy for posttraumatic stress disorder. *American Journal of Psychotherapy, 56*(1), 59–75.

Schoenfeld, F., Marmar, C., & Neylan, T. (2004). Current concepts in pharmacotherapy for posttraumatic stress disorder. *Psychiatric Services, 55,* 519–553.

Schumann, L., & Miller, J. (2000). Post-traumatic stress disorder in primary care practice. *Journal of the American Academy of Nurse Practitioners, 12*(11), 475–482.

Schurr, P., & Friedman, M. (2001, July 9). Posttraumatic stress disorder: Study examines treatment methods, looks for options for military women. *Health & Medicine Week,* 16–17.

Schurr, P., Friedman, M., Foy, D., Shea, T., Hsieh, F., Lavori, P., et al. (2003). Randomized trial of trauma-focused group therapy for posttraumatic stress disorder. *Archives of General Psychiatry, 60,* 481–489.

Taft, C., Stern, A., King, L., & King, D. (1999). Modeling physical health and function health status: The role of combat exposure, posttraumatic stress disorder, and personal resource attributes. *Journal of Traumatic Stress, 12*(1), 3–33.

Women Veterans Working Group. (1995). *She serves too, readjustment counseling service* (pp. 2–32). Washington, DC: U.S. Department of Veterans Affairs.

Zayfert, C., & DeViva, J. (2004). Residual insomnia following cognitive behavioral therapy for PTSD. *Journal of Traumatic Stress, 17*(1), 69–73.

Hormone Replacement and the Treatment of the Transgender Patient: A Critical Literature Review

David Hibbs

The aim of this literature review is to identify transgender-specific healthcare issues that impact primary care delivery and to identify the types of skills and knowledge primary care providers require to deal with these issues. The specific objectives addressed in this review are as follows:

- To define the appropriate and preferred terminology that accurately describes gender variants

- To identify potential barriers to health care that transgender patients face

- To describe specific health effects and outcomes in the transgender population receiving cross-sex hormone therapy

- To summarize how the above impact transgender health and propose treatment guidelines for cross-sex hormone therapy

Definitions

Transgender people are a diverse group of individuals that cross or transcend culturally defined categories of gender. The classification of transgender can include transsexuals, cross-dressers, bigender persons, drag queens, and drag kings (Bockting, 1999). Many people, including healthcare providers, are confused by the abundance of terminology used to describe this particular group of people. There appears to be a lack of standardization in the literature regarding appropriate language and terms to describe the phenomena of men and women who choose to act, dress, or physically alter their bodies to resemble a gender that is opposite of their genetically determined gender. For the purpose of clarity in this literature review, the following terms are defined as follows:

- *Transgender:* An umbrella term that encompasses a variety of people, including transsexuals, cross-dressers, drag kings and queens, and bigender and androgynous individuals. This term comes from the transgender community and is therefore the preferred term in working with transgender people (Gay and Lesbian Medical Association, 2001).

- *Transvestite:* An obsolete term for a person who wears the clothes of and often acts as a member of the opposite gender but has not medically or surgically altered his or her body. The newer and more acceptable term is "cross-dresser."

- *Drag king:* A colloquial term that referrers to a lesbian who cross-dresses for fun but who lives as a female.

- *Drag queen:* A colloquial term that referrers to a gay male who cross-dresses for fun but who lives as a male.

- *Transsexual:* A person who undergoes medical and surgical procedures to remove their genetic sexual characteristics and to gain physical characteristics of the opposite sex.

- *Sexual reassignment surgery:* An elective surgery to alter the gender of an individual. For male-to-female transsexuals it usually involves amputation of testicles and most of the penis, inversion of the penis skin into a vagina, and optional breast implants, tracheal shaves, and labiaplasty. For female-to-male transsexuals it involves mastectomy, hysterectomy, and optional attempts at creating a penis and scrotum.

- *Female-to-male transsexual:* A genetic female who dresses, acts, and alters her body to live as a male.

- *Male-to-female transsexual:* A genetic male who acts, dresses, and alters his body to live as a female.

The Transgender Population

The actual number of people who identify as transgender is unknown. Because of a lack of research focusing on the size of the population and the fear that many transgender people have about revealing their identity, reliable data are difficult to obtain. No probability studies of transgender people are reported in the literature, and no effort is underway to develop measures for inclusion in federal surveys (Gay and Lesbian Medical Association, 2001). Some psychiatric literature estimates that 1% of the population may have had a transgender experience, but this estimate is based only on transgender people who have sought mental health services (Seil, 1996). Although definitive data on the number of transgender persons are lacking in the United States, international estimates are 1 male-to-female transsexual per 11,900 persons and 1 female-to-male transsexual per 30,400 persons (Bakker, van Kesteren, Gooren, & Bezemer, 1993).

The Transgender Patient and Barriers to Health Care

In addition to the various health needs they share with all people, transgender patients may present with specific medical and psychological health issues that are unique to this particular population (Bockting & Coleman, 1992). Transgender patients are among the most stigmatized of sexual minorities (Bockting, 1999). They often face discrimination in healthcare coverage as well as discrimination and insensitivity from ill-informed health-care providers. Transgender-specific health care rarely is a covered benefit, and very few healthcare providers are knowledgeable about transgender health issues. As a result, trans-gender-specific health care is scarce, limiting a transgender patient's choices in accessing health care (Bockting, 1999).

An estimated 30% to 40% of transgender persons in this country do not have a regular healthcare provider and often rely on urgent care and emergency rooms for their imme-diate healthcare needs (Xavier, 2000). In addition, because many transsexuals fear having their transsexual status revealed, they may not receive appropriate and regular screening for certain cancers and diseases that may ultimately lead to increased morbidity and mor-tality, such as uterine, breast, and prostate cancer (Feldman, 2003).

A survey of transgender health seminar participants found that 15% did not have health insurance and 45% of those who reported having a primary care provider did not inform their providers of their transgender identity. This and other current data suggest that transgender patients are a medically underserved population who present chal-lenges for the primary care providers who serve them (Bockting, Benner, Robinson, & Scheltema, 2004).

Transgender-Specific Health Issues: A Concern for Primary Care Providers

Transgender hormone therapy is a medical intervention strongly desired by many trans-gendered persons. Transgender patients desiring hormone therapy may ask their primary care provider to prescribe this treatment (Clements, Katz, & Marx, 1999). Currently, no standardized training in hormone therapy is available to primary or specialty care providers who choose to provide this treatment to their transgendered patient.

Transgender health care involves addressing both general medical conditions and con-cerns related to cross-gender hormone therapy. Because transgender persons often do not have primary care providers, many may present with poorly controlled conditions, such as hypertension and diabetes (Feldman, 2003). Because many transgender people receiving cross-sex hormones are not aware of the serious health risks involved with hormone use, many do not consult with their primary care providers on a regular basis. Similarly, because research on cross-sex hormone therapy is limited or inconclusive, many primary care providers are unaware of the serious health risks related to cross-sex hormone therapy when they prescribe them to their transgender patients. As a result of the lack of research and data available to primary care providers regarding cross-sex hormone administration, many transgendered people receiving cross-sex hormones are not receiving adequate pri-mary care, nor are they being appropriately screened for certain diseases, including breast and prostate cancer (Clements et al., 1999).

Health Outcomes of Cross-Sex Hormone Therapy

Transgender patients' use of hormones necessarily makes their response to some diseases unique. Though the evidence in the literature is sparse, the following examples can be informative on the issue of health affects and outcomes in this population.

Type 2 Diabetes

Feldman (2002) closely monitored 74 male patients receiving feminizing hormone therapy. All patients received a full history and physical including baseline laboratory values for serum glucose and HgbA1C. These laboratory values were tracked every 3 months during the course of hormone treatment. Between 1998 and 2001 three male-to-female patients developed new-onset type 2 diabetes, diagnosed by fasting blood glucose levels greater than 126 mg/dl on at least two occasions (American Diabetes Association 2001 criteria). In the United States the incidence of type 2 diabetes is 3.7 per 1,000 annually (Centers for Disease Control and Prevention, 1997). Thus the appearance of three cases in 3 years in this population is greater than expected.

Feldman (2002) pointed out that male-to-female patients typically begin feminizing hormone therapy after the age of 40, which is an independent risk factor for developing type 2 diabetes; however, Feldman found that feminizing hormone therapy can result in increased weight and body fat, therefore contributing to glucose intolerance. The effect of hormone therapy on glucose tolerance in male-to-female transgender patients has not previously been addressed in the medical literature (Feldman, 2002).

The literature suggests that the introduction of feminizing hormones increases weight gain and body fat, both risk factors in the onset of type 2 diabetes. At the time of writing this literature review no other studies were conducted analyzing the effects of hormone therapy on glucose tolerance. If studies were conducted and showed that diabetes risk lessened in the female-to-male group due to decreased fat levels and weight loss, a more obvious correlation could be drawn independent of other risk factors already present.

As it stands now with a lack of evidence to draw on, primary care providers must be cognizant of the potential increased risk for glucose intolerance patients, particularly male-to-female patients, receiving cross-sex hormone therapy. In addition, cross-sex hormone therapy should be considered a risk factor for diabetes that is equivalent to other risks factors such as obesity, increased age, and a positive family history.

Osteoporosis

Schlatterer, Auer, Yassouridis, von Werder, and Stalla (1998) conducted a study on transsexual patients receiving cross-sex hormone therapy to determine whether and to what extent their regimen of hormone therapy might influence the development of osteoporosis. Researchers included 10 male-to-female and 10 female-to-male transsexuals who were receiving standard doses of cross-sex hormone therapy for at least 1.5 years. The male-to-female subjects were between the ages of 25 and 41 years. The female-to-male subjects were between the ages of 26 and 63 years. The experimental group's bone mineral densitometry was examined using a conventional whole body computed tomography scanner. Researchers compared the bone densities from the experimental group with the bone densities of age-matched healthy individuals published in the Normative Data Base of the University of California, San Francisco. The investigators found no significant difference compared with those of the corresponding biological sex control group. The researchers concluded that for transsexual patients treated with cross-sex hormone therapy the risk of developing osteoporosis is very low (Schlatterer et al., 1998). Data published earlier support the findings that testosterone-treated female-to-male transsexuals have no significant differences in average bone densities compared with an age-matched female control group (van Kesteren et al., 1996).

At the time of this writing no other studies were published regarding a relationship between cross-sex hormone therapy and the development of osteoporosis. Because the effects of cross-sex hormone therapy on bone density remain undocumented, it would be prudent for providers to ensure that all patients, including male-to-female patients, receive adequate counseling and screening regarding calcium consumption, supplementation, weight-bearing exercise, smoking, alcohol use, long-term corticosteroid use, and any other risk factors related to osteoporosis. In addition, providers should consider densitometry screening in those individuals at increased risk for osteoporosis regardless of sex or gender.

Adverse Effects on Liver Function

Tangpricha, Afdhal, and Chipkin (2001) presented a case of a 38-year-old genetic man treated with estrogen therapy. The transsexual patient was initiated on conjugated estrogen, Premarin 0.625 mg daily for the first month. This was increased to 2.5 mg daily by month 3. After 4 months of therapy the patient returned to the clinic with nausea and dark urine for 1 week. Laboratory tests revealed alkaline phosphatase 111 U/l, total bilirubin 3.5 mg/dl, aspartate aminotransferase 1,665 U/l, alanine aminotransferase 3,880 U/l, and gamma-glutamyltransferase 179 U/l. The patient's estrogen therapy was immediately discontinued. A clinical diagnosis of type 1 autoimmune hepatitis was made. The patient was started on prednisone 40 mg daily and azathioprine 75 mg daily. The patient was stable for 11 months. After stabilization the patient requested to be restarted on estrogen therapy despite warnings of the risks involved. A second trial of estrogen therapy was initiated, Premarin 1.25 mg daily, that was eventually tapered up to 2.5 mg daily. Once again the patient's transaminases increased two to three times the normal level, which again resolved after discontinuation of estrogen therapy. The authors pointed out that estrogens may have played a role in triggering autoimmune hepatitis. They also noted the lack of data and research in the area of cross-sex hormone replacement (Tangpricha et al., 2001).

Other literature also suggests that estrogen therapy for the treatment of male-to-female transsexuals is associated with some potential adverse effects on liver function. The treatment of male-to-female transsexuals has been associated with mild elevations in transaminases in the past (Meyer et al., 1986; van Kesteren, Asscheman, Megens, & Gooren, 1997). Although there are no recommendations in the literature regarding specific intervals for testing liver enzymes in transgender patients receiving cross-sex hormone therapy, it may be prudent for the primary care provider to take baseline liver function tests to compare with postadministration follow-up tests. The first scheduled follow-up test could be no later than 6 weeks after the initial administration of hormone therapy. Once serial liver function tests prove to be within normal limits, the provider could consider annual testing in a healthy transgender patient receiving hormone therapy.

Cholesterol

Damewood, Bellantoni, Bachorik, Kimball, and Rock (1989) studied the effects of cholesterol on transsexual men receiving cross-sex hormone therapy. Forty transsexual men, 20 castrated and 20 noncastrated, were included in the sample. The experimental group included transsexuals taking estrogen for at least 3 or more years. The control group consisted of 28 age- and weight-matched genetic men not undergoing hormone therapy. The control group was also matched for alcohol, tobacco use, exercise, and dietary intake. Study subjects were taking Premarin (estrone sulfate 48%, equilin sulfate 26%, 17α-dehydroequilin sulfate 15%) in doses that ranged from 1.25 to 10 mg/day.

For analysis of dose-related variables, patients were divided into low-dose (1.25–2.5 mg/day) and high-dose (5–10 mg/day) groups. After controlling for body composition, age, exercise, and other population factors, the investigators found that estrogen treatment resulted in a significant elevation of high-density-lipoprotein cholesterol levels among transsexual men. Transsexuals who were castrated and took estrogen therapy had an average high-density-lipoprotein cholesterol increase of 66.3% compared with the control group. Transsexual men not castrated had an average increase in high-density-lipoprotein cholesterol of 29.8% compared with the control group. The data demonstrate that exogenous estrogens administered to transsexual males results in a female pattern of lipoprotein cholesterol. The cardiovascular consequences of the female pattern of altered lipoprotein concentrations of transsexual males are unknown (Damewood et al., 1989).

Although the above research demonstrates that male-to-female transgender patients may obtain lower low-density-lipoprotein cholesterol and triglycerides from estrogen and progestin combinations, very little is known about the effects of cholesterol in female-to-male patients receiving testosterone therapy. Because male-to-female patients develop a female pattern lipoprotein profile, which is considered cardioprotective, we may infer that female-to-male patients receiving testosterone therapy develop a male pattern lipoprotein profile, which caries a higher level of cardiovascular risks. As such, primary care providers should be aware of this potential risks factor and screen female-to-male patients appropriately.

Venous Thromboembolism

Although this literature review is focused exclusively on the effects of cross-sex hormone therapy in transgendered patients, most research regarding increased risks of thromboembolic events associated with hormone administration has been conducted in women taking estrogen plus progesterone. However, this research seems to suggest that negative side effects, like venous thromboembolism, can result from hormone therapy. This is a potential risk to transgender patients if we infer that this risk will affect the transgender patient at the same rate.

Gutthann, Rodriguez, Castellsague, and Duque Oliart (1997) evaluated the association between the use of hormone replacement therapy and the risk of idiopathic venous thromboembolism in postmenopausal women receiving hormone replacement therapy. The results showed that the adjusted odds ratio of venous thromboembolism for current use of hormone replacement therapy compared with nonusers was 2.1 (95% confidence interval, 1.4 to 3.2). This increased risk was restricted to first-year users, with odds ratios of 4.6 (2.5 to 8.4) during the first 6 months and 3.0 (1.4 to 6.5) 6–12 months after starting treatment. The risk of idiopathic venous thromboembolism among nonusers of replacement therapy was estimated to be 1.3 per 10,000 women per year. Among current users idiopathic venous thromboembolism occurs at two to three times the rate in nonusers, resulting in one to two additional cases per 10,000 women per year. The investigators concluded that the use of hormone replacement therapy was associated with a higher risk of venous thromboembolism in the first year of use (Gutthann et al., 1997).

Cushman et al. (2004) reported their final data on the incidence of venous thrombosis related to hormone replacement therapy from the Women's Health Initiative Estrogen Plus Progestin clinical trial. The results of the study demonstrated that venous thrombosis occurred in 167 women taking estrogen plus progestin (3.5 per 1,000 person-years) and in 76 taking placebo (1.7 per 1,000 person-years). Compared with women between the ages of 50 and 59 years who were taking placebo, the risk of thromboembolic events associated with hormone therapy was higher with age. Compared with women who were of normal weight and taking placebo, the risk associated with taking estrogen plus progestin was increased among overweight and obese women. The authors concluded that estrogen plus progestin was associated with doubling the risk of venous thrombosis.

van Kesteren et al. (1997) designed a retrospective study at a university hospital to investigate the morbidity and mortality figures in a large group of transsexual subjects receiving cross-sex hormone treatment. Subjects had been treated with cross-sex hormones for a total of 10,152 patient-years. Standardized mortality and incidence ratios were calculated from the general Dutch population. Researchers found that venous thromboembolism was the major complication in male-to-female transsexuals treated with oral estrogen and antiandrogens. The investigators discovered that 36 subjects had suffered from venous thromboembolism that was most probably caused by the treatment with estrogens and antiandrogens. This represented a 20-fold increase in thromboembolism compared with the control group.

According to the literature, patients receiving feminizing hormones are at a significantly increased risk of thromboembolic events. It is important that providers screen transgender patients receiving hormone therapy for a personal or family history of a clotting disorder that may even further increase their risks for developing a thromboembolic event. In addition to screening for risk factors, providers should educate patients on the signs and symptoms of deep venous thrombosis and pulmonary embolus. Those with increased risk factors should be encouraged to quit smoking, exercise regularly, and maintain a healthy weight. In addition, some patients may be considered for daily aspirin therapy.

Breast and Prostate Cancer

Transgender persons who have undergone sex reassignment surgery are often unaware of residual breast or prostate tissue, which can lead to diagnostic delay for breast and prostate cancer. Although no formal studies have investigated the effects of cross-sex hormone therapy on breast or prostate cancer, several cases have been reported. There are at least two reports of male-to-female transsexuals receiving estrogen therapy who developed breast carcinomas. Similarly, there is also a report of a female-to-male patient found to have a breast carcinoma in residual breast tissue after having a complete mastectomy as part of a sex reassignment surgery (Gooren, Asscheman, & Newling, 1997).

Before May 2005 there were at least three reported cases of prostate carcinoma in male-to-female transsexuals on estrogen therapy. It is not clear whether these carcinomas were estrogen sensitive or whether they were present before estrogen administration was started and subsequently progressed to become hormone-independent carcinomas (Van Haarst, Newling, Gooren, Asscheman, & Prenger, 1998).

In May 2005 Miksad and colleagues reported a case of a 60-year-old male-to-female transgendered woman with locally advanced prostate cancer diagnosed 41 years after feminization. The patient presented to her primary care provider with the chief complaint of gross hematuria. She had started feminizing estrogen therapy at the age of 19. After 5 years of weekly estrogen injections (details unknown), she used conjugated estrogen (Premarin 2.5 mg daily) until bilateral orchiectomy at the age of 34 years. After bilateral orchiectomy she took conjugated estrogen (Premarin 1.25 mg) daily except between the ages of 50 and 56 years, when she took no estrogen therapy because of acquisition difficulties (details unknown). Family history was unremarkable for prostate cancer. On examination a large anterior mass was palpated. Her serum prostate-specific antigen level was 240 ng/ml (normal, < 4 ng/ml); no previous prostate-specific antigen level had been measured. The total serum testosterone was 44 ng/ml, a level that is consistent with a feminized male postorchiectomy. Antiandrogenic treatment along with radiation treatment was initiated, and the patient's prostate cancer went into remission (Miksad et al., 2006).

Early castration was thought to protect against prostate cancer because testosterone regulates prostate cancer cell growth; however, the case presented earlier clearly reveals that is not always true. At the time of this writing, no studies investigating the effects of cross-sex hormone therapy related to breast and prostate carcinomas were published. Because cancer risks associated with cross-sex hormone therapy are poorly understood, it is advisable for providers to encourage genetic females receiving masculinizing hormones over the age of 40 to continue annual mammograms, even after complete mastectomy. Likewise, providers should encourage male patients taking feminizing hormones to receive annual mammogram screenings. As noted in the literature, prostate cancer has been reported in both preoperative and postoperative transsexual patients. Prostate cancer surveillance with digital rectal exam and prostate-specific antigen screening should be discussed and offered to all male-to-female patients over the age of 50.

Emotionality and Hormone Therapy

Slabbekoorn, Van Goozen, Gooren, and Cohen-Kettenis (2001) investigated 54 male-to-female transsexuals and 47 female-to-male transsexuals receiving cross-sex hormone treatment to determine whether a cross-sex hormone regimen affected the intensity of negative and positive emotions in general and aggressive and sexual feelings in general. Both groups were administered standard doses of cross-sex hormones. The investigators then used a test battery containing five different questionnaires that were applied twice to all subjects: once before the onset of hormone therapy and once after approximately 14 weeks of hormone therapy.

The results showed that in general male-to-female transsexuals experienced more negative emotions, both before and after hormone treatment, whereas positive emotions and anger readiness seemed to be increased by hormone therapy. Female-to-male transsexuals showed less affect intensity for both negative and positive emotions after testosterone administration but more anger readiness. Comparisons of initial expectations before and actual experienced feelings during hormone therapy revealed that both male-to-female and female-to-male transsexuals changed according to their expectations in feelings of depression, tiredness, tenseness, and changeable mood. However, male-to-female transsexuals experienced these and other negative emotions, such as powerlessness, disappointment, and sadness, more intensely than did female-to-male transsexuals, both before and after 14 weeks hormone therapy.

The authors concluded that both male-to-female and female-to-male transsexuals derived large benefits from hormone treatment. Hormone therapy not only brings about the important physical changes, but also psychological relief. It is the case that these physical and psychological influences have a direct effect on emotional feelings. The investigators found that the intensity of emotions in male-to-female transsexuals appeared to be positively influenced by antiandrogen and estrogen treatment, whereas testosterone treatment in female-to-male transsexuals seemed to result in a reduced emotional intensity.

Although testosterone therapy seemed to stimulate aggression and sexuality in biological women, it seemed to have a dampening effect on their affect intensity in general.

Although female-to-male transsexuals in general derive large benefits from their sex reassignment, testosterone may make them emotionally less susceptible to positive or negative life events but more susceptible to situations with a provocative or sexual content. The start of sex reassignment, initiating the long-wished physical changes, may explain their increased positive emotionality. However, the level of negative emotionality remains high, or is even increased, when they are confronted with aversive emotional events.

These findings are consistent with earlier findings on the influences of estrogen on negative emotionality (Finkelstein et al., 1997; Van Goozen, Wiegant, Endert, Helmond, & Van de Poll, 1997). There is also literature suggesting that emotionality is at least partly sex hormone dependent (Buchanan, Eccles, & Becker, 1992). The results of this study are consistent with an earlier study, namely that cross-sex hormones have a clear effect on the emotional functioning of transsexuals (Van Kemenade, Cohen-Kettenis, Cohen, & Gooren, 1989).

Discussion

The literature suggests that more research needs to be conducted regarding transgender persons undergoing hormone therapy. All the examples above suggest that biological sex influenced by cross-sex hormones produces a unique response to disease and treatment. Because current medical studies focus almost exclusively on traditional biologically assigned gender, the transgender patient's responses to disease and treatments need to be inferred based on that knowledge. For example, if studies show that women who are entering old age begin to show decreased bone density due to hormone shifts that occur in the normal aging process, providers need to remain cognizant of that fact when treating a male-to-female transgender person who is in a similar age group and undergoing hormone therapy.

Another example is a female-to-male transgender person who retained female reproductive organs. Though not recommended, if the patient retained ovaries the patient still needs to be screened for ovarian cancer even though the patient lives life as a man. Like any area of science that lacks sufficient research, inferences have to be drawn from other evidence-based research. Because transgender patients do not neatly fit into one gender classification, guidelines applicable to both genders need to be referenced by the clinician to provide adequate and appropriate primary health care.

Without sufficient research on cross-sex hormone therapy providers must infer treatment guidelines based on research conducted on non-transgendered patients; these inferences may pose serious risks. For example, it was once recommended that postmenopausal women receive hormone replacement. Researchers believed that these replacement hormones would offer the same cardiac protective properties as the naturally occurring hormones that begin to diminish during menopause. Now, however, current research disputes this logical assumption, and it is now believed that hormone replacement therapy negatively affects a postmenopausal woman's cardiac health. This means that clinicians must proceed with caution when using inferences to treat patients when sound evidence is lacking. This is also another example of why more research is essential to effectively and safely treat transgender patients taking cross-sex hormones. Only when enough research has been conducted regarding this phenomenon can clinicians rely on true evidence-based guidelines.

Regardless of the lack of evidence-based research, transgender patients will continue to desire the positive effects of hormone therapy. As such, clinicians should be well versed and prepared for the possible health risks involved with hormone therapy. To treat transgender persons receiving cross-sex hormone therapy, clinicians first need to be cognizant of the medical and social risks and benefits of cross-sex hormone therapy. The provider can then properly meet his or her disclosure responsibility to their transgender patient and obtain informed consent regarding the risks of hormone therapy. Next, the provider needs to examine the eligibility and emotional readiness of patients to participate in cross-sex hormone therapy. Finally, providers need to be aware of ways they can improve their approach in treating transgender patients debating or already undergoing cross-sex hormone therapy.

Provider Knowledge

The first step in treating a patient for hormone therapy is a complete understanding by the provider of the risks and benefits of hormone therapy. The provider does not need to be an endocrinologist but needs to be well versed in the relevant medical and psychological aspects of treating persons with gender identity disorders. For a treatment that carries potentially severe physical and social risks and benefits, a provider must be able to explain these risks in a way that a patient can understand (Harry Benjamin International Gender Dysphoria Association, 2001).

Biological females undergoing treatment could expect a permanent change in vocal timbre, permanent clitoral enlargement, mild breast atrophy, increased upper body strength, weight gain, facial and body hair growth, male-pattern baldness, increased social and sexual interest and "arousability," and decreased hip fat. Biological males undergoing treatment could expect much the opposite; breast growth, redistribution of body fat to more resemble a biological female, decreased upper body strength, softening of skin, decrease in body hair, decreased fertility and testicular size, and less frequent and less firm erections.

The medical side effects in biological females treated with testosterone may include infertility, acne, shift of lipid profiles, and hepatic dysfunction. The medical side effects in biological males treated with estrogen may include increased propensity of blood clotting, infertility, weight gain, and liver disease.

There are social side effects as well that should be addressed with patients including, but not limited to, relationship changes with family and friends as well as new acquaintances. Providers should help their patients explore these social side effects and prepare the patient to appropriately deal with them.

Patient Knowledge

The next step in dealing with transgender patients is determining, along with the patient, what role hormone therapy will play in the care they receive from the provider. Because of the serious potential side effects, age of consent (at least age 18 years) must be met to begin treatment. The next requirement is a full counseling session on the risks and benefits of hormone therapy. To fully trust that the patient understands these risks and benefits, intensive psychotherapy with a trained professional should be undertaken. Only upon completion of a course of therapy followed by other indicators of readiness—such as an increased desire to begin hormone therapy after the counseling regime—should a provider consider undergoing hormone therapy (Harry Benjamin International Gender Dysphoria Association, 2001).

Provider Tools for Treating Transgender Patients

The following are ways in which a provider can promote and improve the health of transgender patients:

- Acknowledge the individual's self-identity
- Promote a nondiscriminatory policy within your practice area
- Promote further studies into transgender healthcare issues
- Promote better access to health care for transgender patients
- Promote an atmosphere that allows all people to explore gender identity

If providers continue to promote better access to care and an environment in which care can be given free of judgment, then all these recommendations will be easier to implement. Once providers as a whole begin to address the critical need for better access to population-specific care for transgender patients, the medical community and research community should begin to follow suit. When this happens providers will no longer be forced to make assumptions from research done on gender-compliant individuals, but instead will be able to look at medical research specifically designed to study and improve outcomes for transgender persons.

Case Study with Clinical Recommendations

A 27-year-old genetic man presents to your clinic wearing women's clothing. He tells you that from a very young age he has believed he was born with the wrong assigned gender.

He also reports that he is most comfortable living life as a woman and that he has done so for the past 6 months. This patient also reports that he is ready for the next step in the process of becoming a woman. He is requesting to be started on female hormones to gain more feminine physical qualities.

1. Legal name of patient _____

2. Name patient prefers to be called _____

3. Pronoun patient prefers   He   or   She

4. Biological sex of patient   Male   or   Female

5. Date of birth ___/_____/_____   Age of patient _____

6. Is the patient at least 18 years old?   Yes   No

Yes: Proceed to next question.	**No:** Explain to the patient that he/she is not eligible for hormone therapy because the legal age of consent is 18. Consider referring to counselor.

7. Has the patient undergone psychotherapy regarding gender dysphoria for more than 3 months?   Yes   No

Yes: Proceed to next question.	**No:** Recommend patient begin counseling or psychotherapy before initiating hormone therapy.

8. Does patient fully understand the medical and social risks and benefits involved in hormone therapy?   Yes   No

Yes: Proceed to next question.	**No:** Recommend that the patient live exclusively as the desired gender before the administration of hormone therapy.

9. Has the patient lived exclusively as the desired gender for at least 3 months?   Yes   No

Yes: Patient is eligible for hormone therapy. Have patient sign consent forms and proceed to hormone administration guidelines.	**No:** Instruct patient on the risks and benefits involved with the administration of hormone therapy. Have patient sign consent form and then proceed to hormone administration guidelines.

Figure 27-1   Hormone Therapy Patient Eligibility Algorithm

This scenario is one that primary care providers will most likely encounter at some point in their careers. The algorithm and guidelines presented in Figures 27-1 and 27-2, respectively, although not scientifically supported, may guide the primary care provider in offering safe, compassionate, and culturally appropriate primary care to a transgender patient desiring cross-sex hormone therapy.

---

1. Has patient signed medical consent form?   Yes   No

Yes: Proceed to dosing regime.

No: Instruct patient on the risks and benefits involved with the administration of hormone therapy. Have patient sign consent form and then proceed to guidelines.

The following regimens should be started at the lowest possible dose and titrated up until serum levels mimic the desired gender's natural level.

Male-to-Female	Female-to-Male
Estrogens	**Androgens**
Estradiol 2–4 mg/day orally *or* transdermal patches 0.025–0.1 mg two patches weekly	Testosterone enanthate 200–250 mg intramuscularly every 2 weeks
Or	*Or*
Estradiol valerate 20 mg intramuscularly every 2 weeks *or* conjugated estrogen 2.5–5 mg/day orally	Testosterone cypionate 200–250 mg intramuscularly every 2 weeks
Antiandrogen	
Spironolactone 100–200 mg/day orally	
Progestogens	
Medroxyprogesterone 5–10 mg/day orally	
Or	
Micronized progesterone 100 mg orally twice daily	

Suggested laboratory studies at baseline, 3 months, 6 months, 12 months, and yearly thereafter:

Free testosterone, Estradiol, Complete metabolic panel, Lipids, Complete blood count	Testosterone, Complete metabolic panel, Lipids, Complete blood count

Figure 27-2 Hormone Administration Guidelines

References

Bakker, A., van Kesteren, P., Gooren L., & Bezemer P. (1993). The prevalence of transsexualism in The Netherlands. *Acta Psychiatrica Scandinavica, 87,* 237–238.

Bockting, W. (1999). From construction to context: Gender through the eyes of the transgendered. *SIECUS Report, 28,* 3–7.

Bockting, W., Benner, A., Robinson, B., & Scheltema, K. (2004). Patient satisfaction with transgender health services. *Journal of Sex and Marital Therapy, 30,* 277–294.

Bockting, W., & Coleman, E. (1992). A comprehensive approach to the treatment of gender dysphoria. *Journal of Psychology and Human Sexuality, 5,* 131–155.

Buchanan, C., Eccles, J., & Becker, J. (1992). Are adolescents the victims of raging hormones: Evidence for activational effects of hormones on moods and behavior at adolescence. *Psychological Bulletin, 111,* 62–107.

Centers for Disease Control and Prevention. (1997). Trends in the prevalence and incidence of self-reported diabetes mellitus—United States. *Morbidity and Mortality Weekly Report, 46,* 1014–1018.

Clements, K., Katz, M., & Marx, R. (1999). *The transgender community health project: Descriptive results. San Francisco Department of Health.* Retrieved August 31, 2007, from http://hivinsite .ucsf.edu/InSite?page=cftg-02-02

Cushman, M. D., Kuller, L. H., Prentice. R., Rodabough, R. J., Psaty, B. M., Stafford, R. S., et al. (2004). Estrogen plus progestin and risk of venous thrombosis. *JAMA, 292,* 1573–1580.

Damewood, M., Bellantoni, J., Bachorik, P., Kimball, A., & Rock, J. (1989). Exogenous estrogen effect on lipid/lipoprotein cholesterol in transsexual males. *Journal of Endocrinological Investigation, 12,* 449–454.

Feldman, J. (2002). New onset of type 2 diabetes mellitus with feminizing hormone therapy: Case series. *International Journal of Transgenderism, 6*(2). Retrieved August 31, 2007, from http://www.symposion.com/ijt/ijtvo06no02_01.htm

Feldman, J. (2003). Transgender health. *Clinical and Health Affairs, 86,* 25–32.

Finkelstein, J., Susman, E., Chinchilli, V., Kunselman, S., D'Arcangelo, M., Schwab, J., et al. (1997). Estrogen or testosterone increases self-reported aggressive behaviors in hypogonadal adolescents. *Journal of Clinical Endocrinology and Metabolism, 82,* 2433–2438.

Gay and Lesbian Medical Association. (2001). *Healthy People 2010 companion document for lesbian, gay, bisexual and transgender (LGBT) health.* San Francisco: Gay and Lesbian Medical Association.

Gooren, L. J., Asscheman, H., & Newling, D. (1997). Prostate cancer in the male to female transsexual. *International Journal of Transgenderism.* Retrieved August 31, 2007, from http://www .symposion.com/ijt/hbigda/vancouver/gooren2.htm

Gutthann, S., Rodriguez, L., Castellsague, J., & Duque Oliart, A. (1997). Hormone replacement therapy and risk of venous thromboembolism: Population based case-control study. *British Medical Journal, 314,* 796–800.

Harry Benjamin International Gender Dysphoria Association. (2001). *The standards of care for gender identity disorders* (6th version). Retrieved August 31, 2007, from http://www.symposion.com/ijt/ soc_2001/index.htm

Meyer, W., Webb, A., Stuart, C., Finkelstein, J., Lawrence, B., & Walker, P. (1986). Physical and hormone evaluation of transsexual patients: A longitudinal study. *Archives of Sexual Behavior, 15,* 12–38.

Miksad, R., Bubley, G., Church, P., Sanda, M., Rofsky, N., Kaplan, I., et al. (2006). Prostate cancer in a transgender woman 41 years after initiation of feminization. *Journal of the American Medical Association, 296,* 2316–2317.

Schlatterer, K., Auer, D., Yassouridis, A., von Werder, K., & Stalla, G. (1998). Transexualism and osteoporosis. *Experimental and Clinical Endocrinology and Diabetes, 106,* 365–368.

Seil, D. (1996). Transsexuals: The boundaries of sexual identity and gender. In R. P. Cabaj & T. S. Stein (Eds.), *Textbook of homosexuality and mental health* (pp. 743–762). Washington, DC: American Psychiatric Press.

Slabbekoorn, D., Van Goozen, S., Gooren, L., & Cohen-Kettenis, P. (2001). Effects of cross-sex hormone treatment on emotionality in transsexuals. *International Journal of Transgenderism, 5*(3). Retrieved August 31, 2007, from http://www.symposion.com/ijt/ijtvo05no03_02.htm

Tangpricha, V., Afdhal, N. H., & Chipkin, S. R. (2001) Case report: Autoimmune hepatitis in a male-to-female transsexual treated with conjugated estrogens. *International Journal of Transgenderism, 5*(3). Retrieved August 31, 2007, from http://www.symposion.com/ijt/ijtvo05no03_03.htm

Van Goozen, S., Wiegant, V., Endert, E., Helmond, F., & Van de Poll, N. E. (1997). Psychoendocrinological assessment of the menstrual cycle: The relationship between hormones, sexuality, and mood. *Archives of Sexual Behavior, 26,* 359–382.

Van Haarst, E. P., Newling, D. W., Gooren, L. J., Asscheman, H., & Prenger, D. M. (1998). Metastatic prostatic carcinoma in a male-to-female transsexual. *British Journal of Urology, 81,* 776.

van Kesteren, P., Lips, P., Deville, W., Popp-Snijders, C., Asscheman, H., Megens, J., et al. (1996). The effects of one-year cross-sex hormonal treatment on bone metabolism and serum insulin-like growth factor-1 in transsexuals. *Journal of Clinical Endocrinology and Metabolism, 81*(6), 2227–2232.

van Kesteren, P. J., Asscheman, H., Megens, J. A., & Gooren, L. J. (1997). Mortality and morbidity in transsexual subjects treated with cross-sex hormones. *Clinical Endocrinology, 47,* 337–342.

Van Kemenade, M., Cohen-Kettenis, P. T., Cohen, L., & Gooren, G. (1989). Effects of the pure antian-drogen RU 23.903 on sexuality, aggression, and mood in male-to-female transsexuals. *Archives of Sexual Behavior, 18,* 217–228.

Xavier, J. (2000). *Transgender needs assessment survey: Final report for phase two.* Washington, DC: Gender Education and Advocacy.

Mustada'afah (Vulnerability) in Arab Muslim Women Living in the United States

Dena Hassouneh

Because this book focuses on vulnerable populations, I searched for a definition of vulnerability that I thought would encompass and articulate well the experiences of Arab Muslim women living in the United States. Unfortunately, despite an extensive review of the literature, I was unable to find a definition of vulnerability that from my insider perspective as an Arab Muslim woman living in the United States expresses the existential aspects of what it means to live from day to day feeling vulnerable. Thus this chapter provides a review of empiric knowledge related to mental health and vulnerability in Arab Muslim women, but it also attempts to convey existential aspects of this phenomenon. As such, I draw on both my personal narrative and empiric knowledge to inform the reader.

This chapter begins with a review of Arab Muslim demographics, Arab and Muslim group differences, and a discussion of anti-Arab and anti-Muslim sentiment in the West. These sections are intended to provide a context for addressing some of the phenomena that may increase vulnerability to stress-related mental illness and/or psychological distress in Arab Muslim women living in the United States. Despite the extreme paucity of knowledge available about mental health in Arab Muslim women in the United States, existing evidence suggests a number of phenomena that likely pose a threat to mental health in this population in both the pre- and post-9/11 eras, including acculturative stress, discrimination, and various forms of trauma. Data specific to Arab Muslim women living in the United States are provided when available. Much of this data comes from a pilot study conducted by Hassouneh and Kulwicki (2007) on 29 Arab Muslim women living in the United States and is preliminary in nature.

Demographic Overview

Information about Arab Muslim women in the United States is lacking for several reasons. The U.S. Census neither includes Arab-American as an ethnic category nor collects information on religious affiliation. Arab-Americans are the only individuals of non-European ancestry who are classified, along with European-Americans, as being white

367

with no qualifying ethnic category (such as the Hispanic white category). The National Institutes of Health requires that researchers use Office of Budget Management ethnic and racial categorizations. Therefore governmental sources of demographic data are extremely limited.

Recognizing that the Census Bureau's use of ancestry as a means of gathering accurate estimates of Arab-American populations in the United States is inadequate, before the 2000 U.S. Census the Arab American Institute petitioned the Office of Budget Management to include an Arab-American ethnic category on the survey (Zogby, 1993). The Office of Budget Management denied the Arab American Institute's request (U.S. Census Bureau, 1997). It is highly doubtful that this will change anytime soon. Given Arab-Americans' current reluctance to identify themselves post-9/11 and the fact that the U.S. Bureau of the Census turned all of its Arab ancestry data over to the Department of Homeland Security in 2004 (Arab American Institute, 2004), the Arab American Institute has now abandoned its efforts to include an Arab-American ethnic category. This set of circumstances has had a drastic effect on the ability to identify potential health disparities in Arab-Americans in general and Arab-American Muslims in particular. From a national perspective the health status of Arab Muslim women in the United States is unknown and virtually invisible.

Given the lack of accurate government statistics, one is forced to turn to nongovernmental sources for demographic data. According to the Arab American Institute there are approximately 3.5 million Arab-Americans living in the United States (Arab American Institute Census Information Center, 2000). However, the percentage of Arab-Americans who are men, women, Muslim, or Christian is a subject of debate. Most sources suggest that most Arab-Americans are Christian, whereas others state that increased Muslim migration has resulted in greater parity among Arab Muslim and Arab Christians residing in the United States (Arab American Institute, 2006; Camarota, 2002). Information related to the gender distribution of Arab Muslims is even harder to find. A study conducted in Illinois reported that 57% of Muslims in the state were men and 43% were women (Ba Yunus, 1997). The extent to which this reflects national figures and represents the Arab portion of the U.S. Muslim population is unknown.

Arabs and Muslims

According to two general U.S. population public opinion polls conducted randomly by the Council for American Islamic Relations (CAIR, 2006), the percentage of respondents who agreed with the statement "Almost all Muslims are Arabs" dropped from 25% in 2004 to 18% in 2006. This finding reflects an increasing awareness in the general U.S. population that although most Arabs in the world are Muslim, most Muslims in the world are not Arab. In a comprehensive study of mosques in the United States, CAIR estimated that 96% of Muslims are of non-European descent, with approximately equal numbers of Arab, South Asian, and African ancestry included in this population (Bagby, Perl, & Froehle,

2001). Although Muslims have a shared faith and common values (Hermansen, 1991), they come from many different ethnic backgrounds.

Among Arab Muslims there are numerous subcultures. For example, the countries of Belaad el Shaam, sometimes referred to as the Fertile Crescent of the Middle East, share much more in common with each other than the gulf countries whose values and customs differ in many ways. The Fertile Crescent comprises Jordan, Palestine, Syria, Iraq, and Lebanon. Among these countries, Jordan, Palestine, and Syria are most alike in terms of dialect, religious affiliations, and local customs. Yet even among these three countries numerous differences exist. These differences are rooted, to some extent, in the tribal history of the region and, to a large degree, in the region's history of European colonization that created new nations, national boundaries, and governments (Hourani, 1991; Said, 1992).

In addition to differences in dialect and customs, religious differences among Arab Muslims, primarily between Shia and Sunni, also exist, with the Sunni being most populous in the United States and worldwide. There are also different levels of acculturation, socioeconomic status, education, religious practice, and Arabic linguistic ability among Arab Muslim women living in the United States.

Anti-Arab and Anti-Muslim Sentiment in the West

Muslims have been continuously subjected to extremely hostile treatment in the United States both pre- and post-9/11. However, in the post-9/11 era public support for infringement on Arab and Muslim civil rights, widespread negative stereotyping, and hate crimes have escalated at alarming rates. Many books provide extensive and well-documented evidence of anti-Arab and anti-Muslim Western sentiment pre- and post-9/11 (Said, 1979, 1997; Said & Barsamian, 2003). See Discrimination Pre- and Post-9/11 for additional information on this topic focusing primarily on post-9/11 events.

The Crusades, as an historical event, have not been forgotten by Muslims across the world, and the specter of Christian fundamentalism under the Bush administration coupled with past and contemporary Western aggression in the region has not escaped many Arab and Muslim Americans. As I write these words I am also celebrating the Eid Al-Adha, the second of two Muslim holidays. The front page newspaper headline today is about the execution of Saddam Hussein which took place on the first day of this holiday. The Eid Al-Adha honors and commemorates the prophet Ibrahim's steadfastness of faith. According to Quranic tradition prophet Ibrahim was asked to sacrifice his son Ishmael but was given a reprieve at the last minute when God sent down a lamb to sacrifice in Ishmael's stead. It has been widely reported that the timing of Saddam's execution on Eid Al-Adha is perceived by many Muslims as a significant religious insult intentionally perpetrated by the U.S. government (Falk, 2006; Khalil, 2006; McDonough, 2006; Morris, 2006; National Public Radio, 2006; Pakistan Times, 2006; Wahab, 2006; Wasey. Regardless of whether one views Saddam's execution as a reason for celebration ness, his execution was not a pleasant addition to the holiday atmospher

Muslim families were trying to achieve for the sake of their children in a country where Eid has no meaning in the dominant culture (Useem, 2005).

I am a Palestinian Muslim woman who was born and raised in the United States, and I have a lifelong personal history of experiencing anti-Arab and anti-Muslim sentiment in both the pre- and post-9/11 eras and a sense of vulnerability. Clinicians need to recognize that this vulnerability, however manifested, large or small, is linked to many of our deepest and most lurking fears: to be taken away, to be locked up, to be invaded, to be dehumanized, to be interned. The popularity of Malkin's 2004 best-selling book, *In Defense of Internment*, along with other publications calling for internment of Muslims in the United States (Malkin, 2004; Pipes, 2004; Shabazz, 2005; Swank, 2005), perhaps provides some credence to our fears.

Acculturation and Acculturative Stress in Arab Muslim Women Living in the United States

Acculturation is a complex process of conflict and negotiation that concerns how ethnic and other cultural minorities adapt to the dominant culture and the associated changes in their beliefs, values, and behavior that result from contact with the dominant culture and its members (Farver, Narang, & Bakhtawar, 2002; Miller & Chandler, 2002). Acculturation may be more stressful for some groups than for others (Berry & Kim, 1988; Keefe & Padilla, 1987). Acculturative stress is a concept that refers to a set of stressors that have their source in the process of acculturation. It is a specific kind of stress that individuals experience over and above general life stress, often resulting in "a particular set of stress behaviors including anxiety, depression, feelings of marginality and alienation, heightened psychosomatic symptoms, and identity confusion" (C. Williams & Berry, 1991). Generally, the greater the difference between the ethnic or other minority culture and the dominant culture, the higher the level of acculturative stress and the more difficulties individuals experience in their psychological functioning (Farver et al., 2002). Studies comparing levels of acculturative stress experienced by immigrant Muslims and their offspring have found no significant differences between these groups (Haque-Khan, 1997; Hovey & King, 1996).

Some of the factors contributing to acculturative stress reported in studies of Muslims living in Western countries include retention of values that conflict with those of the dominant culture, discrimination, intergenerational values conflict, and fragmentation of traditional family social support networks (Haque-Khan, 1997; Hussain & Cochrane, 2002; Sonuga-Barke, Mistry, & Qureshi, 1998). My own experiences as a daughter of Muslim parents provides a personal example of these stressors. I was born and raised in the United States. My parents refused to allow me to date or talk to boys, attend school dances, or socialize outside of the Muslim community. This created some tension in the family during my adolescent years. At the same time I felt alienated from the dominant U.S. culture, having experienced numerous incidents of discrimination and one incident involving a violent hate crime. Our nuclear family lacked an extended family that could have defused these tensions and provided social support.

The few studies of acculturative stress in Arab Muslims living in the West suggest that Muslim populations living in the United States are less likely to assimilate and more likely to experience high rates of acculturative stress than Arab Christians. For example, a non-random survey of 39 Arab immigrants found that compared with Arab-American Christians, Arab-American Muslims faced more discrimination in U.S. society, experienced less satisfaction with life in the United States, and retained their cultural traditions at higher rates, many of which are highly intertwined with Islamic values and practices (Faragallah, Schum, & Webb, 1997). Similarly, in a study of the relationships between acculturation, acculturative stress, religiosity, and depression in 120 individuals from one or more Arab immigrant parents, Amer and Hovey (2005) found that Arab-American Christian participants were more assimilated than Muslims into U.S. society.

These differences in acculturation are not surprising given that the United States is largely a Christian society. Although Muslims and Christians share much in terms of the histories of their faiths, differences in their belief systems, customs, and practices are also significant. Arabs and Arab-Americans who are raised as a practicing Muslims cannot easily abandon or change their Islamic beliefs to ease the process of acculturation. These beliefs are central to personal identity. When living in a society that devalues and villainizes one's faith and spiritual traditions, it is logical to assume that acculturative stress and its associated vulnerability to mental illness and/or psychological distress will occur. Hassouneh and Kulwicki's pilot study provided preliminary evidence of this phenomenon. In this sample high acculturative stress was significantly correlated with depressive symptoms (Hassouneh & Kulwicki, 2007).

Stronger identification with Arab and Muslim values and traditions are likely to be associated with lower levels of acculturation and high levels of acculturative stress regardless of linguistic ability or generational status. As such, it cannot be assumed that an Arab Muslim woman who was born and raised in the United States is highly acculturated. These data have clinical implications for clinicians working in pediatric, adult, mental health, and family practices, requiring the establishment of trust over time, taking into consideration the collectivist nature of Arab and Muslim cultures, and avoidance of stereotyping of Arab or Muslim people during health encounters. Phillips (1999) found that abused American Muslim women who sought help from healthcare providers frequently faced negative stereotyping, and most were reluctant to seek help from non-Muslim mental health clinicians because they feared misunderstanding and stereotyping of their faith. This fear is real given the stereotype among many Americans that Muslims are oppressive to women. CAIR's recent public opinion poll (2006) found that approximately half of all Americans believe that Islam encourages the oppression of women. Although this represents a statistically significant increase in the number of Americans holding this view since CAIR's previous poll (2004), it is consistent with other pre-9/11 opinion polls (Council for American Islamic Relations, 2006; National Conference of

Christians and Jews, 1994). Muslim women are cognizant of this widespread view; therefore Muslim women living in the West who are victims of domestic violence are less likely to seek help out of fear of reinforcing existing negative stereotypes (Hassouneh-Phillips, 1999). The magnitude of this gender-based stereotype on the health of Arab Muslims living in the United States is unknown.

Discrimination Pre- and Post-9/11

Negative stereotypical beliefs about Muslims held by Westerners can be traced back to the Crusades (Said, 1979). In modern history the perceived inferiority of Arab and Muslims was used as a justification for colonialism's "civilizing mission." In the United States this sense of Muslims as "Other" continues and has heavily influenced U.S. foreign policy over the past 50 years. U.S. foreign policy has been and continues to be viewed by most Arab and Muslim populations as discriminatory and oppressive (Bukhari et al., 2004; Gilbert et al., 2002; Haddad, 1991).

As a group whose ancestry is primarily non-European, Muslims in the West face both ethnic and religious forms of discrimination. A 1994 survey conducted by the National Conference of Christians and Jews found that over 40% of Americans viewed Muslims as supporting terrorism and that most saw them as oppressive toward women. Other studies of African-American and Arab Muslims conducted before the tragedy of 9/11 further documented pervasive stereotyping and discrimination toward Muslims in the United States (Al-Shingiety, 1991; Byng, 1998; Haddad, 1991). To some extent these views are reflective of pervasive negative images of Arabs and Muslims that have been promoted in U.S. popular culture and news media for decades (Said, 1997; Said & Barsamian, 2003).

As previously noted, in the post-9/11 era discrimination and stereotyping against Muslims in general and Arab Muslims in the United States in particular has escalated. Nearly 75% of Muslims in the United States have reported that they or someone they know has been discriminated against, harassed, or assaulted since the tragedy (Gilbert et al., 2002). Moreover, "As a result of the post 911 backlash, in 2001, the FBI reported a 1600% increase in anti-Muslim hate crimes and an almost 500% increase in ethnic-based hate crimes against persons of Arab descent" (Zogby, 2003). Muslim women who wear hijab (hair covering) have been particularly visible targets. Ismail (2005) cited a study conducted in 2002 that estimated 13% of all reported discrimination incidents against Muslims involved a woman wearing a head scarf. This kind of targeting may create feelings of vulnerability that influence women's choices regarding wearing hijab. Many women have stopped wearing hijab in the United States because they no longer feel safe to continue this part of their religious practice.

In addition to affecting personal religious practice, this escalation in discrimination and hate crimes post-9/11 has resulted in Muslim families restricting their freedom of movement (Livengood & Stodolska, 2004) and has provided strong support for the ongoing erosion of Arab and Muslim civil rights in the United States. Indeed, a recent survey of public opinion conducted by the Media and Society Research Group at Cornell University found that nearly half of all respondents agreed that at least one form of restriction should be placed on Muslim American civil liberties, including requiring that all Muslims in the United States register their whereabouts with the federal government, close monitoring and surveillance of mosques by U.S. law enforcement agencies, profiling of citizens as potential threats based on being Muslim or having Middle Eastern heritage, and infiltration of Muslim civic and volunteer organizations by undercover law enforcement agents to keep watch on their activities and fundraising (Nisbet & Shanahan, 2004). Because it is known that experiences of racial and ethnic discrimination are detrimental to mental health (D. Williams, Neighbors, & Jackson, 2003), it is logical to suspect that this escalation of anti-Arab and anti-Muslim sentiment poses a significant threat to mental health in U.S. Muslim populations. The gendered nature of this hostility suggests a particularly strong threat to health in Arab-American Muslim women.

Findings from Hassouneh and Kulwicki's pilot study (2007) provide preliminary evidence to support the frequency, severity, and mental health consequences of discrimination against Arab Muslim women. Post-9/11, 63% of women reported experiencing increased discrimination, 67% reported experiencing more overall stress, and 43% indicated that their mental health or the mental health of one or more of their relatives had been negatively impacted by war and/or hate crimes. With regard to discrimination generally, 10% of women reported having been discriminated against in terms of being hit or handled roughly, and 10% had been threatened one or more times. Other forms of discrimination were more common: 53% had been insulted or called names, 67% had been treated rudely, 57% had been treated unfairly, and 27% had been refused service in a store or restaurant or subject to delays in service. Thirty-three percent had been discriminated against in terms of having been excluded or ignored one or more times, and 50% reported that someone in their family had been discriminated against one or more times. Seventy-seven percent of women reported experiencing emotional distress sometimes or most of the time due to incidents of discrimination, and distress caused by perceived discrimination was significantly correlated with depressive symptoms (Hassouneh & Kulwicki, 2007).

War, Torture, Political Adversity, and Violence against Women

Similar to experiences of racial and ethnic discrimination, experiences of violence and trauma have been documented as severe threats to mental health in numerous populations throughout the world (Meichenbaum, 2002). Many Arab Muslims in the United States are refugees who have fled war, torture, or political adversity, suggesting that this population may be at increased risk for psychological distress and psychiatric illness (Hikmet et al., 2002; Kinzie, Boehnlein, Riley, & Sparr, 2002; Weine et al., 2000). Studies conducted with Iraqi refugees in the United Sates and Sweden have documented higher than average rates of posttraumatic stress disorder and depression (Hikmet et al., 2002; Sondergaard, Ekblad, & Theorell, 2001; Sundquist, Bayard-Burfield, Johansson, & Johansson, 2000). Research on the health of Iraqi refugees in Sweden found that mental health in refugees was not only influenced by their own experiences of trauma, but of also by their fear and concern for loved ones back home. Moreover, better health was associated with positive political situations in their home country (Sondergaard et al., 2001). Similarly, Hassouneh and Kulwicki (2007) found significant correlations between the perceived negative mental health impact of war or military occupation on oneself or loved ones with acculturative stress and feelings of guilt and punishment. Thus ongoing war, political adversity, and other forms of violence continue to have an impact on Arab Muslim mental health after migration.

Using a trauma history questionnaire Hassouneh and Kulwicki (2007) found that the number of women reporting any trauma history was extremely high. Ninety-three percent of the sample reported experiencing some form of trauma in their lifetimes. The specific types of trauma reported included crime (23%), general disaster (87%), physical and sexual abuse (30%), and other types of trauma (27%). Although the crime-related events section of the trauma history questionnaire does not ask participants to indicate their relationship to the perpetrator, four women indicated that the crime-related events were perpetrated by husbands or other family members, most often involving actual and attempted robbery (Hassouneh & Kulwicki, 2007).

The cumulative violence experienced by Arab Muslim women as identified by Hassouneh and Kulwicki (2007) was exceedingly high. Therefore health conditions known to be associated with violence exposure, such as depression, anxiety, and posttraumatic stress disorder, may be over-represented in this population (Elliott, March 5, 2006). Information regarding the culturally bound meanings and manifestations of these conditions in Arab Muslim women living in the United States is also unknown. What is known is that Arab Muslim women living in Arab countries often manifest psychological distress somatically (Al-Issa, 2000). Therefore clinicians working with Arab Muslim women should be prepared to gather extensive trauma histories in members of this population and have a high index of suspicion when women come in for evaluation of nonspecific somatic complaints. Given the stigma associated with mental illness in Arab cultures (Al-Krenawi & Graham, 2000; Elliott, March 5, 2006), it is also important to note that primary care is the most likely place that Arab Muslim women with mood disorders will present.

Conclusion

Very little is known about mental health in Arab Muslim women living in the United States, yet existing evidence suggests that this population may be at high risk for a number of stress-related conditions. In the post-9/11 era this risk has likely increased. My own sense of vulnerability is composed of a mixture of feelings including humiliation, denigration, alienation, fear, anger, powerlessness, and fatigue. If I, a U.S. born, highly educated, upper middle class, Arab Muslim woman, am feeling this way, I wonder how deep and painful the vulnerability experienced by less privileged Arab Muslim women must be, how it is managed, and at what price. The clinician can help Arab Muslim women through a kind, respectful, and caring attitude and through acknowledging the deep and personal nature of ongoing societal assaults against oneself, family members, faith, community, and loved ones in ancestral homes. These are important first steps in understanding the vulnerability in Arab Muslim women living in the United States.

References

Al-Issa, I. (Ed.). (2000). *Al-Junun—Mental illness in the Islamic world*. Madison, WI: International Universities Press.

Al-Krenawi, A., & Graham, J. R. (2000). Culturally sensitive social work practice with Arab clients in mental health settings. *Health & Social Work, 25*(1), 9–22.

Al-Shingiety, A. (1991). The Muslim as "Other": Representation and self-image of the Muslims in America. In Y. Haddad (Ed.), *The Muslims of America* (pp. 53–64). New York: Oxford University Press.

Amer, M., & Hovey, J. (2005). Examination of the impact of acculturation, stress, and religiosity on mental health variables for second generation Arab Americans. *Ethnicity & Disease, 15*(S1), 111–112.

Arab American Institute. (2004). *Letter to census director. Re: Data sent to homeland security*. Retrieved August 31, 2007, from http://www.aaiusa.org/issues/1245/081204census_letter

Arab American Institute. (2006). *Arab Americans*. Retrieved August 31, 2007, from http://www.aaiusa.org/foundation/358/arab-americans

Arab American Institute Census Information Center. (2000). *Census Information Center*. Retrieved August 31, 2007, from http://www.aaiusa.org/foundation/34/census-information-center

Ba Yunus, I. (1997). *Muslims of Illinois, A Demographic Report*. Cortland, NY: State University of New York.

Bagby, I., Perl, P., & Froehle, B. (2001). *The mosque in America: A national portrait*. Washington DC: Council on American Islamic Relations.

Berry, J., & Kim, U. (1988). Acculturation and mental health: A review. In P. Dasen, J. Berry, & S. Satorius (Eds.), *Health and cross-cultural psychology: Towards application* (pp. 207–236). London: Sage.

Bukhari, Z., Nyang, S., Zogby, J., Bruce, J., Wittman, R., & Peck, C. (2004). *American Muslim poll 2004: Muslims in American public square*. Washington DC: Zogby International.

Byng, M. (1998). Mediating discrimination: Resisting oppression among African-American Muslim women. *Social Problems, 45*(4), 473–487.

Camarota, S. (2002). *Immigrants from the Middle East—A profile of the foreign born population from Pakistan to Morocco*. Retrieved August 31, 2007, from http://www.cis.org/articles/2002/back902.html

Council for American Islamic Relations. (2006). *American public opinion about Islam and Muslims: Detailed results*. Washington DC: Council for American Islamic Relations.

Elliott, A. (2006, March 5). A Muslim leader in Brooklyn, Reconciling 2 worlds. *The New York Times*. Retrieved August 31, 2007, from http://www.nytimes.com/2006/03/05/nyregion/05imam.html?pagewanted=6&ei=5090&en=b4ea86720c147d39&ex=1299214800&partner=rssuserland&emc=rss

Falk, R. (2006, January 2). The flawed execution of Saddam Hussein. *Waging Peace*. Retrieved August 31, 2007, from http://www.wagingpeace.org/articles/2007/01/02_falkner_saddam.htm

Faragallah, M., Schum, W., & Webb, F. (1997). Acculturation of Arab-American immigrants: An exploratory study. *Journal of Comparative Family Studies, 28*, 182–203.

Farver, J., Narang, S., & Bakhtawar, B. (2002). East meets West: Ethnic identity, acculturation, and conflict in Asian Indian families. *Journal of Family Psychology, 16*(3), 338–350.

Gilbert, D., Kim, A., Atkinson, L., Berbenich, T., Brooks, E., Cornelius, C., et al. (2002). *Muslim American poll—Accounts of anti-Muslim discrimination not exaggerated.* Clinton, NY: Hamilton College.

Haddad, Y. (1991). American foreign policy in the Middle East and its impact on the identity of Arab Muslims in the United States. In Y. Haddad (Ed.), *The Muslims of America* (pp. 217–235). New York: Oxford University Press.

Hagopian, E. (Ed.) (2004). *Civil rights in peril: The targeting of Arabs and Muslims.* Chicago: Haymarket Books.

Haque-Khan, A. (1997). Muslim women's voices: Generation, acculturation, and faith in the perceptions of mental health and psychological help. *Dissertation Abstracts—Section B: The Sciences & Engineering, 58*(5B), 2676.

Hassouneh, D., & Kulwicki, A. (2007). Mental health, discrimination, and trauma in Arab Muslim women living in the U.S.: A pilot study. *Mental Health, Religion, & Culture, 10*(3), 257–262.

Hermansen, M. (1991). Two-way acculturation: Muslim women in America between individual choice (liminality) and community affiliation (communitas). In Y. Haddad (Ed.), *The Muslims in America* (pp. 188–204). New York: Oxford University Press.

Hikmet, J., Hakim-Larson, J., Farrag, M., Kafaji, T., Duqum, I., & Jamil, L. (2002). A retrospective study of Arab American mental health clients: trauma and the Iraqi refugees. *American Journal of Orthopsychiatry, 72*(3), 355–361.

Hourani, A. (1991). *A history of the Arab peoples.* New York: Warner Books.

Hovey, J. D., & King, C. A. (1996). Acculturative stress, depression, and suicidal ideation among immigrant and second-generation Latino adolescents. *Journal of the American Academy of Child & Adolescent Psychiatry, 35*(9), 1183–1192.

Hussain, F., & Cochrane, R. (2002). Depression in South Asian women: Asian women's beliefs on causes and cures. *Mental Health, Religion, & Culture, 5*(3), 285–311.

Ismael, H. (2005, February 24). Modern prejudice: Wearing hijab makes you no less American?? *The Harvard Crimson.* Retrieved August 31, 2007, from http://www.thecrimson.com/article.aspx?ref=505951

Keefe, S., & Padilla, A. (1987). *Chicano identity.* Albuquerque: University of New Mexico Press.

Khalil, A. (2006, December 30). Timing of execution criticized. *Daily Herald.* Retrieved August 31, 2007, from http://www.heraldextra.com/content/view/205086/3/

Kinzie, J., Boehnlein, J. K., Riley, C., & Sparr, L. (2002). The effects of September 11 on traumatized refugees: Reactivation of posttraumatic stress disorder. *Journal of Nervous & Mental Disease, 190*(7), 437–441.

Livengood, J., & Stodolska, M. (2004). The effects of discrimination and constraints negotiation on leisure behavior of American Muslims and the post-September 11 America. *Journal of Leisure Research, 36*(2), 183–208.

Malkin, M. (2004). *In defense of internment—The case for 'racial profiling' in World War II and the War on Terror.* Washington DC: Regnery Publishing.

Meichenbaum, D. (Ed.). (2002). *Trauma, war, and violence—Public mental health in socio-cultural context.* New York: Springer.

Miller, A., & Chandler, P. (2002). Acculturation, resilience, and depression in midlife women from the former soviet union. *Nursing Research, 51*(1), 26–32.

McDonough, C. (2006, December 30). Arab response mixed after Saddam's execution. *Voice of America.* Retrieved August 31, 2007, from http://voanews.com/english/archive/2006-12/2006-12-30-voa19.cfm?CFID=178580949&CFTOKEN=69

Morrison, D. (2006, December 31). The execution of Saddam Hussein—Regional reaction: A martyr was made or justice was cheated. *San Francisco Chronicle*. Retrieved August 23, 2007, from http://www.sfgate.com/cgi-bin/article.cgi?f=/c/a/2006/12/31/MNG2ONAQF91.DTL

National Conference of Christians and Jews. (1994). *Taking America's pulse*. New York: National Conference of Christians and Jews.

National Public Radio, (2006, December 30). Jordanians question timing of Saddam execution. *All Things Considered*. Retrieved August 31, 2007, from http://www.npr.org/templates/story/story.php?storyId=6701098&ft=1&f=1001

Nisbet, E., & Shanahan, J. (2004). *MSRG special report: Restrictions on civil liberties, views of Islam, & Muslim Americans*. Ithaca, NY: Cornell University.

Pakistan Times. (2006, December 30). Saddam Hussein hanged to death. Retrieved August 31, 2007, from http://www.pakistantimes.net/2006/12/31/top.htm

Phillips, D. (1999). *American Muslim women's experiences of abuse: A narrative study of life, meaning, and culture*. Unpublished Dissertation, Oregon Health & Science University, Portland, Oregon.

Pipes, D. (2004). *Why the Japanese Interment still matters*. Retrieved August 31, 2007, from http://www.cnsnews.com/viewcommentary.asp?Page=\Commentary\archive\200412\COM200 41227b.html

Said, E. (1979). *Orientalism*. New York: Vintage Books.

Said, E. (1992). *The question of Palestine*. New York: Vintage.

Said, E. (1997). *Covering Islam*. New York: Vintage Books.

Said, E., & Barsamian, D. (2003). *Culture and resistance—Conversations with Edward W. Said*. Cambridge, MA: South End Press.

Shabazz, S. (2005). *Neoconservatives push internment for American Muslims*. Retrieved August 31, 2007, from http://www.finalcall.com/artman/publish/article_1818.shtml

Sondergaard, H., Ekblad, S., & Theorell, T. (2001). Self-reported life event patterns and their relation to health among recently resettled Iraqi and Kurdish refugees in Sweden. *Journal of Nervous & Mental Disease, 189*(12), 838–845.

Sonuga-Barke, E., Mistry, M., & Qureshi, S. (1998). The mental health of Muslim mothers in extended families living in Britain: The impact of intergenerational disagreement on anxiety and depression. *British Journal of Clinical Psychology, 37*, 399–408.

Sundquist, J., Bayard-Burfield, L., Johansson, L., & Johansson, S. (2000). Impact of ethnicity, violence, and acculturation on displaced migrants: Psychological distress and psychosomatic complaints among refugees in Sweden. *The Journal of Nervous and Mental Disease, 188*(6), 357–365.

Swank, J. (2005). *Internment camps for Muslims*. Retrieved August 31, 2007, from http://www.mich-news.com/cgi-bin/artman/exec/view.cgi/203/8852

U.S. Census Bureau, Office of Budget Management. (1997). *Revisions to the standards for the classification of federal data on race and ethnicity*. Retrieved August 31, 2007, from http://www.census.gov/population/www/socdemo/race/Ombdir15.html

Useem, A. (2005). Adjusting to a less festive Eid. *Religion News Service*. Retrieved August 31, 2007, from http://www.beliefnet.com/story/177/story_17782_1.html

Wahab, S. (2006, December 31). Pilgrims unhappy at Saddam execution on Eid. *Arab News*. Retrieved August 31, 2007, from http://www.arabnews.com/?page=1&section=0&article=90524&d=31&m=12&y=2006&pix=kingdom.jpg&category=Kingdom

Wasey, A. (2007, January 2). Iraqi former president Saddam Hussein executed. *MacNeil Lehrer, Public Broadcasting System*. Retrieved August 31, 2007, http://www.pbs.org/newshour/extra/features/jan-june07/saddam_1-02.html

Weine, S. M., Razzano, L., Brkic, N., Ramic, A., Miller, K., Smajkic, A., et al. (2000). Profiling the trauma related symptoms of Bosnian refugees who have not sought mental health services. *Journal of Nervous & Mental Disease, 188*(7), 416–421.

Williams, C., & Berry, J. (1991). Primary prevention of acculturative stress among refugees. *American Psychologist, 46*(6), 632–641.

Williams, D., Neighbors, H., & Jackson, J. (2003). Racial/ethnic discrimination and health: Findings from community studies. *American Journal of Public Health, 93*(2), 200–208.

Zogby, J. (1993). *Arab Americans seek reclassification as an official minority in the U.S.* . Retrieved August 31, 2007, from http://www.aaiusa.org/washington-watch/1115/w062893

Zogby, J. (2003). *America after 9/11: Freedom preserved or lost? Report to the United States Committee of the Judiciary.* Washington DC: Arab American Institute.

Sample Care Plan for Culturally Competent Care of an Arab Muslim Woman

Carol Vineyard

This short chapter provides a model of one way to concisely present key elements of a care plan and follows the previous chapter by Dr. Hassouneh, who eloquently presented a highly personal description of her perspective as an Arab Muslim woman speaking to her contemporary experience in American society. This care plan serves to operationalize the concepts into a format that nurses and students might use to intervene with an Arab Muslim woman. Not meant to be comprehensive, this chapter serves as a starting point for discussion of many variables nurses might consider when caring for Muslims. I am a senior nursing student speaking as the nurse in this scenario. My purpose is to develop a culturally competent care plan to use as a guide when caring for Ghayda, a hypothetical Arab Muslim woman. The case study instructions were as follows:

> Assume you have passed the NCLEX and are working as a staff nurse during the evening shift on a medical unit of a general hospital. The nurse giving report for the day shift informs your team that a new patient has been admitted and you are assigned to complete the intake assessment. All that is known from the emergency room report is the following: 25-year-old Arab woman named Ghayda . . . admitted with abdominal pain of unknown origin, patient is awake, coherent and appears to speak English; complains of severe "stomach" pain and nausea. She is a graduate student, here in the United States from her home country of Lebanon on a student visa to study art at a local university. She was brought to the emergency department by her aunt and older brother with whom she lives. The emergency department documents indicate that she is Muslim, and you notice the aunt wears a long dress and veil. As she finishes the report, the day nurse comments, "This girl's problem is her brother who is overprotective and won't let the doctor (male physician) examine her." When you enter the room, Ghayda is lying on her side with knees tucked up and the sheet over her. Develop a culturally competent care plan for Ghayda. Limit to one side of one page.

TABLE 29-2 Nursing Care Plan for Ghayda

Assessment	Plan	Interventions	Evaluation
Assess language fluency in English (unfamiliar with medical terms)	Identify resources for Ghayda to communicate (plan to call an interpreter)	Use an interpreter when working with Ghayda	Was the message delivered affectively? Yes
			Did Ghayda understand? Yes
Assess pain level on a scale of 1–10 (reports pain 8/10)	Identify culturally sensitive pain management methods	Ghayda stated she wanted pain medications	Reassess pain level 30 min after medications were given (3/10)
Assess nausea (yes)	Plan to call doctor to have pain medications and nausea relief ordered	Give her the medications to decrease her pain and nausea	Reassess nausea: stated she did not feel nauseated
Head to toe assessment	Identify any problems by system	Run tests to see if she has any abdominal bleeding	Is there (still) blood in her stool? No
			Is her abdomen (still) distended? No
Assess cultural beliefs, and practices (she feels uncomfortable remaining uncovered during an examination and being examined/cared for by male staff members)	Identify culturally sensitive methods to use when doing an examination	Keep her covered and only uncover what needs to be uncovered for the examination.	Is Ghayda more comfortable with the care that is being provided? Yes
	Plan to allow her aunt to remain with her during physical and also have a time that her aunt is not in the room for questions regarding issues that she might not want her family to know	Work to have a female-only staff examine and care for her	Are the necessary tests and examinations being done? Yes
		Explain all procedures before doing them to try to prevent anxiety	
		Allow her aunt to remain with her during physical	
		Have time to question her without family present	

Assessment	Plan	Interventions	Evaluation
Assess Ghayda's religious needs (assume she is a practicing Muslim)	Identify resources	Provide religious materials Plan her care around her prayer time Contact the Imam Provide resources for religious counseling after discharge	Are her spiritual needs being met? Yes Has she requested more spiritual counseling? Yes
Assess Ghayda's family relationship and support system (she is very close to her family and would like her aunt and brother to remain with her)	Plan to let her aunt and brother remain with her during her stay (plan to provide them with chairs and cots)	Provide chairs and cots for her aunt and brother	Are her aunt and brother comfortable and able to remain with her? Yes
Assess economic status and if she has health care insurance	Identify resources to help cover the cost of the hospital stay (limited health insurance from her school) Connect with social services	Social worker will help Ghayda with finding resources to help cover the cost of her health care Provide the number and location of the school clinic for follow-up care after discharge	Is her school healthcare insurance able to cover the cost of her health care, or is a plan in place to help Ghayda cover the cost? Yes, the social worker is currently working with her to find resources to help her cover the cost
Assess the cultural biases with the staff nurses	Develop methods for working with other cultures Plan to meet with the staff nurses	Have the staff nurses identify their biases Discuss culturally sensitive care, and the rational behind it Have scenarios to have the nurses role play	Did the nurses believe they learned something related to providing culturally sensitive care? Yes After the meeting is there an increase in respect for those from other cultures? Yes

Incorporate in the care plan your response to the ideas expressed by the nurse giving the shift report (i.e., incorporate an intervention with the nurse as part of the plan for Ghayda). Do not incorporate literature citations into your care plan, but it is encouraged that you do background reading.

This care plan can be used as an outline for caring for any client who has a different cultural background from the nurse's. Based on the nursing process, the chart is organized on one page to enable staff to see the patient's needs at a glance. Agencies vary in their requirements, and this plan is not meant to be universal. However, the key elements of language fluency, cultural beliefs, and practices should be considered when providing culturally competent care to any patient and family (Table 29-1).

Language Fluency in English

This allows the nurse to provide interpreter services and other resources for Ghayda to ensure that messages are delivered effectively. Just because a client is fluent in English does not mean that he or she knows medical terminology. Be prepared to use interpreter services when working with Ghayda. Services can be canceled if necessary, but even people who are fluent in conversational English might be distracted when in pain. To evaluate if this intervention was successful, ask the following questions: Was the message delivered affectively and did Ghayda indicate that she understood the message?

Pain and Nausea

This allows you to identify culturally sensitive pain management methods, because not all clients want medications to manage their pain. Plan to call the doctor to order pain medications and nausea relief so that it is ready if Ghayda requests the medications. Because Ghayda stated she wanted the pain medications, administer them to help decrease her pain and nausea. Work with Ghayda to establish what she defines as adequate pain relief, for example, she might define adequate relief as 3 out of 10 on the 1–10 scale. Reassess in 30 minutes after medications were administered to see if her pain level is within the preestablished limits as adequate relief and if her nausea is relieved.

Head to Toe Assessment

This is a standard assessment for all patients to identify any problems by system and is performed as traditional physical assessment and through laboratory tests. The important thing to remember is to focus the assessment on the abdomen without neglecting to check all systems. One of the important things to check for is abdominal bleeding. Evaluation is by checking to see if there is still blood in her stool and/or if her abdomen is still distended if she had abdominal bleeding.

Cultural Beliefs and Practices

The purpose of this section is to identify culturally sensitive methods to use when doing the physical examination. Ghayda feels uncomfortable with remaining uncovered during a physical examination and being examined and cared for by male staff members. It would not be culturally appropriate for her brother to be present, and Ghayda could be asked if she wants her aunt to be present. However, it is important for the nurse to have private time with Ghayda to assess for factors she might not want her family to know (e.g., abuse or pregnancy). During any physical examination only uncover what is necessary for the examination and assign only female staff to care for her. Reduce anxiety by explaining all procedures. To evaluate, ask the following questions: Is she more comfortable with the care that is being provided and are the necessary tests being done?

Ghayda's Religious Needs

Confirm whether she is a practicing Muslim to provide religious resources for her. Ask if she would like you to contact the Imam to provide her with spiritual guidance. Evaluation is based on whether she identifies that her spiritual needs are being met.

Ghayda's Family Support System

Ghayda stated she was very close to her family and would like her aunt and brother to remain with her as much as possible during the hospital stay. Plan to provide chairs and cots for them to stay with Ghayda during her stay. Evaluation is whether Ghayda and her aunt and brother indicate they are comfortable during their stay.

Economic Status and Health Insurance

Identify resources to help cover her bills and connect her with social services. The social worker can connect her to resources to cover her hospital bills. Provide Ghayda with the number and location of the school clinic so she can follow up after her discharge. Evaluate by checking to ensure that the social worker is working with Ghayda to find means to cover her bills.

Ethnocentric Biases of the Staff

In this scenario there is evidence that at least one of the nurses may have need for cultural education. Although it was not made clear in the case study whether the problem lies with one nurse or many, it would be useful to provide staff with information about Arab Muslim families to develop nonjudgmental methods of care for patients from other cultures. During the meeting have simulation game exercises and open discussion for the nurses to identify some of the cultural biases they might have and identify ways to work around those to provide culturally sensitive care to their clients. Evaluate by asking the following questions: Did the nurses believe they learned something related to cultural sensitive care and is there an increase in respect for those from other cultures? These outcomes can be measured by simple paper and pencil tests or through focus groups in which staff have a chance to react to the training.

Conclusion

Although this care plan is designed to follow an abbreviated outline, much more could be said about meeting the cultural needs of Arab Muslim women. Readers are encouraged to review the references from Chapter 28 for more detailed information.

Unit Five

Community is a place where therapy and politics meet, for here the health of the individual and the health of the group may be seen for the reciprocal realities that they are.

■ ■ ■

Parker J. Palmer

PROGRAMS

Program Development
for Vulnerable Populations

Mary de Chesnay and Anne Watson Bongiorno

In this book the point is made that vulnerability can be conceptualized both as an individual attribute and a population characteristic. In this unit the focus is on populations, and we provide several examples of how nurses can structure programs to serve large numbers of people. To maximize effectiveness, community health service delivery programs should serve populations by implementing the best practices related to the health issue that is the focus of the program and by doing so in a cost-efficient way. The purpose of this introductory chapter is to provide ideas to consider when designing such programs to maximize their impact with scarce resources.

Focus of the Program

Problem Statement

The problem statement captures the focus of the program and is a clear statement about the purpose of the program, significance of the health issue, and the population served by the program.

Values

The values section is simply a list of the core values held by the designers of the program. For example, for those who work with vulnerable populations, a key value might be social justice and the values section might include the following statements:

- For a program to reduce violence against children: *Every child has the right to live free of abuse.*

- For a public education campaign to prevent HIV/AIDS: *The public has a right to know the risks of sharing needles.*

Mission

The mission statement is an opportunity for the program designers to clearly say what they plan to do and why they believe it is important. An example of a mission statement for a mobile free clinic designed to provide primary care is as follows: *The North Country Mobile Health clinic provides access to affordable primary care for indigent rural residents of the tri-county area.*

Design Process

Recruiting the Team

A useful place to start designing a program is to obtain help from like-minded people who share a concern about the issue and population. It is very important to partner with the people who will be affected by the program. Those who are part of the problem must be part of the solution if program success is to be realized (Ervin, 2002). As part of the community health program in a northern university, nursing faculty identified a need for a nursing presence in congregate, low-income, senior housing. The facilities lacked any onsite wellness resources for its residents, and public transportation to the few outside resources available was limited. Program planning commenced with recruitment of senior residents, staff, local providers, social services, and other stakeholders in local senior health to find out what was of concern or of importance to this aggregate.

The providers in the group identified goals that included improved functioning and quality of life and self-management of health. They recommended exercise, proper nutrition, and foot care activities and programs. Interestingly, the senior residents identified with the goals but believed the main thrust of activities to achieve these goals should focus on objective of decreasing loneliness and increasing socialization. Clearly, a well-rounded group of like-minded individuals should always include representation from the group who will be the recipients of the program.

Feasibility Study

The program must be realistic and cost-effective and have the potential to achieve its goals. The feasibility study defines skills and resources needed to implement the program and offers alternative solutions. It asks, how viable is this program? Need and service are examined for practicality and usefulness. The feasibility study highlights strengths and weaknesses of the proposal and capacity to deliver the program (Stanhope, 2000).

In one rural elementary school the nurse identified that few of the students who failed annual vision screenings subsequently saw an optometrist for follow-up and correction. A student public health nursing project was developed in collaboration with the university, local health department, and area optometrists to examine potential solutions. Although theory and evidence supported the need for a program to provide access to optometry services, the initial solution of providing free transportation, free vision screening at the optometrist, and free glasses was impractical in relationship to the capacity of the community to deliver the program. Alternate solutions are currently being explored. This example highlights the importance of considering how to prioritize scarce resources into programs that are sustainable over time.

Identifying Stakeholders

Programs targeting vulnerable populations implicitly seek to reduce health disparities. The program planner needs to learn how who the stakeholders are and how to identify them. Stakeholders are representative of community engagement in the project. They are those members of the community who function as the power brokers of the program. Stakeholders are often nonprofit organizations or political entities that can help establish and sustain the program or individuals who will be affected by the program or are the target of the program (Issel, 2004).

Stakeholders traditionally are quite invested in the program and should reflect diversity. For example, when one of the authors (Bongiorno) was involved in organizing a statewide coalition for lung health, she looked for a wide variety of representation that would create a powerful basis for action. This included representatives of service organizations, widely respected research scientists in the state, government officials such as the Attorney General, elected local and state level officials, and people with diagnoses of lung illness. She sought to develop a board that was representative of the ethnicity, gender, and geographic location of those with lung disease and those interested in prevention. She recruited a cross-section of heath care providers and human service agency personal who were involved in primary, secondary, and tertiary prevention of the disease and asked media representatives and banking officials to sit on the coalition.

The goal of this stakeholder representation was to create a broad base of scientific expertise and basis for action, human service potential, political will, economic acumen, and media attention to the issue of lung health. Change can only happen when large numbers of people are affected. Programs built with a broad stakeholder base clarify the values and sociopolitical and economic factors as well as the scientific merit of interventions that can make or break a program. A cohesive stakeholder group develops synergy through the influence of its members.

Gatekeepers

Closely related to stakeholders are gatekeepers, people who have power and authority, usually by way of their positions within the setting. They can use this authority to facilitate a project they support or to create barriers to programs they do not support. It does not matter whether the program is a service program or a study. Gatekeepers need to be identified early in the process and persuaded to support the plan of action.

A positive example of gatekeepers was described in the first edition of this book, when the first author and colleagues (Colvin, de Chesnay, Mercado, & Benavides, 2005) designed a research project in a barrio of Managua, Nicaragua. Early in the process of beginning a study on mothers' access to health care in the barrio, the research team met with a key community leader. The woman who was the lead *brigadista* (community health worker) welcomed the team into her home where we described the study and planned how to approach the community. She gave the researchers many helpful tips on the interview instrument, women to invite first, timing, and how to offer culturally appropriate incentives to participate in the study.

In contrast, a negative gatekeeper can effectively halt a program. A doctoral student planned a study in which she would access a rural African-American sample through a local church. She obtained the permission of the pastor, who was enthusiastic in supporting her. However, when she arrived for data collection the deacon told her that he had not given his permission to collect data through the church and he would not allow her to enter. Inability to resolve the power struggle between the pastor and deacon cost the student months of work in that she needed to revise her entire methodology.

Capturing Data

Informal talks and formal interviews yield important data about a particular need in a community and often are the catalyst for action. For example, a tricounty tobacco prevention coalition had a goal to decrease tobacco use in a rural northern state. Part of their strategic work plan was to provide media outlets with brochures about tobacco prevention, such as harm reduction, secondhand smoke, and information about joining the advocacy efforts of the coalition. In an informal discussion the director mentioned that many brochures did not seem to be "moving off the shelves." As consultant to the organization, Bongiorno quickly scheduled a formal interview with the director to discuss a systematic approach to health communication in the organization. The director acknowledged that although the use of the materials fit the organizational goal, the current materials had not been formatively tested. Because the key to effective health communication is to understand your audience, we developed a plan to test the usefulness of current products and develop ideas for greater appeal of print materials.

Surveys and focus groups provide rich data about a population problem from the emic point of view. We determined that with the new tobacco prevention communication brochures we needed to be clear about who we wanted to reach, analyze what we were asking the audience to do, and determine what exchange of benefit for service was being asked of the audience. We also needed to know what was and was not appealing in print media to our target groups. My nursing students used this opportunity to develop a qualitative service learning project. We collaboratively designed a focus group guide and script, recruited participants, and facilitated focus group discussions. In addition, the students developed a written survey and conducted anonymous curbside surveys.

Participant observation is a tool often used by anthropologists and is an important data-gathering technique in vulnerable populations because the data are nonlinear and contextual and provide salient information about a problem that cannot be gleaned from quantitative methods. For example, in a student service learning project about substance prevention, college students smoking behavior was observed by college nursing majors. The nursing students mingled with others outside building entrances that were posted with and without signs prohibiting smoking and with and without ashtrays. They counted how many people in a given period of time were seen smoking, where they smoked, and how they discarded cigarettes. Throughout the semester students also gained information about perceptions of smoking on campus as they participated in various groups. In another project, nursing students involved in sororities and fraternities examined the drinking behavior of college students within the Greek community as participant observers. Nurses have often used participant observation to understand our own practice. Care must be taken to set aside bias and to protect the rights of participants as you record discrete events and observe interactions (Roper & Shapira, 2000).

Good programs directed toward vulnerable populations are built on a foundation of evidence that creates a compelling story of need, gap in service, and the ability to develop an effective strategy to improve the health of the population. Hence, program planners must also create a scientific foundation for their proposal. The epidemiology of the health issue should be clearly and succinctly communicated. Cultural congruence of program interventions needs to be addressed when gathering data as should the biocultural diversity of the program recipients.

A Business Plan

What Is It and Why Is It Important, Especially in Seeking Funding

Grant writers know that funding is only awarded for ideas that are feasible and sustainable. Funding agencies want to know that the grantee is functioning within the limits of his or her ability and experience. A business plan provides funding agencies with valuable information. A business plan is a vital tool in your grant proposal to identify and prioritize the resources needed to implement the program. The plan highlights strengths and weaknesses of the proposal. Business plans project what is ahead and how you plan to allocate resources to meet the current and future needs of your program. At a minimum the plan should define the mission and goals of the program and outline how you plan to conduct business to match the purpose of the program. Traditionally, the business plan describes the program, product, and purpose and discusses the market for the program now and in the future. A solid business plan shares specific market analyses and implementation strategies. The plan also provides a detailed financial analysis, management plan, and a personnel plan with dates and budget.

Business plans range from simple to complex, depending on the scope of your program and request for funding. For example, one school of nursing wanted students to learn first hand the role of advocacy for vulnerable populations. We developed a simple business plan for the program. The mission of the program was to increase nursing students' awareness of advocacy as a nursing mandate for vulnerable populations. Two objectives of the program were to increase knowledge of lobbying practices and to apply knowledge of the legislative process to a vulnerable population. Our market analysis indicated an extreme knowledge deficit of the role of population-based advocacy with students. We outlined a specific strategy and implementation plan to meet the mission of the program.

Students spent a semester investigating a vulnerable population, learning the legislative process, and preparing for a visit to the state capital and their legislator to share their concerns. The management team included faculty and administrators. The financial plan included a detailed budget of costs to the university and student and a projected cash flow from grants and other sources of funds.

Costs and Budget

Anticipating costs is an important part of any business plan. In the financial plan one would identify how to finance the project, accountability and communication regarding costs, and current and projected revenues, surplus, and deficits. It is critical to the success of any budget to project out the cash flow and create a balance sheet. Expenses, personnel costs, indirect costs, and factors such as inflation or market adjustments need to be factored into more complex program plans. Your budget must realistically match the amount of funds a grant agency is willing to award. Your vision of the program and your budget must be realistically aligned for a funding agency to consider your proposal. Matching ideas to funding is a critically important element in grantsmanship.

Sources of Funding

People who believe strongly in the programs they develop can be quite creative at seeking funding. *Grants and contracts* serve as an excellent way to seek funding, though writing and submitting the grant can sometimes take several months. Libraries have grants directories that provide focus of the sponsoring organization, contact information, guidelines for the grant, and much other useful information.

Public campaigns (United Way is one of the best) can generate large amounts of money targeted to the program of interest. Sometimes it is possible to designate a program as a new United Way agency. If not, creating a similar public campaign is not difficult if the team recruits the support of the local media. Walk-a-Thons are a popular way of raising funds. *Grass-roots fund-raising* should not be overlooked if relatively small amounts of funds are needed. Students often use bake sales and car washes to raise funds for airplane tickets to developing countries where they combine learning community health nursing with service. *Formal dinners* with highly visible speakers combined with *raffles* can earn thousands of dollars if the right community leaders are invited. For example, John Walsh (*America's Most Wanted* television program) agreed to be the featured guest at a fundraiser for Prescott House.

Evaluation

Evaluation of programs can be accomplished through traditional research methods. Quantitative measures include tools designed for stakeholder demographic data and satisfaction of participants, such as surveys and questionnaires. Qualitative measures might include interviews and focus groups.

Examples

Tobacco Cessation Program

Clinton County Public Health Department serves high-risk medically indigent pregnant women in a specialized home visiting program (i.e., Maternal Obstetric Medicaid Services [MOMS], operated under the New York State Department of Health guidelines). One aspect of this program is to encourage tobacco cessation. One of the multiple problems facing these women is adverse pregnancy outcomes related to maternal tobacco consumption. Women who smoke during pregnancy have an increased likelihood to deliver low-birth-weight babies. It is extremely difficult to achieve good quit rates with these women, but reduction of tobacco use is more successful. Kallen (2001) linked improved Apgar scores and higher birth weights with reduced tobacco use in pregnancy. The mission of the MOMs program is to promote full-term delivery of infants weighing at least 2,500 grams. Students in the local baccalaureate program were assigned to evaluate the existing rather loosely defined program and develop recommendations for a new program plan. The goal of the program was to improve efforts toward smoking cessation as measured by infant birth weights exceeding 2,500 grams. Students and faculty developed a feasibility report to examine the practicality of completing a program that reviewed the MOMs interventions. This involved an analysis of resources, constraints, and financial issues.

It was determined that this would be a year-long project implemented by sequential cohorts of preselected senior-level clinical students. Stakeholders were identified: pregnant women currently in the MOMs program, graduates of the MOMs program, Clinton County Public Health Department, SUNY Plattsburgh nursing students and faculty, and other area agencies. Interviews were conducted with stakeholders. A survey was developed to collect demographic data, including body mass index scores, Apgar scores of infants, smoking habits, exposure to secondhand smoke, quit attempts, and harm reduction attempts. One hundred fifty charts were randomly reviewed. Outcomes showed that the MOMs program has been effective in decreasing number of cigarettes smoked.

There was little success with quit attempts and reduction in secondhand smoke. Birth weights of infants born to smokers who self-reported decreased use of cigarettes were above 2,500 grams as compared with birth weights of infants born to smokers who did not decrease their smoking. One major problem found during the survey was that the procedure for counseling women was not well documented in the permanent records. The results of the first phase of the program led to the formulation of new policies and forms for documentation and new ideas to increase harm reduction efforts. Information from this year-long project was incorporated into grant proposals for future MOMs funding.

Prescott House

In the mid-1980s the first author was involved in working with the district attorney to set up a children's advocacy center in Jefferson County, Alabama (de Chesnay & Petro, 1989). The focus was to reduce further victimization of child sex abuse survivors through the criminal justice system and to improve prosecution rates of offenders. The team had been concerned about the extreme emotional distress experienced by children and their nonoffending family members as prosecution of the offenders proceeded through the slow-moving justice system. Grant funds became available for a project to model a center after one that had been started by the district attorney in Huntsville, Alabama.

To assess the need for such a program in Jefferson County, the team conducted interviews with a variety of stakeholders and discovered that the most powerful finding was that children were required to tell their stories over and over to many professionals in intimidating circumstances such as police stations and courthouses with big adult furniture. The short-term goal was to require all individuals who needed to interview children to find a quiet private place and the long-term goal was to create a new space with age-appropriate furniture and anatomically correct dolls.

On a short-term basis the team designated a quiet space in the police station with smaller furniture for children. Dolls and coloring materials were brought to the room to enhance the interviews. All interviewers came to the child. However, this plan was limited in that the child still needed to tell the story many times. With each subsequent telling of the story, many children become confused or numb and the story sounds false.

The long-term solution was to acquire a building that would be dedicated to interviewing the children. Funds were raised through private donations, and the house was named Prescott House in honor of the local citizen who donated the building. The house is located away from the courthouse in a residential neighborhood. The former residential space was renovated to accommodate a large conference room upstairs with age-appropriate interview rooms for young children and adolescents. The arrangement of rooms with closed-circuit television enables the child to be in the interview room with one interviewer who wears an earpiece. All other professionals are required to watch from the conference room and feed their questions to the interviewer.

Conclusion

The preceding discussion is meant to provide readers with some basic ideas about program development. Nurses are in a unique position to provide such programs, and the following chapters offer examples of the fine work they do.

References

Colvin, S. P., de Chesnay, M., Mercado, T., & Benavides, C. (2005). Child health in a barrio of Managua. In M. de Chesnay (Ed.), *Caring for the vulnerable: Perspectives in nursing theory, practice, and research* (pp. 161–170). Sudbury, MA: Jones and Bartlett.

de Chesnay, M., & Petro, L. (1989). The accountability of incest offenders. *Medicine and Law, 8,* 281–286.

Ervin, N. (2002). *Advanced community health nursing practice.* Upper Saddle River, NJ: Prentice Hall.

Issel, L. M. (2004). *Health program planning and evaluation: A practical, systematic approach for community health.* Sudbury, MA: Jones and Bartlett.

Kallen, K. (2001). The impact of maternal smoking during pregnancy on delivery outcome. *European Journal of Public Health, 11*(3), 329–333.

Roper, J., & Shapira, J. (2000). *Ethnography in Nursing Research.* Thousand Oaks, CA: Sage.

Stanhope, M. (2000). Program management. In M. Stanhope & J. Lancaster (Eds.), *Community public health* (3rd ed., pp. 416–437). St. Louis: Mosby.

Overcoming Vulnerability: An Evidence-Based Practice Model for Nicaraguan Men

Carl A. Ross

Men as a Vulnerable Population

There is an increasing need to know more about men's health issues. The way men interface with the healthcare system is due to multidimensional factors, such as the way a man may be socialized into the masculine values, beliefs, attitudes, and roles. Many of these factors are culturally rooted. This chapter covers a holistic/transcultural approach to developing a men's health clinic in Managua, Nicaragua.

Men in Nicaragua have a 5-year shorter life expectancy than women and have higher death rates for all the leading causes of death identified by the Pan American Health Organization (1998). According to the Pan American Health Organization (1998) and the Ministerio de Salud (MINSA, 2005), the overall mortality rate estimated for Nicaraguans in 1990 was 10%, which is higher than the Latin American average of 7%. Men are less likely than women to participate in health promotion activities provided by the local clinic. Nicaraguan men appear to be a vulnerable subculture. Nicaraguan men have limited access and limited resources to health care. Healthcare professionals must establish a public health program that focuses on primary prevention for Nicaraguan men. Currently, the model of health care for Nicaragua men falls under the traditional medical model of diagnosing and treating (MINSA, 2005).

The information shared in this chapter can be further used as a model for viewing men as a vulnerable population. Health professionals often treat men and women differently: They tend to perceive men as being less ill, and they tend to perceive women as exaggerating their illness.

The Evidence: Theory of Endurance

As the result of an ethnography conducted in rural Nicaragua a theory of endurance of rural Nicaraguan men emerged, leading to the development of an evidence-based men's health clinic. The men's health clinic has been in operation now for 7 years and has shown a number of positive outcomes related to the health of men in a barrio called Villa Libertad Annex (community) located in Managua, Nicaragua (Ross, 2000).

Ethnography is both the process and product of a formal and systematic qualitative inquiry into the culture and social organization of groups. The purpose of this ethnography was to uncover and explore the cultural meaning of health and well-being among rural Nicaraguan men. The focus was on discovering the emic definition of health, variables that impact the meaning of health, and self-care behaviors used by rural Nicaraguan men to stay healthy.

Informants were Nicaraguan men who lived in a small community in Nicaragua. Both general and key informants participated in the study. Key informants were selected based on their special position of trust, knowledge, and respect within the community. A main role of key informants is to use their own influence to facilitate trust between the local people and the investigator in the community (Ross, 2000).

According to Ross (2000), a theory of endurance emerged from the analysis of this study. It was identified that these Nicaraguan men live in a world of endurance due to the social structure they live under. The main themes that emerged from the data and compose the model are as follows:

1. Health is the ability to function and meet the responsibilities for self, family, and community.

2. Health is believing that you will be cared for by God.

3. Health is composed of five dimensions: spiritual, physical, mental, family, and community.

4. Health is withstanding the hardships of poverty, access to health care, and inadequate healthcare supplies.

5. Economic, environmental, work, and worldview factors guide rural Nicaraguan men's healthcare practices.

The five themes are complex and interrelated. These themes impact the way men define health and well-being and the manner in which they maintain and restore health and well-being.

A cultural example illustrating the use of the model became evident during the fieldwork phase of the study. Nicaraguan men frequently reported they would go to a clinic as a result of experiencing pain and burning on urination and pain located in the flank area lasting approximately 2 weeks. Men would not travel to the clinic immediately because to do so would take them away from their work. When they arrived at the clinic they encountered one of two situations: either the clinic was closed or the antibiotics were not available to treat what was most likely a urinary tract infection. If the physician was at the clinic, the doctor would write them a prescription for the antibiotic, but the men would then need to purchase the antibiotic. Because of poverty, these men did not have the money to purchase the antibiotics. As a result they would return home to suffer further from the symptoms of a urinary tract infection, pray to God for healing and for strength to endure, and use natural medications such as *Llanten* and *Bejuco de Sangre*. *Llanten* is taken to alleviate acidic urine and *Bejuco de Sangre* for alleviating kidney pain.

One can also see how poverty and culture can impact the health and well-being of these men. Nicaraguan men have a strong spiritual dimension of health that gives them faith that God will provide the strength to endure the discomfort to continue to work. These men thank God for the natural medicines He has provided them. A strong cultural value of family is seen when one is ill; the nuclear as well as the extended family and community assist and provide for each other during a time of need. A man's mental health is maintained through knowing that the family and community will assist him until he can return to work (Ross, 2002).

Even though the theory of endurance and model was developed for Nicaraguan men, the concepts of the model may be transferred to a variety of settings involving health care of men, even in the United States. Nurses and especially advanced practice nurses are leaders in primary care and for this reason may help with identifying needs and interventions of this vulnerable population.

The Setting: Villa Libertad Annex, Managua, Nicaragua

This study was conducted in the homes and clinic of the men who live in Villa Libertad Annex, a small barrio that the Universidad Politecnica de Nicaragua (UPOLI) has adopted as a community site for their nursing students. Approximately 2,500 people populate the area. The average family size is about eight members. Thus it can be projected that there are about 300 family units in the district. From local statistics, about half of the population is below age 18 (Cifras Oficiales Censos Nacionales, 2005).

Villa Libertad Annex is typical of the western half of Nicaragua with a population largely of people of mixed Spanish and Indian descent. The main industry is agriculture. This area produces mainly vegetables as cash crops. The residents of Villa Libertad Annex are poor, with an average income of US $1–2/day to equal $300–600 annually (Cifras Oficiales Censos Nacionales, 2005). Most families live below the poverty level, and a few live in extreme poverty (Cifras Oficiales Censos Nacionales, 2005).

Housing is crude and consists of basic plank on frame structures. Roofs are mainly wood and tin sheets. Dirt floors are the norm. Furniture is basic and minimal. Cooking is done in iron pots on primitive clay wood-burning hearths with a simple clay dome as a bread oven alongside the main hearth. There are no chimneys, and smoke is directly vented into the rooms. The kitchen is usually located in the corner of the main family room. This room serves in most cases as the sleeping area, particularly for the children. Hammocks are pulled to the ceiling during the day and lowered at night as the family's beds. Animals are encouraged to stay outside; however, animals ranging from dogs and cats to pigs and chickens run freely through the house, leading to many disease processes. Despite these conditions, the people are very proud and the dwellings are kept as clean as possible.

Water access continues to be a problem in this community. Residents must travel a mile or two to obtain buckets of water for the day's use. Water tends to remain outside the homes in plastic containers, leading to water sources that are invariably contaminated as animals are allowed free access. This problem is further compounded by the generally poor disposal of human waste. Some families have constructed pit latrines, but many have not. Human feces are also used for fertilizer. The problems of water supply and poor sanitation are the most important factors in causing disease.

The nutrition in Villa Libertad Annex is similar to other parts of the country. The staple diet is rice and beans. The blend of nutrition for this community is varied, but the author's initial cursory opinion is that it is suboptimal in general. Some families have a chicken or two that is raised for special dinners such as holidays or birthdays.

According to MINSA (2005) the most important health problems of this barrio mirror those of Nicaragua. Common health problems are cardiovascular, intestinal, and respiratory diseases as well as subtle malnutrition. If problems of childbirth and sexually transmitted diseases are included, then 80% of health issues faced in the region could be accounted for. Other problems include bacterial infections of the skin due to poor cleanliness, accidental injuries, and burns. Hypertension and diabetes exist and need to be dealt with, but these become secondary issues. Dental health and eye problems are poor and need to be addressed (MINSA, 2005).

The Men's Health Clinic

The men's health clinic is housed in the Centro Académico de Enfermería (Academic Nursing Center), a nurse-managed health center run by the faculty of UPOLI School of Nursing. The center was built by UPOLI with monetary assistance from many U.S. and Canadian partners (Universidad Politecnica de Nicaragua: Escuela de Enfermeria, 2007).

The center is situated in the middle of the community with easy access to all residences. The center is open at least 3 days a week if not more depending on the UPOLI schedule. The clinic is well constructed with concrete walls and a tin sheet roof on steel rafters. It consists of four main areas: a central receiving room and three consultation and examination rooms. There is a small area that is used for laboratory specimen analysis and medications, and it houses a rudimentary library system. The faculty of UPOLI School of Nursing are hard working and intelligent and are dedicated healthcare professionals. They rapidly identify community health problems and conduct health education programs addressing these health problems. The faculty work along with their students in providing the services at the center. Visiting nurses, doctors, and dentists from a variety of countries often come to the center to provide additional help with the health care of these individuals.

The author frequently visits the men's health clinic approximately three times a year to work with the men of the barrio. The framework for the men's health clinic is based on the theory of endurance, which emerged from a research project conducted by the author. During each trip to the clinic the author provides content lectures regarding men's health to the faculty of UPOLI. This type of model has two purposes: It allows the faculty of UPOLI to remain competent, and it allows for sustainability of the men's health clinic. This framework is the "train the trainer" approach. These same lecture topics are also presented to the men in a patient education format while they are waiting to be seen by clinicians. Both Nicaraguan and American nursing students do the patient education presentations.

Sustainability of the Men's Health Clinic: A Typical Visit

As mentioned earlier, the UPOLI faculty maintains the men's health clinic in the absence of the author. Below is the process that is used in developing a visit to the men's health clinic:

1. Agree on a common date that works well between the two parties (UPOLI and author).

2. Select nurse practitioner students who wish to travel to Nicaragua and participate in the clinic.

3. Collaborate with UPOLI's faculty and decide on lecture topics and to schedule a classroom.

4. Prepare lectures and have translated into Spanish.

5. Work with students in developing the patient education posters used to present the material to the men.

6. Once in Nicaragua the lectures are presented to the faculty in the morning while the men are at work.

7. The clinicians and students open the men's health clinic in the afternoon because the men are usually done working.

8. UPOLI faculty along with the students obtain each man's chief complaint and vital signs as the men enter the clinic.

9. Students provide patient education material while the men sit on the large front porch waiting for their turn to see the clinicians.

10. Clinicians see men and address their concerns.

11. Health evaluation plans are discussed with each man.

12. If there is an immediate problem to be addressed, the clinicians have a set amount of money used for assisting the men who need it (i.e., laboratory work, diagnostic tests, medications, dressing supplies, etc.)

This process is used before and during a typical trip to the men's health clinic.

Conclusion

This chapter has presented an evidence-based practice model for establishing a men's health clinic. The clinic was generated and grounded from the data obtained through qualitative research using ethnography. The goal of these men, despite the inherent social and cultural limitations, is to maintain an optimal level of health and well-being. The author remembers the UPOLI faculty's response when he informed them of his wishes to establish a men's health clinic. The consensus was that it was a great idea *but* men do not participate in healthcare activities. However, their support was present. Currently, there are approximately 200 men who participate in the activities of the men's health clinic. The men have developed a healthcare group and elected officers to serve as leaders in the community regarding health care of men. They have also developed a motto and logo for the men's health clinic, which is "Healthy Men Make a Healthy Community."

References

Cifras Oficiales Censos Nacionales. (2005). *Informe annual.* Managua, Nicaragua: Cifras Oficiales Censos Nacionales.

Ministerio de Salud (MINSA). (2005). *Situación de Salud en Nicaragua.* Fuente: MINSA.

Pan American Health Organization. (1998). *Health in the Americas.* Washington, DC: Author.

Ross, C. (2000). *Caminando mas cerca con Dios. [A closer walk with thee]: An ethnography of health and well-being of rural Nicaraguan men.* Published doctoral dissertation, Duquesne University, Pittsburgh.

Ross, C. (2002). The theory of endurance of Nicaraguan men. *Home Health Care Management Practice, 14*(6), 448–451.

Center for Reducing Risks in Vulnerable Populations

Julie Johnson Zerwic, Linda Graham, JoEllen Wilbur, and Janet L. Larson

The advancement of nursing science as it relates to the health of vulnerable populations has traditionally been accomplished by the work of small teams of nurse researchers working in isolation and/or in collaboration with individual scientists from other disciplines. But with recent advances in scientific knowledge at the molecular and genetic levels as well as at the physical and behavioral levels, it has become clear that greater progress will be accomplished by teams of researchers from multiple disciplines working together on related projects, each bringing a unique perspective to the team. This approach is strongly encouraged by the National Institutes of Health, the primary source of support for health-related research in the United States, and it is embodied by the Center for Reducing Risks in Vulnerable Populations at the University of Illinois at Chicago.

Center for Reducing Risks in Vulnerable Populations

The University of Illinois at Chicago College of Nursing (CON) established the Center for Reducing Risks in Vulnerable Populations (CRRVP) to address the health needs of vulnerable people with chronic diseases, specifically cardiorespiratory, neurobehavioral, and cancer-related health problems. We united the many investigators at University of Illinois CON already conducting research in these areas (see Boxes 32-1 and 32-2 for two examples), established a biobehavioral framework to organize the science, and created the CRRVP to serve as an incubator for this type of research.

The CRRVP is supported by the National Institute of Nursing Research at the National Institutes of Health (P30 NR009014). The overall purpose of the CRRVP is to advance the science of biobehavioral health for vulnerable populations with chronic disease, to support research development and training by providing core services and resources to investigators, and ultimately to reduce disparities in disease/illness. Consistent with the biobehavioral focus, the CRRVP supports research that reduces disparity and promotes healthy

Box 32-1

Dr. Marquis Foreman's research program addresses the health needs of vulnerable people with chronic diseases, specifically the elderly experiencing delirium, a neurobehavioral health problem. Dr. Foreman's research program has focused on describing the natural history of delirium and delineating its pathogenesis and outcomes. He is currently conducting a study using a prospective, longitudinal, cohort design with 3 years of follow-up to examine long-term outcomes. The aims of this study are to evaluate the long-term effects of delirium on health outcomes, specifically functional and cognitive status, mortality, and utilization of healthcare resources; document the effect of continued care on the severity, duration, and reoccurrence of delirium; and describe the natural course of delirium beyond an episode of hospitalization.

Box 32-2

Carol Estwing Ferrans has been conducting studies examining the effects of illness and treatment on quality of life in cancer and other chronic illnesses. Early in her career Dr. Ferrans developed the Ferrans and Powers Quality of Life Index and has contributed to the development of the field of quality of life research through her conceptual work focused on clarification of the construct. An important part of her research has focused on cross-cultural issues, including approaches to increase validity of data and participation in research in minority populations. This has included the development of culturally specific measures for African-Americans and Hispanic-Americans. Dr. Ferrans' current research examines cancer survivorship issues for African-Americans, focusing on the impact on quality of life and barriers to cancer screening. In addition, she is examining issues surrounding delay in seeking treatment for breast cancer in African-American, Hispanic, and white women.

life-styles for vulnerable populations; elucidates underlying physiological and psychological mechanisms that contribute to symptoms, functional status, perceived health status, and quality of life; and tests interventions to minimize symptoms and enhance functional status, perceived health status, and quality of life. The services of the CRRVP are provided through three research core facilities: (1) Multiethnic Emphasis Core, (2) Biobehavioral Methods Core, and (3) Development and Dissemination Core. They are described later in this chapter.

Figure 32-1 shows the framework that the CRRVP uses to guide biobehavioral research and positively impact health-related quality of life. Key elements in this framework include personal (individual) factors, environmental factors, physiological and psychological variables, symptom status, functional status, general health perception, and quality of life. Personal factors contribute to the vulnerability or resilience of the individual: for example, age, genetic composition, and knowledge. Environmental factors are either risk factors or resources that exist outside the person and can influence health outcomes (Shaver, 1985). Resources in the local community are a part of the environment and could include a neighborhood health clinic, a grocery store with reasonable prices, and a

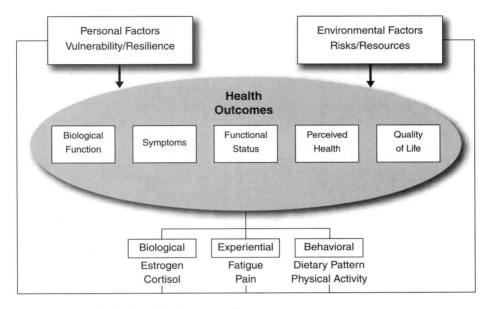

Figure 32-1 Model of Health Outcomes Factors

community center or seniors' center with educational programs. Physical environmental factors might include an unsafe neighborhood with no place to exercise, whereas social environmental factors might include availability of education, level of income, availability of paid work, social support for being physically active, and cultural expectations/norms for diet. These factors all interact to influence health outcomes. Although some of these factors cannot be modified, nursing practice is directed toward assessing and changing factors that are modifiable, such as motivation, attitude, and knowledge. Nursing then aims to help individuals to manipulate those factors in an effort to improve health-related quality of life.

The CRRVP emphasizes the use of biological measures and experiential and behavioral measures to enhance the understanding of phenomena from a biobehavioral perspective. For example, one researcher studies cardiovascular risk factors in non–English-speaking immigrant and minority women. Her work focuses on individual, family, and community factors that contribute to behavioral patterns. She includes salivary cortisol as a *biological* marker of stress and self-report questionnaires as an *experiential* marker of stress. Another researcher who is testing the effectiveness of an upper body strength-training program for patients with chronic obstructive pulmonary disease uses dual-energy x-ray absorptiometry to measure changes in muscle mass and self-report measures of physical activity.

To achieve its goals, the CRRVP brings together researchers with diverse and complementary expertise under a single umbrella and offers resources and experiences that take

TABLE 32-1 Aims and Activities of the CRRVP Research Cores

Core	Specific Aims	Activities
Multiethnic Emphasis	Facilitate research with ethnic minorities by nurturing community partnerships and preparing culturally competent nurse researchers.	Expand community collaborative multiethnic research related to health disparities among vulnerable groups. Optimize recruitment and retention of multiethnic research participants, particularly Blacks and Hispanics, who represent vulnerable groups most at risk for health disparities. Foster the development of culturally sensitive, tailored, individual, group, or system interventions. Build collaborative community relationships with the multiethnic community-based advisory board.
Biobehavioral Methods	Strengthen the methodologies used by CRRVP investigators/affiliates and train novices regarding the measurement of biobehavioral (biological, behavioral, and experiential) variables, management of data, and analysis of data.	Provide consultation and data collection support for measures of health and function: (1) instrument bank, (2) expert consultations for qualitative research methods, (3) evaluation and adaptation of instruments for specific ethnic groups, (4) general research design and measurement issues, and (5) interviewer training for project staff. Provide consultation and services to support data collection, management, analysis, and sharing: (1) DataBANK to house data sets available for secondary analysis, (2) data management services, (3) statistical consultation, (4) computer programming consultation, and (5) computerized data collection systems that can be readily used in the field setting. In conjunction with the Development and Dissemination Core, (1) provide programs for development of investigators and project staff with an emphasis on methodological issues related to the study of vulnerable populations, (2) organize/support the research interest groups, (3) organize research seminars related to data management and statistical analysis, (4) organize annual colloquia, and (5) support the development of special research projects that promote new collaborations among investigators for the purpose of advancing the scientific basis for reducing risks in vulnerable populations.

Core	Specific Aims	Activities
Development and Dissemination	Development: Advance nursing science related to reducing risks in vulnerable populations.	Award pilot study funding to promote research focused on reducing health risks in vulnerable populations.
		Facilitate the development of successful investigator-initiated programs of research.
		Link novice investigators with available resources (people, technology, programs) that facilitate their successful development as independent researchers.
	Dissemination: Facilitate the dissemination of research findings to the scientific and clinical communities and to the general public.	Facilitate development and presentation of symposia focused on reducing health risks in vulnerable populations.
		Facilitate translation into practice of research findings in venues suitable for and accessible to nursing clinicians in direct practice.
		Publicize results of the science performed by CRRVP investigators/affiliates to the general public.
		Enhance successful publication of databased manuscripts.

Source: Center for Reducing Risks in Vulnerable Populations.

advantage of this synergy and strengthen it. This promotes novel insights and collaborations that move the science forward in new and exciting directions. One researcher specializing in fatigue in stem cell transplant patients was searching for an intervention that might reduce this symptom and improve their quality of life. The CRRVP facilitated a collaboration between her and a researcher highly experienced in using exercise to reduce symptoms and improve functional status in persons with chronic disease. This collaboration resulted in the novice researcher receiving funding to examine the effectiveness of exercise in reducing fatigue and enhancing quality of life in stem cell transplant patients (a new population in which to study such exercise programs' outcomes). This collaboration also led to the experienced researcher incorporating the measure of fatigue into her studies, where she was surprised to find that the exercise intervention was having a bigger impact on reduction of fatigue than on other symptoms. Such collaborations are facilitated often through the CRRVP's three research cores (Table 32-1).

Multiethnic Emphasis Core

The CRRVP established as one of its three cores the Multiethnic Emphasis Core to provide resources and skills to enhance health and reduce health disparities in multiethnic groups. Scientists accomplish the work of the Multiethnic Emphasis Core with expertise in public health, community organization, and nursing. Through this core the CRRVP developed the infrastructure to facilitate research with ethnic minorities by nurturing community partnerships and preparing culturally competent nurse researchers.

The Multiethnic Emphasis Core's community advisory board was established to address health disparities through collaboration and partnership with the African-American and Hispanic communities of Chicago. The board includes professionals serving and working in low-income ethnic minority communities and religious leaders and community residents. The Multiethnic Emphasis Core builds continuing collaborative community relationships by maintaining and expanding the multiethnic community advisory board of experts to include representatives from groups targeted by CRRVP researchers. The board offers a forum for both community members and researchers to discuss planned and ongoing projects and to elicit input. The board's partnership is promoted through its active involvement in key stages of the research plans: objectives and design, recruitment strategies, and implementation. The community advisory board is often consulted for their perspective on results and plans the most appropriate format in which to communicate those results to the community.

The work of the community advisory board is predicated on the development of partnerships between the community representatives and the CRRVP investigators. To develop research-based interventions that are driven according to community needs and participation (rather than imposed on the community), faculty researchers must work collaboratively as committed partners. Relationship-building based on trust, power sharing, dialogue, and collaborative inquiry is an imperative for deriving knowledge and interventions that will reduce or eliminate health disparities (Minkler & Wallerstein, 2003).

Other ways that the Multiethnic Emphasis Core helps ensure the preparation of culturally competent nurse researchers include a seminar series and expert consultation. Each year, the Multiethnic Emphasis Core identifies an area of concentration for a series of seminars. Examples include conceptualization and measurement of socioeconomic status, acculturation, geographic information systems as objective measures of the built environment, community participatory research methods, and racism/discrimination. Expert consultation is provided on appropriate measures, research design, and analysis.

One of the CRRVP researchers has used the community advisory board extensively to obtain advice on issues of recruitment of African-American women, such as the use of incentives and appropriate venues for advertising. This researcher has also benefited from the Multiethnic Emphasis Core's seminar series. For example, one seminar series focused on measures of socioeconomic status. This researcher benefited from the series and has expanded beyond the traditional measures of socioeconomic status to include a measure of hardship that captures participants' ability to meet expenses for housing, telephone, food, and medical care.

Biobehavioral Methods Core

The Biobehavioral Methods Core was established to strengthen the infrastructure for research methodology in the CON, particularly for research that focuses on reducing risks in vulnerable populations with chronic disease. The activities of the Biobehavioral Methods Core are implemented by scientists with expertise in pharmacology, physiology, information technology, nursing, and statistics. Activities of the Biobehavioral Methods Core include the development and support of research interest groups, core biological and performance laboratories, and the instrument bank.

The research interest groups sponsored by the core bring together researchers who have a common interest in a measure, intervention, research design, patient population, or statistical analysis. For example, a number of investigators in the CON were using exercise as a research intervention for people with chronic disease. These researchers perceived themselves to have little in common because they were working with diverse populations. The core brought together this interdisciplinary group of individuals (faculty and students), and they formed the exercise research interest group. Within this group they explored issues of exercise adherence, exercise safety, and measurement using the latest technology.

The core biological laboratory consults with researchers on the most appropriate methods to sample and measure biological signals such as neurohormones and inflammatory markers. The core lab develops commercially available assays and analyzes biological samples collected by the investigative team. For example, one researcher consulted with the biological core lab on the best method for measuring salivary cortisol in infants and breast-feeding women. Commercial assays were available for serum cortisol but not saliva. Therefore the laboratory modified the serum assay to measure low levels of cortisol found in salivary samples. Since that time, a commercial enzyme-linked immunoassay was developed to measure salivary cortisol. It has the advantage of using very small sample volumes. The new method was validated against our method and is currently in use in the laboratory.

The core sponsors an instrument bank that facilitates access to reliable and valid measures appropriate for biobehavioral research in vulnerable populations. The instruments are organized according to the biobehavioral model that organizes the science of the CRRVP. Supporting documentation is collected for the instruments. For example, the instrument bank has a large collection of measures of fatigue. Recently, a group of investigators designed a study on fatigue experienced in older adults. They accessed the instrument bank to identify the most appropriate measures of fatigue in an older adult population.

Development and Dissemination Core

As an incubator, the CRRVP supports the development and training of researchers studying vulnerable populations with or at risk for chronic disease. The goal of the Development and Dissemination Core is to nurture and develop investigators throughout the research process. Each year four pilot studies that focus on reducing risks in vulnerable populations are funded. Individuals who receive pilot funding meet with center investigators to discuss any issues that arise in conducting the pilot study and to map out plans for manuscript submissions and future grant applications. Pilot investigators are strongly encouraged to take advantage of all services provided by the CRRVP, such as editorial assistance, expert reviews, and consultation with the community advisory board.

Pilot Studies

The goal of funding the pilot studies is to stimulate research that addresses the needs of vulnerable populations that include ethnic minorities and people with chronic disease, specifically cardiorespiratory, neurobehavioral, and cancer related. The CRRVP supports the research of novice investigators and midcareer investigators who are shifting their focus to vulnerable populations. These pilot studies enable investigators to submit competitive grants to the National Institutes of Health. Provided below are three examples of studies funded by the CRRVP.

Eileen Collins' research program analyzes exercise as an intervention to promote cardiorespiratory fitness and health in people with chronic disease. The CRRVP funded Dr. Collins to tailor and test the psychometric properties of a questionnaire to assess the level of physical activity in persons with spinal cord injury (SCI). This instrument will be used in subsequent research studies to determine the effect of physical activity interventions on quality of life as well as secondary complications of SCI. The sample of men was recruited from a Veterans Administration Hospital and included 40% African-Americans and Latinos. Dr. Collins' interdisciplinary research team includes an exercise physiologist, statistician, and research methodologist. Dr. Collins received editorial assistance from the CRRVP both in manuscript and subsequent grant submissions. In addition, the CRRVP arranged for both researchers internal to the CON and external experts to provide critiques and suggestions before her federal grant submission.

Sandra Burgener's program of research focuses on improving neurocognitive and physical functioning of persons with dementia. The CRRVP funded Dr. Burgener to develop and test the effectiveness of a wellness intervention for persons with dementia. The intervention includes a combination of Taiji exercises focusing on strength, balance, and fall prevention; cognitive-behavioral therapies addressing memory, social functioning, and mental and emotional well-being; and support group participation addressing self-concept, social isolation, and self-esteem. Dr. Burgener's interdisciplinary research team includes an exercise physiologist, an expert in Taiji and a statistician. Dr. Burgener received consultation from the CRRVP Biobehavioral Methods Core regarding the research design and editorial assistance from the CRRVP Development and Dissemination Core.

Lorna Finnegan studies survivors of childhood cancer with the goal of improving their health and minimizing the late effects of cancer and cancer treatment. Life-style choices in combination with late effects put this vulnerable population at risk for premature development and accelerated progression of diseases associated with aging, such as hypertension, diabetes, coronary artery disease, and osteoporosis. The CRRVP funded Dr. Finnegan to evaluate the psychometric properties of four rating scales that measure important determinants of physical activity adoption (self-determination, self-efficacy, decisional balance, and health-related worries) in young adult survivors of childhood cancer. This study is part of a series of investigations that will lead to the development and testing of a computer-tailored physical activity assessment and intervention system designed for young adult survivors of childhood cancer. Dr. Finnegan's interdisciplinary research team includes a disability expert who provides statistical consultation.

Dissemination

All this work to nurture and improve research related to vulnerable populations would be futile if it did not make an impact on the larger world. Thus this core is also charged with disseminating research findings. It has the task of making known to the larger scientific community and the lay public the importance and implications of vulnerable populations research. For example, disseminating research findings to nurses who work primarily in nonresearch-intensive environments has been an important initiative of the CRRVP. Nurse researchers typically publish their research in journals that are primarily accessed by other researchers. Although this outlet is important, nurses in clinical settings do generally not read these journals. The Development and Dissemination Core successfully contracted with the *American Journal of Nursing* to publish a quarterly column that highlights the research of a CRRVP investigator and translates the results for the clinical audience. The column is entitled "Reducing Risks," and one of the columns published was "Recognizing 'Quiet' Delirium" by Forrest et al. (2007).

A second dissemination focus for the CRRVP has been to share research with the general public. The CRRVP coordinates a health column that is published in the *Gazette,* a free monthly newspaper that serves a diverse ethnic readership with a circulation of 17,000. These columns have included vital information for the public regarding such health concerns as stroke, influenza, and HIV. Another activity is that the CRRVP works with the university's media relations to disseminate to major media outlets. Catherine Ryan's funded pilot study found that sweating may be a key symptom in how quickly people seek treatment for acute myocardial infarction, a finding that was covered in the *New York Times* and dozens of other media outlets.

Conclusion

The CRRVP aims to move forward the science in vulnerable populations with chronic disease. This is accomplished by providing facilities and activities to investigators that help them to recruit diverse samples, measure appropriate outcomes, develop their long-term research programs, and disseminate information to scientific, clinical, and lay audiences. Crucial to achieving these goals are the CRRVP's three research cores: Multiethnic Emphasis Core, Biobehavioral Methods Core, and Development and Dissemination Core. Vulnerable populations research is an important area of study. The University of Illinois at Chicago CON's CRRVP serves as a model of interdisciplinary research that brings together the expertise of many disciplines to advance scientific knowledge with respect to the health of vulnerable populations.

Acknowledgment

Manuscript preparation was supported in part by the Center for Reducing Risks in Vulnerable Populations (NIH/NINR no. P30 NR009014, University of Illinois at Chicago College of Nursing). We thank Kevin Grandfield for editorial assistance.

References

Forrest, J., Willis, L., Kwon, M. S., Holm, K., Anderson, M. A., & Foreman, M. D. (2007). Recognizing "quiet" delirium. *American Journal of Nursing, 107*(4), 35–39.

Minkler, M., & Wallerstein, N. (2003). Introduction to community-based participatory research. In N. Wallerstein (Ed.), *Community-based participatory research for health* (pp. 3–26). San Francisco: Jossey-Bass.

Shaver, J. (1985). A biopsychosocial view of human health—Relevance for nursing. *Nursing Outlook, 33,* 186–191.

Reducing the Vulnerability of Nurses

Elaine Goehner and Pamela A. P. Smith

Nurses care for vulnerable populations on a daily basis. Yet, as caregivers, they are a vulnerable population. The American Association of Critical-Care Nursing (AACN) Synergy Model identifies vulnerability as a patient (not a nurse) characteristic. In this model vulnerability is defined as a "susceptibility to actual or potential stressors that may adversely affect patient outcomes" (Hardin & Kaplow, 2005, p. 227). Although this definition is in relationship to patient care needs, the concept of vulnerability may also be applied to nurses.

Nurses are vulnerable because they are subject to many stressors that may adversely affect outcomes for their patients, families, and themselves. For example, stressors in the environment include staffing shortages, recruitment and retention challenges, new technology, and patients with highly complex problems. This chapter addresses how and why nurses are vulnerable and how this vulnerability can be reduced or mitigated within the work environment. We apply both the Synergy Model and Swanson's Caring Theory to explain the impact of work by clinical nurse specialists, professional development specialists, and others on nurses, as a vulnerable population, within a center for nursing excellence.

Swedish Center for Nursing Excellence

Founded in 1910, the Swedish Medical Center (SMC) in Seattle, Washington, has become the region's hallmark organization for excellence in health care. In an independent research study conducted by the National Research Corporation, SMC is consistently named the area's best hospital, with the best doctors, nurses, and care in a variety of specialty areas. SMC is also the largest, most comprehensive, nonprofit healthcare provider organization in the Pacific Northwest, with three hospitals, a community-based emergency department and specialty center, home-care services, multiple primary care and specialty clinics, and physician groups (SMC, 2006). In February 2005 a new nurse executive began her tenure as the leader for the department of nursing. After an assessment of nursing needs, the nurse executive identified an opportunity to use resources differently to support professional development of the nurses. During her first year in the role, she mobilized an increase of $12 million to supplement nursing resources at the bedside and to create the Center for Nursing Excellence (CNE).

The conceptual model of the CNE, in applying concepts from the Caring Theory to the work of the Swedish CNE, assumes the staff nurse as the *care-receiver* and the CNE staff as the *care-providers*. Swanson (1991) defined caring as a "nurturing way of relating to a valued other toward whom one feels a personal sense of commitment and responsibility" (p. 162). The benefits of caring, as described by Swanson, are consistent with the CNE mission and the department of nursing philosophy. Care-receivers/nurses report enhanced self-esteem, self-worth, knowledge, coping, positive mental attitude, and sense of dignity and trust. Later in the chapter we provide specific examples of how the CNE addresses these issues with staff nurses.

Swanson (1991) linked increasing vulnerability with a noncaring relationship. In addition, she identified a sense of fright, despair, helplessness, and the occurrence of lingering bad memories. Although Swanson used the model to describe the care-receiver as patient, we believe this outcome of noncaring also applies to the nurse. When support is not adequate to provide a caring environment, nurses may experience dissatisfaction with work and feelings of vulnerability. Additionally, the effects of not caring are similar to the characteristics of an oppressed and vulnerable population.

The Synergy Model, drafted by the American Association of Critical-Care Nursing in the 1990s, states a synergistic relationship of patient, nurse, and environment creates the power of nursing (Hardin & Kaplow, 2005). The work of Virginia Henderson (2006) and Patricia Benner (1984) also serves to inform theory to explain the application of this model in nursing practice. At the CNE these frameworks have been merged to describe the model of nursing service delivered at SMC (Figure 33-1).

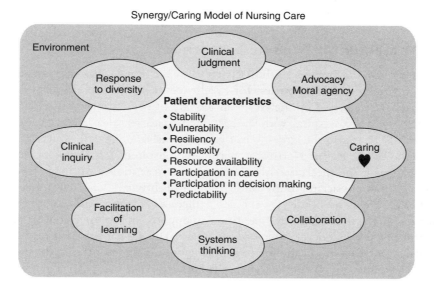

Figure 33-1 Model for Nursing Service Delivery

TABLE 33-1   Role of the CNE Based on Caring and Synergy Concepts

Competencies	Knowing	Being With	Doing For	Enabling	Maintaining Belief
Caring	Assess the individual and groups: cognitive, affective, psychomotor practice Engage w/ staff by inviting them to work together on projects Creating intentional relationships	Emotionally entering their practice environment; modeling at the bedside Being there: PDS & educator on day, evening, and night shifts	Recognition: awards, promotional opportunities Ethics Fellowship for staff nurses	Coaching: allowing with support; giving feedback Instructing: to increase self-reliance	Finding ways to explore meaning in work; highlighting storytelling Offering realistic optimism Provide support to "go the distance"
Advocacy	Who is the nurse personally and professionally?	Standing next to Helping give voice; use of language to lift people up	Anticipate and advocate for resources they need such as unit moves, transitions Protecting from needless work such as with interpretation of standards, regulations	Building shared leadership groups Supporting clinical practice teams	Build confidence in the future of individual nurses and nursing as a profession

TABLE 33-1 Role of the CNE Based on Caring and Synergy Concepts *(Continued)*

Competencies	Knowing	Being With	Doing For	Enabling	Maintaining Belief
Clinical inquiry	Identify researchable clinical questions Apply various ways of knowing to inform practice	Clinical nurse specialist: expert bedside consultation	Measure and providing graphic representation of work Gathering info from various sources (lit review)	Developing standards to be used by nurses Coach w/ research methods, internal review board procedures	Helping staff stay engaged in long difficult processes such as research
Clinical judgment	Teaching the science and techniques of critical reasoning and how to apply to specific situations Support when conflicting data require additional objective review to understand a problem	Witnessing the use of clinical judgment; affirm and confirm their use; validating Available to debrief as a way of sharing feelings and conveying availability	Seeking out opportunities to model Providing feedback while preserving dignity	Provide ways to document clinical judgment (patient records) Supports use of tools (clinical pathways, research)	Believing in the nurse's knowledge and experience
Diversity	Asking questions to identify differences Honor variation in experience	Model acceptance of diversity Avoid over-simplifying or redundant training	Supporting differences in approaches while focusing on the goals/results	Provide multiple approaches to learning (online, classroom) Validate skills and knowledge and allow nurses to "test out"	Search for diverse opinions and help others find value and meaning

Competencies	Knowing	Being With	Doing For	Enabling	Maintaining Belief
Systems thinking	Provide info to the nurse from a system point of view: bedside to board room	Reinforce the values of relationship with other departments and people Illustrate relationship of nurses to others in the organization	Model collaboration and participation at various levels of decision-making	Providing info for effective involvement Identify the motivated nurse and get them involved in the right work	Creating sustainable change within nursing
Learning	Use of evidence/scholarly work to develop teaching plans and to set educational goals	Give emotional and other forms of support learning	Relating to each registered nurse as a professional Pilot learning strategies; programs (documentation)	Testing/validating Encouragement Scholarship	Providing prep classes for cert exams
Collaboration	Who should be involved Play to strengths Demonstrate motivation	Providing adequate time for assessment and planning together	Bring/selecting the right people to do the right work Provide with needed resources (time, tools, expertise)	Reinforcing effective behaviors Giving critical feedback and coaching	Group involvement results in better outcomes and staff being heard Everyone has something to contribute

The medical model, although helpful to the nurses in understanding the human body and disease, does not capture the complete essence of nursing and leaves nurses dependent on others to describe the profession of nursing. Nursing practice is a complex and continual synthesis of art and science (Chinn & Kramer, 2004). Explaining, documenting, and articulating the full range of nursing practice is a crucial step needed to alleviate the vulnerability of nurses by articulating nursing practice.

SMC has adopted the Synergy Model and Swanson's mid-range theory of caring to enlighten leading, transforming, and informing nurses' decisions and authority over their practice. The models extend the nursing department philosophy as well as the organizational values and beliefs. For example, the SMC values of patient-centered care, respectful relationships, and service are all consistent with the synergy and caring concepts. The adoption of these models advises and explains nursing practice at SMC, and we predict it will result in both advancing nursing practice and reducing nurse vulnerability at SMC. These models of caring and synergy are operationalized through the competencies the CNE staff has identified to reduce nurse vulnerability (Table 33-1).

Environment and Nurse Vulnerability

The physical work environment influences nurse vulnerability. Physical demands, an aging workforce, and aging hospital facilities are common characteristics of today's healthcare delivery organizations. Many hospitals were built in the mid-1900s, and the design of nursing units is not conducive to the higher physical and technological demands of taking care of today's complex patients. For example, the physical arrangement on nursing units often requires nurses to walk long distances to get supplies, equipment, and medications needed to provide patient care. The Institute of Medicine (2004) report, *Keeping Patients Safe,* recommended redesign of patient rooms toward greater efficiency, placing necessary items close to the bedside.

The nurse is also affected by a work environment that contributes to feelings of inadequacy, lack of confidence, and low self-esteem. For example, increases in patient acuity and budgetary reductions for bedside care sets the expectation that the nurse should constantly adjust and assimilate to these changes quickly, often without input or control. An example is learning to use an automated patient information system, a challenge for many Baby Boomer nurses (Kupperschmidt, 2006). These rapid changes may contribute to feelings of inadequacy and a sense of failure.

Nurses are vulnerable due to the real or perceived lack of resources in providing patient care. They may feel angry and unsupported when working under pressure without adequate staff, supplies, or equipment.. When nurses believe they are not heard, they may feel vulnerable and experience low morale. When nurses believe they are continually under-resourced, they may respond to any changes in the environment with anger and criticism. To handle these negative feelings, nurses may withdraw from other staff, patients, and their families to cope. Interdisciplinary tension and a reluctance to collaborate with other team members result when nurses believe they lack control of their environment, are unprotected by leadership, and feel unsupported in times of change. This isolation is detrimental to providing a caring and safe relationship with patients.

Over the past 100 years the work environment and nursing practice has steadily been transformed by societal changes, research, technology, and government policy. Throughout these changes nurses remain challenged to control their practice. Historically, nursing has its roots in religious orders and in the military, both known for reliance on hierarchy, power, and control over their members. This undeniable past has contributed to a sense of oppression that exists within the nursing profession today.

Roberts (1983) stated a group is oppressed if they view themselves as controlled by others with greater prestige, power, and status. In another sentinel article, Freire (1971) proposed oppression results from the ability of the dominant group to identify their norms and values as the "right" ones and uses power to enforce these beliefs on others. Those who do not belong to the dominant group try to assimilate and internalize the dominant group's values, while knowing they do not agree. This leads to self-hatred and low self-esteem, according to Miller (1976).

Friedson (1970) defined nursing as an oppressed population based on a lack of autonomy, accountability, and control over their profession. Indeed, nurses often do describe feelings of oppression because of the heavy weight of accountability for patient care with little control over the environment. This sense of oppression may be particularly true for nurses practicing in hospitals with 24-hour responsibility for patient care.

Conversely, we live in the information age, characterized by the need to recognize the "knowledge worker," a term coined by Peter Drucker in 1960 to describe various professionals, including nurses (Drucker, 1993, 2002). The impact of the information age has brought "instant communication, boundary-less relationships, the globalization of economics and politics, Internet interaction, and knowledge that exceeds our capacity to assimilate it" (Porter-O'Grady, 2003, p. 1). Knowledge rapidly becomes obsolete; therefore the knowledge worker needs formal education and continuing education. In addition, the knowledge worker, the nurse, is highly mobile, carries multiple "intelligences," and practices well as part of a team (Drucker, 2002). These characteristics are often in conflict with roles within complex and highly regulated healthcare delivery organizations. Environments where nurses are overmanaged and feel powerless over their practice do not support them as knowledge workers and contribute to vulnerability.

> The best trained people in the world are American nurses. Yet whenever we make a study on nurses, we find that 80 percent of their time is spent on things they aren't trained for. . . . How to make the knowledge worker more appropriately productive is a challenge we will need to face seriously over the next twenty years (Drucker, 2002, pp. 88–89).

Effect of Vulnerability on the Behavior of Nurses

How vulnerable nurses feel has an impact on their ability to advocate for the patients, families, other nurses/staff, or themselves. Nurses often question their own clinical judgment, knowledge, and adequacy, fearing the reaction of others. The threat of negative responses and criticism, either real or perceived, is sufficient to keep many nurses from speaking up for what they believe is right on behalf of the patients, families, or themselves. This behavior creates a threat to patient safety, among other hazards, and leads to hostile behavior.

Hostility often emerges within a nursing peer group because it is safer for the nurses to express anger and hostility toward each other than toward those viewed as having more power and control (Bartholomew, 2006). Roberts (1983) identified a concept labeled "submission aggression syndrome" (p. 23). Although members of an oppressed group complain, self-hatred and low self-esteem create submissiveness when confronted with the more powerful person. This submissiveness places the person at a disadvantage in the relationship and reinforces low self-esteem. This syndrome is also known as "horizontal violence" (Bartholomew, 2006). Nurses are known to exhibit horizontal violence toward each other at times because it is usually dangerous to voice anger or frustration toward physicians or administrators (Roberts, 1983). This negative energy can significantly damage relationships with other nurses, physicians, and patients.

Relationships on multiple levels are fundamental to nursing practice: nurse to patient, nurse to nurse, and nurse to physician. DeLellis (2000) stressed the importance of respect in professional relationships. When nurses are not respected or lack effective relationships with peers, horizontal violence may exist. In some work groups horizontal violence and other damaging behaviors become the norm, emulated by new staff as a way to "fit in," further passing along this destructive phenomenon within the nursing profession. The damage done by this legacy is unavoidably transferred to patients.

To assert personal power and avoid perceived control and criticism by others, nurses resort to lashing out toward their peers, behavior that deprecates, devalues, and disrespects others (Bartholomew, 2006). Horizontal violence is grounded in the need to feel powerful and in control. To counter the damage done through horizontal violence, nurses need to recognize and consciously adopt behaviors to reduce feelings of vulnerability.

Nurse leaders are not immune to vulnerability. This can be observed when nurse leaders experience

- Eroding of resources (i.e., reduction of nursing positions, loss of clerical support)
- Undercutting of the leadership role by staff, administration, or physicians
- Limited voice in decision-making
- Tolerance for lateral violence (Bartholomew, 2006)

Addressing Nurse Vulnerability through a CNE

Assessment of nursing at SMC identified numerous resources such as clinical nurse specialists and nurse educators who were sparsely distributed throughout the organization in departments that did not report directly to the nursing department, thus fragmenting nursing resources. In an effort to maximize the impact of these resources, the SMC CNE was established, bringing people and resources together in an effective visible entity responsible for enhancing professional nursing practice. Structuring a wide variety of resources into a single entity allowed the CNE staff to collaborate more effectively and gain momentum through close alignment of mission, vision, and available resources.

The purpose of a CNE is to provide a structure for organizing professional nursing within a healthcare organization, giving leadership a way to explain, demonstrate, and showcase nursing and nurses (Knox & Gharrity, 2004). The CNE provides support and direction for nursing in the areas of education, research, staff development, nurse recruitment and retention, and leadership development. The mission of the SMC CNE is to deliver comprehensive, innovative, and professional resources to nurses as they deliver exceptional care for patients and families at SMC and in the community. Included in the CNE are advanced practice nurses such as clinical nurse specialists, professional development specialists, clinical educators, nurse researchers, patient/family educators, communication specialists, standards/quality directors, and project specialists (Figure 33-2). Each of these roles contributes to decreasing nursing vulnerability, enhancing nursing development, and helping sustain a healing environment for both the patient and nurse.

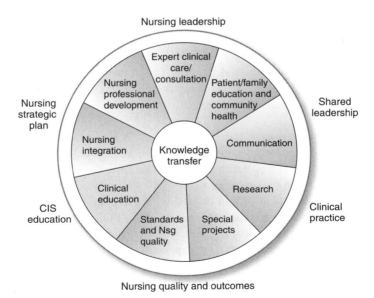

Figure 33-2   Center for Nursing Excellence Resource Groups

When the CNE opened in February 2006, the Executive Director began formulating a vision and goals for the CNE. The goal of the Center is to provide the structure needed to support nurses in their ability to provide quality care to patients through reducing their vulnerability. Although the general functions of the CNE were clear to the nurse executive team, the task of moving departments or resource groups into new cost centers and locating most staff in a single physical location took several months to complete. Between February and September 2006, the majority of staff was hired. Five of the CNE leadership team members have doctoral degrees, and all nurses hired have master's degrees in nursing or are currently pursuing advanced degrees in nursing. Of the nurses hired into clinical nurse specialists, professional development specialists, and educator roles, all but two were internal transfers. The fact that SMC had already employed many advanced practice nurses at the bedside promoted retention while enhancing opportunities for utilization of talents applied to a larger audience.

The Director for Nursing Integration, Assimilation and Retention, hired February 2006, is responsible for creating a "pipeline" for the nursing workforce, working with nursing leadership and human resources directors to design processes and strategies for recruitment. The "re-recruitment" of long-tenured nurses is also a priority, based on the belief that nurses, rich in experience and knowledge, are ready to participate with innovative strategies to help nurses entering practice or the facility.

The nurse assimilation coordinator is responsible for building and maintaining relationships with school of nursing faculty and representatives, organizing clinical placement of over 500 nursing students a year, managing contracts and agreements, and orienting faculty and students. Other duties include connecting with staff nurses to identify "the best and the brightest" students who are interested in nursing technician positions and subsequently to identify the most qualified nurse technicians for new graduate nurse positions. This creates a pipeline for the nursing workforce. The coordinator's ability to build relationships with students and staff nurses helps them work effectively as a team, makes recruiting nurse technicians easier, and enables a smoother transition from nurse technicians to staff nurse positions—all factors that decrease vulnerability among the nursing staff.

The professional development specialist (PDS), with expertise in both education and clinical roles, focuses on professional nursing development. The PDS works directly with staff nurses and nurse managers, while building alliances with the clinical nurse specialist and clinical educators. The PDS decreases nurse vulnerability by building strong nursing teams, by supporting the manager and individual nurses, and by career advisement, goal setting, and education. Another primary function of the PDS is to assist preceptors in the integration and transition for new nurse employees, including new graduates and experienced nurses new to the organization or the specialty area.

New staff, especially new graduates, experience significant stress during the first 6 months in a new job (Duchscher, 2001). The PDS provides support and guidance for preceptors while being careful not to interfere with the relationship between the preceptor and new nurse. New graduate nurses require support and guidance for up to 18 months to complete a smooth transition from student nurse to staff nurse (Duchscher, 2001). Long after the preceptor relationship is concluded, the PDS maintains contact with new nurses to ensure small problems are addressed quickly and effectively. This level of support, provided on all shifts, is a significant step in decreasing nursing vulnerability.

Clinical educators, another role in the CNE, provide programs for new employee orientation, expanded knowledge acquisition, preceptor development, and nursing assistant and patient transporter orientation. These programs are critically important to provide structure, information, and outline expectations for new employees. This phase of the pipeline ensures new employees have the "starter set" of skills, the help of the preceptor, and the guidance of the PDS, thus reducing their sense of vulnerability as they verify their skills and knowledge. A purposeful and effective introduction to the organization is critical to the new employee's future satisfaction and sense of confidence. Effective onboarding processes reduce vulnerability by setting a tone of caring about the individual nurse and empowerment to provide excellence in nursing care.

Another key partner in this process is the support of expert support staff, including a person with excellent computer and communication skills. One of the most complex challenges in a large and multicampus setting is communication. It affects the morale of staff and the ability to standardize practice patterns. The CNE is consciously working on multifocal methods of communication with nursing staff. An example of this is the recently updated and comprehensive internal website called *FirstSource*. Other strategies are the use of e-mail and other online methods, brochures, flyers, rounding, and telecommunicated messages. This will continue to be an ongoing challenge for the Center to face.

Conclusion

The CNE at SMC is an innovative model program committed to reducing the vulnerability and increasing the resiliency of nurses by an active engaged approach that values the nurse–patient relationship and supports the nurse in the caregiving role. The mission is "to inspire clinical excellence by providing comprehensive, innovative resources and services to nurses, patients/families, and the community." The CNE strives to lift nurses up to their highest level of performance as a way to retain quality staff within a caring environment. Finally, the application of theory and conceptual models to design the work of the CNE staff is an effective way to embed the use of nursing theory into practice.

References

Bartholomew, K. (2006). *Ending nurse-to-nurse hostility: Why nurses eat their young and each other.* Marblehead, MA: HCPro.

Benner, P. (1984). *From novice to expert: Excellence and power in clinical nursing practice.* Menlo Park, CA: Addison-Wesley.

Chinn, P., & Kramer, M. (2004). *Integrating knowledge development in nursing* (6th ed.). St. Louis, MO: Mosby.

DeLellis, A. (2000). Clarifying the concept of respect: Implications for leadership. *Journal of Leadership Studies, 7*, 35–49.

Drucker, P. (1993). *Post-capitalist society*. New York: Harper Business.

Drucker, P. (2002). *Managing in the next society*. New York: Truman Talley Books St. Martin's Press.

Duchscher, J. B. (2001). Out in the real world: Newly graduated nurses in acute-care speak out. *Journal of Nursing Administration, 31*(9), 426–439.

Freire, P. (1971). *Pedagogy of the oppressed*. New York: Herder & Herder.

Friedson, E. (1970). *Profession of medicine*. New York: Harper & Row.

Hardin, S., & Kaplow, R. (Eds.). (2005). *Synergy for clinical excellence: The AACN synergy model for patient care*. Sudbury, MA: Jones and Bartlett.

Henderson, V. (2006). The concept of nursing. *Journal of Advanced Nursing, 53*(1), 21–34.

Institute of Medicine. (2004). *Keeping patients safe: Transforming the work environment of nurses*. Washington, DC: The National Academies Press.

Knox, S., & Gharrity, J. (2004). Creating a center for nursing excellence. *JONA'S Healthcare Law, Ethics, and Regulation, 6*(2), 44–51.

Kupperschmidt, B. R. (2006). Addressing multigenerational conflict: Mutual respect and care-fronting as strategy. *OJIN: The Online Journal of Issues in Nursing, 11*(2), 1–14.

Miller, J. B. (1976). *Toward a new psychology of women*. Boston: Beacon Press.

Porter-O'Grady, T. (2003). *Quantum leadership: A textbook of new leadership*. Sudbury, MA: Jones and Bartlett.

Roberts, S. J. (1983). Oppressed group behavior: Implications for nursing. *Advances in Nursing Science*, July, 21–30.

Swanson, K. M. (1991). Empirical development of a middle range theory of caring. *Nursing Research, 40*(3), 161–166.

Swedish Medical Center (SMC). (2006). *Home Page*. Retrieved September 13, 2007, from http://www.swedish.org

U.S. Department of Health and Human Services. (2000, March). *The registered nurse population: Findings from the National Sample Survey of Registered Nurses* (pp. 1–135). Retrieved September 13, 2007, from http://bhpr.hrsa.gov/healthworkforce/reports/rnsurvey/rnss1.htm

Opening a Clinic: A Far-Off Dream Becomes a Reality

Rebecca K. Conte

This chapter describes the inspiration behind New Seed International USA, a foundation created for the purpose of opening a clinic in Ghana. Although nursing is an international profession, practices vary drastically among countries. As a nursing student at Seattle University in Seattle, Washington, I viewed nursing as a transcultural practice, changeable according to cultural beliefs but generally practiced in a similar manner. When walking into the regional hospital in Ghana after my junior year of nursing school, my eyes were opened to a different way of practicing nursing, a way that was both novel and foreign to me. I spent 6 weeks experiencing firsthand the people, culture, environment, education, and politics and how all of these affected the delivery of health care. After completing my time in Ghana, I could not forget this experience and wanted to stay connected with this beautiful country in any way possible.

Vulnerability in the United States occurs usually at a time when one is susceptible to negative health outcomes; however, in other parts of the world vulnerability is a life-long reality. The individuals with whom I worked face healthcare obstacles daily. This chapter provides a glimpse into my experience in this beautiful West African country, and I hope to help the reader connect with the vulnerability and adversity these people face daily. More importantly, this chapter is designed to encourage others to make a change in this world—to take action when they see a need. Many times throughout the establishment of New Seed International USA, I was reminded of my age. I was 21 and trying to do something to help those I cared about, but age does not matter if one cares about an issue and is willing to take action. I hope this chapter will provide a basic framework that others can use, if not to establish an organization, then at least to follow passions of their own in whatever way seems appropriate.

Setting

Life in Ghana

Ghana is a small country located along the Atlantic Ocean in West Africa. Roughly equivalent to the geographical size of Oregon, Ghana has a population of 22.4 million (Central

Intelligence Agency, 2007), compared with Oregon's state population of 3.6 million (U.S. Census Bureau, 2007). Ghana was the first sub-Saharan African country to gain independence in 1957 (Central Intelligence Agency, 2007). Since it was first an English colony, English is still the primary language. However, there are up to 80 African dialects found throughout the country, with nine main spoken languages (Central Intelligence Agency, 2007). Ghana is divided into 10 different regions. One of the largest artificial lakes in the world, Lake Volta is in the east and runs from north to south. I resided in Volta Region, surrounding Lake Volta, in one of its 15 separate districts (Central Intelligence Agency, 2007). Ho, the capitol of Volta Region, is a larger district called home by over 76,000 people (Makafui Amenuvor, personal communication, June 17, 2006).

Slave Trade

With its location along the coast easily accessible to the New World, Ghana was the second largest slave transporter in the world. The 300-mile ocean coast became the home for over 300 slave forts, including the two largest ever to exist, Elmina Castle and Cape Coast Castle (Embassy of Ghana, 2007). I became physically sick as I saw the living quarters of the slaves at Cape Coast Castle, the second largest slave fort. Lines are drawn 10 inches above the ground, showing where ground level used to be. When the slave forts were excavated in 1979, the ground level was 10.5 inches higher because of excrements from the slaves, so packed down that it become a new floor level (Cape Coast Castle Tour Guide, personal communication, July 1, 2006). Millions of Africans were sent to Cape Coast Castle, but not all were shipped out of Ghana because many did not survive the miserable living conditions in the forts.

Although the living conditions were terrible in the fort, these conditions did not improve once the slaves were shipped off as laborers to a new country. As slaves were leaving Ghana, they traveled through underground tunnels that led to the "door of no return." This door signified the leaving of their country, boarding a ship, and being sent to a new world where they were sold for labor. After the slave trade had officially ended, the British returned, sealing shut the tunnel to the door of no return. This closing signified that no individual would ever walk that path again.

Unfortunately, slavery still exists in Ghana. Today, trafficking children into forced labor or sexual exploitation happens all over the country (U.S. Department of Labor, 2007). Parents are told stories of how their children will become apprentices in fishery or other vocational skills. Parents sell their children, thinking they are providing a better life for them, but they never see their children again and often do not receive payment. According to the U.S. Department of State's Trafficking in Persons Report (2006) the International Organization of Migration estimates that thousands of children are sold to work in fishing villages around Lake Volta alone, excluding other forced labor and sexually exploited children. If sold into sexual exploitation, women and children are usually sent out of the country, either to Europe or Nigeria.

Health Care in Ghana

The healthcare system in Ghana is divided into four sectors: national, regional, district, and private. At the national level are the Ministry of Health and Ghanaian Health Services. The Ministry of Health's primary purpose is for policy formation and determining the responsibilities of each branch of health care throughout the country. Ghanaian Health Services implements that which is determined by the Ministry of Health. Ghanaian Health Services is the allocation of the resources provided to and by the Ghanaian government to public facilities while also partnering with the private sector healthcare services.

Below the national level is the regional level. The primary responsibility of the regional level is to implement the national level policies with the district level. The regional level serves as the primary link between the national and district level. Regional healthcare facilities usually provide better care. While working at a regional hospital many patients I encountered were transferred from other district hospitals and other regions. This is similar to health care in the United States when an individual can be transferred to receive a higher level of medical care and at a level 1 medical center.

Although some regional facilities exist, primary care is usually provided by the district. Within each district in Ghana (which could serve one to several villages), services are implemented. This is where most individuals seek health care. Services provided are usually for tertiary or emergency care, although community health nurses are provided by Ghanaian Health Services. These community health nurses primarily go into villages and provide immunizations and height, weight, and other assessments when necessary (assessments are usually only provided for children in need of referral to a hospital or private clinic). When cases are in need of more medical attention than that provided by a district facility, some individuals seek services from the regional facility (which could be hours away from their village). Private sector facilities are also available but are often unaffordable to individuals. Although private clinics provide services that for some are unaffordable, these are less expensive than going to a hospital where a patient would need to be admitted for a minimum of 24 hours.

HIV Infection in Ghana

Overall statistics that give HIV infection rates for the entire country are unfortunately an inaccurate portrayal of the HIV rate in Ghana. With such a large population and infection rates varying drastically between regions, it is more accurate to view HIV infection rates by separate regions or districts.

Many Ghanaians have different views as to why rates vary between regions. Some Ghanaians believe that when Africans were enslaved they were taught how to behave by their masters. For example, the French were viewed as promiscuous, having many sexual partners, and the African nations that were French colonies have high HIV rates (Dr. Joe Appiah-Kusi, personal communication, November 15, 2006). For example, according to

UNICEF (2005a, 2005b), Togo has an estimated adult transmission rate of 3.2%, whereas Ghana's adult transmission rate is 2.3%.

Other Ghanaians explain that sex trafficking is more prevalent along the border with Togo (coinciding with the previous French promiscuity theory), which might explain why HIV rates are higher among border regions, especially the Volta and Eastern regions. Sex trafficking is also believed to be more common in the country's capitol of Accra, explaining the higher HIV transmission rate in the Greater Accra region. Although these theories are not supported by data, this is the view of some Ghanaians regarding HIV transmission in their country.

My Experience

New Seed International

While living in Ho I worked at the Volta Regional Hospital and with a nongovernmental organization called New Seed International (NSI). NSI was founded by Livinus Acquah-Jackson, a Ghanaian whose original intention was to build a community center for youth. Once Livinus realized the devastation of AIDS in his community, his passion quickly changed to caring for those infected with the deadly virus. Working out of a small 8-by-12 foot office, NSI impacts the lives of those living with HIV/AIDS daily. Patients travel from as far away as Togo to seek assistance from NSI in hopes that as patients they will receive appropriate health care if NSI fights for them.

NSI's primary activities include, but are not limited to, educating communities on HIV/AIDS, understanding stigmas, teaching how it is transmitted, and how to care for a loved one infected with the virus. NSI also works on preventing the spread of HIV/AIDS by supporting vulnerable individuals at risk for contracting the virus, especially young women who are likely to enter into prostitution if unable to get a job to financially support their families. In these cases NSI helps individuals find jobs to financially sustain their families. NSI advocates for patients in a healthcare setting and completes home healthcare visits for individuals who are infected and unable to leave their homes to seek medical assistance. (If hospitalization is needed, NSI transports the patient to the local hospital.) NSI also provides family support to those caring for someone infected with HIV/AIDS (including counseling, education, financial support, and any other means requested by the family).

Working with NSI changed my life. Patients that I worked with on a daily basis, most of whom are no longer living, will remain in my heart forever. When going for a home health visit, I would sit on a patient's bed and watch his or her respiration rate decrease as he or she struggled with each breath and fought to stay alive. Sometimes we rushed individuals to the hospital, where more often than not they would just wait for medical care that was never given. At some point they would give up and die. This was the routine for all patients infected with HIV. Almost all seroconvert to AIDS because of a lack of appropriate healthcare treatment. Although I do not have the answers as to why treatment was not provided (my thoughts are that it is either because the healthcare professionals are uneducated about the HIV virus or the stigma associated with the disease leaves them not wanting to treat these individuals), I do know that antiretroviral medications are available in Ghana but are often not prescribed, especially in the Volta Region. NSI fights for these patients and hopes that one day the death rate will decrease from its current 73%.

Opening a Clinic

After my experience in Ghana I came home emotionally drained. I continued my contact with Livinus, only to hear e-mail after e-mail that more patients that changed my life were now dead. I got to the point where I was crying almost every day because of my heartache for my new home in Ho, which was thousands of miles away. I believed that no matter how much I longed to make a change, it was impossible while I remained in Seattle. I was wrong.

Livinus had an idea to open the "Save More Lives Project," a mix between a community center, clinic, and hospital. I knew the original idea was a little unrealistic but that there was a way to make it more feasible. After brainstorming, I realized that what was really needed was a clinic where healthcare professionals were adequately educated about HIV/AIDS. Patients could come into the clinic and receive education, counseling, and treatment and medication as needed. The latter was the most important aspect of building the clinic, because if treatment was going to be provided in the same way that it was at Volta Regional Hospital, there was no reason for a new building.

My plan is to return to Ghana after graduation and oversee the process of this project. With many potential builders already wanting to help, my goal is that construction will begin this summer so I can start educating possible employees on how treatment will be provided at our clinic. Some question my ideas for change and believe that the present type of care provided to these patients is simply appropriate within the culture, but through my work with Livinus and many others in the community I am well aware that this is not the case. With sufficient education about the virus, best practices in treatment and holistic nursing care, and outreach work for those infected, the outlook of a patient with AIDS in this community can drastically improve.

While in Ghana I sent e-mails home regularly to share my experiences and emotional challenges of watching lives disappear in front of me. Upon my return I discovered that a family friend had sent my e-mails to the *Seattle Post-Intelligencer*, a local newspaper, sharing with them what I had experienced. The newspaper later contacted me because they were interested in writing a story on my future aspirations in Ghana. "Nursing Student on a Mission to Build a Hospital in Ghana" (Black, 2006) hit the stands, and my faint dream of someday seeing this come to life instantly became a reality.

My e-mail inbox was flooded by people from around the world who were inspired or wanted to help in any way they could. I was overwhelmed by the response. I was given multiple opportunities to share my story through presentations. Along with sharing my story I was able to put a face to AIDS in Africa for many who did not know much about the devastation. Many believe that the lack of treatment is because of the lack of resources, so time and energy is placed in sending medications over. Although that is a problem in many other African countries, Ghana has appropriate resources but is not allocating those resources effectively.

By educating others I was able to share my opinions on how one person can make a difference, without having to move to Ghana to change outcomes. We can make differences through the way we vote, what policies we support, the organizations we become involved in, and by simply being educated on how to help make a change. Through all these opportunities I encountered doors continued to open, making everything come together in a very short time. As a result, New Seed International USA was born.

Procedure for Establishing New Seed International USA

An acquaintance from my years as a high school athlete contacted me saying that he could help start the nongovernmental organization. As a lawyer who had helped many individuals start a nongovernmental organization, he offered to help me complete the paperwork needed to qualify for state recognition as an organization and tax-deductible status from the Internal Revenue Service (IRS). My acquaintance advised me on most of the process for setting up the organization and served as the main resource for the information to follow. The process included developing Articles of Incorporation, Directors and Officers, Bylaws, applying to the state for organization status, and applying to the IRS for tax-deductible status. Although this quantity of paperwork can be intimidating, most of the information needed is not complex. I describe the various components below.

After deliberation with family and a few close friends, I realized this was the right long-term decision for NSI. The resources provided to me by the law firm and other members of the community gave me the comfort I needed to know that I could take on this challenge. Although it did not happen overnight, the law firm compiled all the appropriate paperwork in a matter of weeks.

Articles of Incorporation

First we had to develop Articles of Incorporation, which are the primary rules or guidelines used to run a corporation. All necessary information regarding the corporation is needed in this document. For instance, we first had to select a name. Because the primary goal of this organization was to financially support NSI in Ghana, I decided to create the sister organization, NSI USA (USA is added for identification purposes only—the legal name used for our organization is New Seed International). Other information includes the duration of our existence as a corporation (perpetual), the registered office and agent (the registered office is my home address and I am the agent), the incorporator (myself), and purposes and powers. The purposes and power section describes our reason for forming this organization. In this section I explained how NSI USA primarily will focus on supporting NSI Ghana by funding the construction of a clinic and helping financially maintain services needed for the clinic to serve the HIV/AIDS population in Volta Region.

Directors and Officers

After developing the basic guidelines or rules for NSI USA (by writing the Articles of Incorporation), NSI USA then needed to establish leadership in the form of directors and officers. A director or board of directors serves as the executive counsel of the corporation. For NSI USA I am the sole director. As the director I am in charge of managing all affairs. Generally, for large companies power is split between the board of directors and shareholders. To keep the establishment of NSI USA simple, one director was established with many officers. Offices are held by individuals to help run internal operations or the day-to-day aspects of the company. Positions held by officers include president, vice president, secretary, and treasurer. For NSI USA these positions are held by other individuals devoted to a positive outlook for those infected with HIV/AIDS in Volta Region and surrounding areas.

Bylaws

Bylaws are the set of rules used to govern internal affairs and management of an organization. The bylaws are drafted according to what the Articles of Incorporation document determines. For NSI USA I drafted the bylaws as the director. Bylaws can include information ranging from how directors are elected, how meetings for the directors and officers are to be conducted and for what purposes, and what offices will be held as well as the description of each office role. NSI USA's bylaws contain articles regarding information on our organization: name and location of officers, purpose, information regarding the board of directors, how officers will be elected and a description of each office, administrative provision, and how any future amendments will be made.

Application to the State

To be recognized as a charitable organization, the organization must go through the application process in any state in which it wishes to be recognized. To become NSI USA I had to apply to Washington State to receive a certificate of recognition under our organization name. The application is very short and includes general information about the organization including background information, organizational structure, purpose of this organization, basic financial information, administrative information, and fundraising information.

Form 1023: Application to the IRS

Form 1023 is filed for the purposes of receiving tax-exempt status from the government. Some nonprofit organizations can appeal to the government for this status. Not only would this excuse NSI USA from filing taxes, it would also allow large donors to give tax-deductible contributions to our organization. The application to the IRS for this tax-exempt status was the longest part of the process to establish NSI USA. This process has become more challenging since September 11, 2001, in order for the government to better monitor finances sent to other organizations outside of the United States (Julie Yee, personal communication, November 30, 2006).

Form 1023 includes information from all previous paperwork needed as well as additional information in greater detail. The form is 28 pages long, but also asks for additional attachment information where more than a sentence answer is needed (some answers require multiple paragraphs of detailed information). After the general information needed is supplied, the application goes into specific activities of the organization. This includes any information regarding involvement with other organizations, any housing or age-specific requirements, working location, how our clients will benefit from our establishment, whether we provide education through our program, and so on. Although this process seems tedious, it is vital to the acceptance of our tax-exempt status.

The key part of this application process for NSI USA was the detailed financial data outlook for the next 4 years. When I first started this process the lawyer informed me that any projected income over $25,000 in one fiscal year would require the assistance of a certified public accountant. Having a certified public accountant shows the government an accurate account of all expenses, therefore making the organization more trustworthy. With the help of my certified public accountant, we projected our future financial income and expenses. Because my goal is to receive all the funds for the clinic by the end of 2007, we hope our income will be $50,000 for our first year. While we acquire this significant amount of money, we also plan to have $50,000 of expenses because we hope to start building. This made the financial data on the application easier to complete because we plan for our expenses every year to match our income of that same fiscal year.

Long-Term Plans

Since NSI USA has begun, I have been playing catchup. After the newspaper article brought attention to the public, I started NSI USA, filed all necessary paperwork, opened a bank account, gave numerous presentations, and started a website. Although this has been an important process, it has been overwhelming in my senior year and I look forward to graduation and being able to dedicate more of my time to NSI USA.

As for the future of NSI USA, the first project is to continue to raise funds for building the clinic in Ghana. As director I plan to return to Ghana after graduation. Among other things, this trip will include gathering data for future projects, fundraising, checking the status of the building project (whether it is already underway or if more information needs to be gathered before construction), and beginning to educate staff on appropriate care for those infected/affected by HIV/AIDS. My goal is for all funds needed for the construction of the clinic to be raised by the time of construction, which hopefully will occur within the year 2007.

Once the building of the clinic is done, the first initial years of the incorporation of NSI USA will continue to include fundraising. As of today, those couple of years will focus on financially supporting the clinic until it is able to sustain itself. Once the clinic is self-supporting, my goal for NSI USA is to find other ways of improving rural HIV/AIDS care, in Ghana as well as in other countries in Africa. While I continue to learn about running an organization, I look forward to the doors that NSI USA will continue to open on behalf of vulnerable populations in the future.

Conclusion

This chapter describes the process to start New Seed International USA as a tax-deductible organization in the state of Washington, but the process might be different in other states. Although this chapter does not cover every bit of information needed to become an organization, it provides some of the basic information. For those who are not planning to do anything as complex as starting an organization, I hope that my story proves that anything is possible with passion, determination, and some hard work.

References

Black, C. (2006). Nursing student on a mission to build a hospital in Ghana. *The Seattle Post-Intelligencer*. Retrieved September 4, 2007, from http://seattlepi.nwsource.com/local/290693_nurse01.html

Central Intelligence Agency. (2007). *The world factbook*. Retrieved September 4, 2007, from https://www.cia.gov/cia/publications/factbook/geos/gh.html

Embassy of Ghana. (2007). *Ghana tourism*. Retrieved February 13, 2007, from http://www.ghanatourism.gov.gh/regions/region_detail.asp

UNICEF. (2005a). *At a glance: Ghana: Statistics*. Retrieved September 4, 2007, from http://www.unicef.org/infobycountry/ghana_statistics.html

UNICEF. (2005b). *Togo: Statistics*. Retrieved September 4, 2007, from http://www.unicef.org/infobycountry/togo_statistics.html

U.S. Census Bureau. (2007). *State & county quickfacts*. Retrieved September 4, 2007, from http://quickfacts.census.gov/qfd/states/41000.html

U.S. Department of Labor: Bureau of International Labor Affairs. (2007). *Ghana: Incidence and nature of child labor*. Retrieved September 4, 2007, from http://www.dol.gov/ilab/media/reports/iclp/tda2004/ghana.htm

U.S. Department of State. (2006). *Trafficking in persons report*. Retrieved September 4, 2007, from http://www.state.gov/documents/organization/66086.pdf

Chapter 35

Program Proposal for Native American/Alaskan Native Community Organization

Charee L. Taccogno

This chapter provides an example of a community need, analyzes a relevant nursing theory, and translates the need and theory into a community-based program proposal. This program is further described by its staff, staff functions, and role in the community. The program's underlying assumption is that the participation of community members promotes change and empowers individuals and community (Anderson, Guthrie, & Schirle, 2002).

Background

I wanted to create a program that would target those living in isolated areas on the Navajo reservation. I have witnessed the solitary life-style of a traditional 80-year-old woman who speaks only Navajo, weaves rugs, and raises sheep. She does not have indoor plumbing, electricity, or means of transportation. Like many others within this population she has diabetes and hypertension. Her way of life can be problematic because she cannot read the labels on her prescribed and over-the-counter medications and has to travel 45 miles to the nearest clinic. Although this case is emotionally compelling, I have discovered other pressing needs within this community. I provided this example as an illustration of the unexpected outcomes or assessments in program development.

In reference to the health status of the general U.S. population, the previous Surgeon General, David Satcher, commented, "over half of the deaths that occur in this country in any given year are caused by human behavior" (Johnson & Rhoades, 2000, p. 81). On Native American/Alaskan Native reservations this statement is especially true. Johnson and Rhoades (2000) further elaborate that any behavior change depends on the individual and that the medical system can only provide information and create environments to promote healthy life-styles. This belief is challenged by an alternate view that behavioral change is not dependent on the individual because the individual responds to the environment and then acts on the environment. Thus behavioral change can occur and can be based on an intervention from the surrounding community or environment.

Conceptual Framework: Community Organization for Change

The nursing model of community organization for change is a framework that uses the theories of ecology, systems, diffusion, social support, and social learning to assist the community health nurse to develop appropriate interventions for community change (Anderson, Guthrie, & Schirle, 2002). A common theme is that there are continuous inputs and outputs that interact with and influence the individual, family, neighbors, schools, churches, city, and government. Thus a community-based program is appropriate to create individual behavioral change because it is the environment that has already influenced and perpetuated the current use of risky behaviors. Per Benner, the individual, or person, is not born with a set of ingrained behaviors or personality traits but through life's experiences an individual's behavior and personality take shape (Brykczynski, 2006). In community program planning it is important to note this theory as part of different interpretations of self; King stated that individuals have differences in needs, wants, and goals (Sieloff, 2006). Therefore the success of any community intervention depends on the participation of the community, but it must also value the individuality within that community.

The other components of the theories of ecology, systems, diffusion, and social support can be generalized as being the environment. The environment contains all the physical and nonphysical components that surround the individual. Physical components of the environment include the individual's immediate surroundings and supplies: shelter, food, water, clothing, transportation, and so on. The environment is further defined by geographical region that is composed of services, terrain, climate, and population. As the individual is inherently different, so is each environment that can be used to help or hinder the person. The environment changes from city to city and from neighborhood to neighborhood, house to house, and room to room.

There are also nonphysical components to the environment, which is especially true when attempting to define a community. As previously stated, persons make up part of the physical environment. It is their attitudes, beliefs, and interactions with the individual that create an intangible environment. A community is a group of any size and can be defined in different aspects relating to its government, locality, culture, heritage, religion, occupation, and common interests (Baker & Brownson, 1999; Dictionary.com, 2007; Issel, 2004). Primarily, the community members have the potential for interaction, an emotional connection, and accepted values and norms (Baker & Brownson, 1999; Issel, 2004).

In Anderson's, Guthrie's and Schirle's (2002) model, the community health nurse (CHN) and the community are at the center and interact at all stages of program development (assessment, planning, implementation, and evaluation). The CHN and community interactions are in the form of empowerment, partnership, participation, community competence, and cultural responsiveness. However, these interactions have also been described as key objectives of community-based participatory action research. Teufel-Shone, Siyuja, Watahomigie, and Irwin (2006) illustrated that community-based participatory research is an acceptable and valuable tool in Native American/Alaskan Native communities. This framework acknowledges the high distrust of Native American/Alaskan Natives toward government and research, that within their community community members are culturally competent, and the community members are given the opportunity to make decisions in their community.

The frameworks of participatory action research and community organization for change are closely related. The outcomes of participatory action research are generally measured by the community's interactions and capacity building; however, Minkler (2000) discussed the lack of consensus in what constitutes participatory action research. For some researchers it was the ability to have the community involved only in the assessment phase, whereas for others it was to have the community members involved at all program phases. The lack of consensus is also evident in the various terminology used as in community-based participatory research or community engagement. These processes lack an *action* component. Without action the community does not witness the outcome of an assessment as scholars and researchers do in the form of a journal article or conference presentation. A more tangible and measurable outcome is needed. Future communities may be hesitant to assist in any future research or health promotion endeavors if there are only continual assessments and no action. For this reason, the organization for change model is a valuable framework because it also incorporates the most outer layer, the program.

The organization for change model has several assumptions: (1) improvements in community health result from increased community competence, (2) individuals learn from participating, (3) a program is more likely to succeed and be sustainable if the community participates, and (4) health-seeking and health-promoting behaviors are influenced by culture (Anderson et al., 2002).

Sample Case

A program was developed with the modified organization for change model as a guiding framework. Following is a description of a program envisioned for the Navajo community to improve health outcomes and to increase the quality of life.

Setting and Population

To decrease the mortality rates due to human behavior, a community-based program will be created that uses community health representatives (CHRs) and CHNs to assist the community. The program will be based on the Navajo Reservation, which is in Arizona, Utah, New Mexico, and Colorado. The Navajo Reservation has 110 chapter houses, places that have a community-appointed board, are used for community gatherings, and provide supportive services. Each chapter house reports to a larger program, or agency, of which there are five. These agencies then represent the communities at the Navajo government in Window Rock, Arizona, and the target population includes the Navajos that use the Indian Health Services programs.

Relevance and Significance

Per Stanhope and Lancaster (2006), the program is relevant and significant to the role of a CHN and in fulfilling the goals of *Healthy People 2010*. The CHN works toward promoting a healthy life-style, providing targeted outreach, and forming partnerships. In addition, the overall goals of *Healthy People 2010* are to increase the quality and years of healthy life and to eliminate health disparities. This program will address the more focused objectives to prevent secondary illnesses and increase community education programs through the roles of the CHN. Currently, the Indian Health Service (2006) has three divisions that can work together to accomplish these goals: Information Technology, Partnership, and Health. Having the need for increased CHRs and CHNs will increase the need for schools or local training centers. Also, the increased visibility of Navajo workers will serve as role models for those in the community, perhaps increasing the numbers of those receiving secondary education.

In addition, the 1976 Indian Health Care Improvement Act (Public Law 94-437) established two national goals: to ensure that the health status of Native Americans is elevated to the highest possible level and to achieve the maximum participation of Native Americans in Native American health programs (Johnson & Rhoades, 2000). These health programs can include inpatient or outpatient care, dental services, preventative services, mental care, and alcohol abuse treatment. This law also provides for scholarship money to be used in increasing health-trained professionals to work with Native American and Alaskan Native populations. This is part of the effort to reduce the proportion of families that experience difficulties or delays in obtaining health care or who do not receive needed care.

Program Goals

The goals of the program are to promote community capacity through education and empowerment and to decrease the mortality rates influenced by human behavior.

Program Staff and Functions

Each chapter house will have a designated CHR. According to the World Health Organization definition, the CHR lives in and is reportable to the community of service (Swider, 2002). All members within the community will be urged to apply, and each chapter house community will vote to select the CHR. This aids in empowering the community and in providing job opportunities in a destitute area, but it is most important in that the community knows the CHR will share the tribe's culture and beliefs (Belone, Gonzalez-Santin, Gustavsson, MacEachron, & Perry, 2002).

Upon selection the CHR will receive training in first aid, basic life support, social services, and information technology. In an extensive literature review, Swider (2002) identified the vast functions of a CHR for the individual and community: an advocate, mediator, educator, and provider. Further, the CHR will be highly encouraged to make his or her own life-style modifications to promote health and decrease risky behavior, such as cigarette smoking cessation, healthy eating, exercising, participation in community activities, and participation in traditional healing exercises. The CHR will have office days at the chapter house and provide services in an individual's home.

The CHR is part of a larger healthcare team; 22 CHNs will also provide services among the 110 chapter houses. The nurse will perform nursing services and also serve as a case manager. The CHN and CHR will both be trained to use information technology for communication, documentation, and evaluation purposes. Within this informatics system will be a database that contains the enrollment numbers, demographics, and electronic medical record of the individuals in the community. As case manager the nurse will monitor, assess, plan, and coordinate services for the client. This nurse will depend on the communication from the CHR and medical provider to guide field visits. By visiting the client at home, the CHN is able to make appropriate home assessments, evaluate medications, change dressings, and provide other necessary follow-up. It is desirable that the CHN is also from the same community.

The CHR and CHN roles have only been described as providing health care; however, both the CHR and CHN will serve as catalysts within the community to achieve the goals of changing behavior and empowering the community. In addition, the CHR and CHN will also serve as change agents as the face-to-face contacts are instrumental in changing patient behavior (Swider, 2002).

Another team member is the advanced practice nurse (APN). The APN, with expert knowledge in community assessment, program planning, and evaluation, will serve as a resource person in guiding representatives and nurses in the community. The APN will also have relationships with tribal, federal, state, and other local governments to affect policy and advocate for the Native American and Alaskan Native populations. Within each phase of the model, it is optimal that the community individuals assist to increase the sustainability of the program and empower the community. Eventually, the CHN will mainly serve as a technical assistant in the community's programs. This makes it difficult to outline the exact interventions of the program, because eventually the community determines interventions.

An important first step for the nursing and representative staff is to establish rapport with community members. Each chapter house will hold a large informal gathering so that the CHR, CHN, and APN can all mingle and meet with the local community. This should happen at each site, and the overall relationship-building phase should be a slow introductory process. Also, Chino and DeBruyn (2006) sited that Western frameworks used in Native American/Alaskan Native communities often fail because they do not allow sufficient time for relationship building. This is a vital step because the opinions, perspectives, and behaviors of willing participants and hesitant community members are likely to vary greatly but can be equally important and informative (Teufel-Shone et al., 2006). Further, community members should not be made to serve as translators or appointment makers but should be collaborators.

Organizing Change: Program Design

This program is being presented as a proposal and requires the collaboration of the community to assess, plan, implement, and evaluate. Thus it is impossible to outline the exact steps and rationale for interventions.

Assessment

The first step in organizing for change is to conduct an assessment or reassessment of the community. This assessment data consist of demographics, the community's culture, available social networks or organizations, and needs wanted by the community. The CHR and CHN perform assessments in formal settings, such as a chapter house meeting or survey, and informally at social events. Teufel-Shone et al. (2006) argued that formative assessments are a necessary phase because Native American/Alaskan Native communities are not homogenous entities. It also shows the community that the individuality within the community is valued. Further, an effective assessment determines whether qualitative or quantitative data will be collected and the methods in which data collection will proceed.

Planning

Program planning is the second step. Although the program goals have already been identified, the community has the power to determine the objectives and interventions to meet those goals. The early objectives should be specific and easily obtainable to increase morale and community participation (Anderson et al., 2002). At this point the plans for evaluation should be clearly outlined so that appropriate documentation occurs. At this time it is seen whether there are training needs for the community or whether outside funding is needed.

Specific program activities can be designed to meet each goal and objective. First, regular visits within a person's home or at social events may reach persons at various stages of the change continuum described by Prochaska, DiClemente, and Norcross (as cited in Anderson, 2005): precontemplation, contemplation, preparation, action, and maintenance. Second, each chapter house elects the CHR to further build community empowerment and capacity to plan. Third, community members are asked to assist in ways that highlight the members' talents or areas of interest. For example, an artist can be encouraged to design a pamphlet or advertisement about the health program. Fourth, traditional healers can be asked to provide a prayer or blessing for the program and should be consulted regarding what is hindering or promoting the community's health. Finally, electronic media should be used. The use of video can be a great asset because Native American/Alaskan Natives are visual learners, and other community members can see the support and involvement of other Native American/Alaskan Natives. It is also important to continually support the community by praising efforts to make change and to advertise these efforts. Anderson (2005) reported that the themes of hopelessness and helplessness plagued vulnerable communities because media reported only on the negative behaviors of these communities. The study participants asked that successes also be acknowledged so they will want to try to make improvements.

Implementation

The next step is to implement the community's developed plan. The community, with the assistance of the CHN, needs to decide on an appropriate time frame for each part of the plan to be initiated and completed. All the community members need to be made aware of the goals, plan, and program end date.

Evaluation and Dissemination of Results

Evaluation of the plan occurs continually and also every project's end. Also called summative evaluation, process evaluation identifies interventions that are working and are not working. The plan then can be altered as necessary. Being able to adjust the project based on the community's feedback is a way in which community competence can be increased. The formative, or outcome, evaluation is used at the end of the program to determine how effective the program was and if there was any unexpected outcomes. Results can be shared at conferences or pow-wows where other tribes may benefit from the knowledge gained in these Navajo communities. Radio stations, local newsletters, and national magazines and newspapers can tell of the actions and results of the community.

Each type of evaluation needs to occur at the APN and community level. The APN needs to be aware if the model is working, which can be done in part by monitoring the presence at chapter house or agency meetings, decreased use of the CHN in project assistance, monies or resources gained, or partnerships formed. The APN can also use anecdotal evidence and data from hospitals or community health centers about number of visits, reasons for visits, and the patient's views of the programs. Each community would want to see the impact of their work, which can be done with qualitative and quantitative tools. Each chapter house or agency could disseminate the results, tools, and procedures on the Internet to prevent duplication of work. Video sharing is a way in which community members can increase self-esteem and make community connections to large institutions (Anderson, 2005). This type of reporting also gives the community some control over what is being reported to the world about them.

Conclusion

This chapter's focus was to identify a community need, analyze a relevant nursing theory, and translate the need and theory into a community-based program. A program was created and staffed so that a community can determine its methods of increasing positive health outcomes. The program did not address exact mechanisms in which it will change individual health behaviors, but it did address that a change in an individual's environment will influence the individual.

References

Anderson, D., Guthrie, T., & Schirle, R. (2002). A nursing model of community organization for change. *Public Health Nursing, 19*(1), 40–46.

Anderson, J. B. (2005). Unraveling health disparities: Examining the dimensions of hypertension and diabetes through community engagement. *Journal of Health Care for the Poor and Underserved, 16*(4), 91–117.

Baker, E., & Brownson, C. (1999). Defining characteristics of community-based health promotion programs. In R. Brownson, E. Baker, & L. Novick (Eds.), *Community-based prevention: Programs that work* (pp. 7–19). Gaithersburg, MD: Aspen.

Belone, C., Gonzalez-Santin, E., Gustavsson, N., MacEachron, A. E., & Perry, T. (2002). *Social services: The Navajo way* (pp. 773–769). Arlington, VA: Child Welfare League of America.

Brykczynski, K. A. (2006). Patricia Benner: From novice to expert. Excellence and power in clinical nursing practice. In A. M. Tomey & M. R. Alligood (Eds.), *Nursing theorists and their work* (pp. 140–166). St. Louis, MO: Mosby.

Chino, M., & DeBruyn, L. (2006). Building true capacity: Indigenous models for indigenous communities. American Journal of Public Health, *96*(4), 596–599.

Dictionary.com (2007). Definition of "community." Retrieved, March 11, 2007, from http://dictionary.reference.com/browse/community

Issel, M. L. (2004). *Health program planning and evaluation: A practical, systematic approach for community health.* Sudbury, MA: Jones and Bartlett.

Johnson, E. A., & Rhoades, E. R. (2000). The history and organization of Indian health services and system. In E. R. Rhoades (Ed.), *American Indian health: Innovations in health care, promotion, and policy* (pp. 74–92). Baltimore: The Johns Hopkins University Press.

Minkler, M. (2002). Using participatory action research to build healthy communities. *Public Health Reports, 115*, 191–197.

Sieloff, C. L. (2006). Imogene King: Interacting systems framework and middle range theory of goal attainment. In A. M. Tomey & M. R. Alligood (Eds.), *Nursing theorists and their work* (pp. 297–317). St. Louis, MO: Mosby.

Stanhope, M., & Lancaster, J. (2006). *Foundations of nursing in the community: Community-oriented practice* (2nd ed.). St. Louis, MO: Mosby.

Swider, S. M. (2002). Outcome effectiveness of community health workers: An integrative literature review. *Public Health Nursing, 19*(1), 11–20.

Teufel-Shone, N. I., Siyuja, T., Watahomigie, H. J., & Irwin, S. (2006). Community-based participatory research: Conducting a formative assessment of factors that influence youth wellness in the Hualapai community. *American Journal of Public Health, 96*(9), 1623–1628.

Mobile Care Clinic: An Integrated Program for the Homeless

Linda Frothinger

On any given day in the United States approximately 1% of the population is homeless. Defining homeless as one who lives without a permanent resident, this person may sleep in a shelter, transitional housing, an abandoned building, vehicle, outdoors, or any other nonpermanent location (Griner, 2006). In January 2007 2,140 homeless were counted in the greater Seattle area during King County Public Health's "One Night Count." These numbers, however, do not reflect the number of people staying in emergency shelters or transitional housing, in which case the total homeless population is estimated at more than 5,000. This brings Seattle's homeless percentage closer to 1.5%, with the Seattle area population estimated at 3.4 million (King County Public Health, 2005).

Health care for this population is a significant issue in Seattle, where nearly 100% of Seattle's homeless rely on community health clinics and hospital emergency departments for primary health care (King County Public Health, 2005) because of a lack of a place to go, referral, transportation, and insurance. This reflects the root causes for homelessness, as discussed by Aday (2001) in *At Risk in America*, who suggested economical, social, and political structures as basic and essential to individual well-being. When these structures do not adequately support an individual, poor outcomes in health and daily sustenance are compromised. Simply lacking the basic essential resources puts an individual at risk for health and wellness (Aday, 2001).

Presented here is a proposed model to address the homeless population's need for health care. A theoretical approach of care designed to address the numerous mental and physical issues prevalent in the homeless population is central. A proposed model directed at behavior and integration of healthcare disciplines provides a framework upon which a mobile care unit may address the multiple healthcare needs of the homeless population. The outcome proposing that the homeless person's reliance on the emergency department for primary care may decrease as a multidisciplinary approach to health care begins to address the economic, social, and political structures of support for this individual, ultimately empowering the homeless person to become self-sustaining.

Background to Increase in Population Disparity and Health Care

Health care for the homeless population is not a new idea. The 1980s prompted the American government to initiate investigations into the growing disparities in our country's population, resulting in publicly and privately funded projects. In the 20 plus years since this "campaign," disparities continue to exist, with the gap widening between upper middle class and poverty.

The 1990s investigation into health disparities realized by an increasingly growing number of vulnerable individuals prompted initiatives to focus on basic provision of care. However, for the homeless care is not basic. Care not only includes primary medical but also mental health, substance abuse, dental, optometry, and podiatry (Aday, 2001). The mobile healthcare clinic in Seattle proposes to address the multiple health concerns of this population through the integration of healthcare provision by a physician, a nurse practitioner, an occupational therapist, and a behavioral master's prepared nurse.

Case Study

Sunday morning a college student rides through downtown Seattle on the metro (public bus transportation). The streets are quiet but not without the form of someone curled up in a building entryway, attempting to sleep and stay warm. Transferring to another bus, the student gets off the bus and walks to her next bus stop. She eyes another individual staring and seemingly unaware. He falls, hitting his head, triggering a seizure. She calls 911.

The patient is a 39-year-old homeless man, known as C.T. Admitting diagnosis is generalized seizure, comorbidity, upper respiratory infection, and questionable alcohol withdrawal. Testing includes a magnetic resonance image to rule out brain tumor and hemorrhage and lumbar puncture to rule out bacterial meningitis. Complete blood count and arterial blood gas indicate elevated white blood cell count and trace of Phenytoin, 2 μm/ml, which is a subtherapeutic level. C.T. spends the next 3 days in the hospital on a medical/surgical unit visited daily by a hospitalist.

Four days into his hospital stay a nurse practitioner enters C.T.'s room, introducing herself as the nurse who will help C.T. with his follow-up care after leaving the hospital in the next couple of days. The nurse practitioner comes to learn that C.T. developed a seizure disorder after his Gulf War deployment. After suffering a brain injury C.T. began experiencing headaches and dizziness. After returning home he found it difficult to hold a job, resulting in the end of his 2-year marriage. He was then 24 years old. The past 15 years C.T. has spent moving from job to job, each one ending with the onset of a seizure. C.T. normally does well with his daily 400 mg of Dilantin and for a few days after he runs out. However, after going without medication for more than 3 or 4 days C.T. usually experiences a generalized seizure, followed by a hospital emergency department visit to refill his Dilantin. His primary care provider left a few months back, and he hasn't found another. The nurse practitioner listens intently, understanding that the mobile clinic she volunteers in may be able to help C.T. address his health needs.

Comorbidities including depression and stress related to C.T.s homelessness exacerbate his seizure disorder. Stress often acts as a precursor to the onset of a seizure, with the seizure itself putting undo stress on the brain. Aggravation of one only serves to intensify the other, ultimately influencing C.T.s behavioral responses. This is observed during C.T.'s hospital stay as the hospitalist attempts to get C.T.'s Dilantin levels within a therapeutic range of 10–20 μm/ml. C.T. experiences two additional generalized seizures during the time that he is put back on Dilantin until a therapeutic range is achieved. This adds to C.T.'s level of stress, which only aggravates his situation. By C.T.'s fourth hospital day he has experienced two generalized seizures and several partial seizures. By day 5 a therapeutic Dilantin level of 14 μm/ml is achieved, and C.T. is nearing the end of his stay. What will happen to him when he leaves?

Mobile Health Clinic

Addressing the challenges of homeless individuals who leave Seattle's area hospitals prompted the nurse practitioner to investigate the feasibility of initiating a mobile care clinic to meet this population's needs. Homeless individuals' needs surpass those who live in a group or family environment where emotional needs are more likely supported. Beyond the emotional needs of the homeless individual, there are also issues focusing on simple sustenance, resources, and continuity in basic health care. Working within the homeless individual's present-time orientation, demographics, and emotional and physical needs becomes the vehicle from which teaching health care and health promotion may transpire (Green, Green, & Dufour, 1994). Ultimately, this teaching results in fewer emergency department visits and hospital readmissions. The cost-effectiveness of such an approach is estimated at a "$3–4 savings for Medicaid for every incremental dollar spent providing disease management support" (Health Care for the Homeless, 2004), suggesting an ultimate saving of governmental dollars.

The implementation of a Seattle mobile clinic started a few years before C.T.'s hospital stay following this nurse practitioner's documentation of homeless patients at a Seattle hospital. She observed that every 1–2 weeks the unit she works on had at least one homeless patient. Lacking primary health providers and/or insurance, these individuals usually came through the emergency department for care, often admitted to the hospital for lengthy stays related to severe infections requiring intravenous antibiotic treatment and/or other health concerns. The cost to care for these homeless individuals became the impetus and foundation of a proposal to three area hospitals to implement a mobile clinic. Each institution employs a nurse practitioner, an occupational therapist, and a behavioral nurse who willingly volunteer one evening weekly. One physician is available one evening each week. The clinic also uses students from area university nurse practitioner programs, occupational therapy programs, and medical residency programs. The premise of the mobile clinic is a multidisciplinary approach to care, addressing physical, behavioral, and psychosocial needs of the individual (National Health Care for the Homeless Council, 2006).

The development of an integrated healthcare program for this population is based on the understanding that the demographic, emotional, and health needs of many homeless people differ from the person with permanent housing and stable income. Considering many homeless individuals are "present-time" oriented suggests the need for a clinic to operate outside the realm of "normal" business hours, able to self-locate to meet the needs of both patient and care providers. This enables the clinic to determine locations in Seattle that might best serve this group of individuals. The clinic also addresses the difficulty many homeless individuals face in traversing the multiple services they may require and the knowledge that nearly 70% of all healthcare visits by the average person carry a psychosocial component. Addressing basic needs complicated by compromised health sets the foundation upon which these four care providers direct their energies (National Health Care for the Homeless Council, 2006). The mobile clinic's provision of care two nights per week becomes a perceived sense of continuity in care, allowing for appropriate follow-up, referrals, and health promotion education. In the eyes of the homeless person where continuity is often missing; weekly clinic visits introduce this concept into their life patterns.

Integration of Care

An integrated care model meets basic medical, physical, and emotional needs within the homeless population by using four goals: meeting immediate physical needs, building a trusting relationship, assimilating the homeless individual into potential service areas with the appropriate resources available, and addressing behavioral issues as they pertain to the physical and psychosocial health of the individual. The nurse practitioner and physician play an essential role in meeting immediate physical needs and building a trusting relationship. The behavioral nurse is integral to establishing a connection across all areas of care and building trusting relationships. They play a leadership and consultant role, coordinating clinical team practices with patient behavior and health promotion. The occupational therapist assists in incorporating real life practices of the patient while addressing their healthcare needs. All providers practice sensitivity to the individual's medical and social implications. Although each of these areas of focus are somewhat defined, a team approach to care enables cross-care teaching and cross-care evaluation to occur between providers (Figure 36-1).

The premise for the clinic's success lies in the team-building concept. Weekly meetings among providers focus on administrative business, case management, observed clinical issues, and individual frustrations. Frustrations are viewed in a supportive environment where value is placed on peer-provided feedback. Evaluation of individual patient programs and the overall clinic program are done monthly with quarterly reports. Data a compiled semiannually into reports, including patient demographics (age, gender, ethnicity, living arrangements, employment/work placement, and/or healthcare coverage or

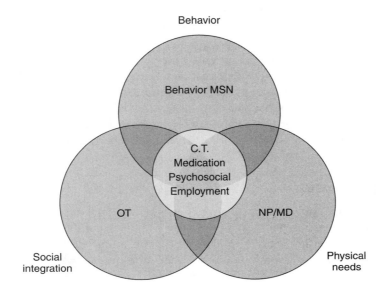

Figure 36-1   Integrated Health Model

MSN, master's prepared nurse; NP/MD, nurse practitioner/medical doctor; OT, occupational therapist.

lack thereof), budget and cost analysis, services provided, student practitioners, number of patient visits, and number of individual repeat visits. These data are also available as monthly or quarterly printouts for review.

Case Study: Integrated Care

Application of C.T.'s case to an integrated healthcare program enables each care provider the opportunity to understand the multiple facets of C.T.'s health. Cross-training is an essential component of the follow-up reports between providers to understand the intertwining health needs of C.T. The interrelationships in C.T.'s health may be understood when we look at his physical health and psychosocial behavioral responses.

Nurse Practitioner and Physician

C.T.'s physical health includes his need for medication to control his seizures, which in turn impacts his psychosocial behavior and subsequent inability to maintain employment, resulting in his homelessness. Addressing his need for medication is central to this team's integrated care approach, including educating C.T. to understand how his medication impacts his total health and function in society. The team understands that his medication can be maintained by the physician and/or the nurse practitioner; however, the behavioral nurse is central to ensuring the nurse practitioner and/or physician intervene effectively. Discussing C.T.'s medication compliance becomes their central focus with the understanding that their cross-training of the other healthcare providers will also become integral in each of their realms of care. In turn, each member of the team incorporates the medication regimen into his or her own plans of care. As comprehension and achievement by C.T. of his daily need for Dilantin become a customary part of his daily routine, addressing C.T.'s other components of health may also become integrated into each provider's plan of care.

Occupational Therapy

The role of an occupational therapist becomes essential to C.T.'s success with the understanding that the profession has moved from early proponents of a mind–body approach, which has reemerged in the past century. The concept of "moral" treatment introduced in the 1700s has evolved into a combination of science and human value prompting occupational therapy to include "meaningful activity" into provision of care and proposing that in conjunction with science, occupational therapists should promote "physical, social and economic rehabilitation of the patient" (Bing, 1981). Occupational therapy's focus on activity in combination with treatment results in a self-actualization process, ultimately preparing the individual for reentrance into society (Griner, 2006).

Occupational therapy will integrate the role Dilantin plays in C.T.'s daily activity, considering the necessity of this medication to manage his seizures, educating C.T. on how this affects his daily activities and psychosocial achievements. The occupational therapist's plan incorporates the medical and nursing practice of medication administration and education, understanding that communication plays an integral part in C.T.'s behavioral responses so that medication adherence may be achieved. C.T. becomes empowered to combine his knowledge and skills with behavioral practices to promote his reentrance into society and self-sufficiency.

Behavioral Nurse

The behavioral nurse continues to implement strategies of communication for each of the providers. Discussion centers on individual plans of care with long-term goals of medication adherence and eventual employment for C.T. Educating C.T. on the interrelationships between his behavior, actions, and health suggests that he will be accountable for understanding these actions. This is fundamental yet crucial to continued care and positive outcomes for C.T. The basis to initiating this process requires C.T.'s willingness to become and remain involved in his care. Starting with weekly clinic visits focusing on medication education and adherence sets the foundation for future success. The frequency of visits in the initial stages of care allows C.T. to begin reframing from a present-time only point of reference to focused reference points in time—the weekly visits. It is here that he begins to take responsibility with the integrated health care, gradually empowered by his physical wellness and continued involvement (National Health Care for the Homeless Council, 2006).

Conclusion

Integrated care has its barriers, including funding, reimbursement limitations, and lack of resources and experience. Yet the advantages cannot be overshadowed by these barriers when indicators point to decreased emergency department visits and an increase in primary and specialty care by homeless populations when given opportunities for health care (Whitley, Everhart, & Wright, 2006). This empowerment has the potential for increased social functioning and an understanding of the connection between behavior and health. Ultimately, personal accountability for connecting behavior with health may be considered an essential foundation for any individual to achieve positive outcomes.

References

Aday, L. A. (2001). *At risk in America: The health and health care needs of vulnerable populations in the United States* (2nd ed.). San Francisco: Jossey-Bass.

Bing, R. K. (1981). Occupational therapy revisited: A paraphrastic journey. *American Journal of Occupational Therapy, 35,* 499–518.

Green, R. D., Green, L., & Dufour, L. T. (1994). Health needs of homeless clients accessing nursing care at a free clinic. *Journal of Community Health Nursing, 11*(3), 139–147.

Griner, K. R. (2006). Helping the homeless: An occupational therapy perspective. *Occupational Therapy in Mental Health, 22*(1), 49–61.

Health Care for the Homeless. (2004). *Outcomes for primary health care programs.* Retrieved September 4, 2007, from http://bphc.hrsa.gov/hchirc/pdfs/bibs/16%20outcomes.pdf

King County Public Health. (2005). *Health care for the homeless network: Community survey summary.* Retrieved September 4, 2007, from http://www.metrokc.gov/health/hchn/survey-summary.htm

National Health Care for the Homeless Council. (2006). Integrating primary and behavioral health care for the homeless people. *Healing Hands, 10*(2), 1–6.

Whitley, E. M., Everhart, R. M., & Wright, R. A. (2006). Measuring return on investment of outreach by community health workers. *Journal of Health Care for the Poor and Underserved, 17,* 6–15.

Unit Six

"Every problem has a gift for you in its hands."

■ ■ ■

Richard Bach

TEACHING–LEARNING

Teaching Nurses about Vulnerable Populations

Mary de Chesnay

There are many ways to teach nursing students how to work with vulnerable people, and there are numerous activities students can engage in to gain practice in providing culturally competent care. The purpose of this unit is to present faculty with strategies or to inspire them to devise similar learning activities for their own students. It is hoped that students who read this unit will find some of the experiences presented inspirational with regard to their own fieldwork.

For any activity designed to prepare nurses to provide culturally competent care, it is critical to emphasize two things: to know oneself and to show respect for others. First, the best thing nurses can do to prepare for working with vulnerable people is to know themselves. The more a person knows and acknowledges his or her own biases, the more easily that person can put these aside and concentrate on the patient as a person instead of a stereotype. *Ethnocentric bias* is a term derived from anthropology and refers to the notion that one's own cultural beliefs, practices, folkways, values, and norms are the right ones. Ethnocentric biases develop from our experience of living within our own cultures: growing up in families, attending educational institutions with certain emphases, and interacting with people we like or do not like. Ethnocentrism is neither good nor bad, it just is. To acknowledge that we all have biases simply indicates that we are human. Human beings tend to get in trouble when they act toward others as if their own way is the only right way or when they confuse bias with truth.

How do we learn to deal with ethnocentric bias? It is essential to recognize a particular feeling or attitude as bias and then critically examine our own values and beliefs, particularly in terms of how we see others who are different from ourselves. This principle of self-examination relates to everyone, not just to members of majority groups. It might be helpful to apply the general system theory concept of multifinality, which holds that there are many ways to the same end. Appreciating that other ways of achieving the goal might be equally effective and valid is a key component of self-awareness.

The second thing nurses can do to prepare for working with vulnerable people is to learn to show respect. Novices tend to expend large amounts of time and energy trying to learn cultural material quickly so they can interact "appropriately" in terms of superficial gestures, such as making eye contact or not, shaking hands or not, or touching arms. Yet, despite the best of intentions, these actions can sometimes be interpreted as mocking the group. Being yourself yet doing your best in terms of showing the most respect according to your own cultural standards is more likely to be understood by the patient as respectful.

Another key point in providing culturally competent care is to reframe compliance or adherence in light of the patient's or group's cultural norms, values, and folkways. For example, students might not understand food taboos and offer pork to a Muslim or Jewish patient and then wrongly interpret the patient's rejection of pork as loss of appetite. Many Arabs and Jews do not observe the dietary laws, but many do, and it is important to ask. The patient and family are the best teachers of their culture. The point is to ask and not to assume.

Why Teach Nursing Students about Vulnerable Populations?

Global demographics are changing as populations evolve into ever more complex societies. Demographics of individual countries change rapidly as people move within their countries or from one country to another to find food, jobs, or simply better lives for their families. As the costs of living and health care spiral higher, the most vulnerable members of the population become even more entrenched in the daily ordeal of living. The nursing profession cannot afford for its practitioners to be isolationist in the way they treat patients and families. Neither can we afford to ignore communities. Community-based care and focus on populations are aspects of nursing that students need to learn to provide cost-effective culturally competent care.

The kinds of experiences students have in their basic educational programs can improve their confidence. In this chapter two models from different universities are presented. Although both universities happen to be private, the strategies and activities are universal and can be adapted by anyone interested in helping students develop or improve cross-cultural interpersonal relations. In Chapter 39, "Preparing Nursing Professionals for Advocacy: Service Learning," a third service learning model is presented from a different point of view. Many schools have implemented similar programs on behalf of the vulnerable populations of their own or international communities. Websites for the schools are a good source of information.

What Should Students Learn?

Nurses need experiences that teach them to be comfortable with people different from themselves, and this requires interaction with many kinds of people. It is not sufficient to review the literature and write papers on vulnerable populations. Writing papers is useful but can be an empty intellectual exercise if not combined with developing competence in talking with people. Fieldwork is an excellent way to develop interaction skills.

Students need to develop an understanding of culture and become aware of their own ethnocentric biases. They need to do so within a safe context in which they will not be criticized by their faculty for attitudes they hold but rather coached to develop new ideas or views about the vulnerable. For example, it is not useful to berate students who believe that all homeless people should take menial jobs to get off the street. Instead, they should be guided to understand the complexities of homelessness and why even menial jobs are not an option for many people.

Even though the statistical information on vulnerable populations often becomes obsolete before it is printed because the health disparities in this country increase with population increases, students still need to know who the vulnerable are and recognize the health disparities of the vulnerable populations in their communities. Students should be encouraged to review the literature critically for applicability to vulnerable populations and to formulate practices that better serve the vulnerable.

Finally, students should learn how to reverse vulnerability. Nursing means not only curing and preventing illness but also strengthening the patient's resources so that the patient becomes less vulnerable. Once trendy, the term *empowerment* has fallen out of favor because it has a patriarchal connotation, but the notion that people can be helped to attain autonomy is still useful in teaching students to care for the vulnerable. Perhaps a more appropriate intervention is helping the patient develop or increase resilience. Everyone has strengths, and focusing on strength rather than weakness is a good therapeutic technique.

Models of Experiential Learning

Duquesne Model

Duquesne University is a small liberal arts institution founded in 1878 and operated by the Spiritans, an order of priests with strong service ties to developing countries in Africa and South America. Through its school of nursing, Duquesne confers undergraduate and graduate degrees, including the PhD, and a variety of certificate and continuing education programs. During the author's tenure as dean of the school from 1994 to 2002, the faculty created a variety of programs and experiences for students and faculty to operationalize the service mission of the university. Two major outreach programs (local and international) are particularly relevant to the education of nursing students in caring for people from vulnerable populations, and these programs involved students at all levels: baccalaureate, master, and doctoral.

Nurse-Managed Wellness Centers

The first outreach program was initially funded by the School of Nursing and later by a grant from the U.S. Department of Housing and Urban Development. The faculty member who coordinated the gerontological clinical nurse specialist track in the Master of Science in Nursing program created a model for outreach into the community by starting a wellness clinic in a high-rise apartment building designated for senior citizens (Taylor, Resick, D'Antonio, & Carroll, 1997). Students and faculty conducted many health-screening and health-promotion activities. The model was evaluated as successful by residents, staff, faculty, and students, with the result that the clinic was replicated later in a federally funded project to expand services to African-Americans in the poor neighborhoods near the university.

With the success of the prototype center, two additional centers were opened in the African-American communities called the Hill District and East Liberty (Resick, Taylor, & Leonardo, 1999). Later, the Visiting Nurse Association in Butler County, Pennsylvania, adopted the model for a rural community north of the city. To prepare for the expansion of the clinic, the faculty used ethnographic methods to gain access to the community, to establish rapport with civic leaders and community residents, and to identify areas of need that the School of Nursing could fulfill (Resick, Taylor, Carroll, D'Antonio, & de Chesnay, 1997). The community members initially had reservations about the proposed clinic because they perceived previous experiences, when outsiders had come into the community for various research projects, as disrespectful to them. However, by using the principles of ethnographic research and the methods of participant observation and interviewing, the faculty found ways to involve the community in planning so that when the second clinic opened the community members reported that they felt a sense of ownership.

As of this writing, the original clinic and the Hill District clinic are thriving and provide a continuous educational experience for students and a practice setting for the nurse practitioner faculty. Faculty and students conduct health assessments, medication evaluations, teaching presentations, exercise classes in the form of dance therapy, and other health promotion activities. One of the projects at the clinics involved creating a chart audit system for measuring outcomes. This experience provided graduate students with the opportunity to apply theory to the practice of nursing in a functioning practice setting and allowed them to test the validity and reliability of the audit tool in a real setting in a way that would be used by the staff (Resick, 1999).

When necessary, staff members refer residents to their primary care providers and, in some cases, directly to the emergency room. Students who rotate through the clinics obtain a sophisticated understanding of the healthcare issues of the elderly in the two independent-living high rises, one predominantly white and the other predominantly African-American. Through the clinics students learn firsthand the issues of the elderly as a vulnerable population.

Other activities in the local communities were initiated at the request of the community leaders, who had identified problems. One highly successful program taught cardiopulmonary resuscitation (CPR) to residents of all ages. A research project was conducted by faculty to examine community knowledge about CPR, and the results were helpful in developing the CPR programs (Winter, 2001). Classes were conducted by certified faculty in the community centers, and people of all ages completed the course.

Center for International Nursing

The Center for International Nursing was created in 1992 (Carty & White, 1993; White & Smith, 1997) to provide an administrative structure within which students and faculty could conduct educational programs, service projects, and research abroad. Initially, the Center's focus was Nicaragua, but later the Center expanded to South America, Africa, and Europe to complete specific initiatives. From 1994 to 2002 over 130 students at all levels completed international projects, and every year 6 to 10 undergraduate students completed part of their community health nursing clinical requirement in a barrio in Managua in conjunction with Duquesne faculty and faculty in the sister school, Universidad Politecnica de Nicaragua (UPOLI) (L. Cunningham and S. Colvin, personal communication, August 2000). The students conducted community assessments, performed health assessments, intervened in referrals to the community health clinics, and conducted health fairs to teach the community residents a variety of health promotion techniques. On another project one of the critical care faculty taught part of the trauma content to students in a hospital in Managua (C. Ross, personal communication, September 1999).

Largely due to the publicity about the activities of the Center, the nursing school was approached by the Pittsburgh Rotary Club, who wanted to begin an international health project. They built a clinic in partnership with the Rotary Clubs of Managua and Jinotega in a northern community of Nicaragua near the city of Jinotega. Community residents wanted to name their clinic for the late member of the Pittsburgh Pirates baseball team, thus La Clinica de Roberto Clemente. Clemente died in a plane crash while trying to deliver medical supplies after the Managua earthquake of 1972 and is still revered in Nicaragua. This clinic is used by nurse practitioner faculty as a clinical site for graduate students, and the community was the site of an ethnographic study on men's health conducted as dissertation research by a doctoral student, as described in Chapter 34 of the first edition of this book (Ross, 2000).

A second international study was conducted as action research by a doctoral student who worked in Peru on the clean water project run by the Sisters of Mercy (Zolkoski, 2000). Other doctoral students have conducted independent studies in Nicaragua and served as teaching faculty for some of the programs offered to the local nurses and physicians.

Faculty made a commitment to the sister school (UPOLI), and many other projects were conducted with the poor of Nicaragua. Emphasis on the "train the trainer" approach meant that the faculty tried to work with the local nurses as much as possible; many projects were accomplished with the support of the sister school faculty. The study described in Chapter 17 of the previous edition of this book, "Child Health in a Barrio of Managua," was an outcome of the work conducted under the auspices of the *hermanamiento* (sister school relationship) (Colvin, de Chesnay, Mercado, & Benavides, 2005). Many other projects and programs have been conducted and are too numerous to mention here.

Online Doctoral Program

Concurrent with the increasing international visibility of the Duquesne University School of Nursing, the faculty became aware of the desire of nurses in developing countries to improve nursing education for their people. Dr. John Murray, the university president, challenged the deans to experiment with distance learning strategies, and the faculty chose to meet his challenge by creating opportunities for nurses in developing countries to earn Duquesne's PhD in nursing through synchronous web-based courses, coupled with residency on campus during the summers. The first course was taught by Dr. Jeri Milstead in summer of 1997 (Milstead, 1998). Although some international nurses applied to the program, we as faculty were surprised at the popularity of the program among nurses who lived within driving distance of the university. Many lived in medically underserved areas where they needed to continue working because there was no one to replace them or because they still had children at home, but they were highly motivated, and the program became extremely competitive.

Seattle University Model

The Seattle University College of Nursing has demonstrated a long tradition of consistent fit with the mission of the university to promote social justice by serving the poor. In response to changes in health care during the 1980s, faculty revised the master's degree program to teach advanced practice nurses to work with vulnerable populations (Vezeau, Peterson, Nakao, & Ersek, 1998). Originally developed as a clinical specialist program, the faculty recognized the need for nurse practitioners and added a family nurse practitioner track and, more recently, an innovative second-degree immersion track for people with college degrees in other disciplines who wish to be nurses.

Many experiences in other courses (e.g., the clinical courses and the thesis/scholarly project) enable the students to develop comfort and skill at working with diverse patients, families, and communities. For the thesis or scholarly project, the students are expected to develop projects significant to their own future roles as advanced practice nurses and to vulnerable populations. Chapters 18 and 19 are reports of research with implications for vulnerable populations in Africa and the United States, respectively.

For the bachelor's program students work in the poor neighborhoods, called garden communities, located near the university. Garden communities are scattered around the city, and students spend a good bit of clinical time there. Faculty are assigned to each community and provide clinical supervision and support. The undergraduate course on vulnerable populations is a two-credit required course in which the students conduct fieldwork by interviewing persons different from themselves to develop comfort with and competence at interacting with culturally diverse people and groups. Students discuss their fieldwork in a variety of settings in the United States and Belize.

Key Components of Educational Experience

A plan for teaching nursing students how to care for vulnerable populations might include the following:

- Identify the vulnerable populations within the community. If international nursing is an interest of the school, then faculty might capitalize on their own international research or service experiences. Sister school relationships, such as the Duquesne *hermanamiento,* could provide wonderful opportunities for faculty and student exchanges, service learning projects, or collaborative research with nursing faculty in other countries.

- Develop a set of guidelines for students to follow for their fieldwork with the expected outcomes clearly stated. (The Instructor Manual for this book has sample syllabi and detailed guidelines.) Outcomes should include an expectation for improved self-awareness.

- Designate key faculty to coordinate or guide the process. Not every faculty member will want to be involved, but it is essential to have at least one faculty champion for each project.

- Establish the need for specific projects in concert with stakeholders who are key members of the population.

- Decide whether service learning projects will be part of the curriculum and conducted within specific courses or whether they will be freestanding as people express interest. One way to focus on vulnerable populations without major curriculum changes is to allow students to use independent study courses for fieldwork.

- Design and implement a small-scale project that can be funded through existing resources. Later, after individual faculty have established a track record, more sophisticated projects can be funded through grants and contracts.

- Evaluate the projects not only in terms of student satisfaction and learning but also in terms of benefits to the population.

- Consider evaluation data carefully before designing subsequent projects.

Conclusion

The models presented here have several characteristics in common that contributed to their effectiveness in meeting the objectives of the courses and programs. Characteristics of successful experiences for students include opportunities for developing self-awareness, fieldwork that enables them to develop communication skills and exercises in interacting with people different from themselves, and review of available literature on the population of interest. Although these experiences are challenging, the students generally rate them as positive. In many cases in which students have traveled to be immersed in another culture, they indicate that their experiences were life-changing. The success of these service learning programs demonstrates that providing such opportunities at undergraduate and graduate levels is a crucial aspect of nursing education with regard to vulnerable populations.

References

Carty, R., & White J. (1993). *Nicaraguan-American nursing collaborating project* (pp. 37–38). Washington, DC: American Association of Colleges of Nursing.

Colvin, S. P., de Chesnay, M., Mercado, T., & Benavides, C. (2005). Child health in a barrio of Managua. In M. de Chesnay (Ed.), *Caring for the vulnerable: Perspectives in nursing theory, practice, and research* (1st ed., pp. 161–170). Sudbury, MA: Jones and Bartlett.

Milstead, J. (1998). Preparation for an online asynchronous university doctoral course: Lessons learned. *Computers in Nursing, 16*(5), 247–258.

Resick, L. (1999). Challenges in measuring outcomes in two community-based nurse-managed wellness clinics: The development of a chart auditing tool. *Home Health Care Management and Practice, 11*(4), 52–59.

Resick, L., Taylor, C., Carroll, T., D'Antonio, J., & de Chesnay, M. (1997). Establishing a nurse-managed wellness clinic in a predominantly older African American inner-city high rise: An advanced practice nursing project. *Nursing Administration Quarterly, 21*(4), 47–54.

Resick, L., Taylor, C., & Leonardo, M. (1999). The nurse-managed wellness clinic model developed by Duquesne University School of Nursing. *Home Health Care Management and Practice, 11*(6), 26–35.

Ross, C. (2000). Caminando mas cerca con Dios [A closer walk with Thee]: An ethnography of health and well-being of rural Nicaraguan men. Unpublished doctoral dissertation, Duquesne University, Pittsburgh, PA.

Taylor, C., Resick, L., D'Antonio, J., & Carroll, T. (1997). The advanced practice nurse role in implementing and evaluating two nurse-managed wellness clinics: Lessons learned about structure, processs and outcomes. *Advanced Practice Nursing Quarterly, 3*(2), 36–45.

Vezeau, T., Peterson, J., Nakao, C., & Ersek, M. (1998). Education of advanced practice nurses serving vulnerable populations. *Nursing and Health Care Perspectives, 19*(1), 124–131.

White, J., & Smith, C. (1997). Developing an international nursing partnership with Nicaragua. *International Nursing Review, 44*(1), 13–18.

Winter, K. (2001). Bystander CPR in two Pittsburgh communities. *Cultura de los Cuidados, 5*(9), 82–89.

Zolkoski, R. (2000). Clean water for Chimbote, Peru: Transcultural nursing in participatory action research. Unpublished doctoral dissertation, Duquesne University, Pittsburgh, PA.

Healthy Communities: A Framework for Experiential Learning in Community Health Nursing

Barbara A. Anderson and Amanda B. Frye

Vulnerability is a concept that may be applied to either individuals or populations at risk. Frequently, vulnerability refers to an aggregate group. Vulnerable populations are often described as helpless, susceptible, at risk, or marginalized, rarely referring to their resilience or strengths. Individuals within the specified group may not feel vulnerable, resisting categorization as prejudicial or as a deflection from their strengths (de Chesnay, 2005)

Vulnerable populations are frequently strong people facing difficult circumstances. They usually have the potential for resilience when their strengths are mobilized. Resilience, "the process of adapting well in the face of adversity, trauma, tragedy, or even significant sources of stress" (Newman, 2003, p. 42), is characterized by hope, positive action, and movement toward wholeness (de Chesnay, 2005). Powerful factors influencing resilience are family strengths, religious systems, and individual personality characteristics (Greeff & Human, 2004). The influence of a healthy community on vulnerable populations is a factor that has rarely been addressed in the resilience literature. Does a healthy community make vulnerable populations less vulnerable? More resilient? What does a healthy or an unhealthy community look like? Does an unhealthy community lessen resilience or increase susceptibility to adverse outcomes among vulnerable populations?

Conversely, the influence of vulnerable populations on the health of the community is rarely addressed. There is lip service paid to the belief that immigrants (as an example of a vulnerable group) build healthy communities. Yet immigrants are often marginalized by the community. They may be targeted as the root cause of community problems. Acceptance may occur over time, providing they accommodate to mainstream norms. The homeless, as a vulnerable population, are almost always viewed as eroding to the health and well-being of a community. What is the impact of vulnerable populations on the community? Do they make the community a healthier or an unhealthier place to live? Do they bring strength, resilience, and different paradigms or do they create uncomfortable questions, economic instability, and social disruption in the community?

These are critical questions facing both students studying community health nursing and the nursing educators who teach them. The prevailing paradigm is that vulnerable populations bring problems and that the community, if mobilized and as a reservoir of programs, holds solutions to the problems. This perspective assumes a problem-based assessment, active interventions for solutions to problems, and evaluation of outcomes for problem resolution. Educational approaches use this perspective in problem-based learning. In fact, problem-based learning begins with the word *problem*. Health professional students quickly adapt to a problem-oriented paradigm, perhaps failing to assess initially for individual or aggregate strengths among vulnerable populations or to define the indicators of an integrated healthy community. Further, they frequently overlook the dynamics of interface between vulnerable peoples and their community.

Vulnerable populations can mobilize their strengths in facing difficult circumstances if supported by a healthy community. Likewise, communities can become healthier and more whole as they learn from and incorporate the strengths and knowledge of vulnerable populations. Educators need to help students to seek out strengths rather than problems, indicators of a healthy community rather than a laundry list of community services, and evidences of interface between vulnerable populations and their community. This approach helps students to develop an integrated framework of community assessment. The ecological model of health, as described by the Institute of Medicine (IOM), is a strong foundational theory for educating students in this approach.

Ecological Model of Health

The nation's blueprint for health, *Healthy People 2010: Understanding and improving health*, links the nation's health to the health of each state and territory, which, in turn, is almost inseparable from the health status of individuals (U.S. Department of Health and Human Services, 2000). Individual health, likewise, is linked with social and environmental influences: the *social ecological model* (Skokols, 1996). The IOM (2003b) proposed this model as a comprehensive framework for understanding the determinants of the nation's health. The *ecological model of health* assumes the interaction of individuals and populations with biological, sociocultural, and environmental determinants and suggests that individual and aggregate health status are a function of daily and lifetime interaction (IOM, 2003b) (Figure 38-1).

Using the ecological model as the basis for national health planning necessitates integrated holistic strategies aimed at individual, family, and community levels. "Public health professionals must be aware of not only the biological risk factors affecting health; they must also understand the environmental, social, and behavioral contexts within which individuals and populations operate in order to identify factors that may hinder or promote the success of their interventions" (IOM, 2003b, p. 34). The ecological model of health is a framework for studying the interface of vulnerability and community. The following example demonstrates this interface.

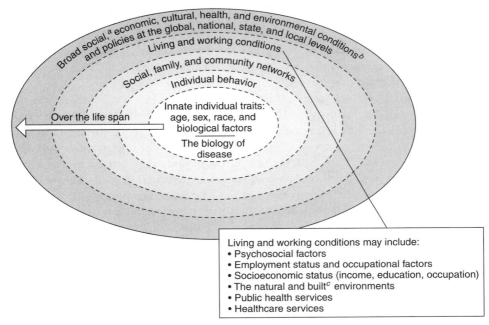

Figure 38-1 Ecological Model of Health (IOM, 2003a)

The dotted lines between levels of the model denote interaction effects between and among the various levels of health determinants (Worthman, 1999).

[a] Social conditions include, but are not limited to economic inequality, urbanization, mobility, cultural values, attitudes, and politics related to discrimination and intolerance on the basis of race, gender, and other differences.

[b] Other conditions at the national level might include major sociopolitical shifts, such as recession, war, and governmental collapse.

[c] The built environment includes transportation, water and sanitation, housing, and other dimensions of urban planning.

Source: Adapted from Dahlgren and Whitehead, 1991.

Vulnerability to cervical cancer can be explained within the ecological framework. Innate individual characteristics (age, sex) are modified by individual sexual behavior. Primary prevention (vaccination, health behavior messages), secondary prevention (Pap smears), and tertiary care (medical interventions) are mediated by cultural and family values and community resources. Living and working conditions affect individual susceptibility to illness and accessibility to intervention. Social, economic, and environmental conditions at local, national, and global levels drive policy and programs. Ultimately, these factors determine who is most likely to be vulnerable.

Case Study 1: The Ecological Model—The Story of a Life

Teresa never traveled further than a few miles from her rural village in eastern Honduras, although her husband occasionally traveled to the regional trading center to sell the corn they raised and to obtain supplies for the family. He also purchased local whiskey and the services of women practicing survival sex.

Married at the age of 14, Teresa bore four children in rapid succession as sexually transmitted human papilloma virus eroded her cervix and developed into cancer. Primary health care was available at regional clinics, but she had no way to get to the clinic except on foot over rugged terrain. Besides, she had no information about the importance of preventive care. Secondary care (e.g., Pap smears) was available in some sites, but because of a lack of resources there was no follow-up of positive results. Once cancer developed there was limited and expensive palliative care in the regional hospital. Until pelvic pain was intense, Teresa never saw a healthcare provider. By then, the cancer had metastasized to her pelvic region. At the age of 28 Teresa died, leaving behind four young children and an alcoholic husband.

Discussion Questions for Case Study 1

- What were the innate characteristics, individual behavior factors, community networks, and the living conditions acting as determinants of health for Teresa?

- Discuss the local, state, and global conditions and policies that surround this story. At each level of the ecological model, what were the primary, secondary, and tertiary strategies that could have modified the outcome for Teresa?

- Using the ecological model, describe the determinants for health for the children and the husband.

- How would national policy to vaccinate all adolescent women have modified this story?

Vulnerability and the Ecological Model

The ecological model of health is a framework for assessing the strengths and resilience of vulnerable populations. Innate personality characteristics, the first level of the model, may affect resilience (Greeff & Human, 2004), whereas individual behavioral responses, the next level, affect outcome. Behavioral responses are learned within the context of family and community. Family norms, social messages, and community networks provide the external structure for individual behavior. As an example, the Yup'ik people of the Russian Mission, an indigenous Native American group in rural Alaska, are a vulnerable group facing cultural loss. At the same time they have demonstrated resilience and strength. Using tribal knowledge, as described below, in the design of environmental education programs, this population focused on subsistence and survival skills. The educational programs impact individual behavior through imparting community expectations: honoring the natural world, respecting the principles of Yup'ik ecology, assuming tribal identity, and acknowledging the power of the community over individual behavior. Tribal knowledge is a determinant in decreasing individual and aggregate vulnerability through defining individual behavior (Takako, 2006).

Community networks, a link in the ecological model, are powerful determinants of health. LA VIDA, a community-based partnership in Detroit, used the ecological model of health in identifying abused Latina women as a vulnerable population. Applying the ecological framework, it identified the living conditions of these women as a powerful determinant of health and built family and community safety networks within the Latino community (Maciak, Guzman, Santiago, Villalobos, & Israel, 1999). Likewise, the Gathering of Native Americans (GONA) used the ecological model to intervene at the level of living and working conditions. GONA is a national educational curriculum addressing outcomes with substance abuse among Native Americans. Using the GONA curriculum, tribal consortiums in the Southwest initiated a community development program entitled Community Involvement to Renew Commitment, Leadership, and Effectiveness, or CIRCLE. CIRCLE identified the signature strengths of the tribes in the consortiums: belonging, honoring skills, working together, and sharing knowledge. It used the ecological approach in addressing the living and working conditions affecting intimate partner violence and health disparities (Chino & DeBruyn, 2006).

Individual behavior, family, community networks, and living–working conditions are strong determinants of vulnerability. Broader social and environmental conditions are also strong determinants of health and vantage points for policy. The Road to Maternal Death paradigm, identifying social and environmental factors as health determinants to maternal mortality, contributed to the development of the international Safe Motherhood Initiative, a policy response and blueprint for action that addresses not only the individual determinants of maternal mortality, but also the broader social and environmental conditions affecting the low status of women and its impact on maternal mortality (World Health Organization [WHO], 2004). The Safe Motherhood Initiative is an example of policy for a vulnerable population framed by the ecological model of health. The ecological model, as a theoretical framework, identifies health determinants and interventions for vulnerable populations at varying levels of impact.

Community as Determinant of Health

The community can be a healthy environment for its citizens, including those most vulnerable, or it can be a place that destroys the health and spirit of the people. An urban environment with sprawl, poor hygiene, and inadequate planning creates conditions that encourage sedentary life-styles, development of illnesses linked to environmental pollutants, and conditions of mental stress, social division, and alienation (Franklin, Frank, & Jackson, 2004). On the other hand, a community characterized by citizen empowerment, including those who are most vulnerable, creates conditions for citizen engagement toward building the health of the community (Diers, 2004). The IOM (2003a) defines community as a group of people who share interests, values, culture, and common risks or who live in the same geographical region. The key operative is that community is a shared experience, positive or negative. The ecological model of health identifies and links factors that communities share in the determination of their health.

What does a healthy community look like? Urban migration is a global trend, and most of the world's people now live in urban communities, many of them living in the developing world. The WHO identified urban health as a leading public health priority. The "Healthy Cities" initiative was designed to set standards promoting health at all levels of the ecological model. It recognized that the environment of the city is a powerful determinant of human health. In October 2003 political leaders throughout Europe convened in Belfast, Ireland, to draft a strategic plan and call for action. "The Belfast Declaration for Healthy Cities: The Power of Local Action" is a blueprint that has been widely accepted as definitive of the healthy city (WHO, 2003). According to the Belfast Declaration, a healthy city is an urban environment that promotes human health by

- Reducing inequalities and addressing poverty
- Building strategic partnerships for human health
- Considering health impact in urban planning
- Including citizens in planning and policy decision making
- Working toward the UN Millennium Development Goals
- Strengthening linkages with other cities nationally and globally
- Sharing resources and lessons learned with other cities

In September 2005 mayors and political leaders in the WHO Healthy Cities Network met in Bursa, Turkey, to draft a guiding statement on the environmental design of urban environments that promote healthy cities. Bursa was a symbolic place to hold the planning conference. Recently, it was the site of a devastating earthquake. Earthquakes may be predicted in geographically unstable regions, but predicting the timing is not possible. The huge earthquake in Bursa was predicted, but no one knew when it would happen, and Bursa was particularly unprepared. We visited Bursa shortly after the earthquake and were able to assess how lack of urban planning had adversely affected the health and well-being of the populace.

The Bursa statement, "Designing Healthier and Safer CITIES: The Challenge of Healthy Urban Planning," acknowledges that urban policies and planning can affect the physical and mental health of citizens (WHO, 2005). Referring to the principles of the ecological model of health, the statement affirms that urban environments are powerful determinants of health. It calls for health impact assessment in all urban planning. Affirming the Belfast Declaration, the Bursa Statement identifies specific indicators of a healthy urban environment (WHO, 2005). These indicators are the assessment criteria for a healthy city (Table 38-1).

TABLE 38-1   Indicators of a Healthy Urban Environment

- Adequate space for exercise, active life-style, and cultural events
- Promotion of social networks
- Affordable high-quality housing
- Equity and programs for poverty reduction
- Opportunities for local food production and healthy food outlets
- Diverse employment opportunities
- Accessible, ecological, safe transport systems
- Reduction in emissions that threaten climate stability
- Acceptable noise levels
- Good air and water quality
- Good sanitation and waste disposal
- Adequate planning for community safety and disaster management

The Healthy Hawaii Initiative (HHI), based on the ecological model and the principles in the Healthy Cities initiative, has made progress toward building a healthier community. The initiative focuses on individual behavior (smoking, nutrition, physical activity) while concurrently addressing other levels of the ecological model: utilizing community networks, designing healthy living and working environments, and formulating supportive policy (Nigg et al., 2005).

While recently at a professional conference in Honolulu, I (B.A.A.) noted widespread social marketing about the HHI. Hawaiian health professionals were well aware of the initiative but so were residents in multiple walks of life with whom I talked. Nigg et al. (2005) reported that the initiative was well received by the citizens of Hawaii and that the analysis of the process and outcomes measures were promising. The HHI is an example of integrated community development applying the ecological model and the principles of the Healthy Cities initiative.

Although the HHI is a government public health initiative, private and locally based initiatives are also pivotal in promoting healthy communities. Faith-based communities often prioritize both healthy communities and reaching vulnerable populations (Goldman & Roberson, 2004). Neighborhood-focused citizen-led organizations have the advantage of local commitment (Diers, 2004; Sarriot et al., 2004). Community–academic partnerships can be powerful as they bring together local perspectives and scholarly methods (Adams, Miller-Korth, & Brown, 2004; Brugge & Cole, 2003). As an example, the Boston Healthy Public Housing Initiative, a community–academic partnership, joined professors, students, and vulnerable populations in poverty in a collaborative project to assess the conditions of public housing as a determinant of childhood asthma (Brugge & Cole, 2003).

Community initiatives in rural areas can profoundly improve health across levels of the ecological model. For instance, the Andean Rural Health Care project in Bolivia, South America, demonstrated the effectiveness of local community partnerships with private nongovernmental organizations. This project developed a system of accessible primary health care built on principles of the ecological model. It targeted individual health through developing local talent and culturally acceptable community networks (Perry et al., 1991).

Likewise, community–academic partnerships can build healthy communities by working together to address factors contributing to vulnerability. The Del Rio Project demonstrated that partnerships can promote community solutions along all spectrums of the ecological model of health. Students and faculty of East Tennessee State University, representing public health, nursing, and medicine, in collaboration with citizens of this isolated Tennessee community effected change at the individual level (building and staffing a primary healthcare center), the community networks level (the development of a Community Partnerships Initiative), and the living/working level (assessment of local concerns about water quality) (Goodrow & Meyers, 2000).

A healthy community has the potential to make the general population less vulnerable and to promote resilience among those who are most vulnerable. Conversely, a population striving for health, including those who are most vulnerable, contributes to building a healthy community. The case study below exemplifies different approaches to community development, the impact on vulnerable populations, and the effect that vulnerable populations have on the health of the community.

Case Study 2: A Tale of Two Cities

City A

City A is a medium-sized city in a temperate region. It has a diverse population with moderate levels of homelessness, drug traffic, and crime. The city has a recently renovated downtown area fringed by urban blight and suburban flight. Citizens express concern about the quality of the schools, urban congestion, safety on the streets, and the unsightly appearances of homelessness. Efforts to involve citizens in community action programs to solve these issues have had limited success. Most people say they are working long hours, have long freeway commutes, and do not have time to be involved. Healthcare providers are concerned about the growing rates of type 2 diabetes and obesity. The health indicators are average compared with national norms.

City A has a strategic plan for development supported by local public policy and ordinances. Favorable business lending practices, cheap land in the business districts, low taxes, liberal zoning regulations, and a good freeway system make City A an attractive place in which to work and to purchase real estate. Employment opportunities abound in two powerful industries, and the population is growing.

City B

City B is a medium-sized city in a colder climate. The population is diverse with many new immigrants, primarily refugees and migrant workers. The city is a magnet for the homeless as it provides a range of services, including job training. Drug traffic and crime are moderate. The central area has been renovated while maintaining historic sites. Expensive high-rise condominiums are replacing much of the low-income housing in the downtown. The take-over of land in this area is resented by lower income families forced to move from the area. Low-interest home loans and planned development of medium-priced single family homes are helping these working poor to achieve decent housing, but the very poor and homeless are on the streets. Throughout the metropolitan region green spaces are abundant for recreation, exercise, and urban gardening. Farmer's markets are a local tradition. The health indicators of the population are above the national norm, with less obesity, more active life-style, and relatively good access to healthy foods.

Citizens express concern about the rapid growth of the city, the quality of the schools, freeway congestion, inadequate public transportation, and lack of city services when weather conditions are adverse. There is considerable civic activism and energy generated around these issues. The homeless have formed an association that produces a local newspaper addressing housing and social issues. The city government provides matching funds for locally identified community development projects to various civic associations and neighborhood organizations, including the Homeless Association.

Discussion Questions for Case Study 2

- Based on the ecological model of health, the Belfast Declaration, and the Bursa Statement, are City A and City B healthy cities?
- Do they exhibit the ability to care for vulnerable persons in the community?
- Do those vulnerable persons living in these cities have an opportunity to contribute toward making their environments a healthier place to live?

Healthy Communities and Vulnerability: Framing the Learning Experience

Who Will Keep the Public Healthy?

The ecological model of health helps students to develop a contextual framework for community and vulnerability by linking environment and health. Experiential learning occurs as a centered activity involving observation, participation, and reflection (Dyjack, Anderson, & Madrid, 2001; Gofin, 2002; Scott, Harrison, Baker, & Wills, 2005; Tanner, 2006). It is "the process by which the learner reflects on his or her experience and draws significance and meaning from such reflection" (Strauss et al., 2003). Experiential learning applying the ecological framework is a powerful approach to understanding the community–vulnerability interface.

Do community health nursing students know what a healthy community looks like? One approach to building this knowledge is to apply the healthy city indicators to the assessment of the community. Does the community meet the criteria for being "healthy" along the varying levels of the ecological model? Can nursing students identify vulnerability? In what context is a population vulnerable? Who within a defined vulnerable aggregate is vulnerable or not vulnerable? What variables contribute to vulnerability? What variables contribute to resiliency? Framed within the ecological model, resilience and vulnerability become tangible and identifiable responses to internal and external environments.

Can students identify the impact of the community on exacerbating vulnerability or building resiliency? Through guided community assessment in an experiential milieu, students can learn to identify how the community contributes to levels of vulnerability or resiliency. Examples include how the community addresses homelessness or violence. This educational approach builds an understanding of the community as a therapeutic agent in decreasing vulnerability. It teaches community health nursing as "deep smarts," that is, competency and emotional intelligence (Leonard & Swap, 2004), learned through direct observation, engaged immersed participation, and deep introspection.

Are students encouraged to reflect on how vulnerable populations affect the community? The focus in addressing vulnerability is generally on problems rather than the strengths, but one cannot see strengths if one is not looking for them. What if community health nursing students were guided away from looking at the "problems" of vulnerable populations and were encouraged to identify signature strengths and evidences of resiliency in managing problems before the word *problem* was even introduced? What if students were encouraged to participate in community organization and development from the rubric of how vulnerable populations strengthen the community across the levels of the ecological model? Would it take the "problem" out of problem-based learning and substitute an ecological model of learning that acknowledges multiple levels of health determinants and the dynamic interface between communities and vulnerable populations?

Educating community health nursing students toward "deep smarts" involves using an educational model that acknowledges the ecology of health coupled with an experiential methodology that deeply interfaces with vulnerability in the community. It proposes that healthy communities make vulnerable populations more resilient and that vulnerable populations bring strengths and paradigms to build healthy communities.

References

Adams, A., Miller-Korth, N., & Brown, D. (2004). Learning to work together: Developing academic and community research partnerships. *Wisconsin Medical Journal, 103*(2), 15–19.

Brugge, S., & Cole, A. (2003). A case study of community-based participatory research ethics: The Healthy Public Housing Initiative. *Science and Engineering Ethics, 9*(4), 501–581.

Chino, M., & DeBruyn, L. (2006). Building true capacity: Indigenous models for indigenous communities. *American Journal of Public Health, 96*(4), 596–599.

Dahlgren, G., & Whitehead, M. (1991). *Policies and strategies to promote social equity in health.* Stockholm, Sweden: Institute for Future Studies.

de Chesnay, M. (Ed.). (2005). *Caring for the vulnerable: Perspective in nursing theory, practice, and research* (1st ed.). Sudbury, MA: Jones and Bartlett.

Diers, J. (2004). *Neighbor power: Building community the Seattle way.* Seattle: University of Washington Press.

Dyjack, D., Anderson, B., & Madrid, A. (2001). Experiential public health study abroad education: Strategies for integrating theory and practice. *Journal of Studies in International Education, 5*(3), 244–254.

Franklin, H., Frank, L., & Jackson, R. (2004). *Urban sprawl and public health: Designing, planning and building for healthy communities.* Washington, DC: Island Press.

Gofin, J. (2002). Planning the teaching of community health (CPOC) in an MPH program. *Public Health Reviews, 30,* 293–301.

Goldman, M., & Roberson, J. (2004). Churches academic institutions, and public health: Partnerships to eliminate health disparities. *North Carolina Medical Journal, 65*(6), 368–372.

Goodrow, B., & Meyers, P. (2000). The Del Rio Project: A case for community-campus partnership. *Education for Health, 13*(2), 213–220.

Greeff, A. P., & Human, B. (2004). Resilience in families in which a parent has died. *American Journal of Family Therapy, 37*(1), 27–42.

Institute of Medicine (IOM). (2003a). *The future of the public health in the 21st century.* Washington, DC: The National Academies Press.

Institute of Medicine (IOM). (2003b). *Who will keep the public healthy? Education public health professionals for the 21st century.* Washington, DC: The National Academies Press.

Leonard, D., & Swap, W. (2004). Deep smarts. *Harvard Business Review, 82*(9), 88–97, 137.

Maciak, B., Guzman, R., Santiago, A., Villalobos, G., & Israel, B. (1999). Establishing LA VIDA: A community-based partnership to prevent intimate violence against Latina women. *Health Education & Behavior, 26*(6), 821–840.

Newman, R. (2003). Providing direction on the road to resilience. *Behavioral Health Management, 23*(4), 42–43.

Nigg, C., Maddock, J., Yamauchi, J., Pressler, V., Wood, B., & Jackson, S. (2005). The Healthy Hawaii Initiative: A social ecological approach promoting healthy communities. *American Journal of Health Promotion, 19*(4), 310–313.

Perry, H., Robison, N., Chavez, D., Taja, O., Hilari, C., Shanklin, D., et al. (1991). Attaining health for all through community partnerships: Principles of the census-based, impact-oriented (CBIO) approach to primary health care developed in Bolivia, South America. *Social Science Medicine, 48*(8), 1053–1067.

Sarriot, E., Winch, P., Ryan, L., Bowie, J., Kouletio, M., Swedberg, E., et al. (2004). A methodological approach and framework for sustainability assessment in NGO-implemented primary health care programs. *International Journal of Health Planning and Management, 19,* 23–41.

Scott, S. B., Harrison, A. D., Baker, T., & Wills, J. D. (2005). An interdisciplinary community partnership for health professional students: A service-learning approach. *Journal of Allied Health, 34*(1), 31–35.

Skokols, D. (1996). Translating social ecological theory into guidelines for community health promotion. *American Journal of Health Promotion, 10,* 282–298.

Strauss, R., Mofidi, M., Sandler, E. S., Williamson, R., III., McMurtry, B. A., Carl, L. S., et al. (2003). Reflective learning in community-based dental education. *Journal of Dental Education, 67*(11), 1234–1242.

Takako, T. (2006). Building a bond with the natural environment through experiential engagement: A case study of land-based education curriculum in rural Alaska. *Journal of Experiential Education, 28*(3), 281–284.

Tanner, C. (2006). The next transformation: Clinical education. *Journal of Nursing Education, 45*(4), 99–100.

U.S. Department of Health and Human Services. (2000) *Healthy people 2010: Understanding and improving health* (2nd ed.). Washington, DC: U.S. Government Printing Office.

World Health Organization (WHO). (2003). *Belfast declaration for healthy cities: The power of local action.* Retrieved November 1, 2007 from http://www.euro.who.int/document/Hep/Belfast_DEC_E.pdf

World Health Organization (WHO). (2004). *Making pregnancy safer: the critical role of the skilled attendant: A joint statement by WHO, ICM and FIGO.* Geneva, Switzerland: World Health Organization.

World Health Organization (WHO). (2005). *Designing healthier and safer CITIES: The challenge of urban planning.* Retrieved September 17, 2007, from http://www.sagliklikentlerbirligi.org.tr/eng/pdf/bursa_statement_E.pd

Worthman, C. M. (1999). Epidemiology of human development. In C. Panter-Brick & C. M. Worthman (Eds.), *Hormones, health, and behavior: A socio-ecological and lifespan perspective* (pp. 47–104). Cambridge, UK: Cambridge University Press.

Chapter 39

Preparing Nursing Professionals for Advocacy: Service Learning

Lynda P. Nauright

Advocacy as a Nursing Ethic

Paralleling the women's movement, nursing in the 1960s and 1970s was evolving from the ethic of loyalty to the physician and hospital to a new ethic of patient advocacy. Modern nursing, which began on the battlefield of the Crimea, had been ingrained with a military metaphor. Nurses wore uniforms, caps, and cloaks. Different schools had unique insignia. Stripes were added as the student progressed up the ranks (Winslow, 1984).

Consistent with the military theme, loyalty to the commanding officer and strict obedience to his orders were a major part of the nursing ethic. The Nightingale pledge, written in 1893, states, "with loyalty, I will endeavor to aid the physician in his work" (Davis & Aroskar, 1978, pp. 12–13). The following is from Charlotte Aiken's classic text on nursing ethics (1916, p. 44):

> Loyalty to the physician is one of the duties demanded of every nurse, not solely because the physician is her superior officer, but chiefly because the confidence of the patient in his physician is one of the important elements in the management of his illness, and nothing should be said or done that would weaken this faith or create doubts as to the character or ability or methods of the physician.

The moral power of this reasoning was compelling. Nurses were concerned about their patients' well-being and were taught repeatedly that the "faith" that people have in a physician is as much a healing element as any medicinal treatment. Thus even if the physician blundered the patient's confidence was to be maintained at all costs. Another statement from Parsons (1916, p. 32) asserts this concept:

> If a mistake has been made in treating a patient, the patient is not the person who should know it if it can be kept from him, because the anxiety and lack of confidence that he would naturally feel might be injurious to him and retard his recovery.

473

From the beginning of the 20th century some thoughtful nurses questioned and debated among themselves where such loyalty should end (Letter to the editor, 1910), and as early as 1932 Annie Goodrich spoke of modifying, if not abolishing, nursing's militarism (Goodrich, 1932). But the code for nurses, accepted by the American Nurses Association (ANA) in 1950, and a similar one accepted by the International Congress of Nursing in 1953 called for nurses to verify and sustain physicians' orders, sustain confidence in the physician, and report incompetence or unethical conduct "only to the proper authority" (ANA, 1950, p. 196; International Congress of Nursing, 1953).

But in the turbulent 1960s and 1970s a diminishing confidence in the medical profession, or perhaps just a more realistic view of it, coupled with rising consumerism and feminism brought about changes in perspective by both nurses and patients. Leaders of the patients' rights movement turned to nurses for assistance in securing fundamental rights of patients for informed consent, the right to refuse treatment, and the right to have full information about diagnosis and prognosis. George Annas (1974), an attorney and author of *The Rights of Hospital Patients* (1975), explicitly attacked the military metaphor and called for nurses to accept the new role of patient advocacy. He was not disappointed. Nurses enthusiastically embraced, and continue to embrace, the role of patient advocate.

Nursing codes of ethics were revised as well. In 1973 the International Congress of Nursing dropped all mention of loyal obedience to physicians' orders and said that "The nurse's primary responsibility is to those people who require nursing care" (Davis & Aroskar, 1978, pp. 13–14). The 1976 revision of the ANA code for nurses specifically requires nurses to protect the "client" from the "incompetent, unethical or illegal practice of any person" (ANA, 1986, p. 8). Gone from the revised code are rules obliging the nurse to maintain confidence in physicians or obey their orders. In fact, the word *physician* does not even appear in the code. Given that patient advocacy is a nursing value, how then do we prepare students to be patient advocates, to care about advocacy, and to exercise social responsibility? One method is through learning strategies such as experiential and service learning.

Service learning is defined as educational experiences in which students participate in a service activity that meets community needs within the framework of a specific credit bearing work. Service learning evolves from a philosophy of education that emphasizes active learning and is directed toward encouraging social responsibility (Mueller & Norton, 1998). Service learning connects thought and feeling in a deliberate way, creating a context in which students can explore how they feel about what they are thinking and what they think about how they feel. A variety of service learning opportunities, in which students are able to use their skills and knowledge to help the community while furthering their learning, is a powerful tool for teaching students to be advocates.

The concept of service learning is based on Kolb's (1984) theory of experiential learning. Kolb's model outlines an immediate *concrete experience* during and after which a person makes observations and reflections. Out of these reflections comes an abstract theory of why things are as they are, which leads to ideas on how to address the situation experienced. This, in turn, leads to active experiments and thus learning.

Other educational theories and principles support the teaching–learning strategy of service learning. Malcolm Knowles (1984) in his adult learning theory proposed that adults are motivated to learn when they experience a need to know something to deal with a particular situation or problem. Finally, it is generally accepted that the more interactive the education experience, the greater the likelihood of success.

After participating in a course using service learning, one student wrote, "Before taking this class, I did not have any idea of the importance of personal involvement. Having graduated 20 years ago, I was "trained" to do tasks, not think too much, and be a good girl. Thank God times have changed. I have been helping myself as well as others by volunteering. The time that I have spent at [a homeless shelter] has given me a broader understanding of the word 'care'."

Benefits of Service Learning

One obvious benefit of service learning is that it meets actual community needs, but there are many other benefits. Service learning fosters caring for others, allows students to experience firsthand how vulnerable populations are affected by public policy, and helps students develop empathy with diverse individuals. Reflection about the experience is a critical component of service learning and fosters moral development and enhances moral decision making. This direct participation with vulnerable populations often causes students to develop a better understanding of self and their own strengths and weaknesses. They develop skills in problem solving, critical thinking, leadership, and ethical decision making. An increased sense of civic responsibility, increased political/global awareness, and development of cultural competence may also be outcomes (Mueller & Norton, 1998).

Benefits also accrue to the institutions who engage in service learning. The foundation of an effective service learning program is a balanced long-term partnership between communities and institutions of higher education. This "hands-on" community involvement enhances institutional visibility, may appeal to potential donors, and helps to minimize the traditional separation between "town and gown" (Pellietier, 1995).

Experiential and Service Learning: The Emory Model

The Nell Hodgson Woodruff School of Nursing at Emory University, ranked sixth among U.S. private schools of nursing, is recognized as a leader in the preparation of students for beginning and advanced practice in nursing. The School of Nursing is committed to improving care and nursing leadership through its key values of scholarship, leadership, and social responsibility. An important component of the curriculum for both the baccalaureate and graduate programs is the opportunity for experiential and service learning. This chapter describes some of the opportunities made available to students.

The outreach activities of the School of Nursing are coordinated through the Office of Service Learning. Service learning is a teaching and learning strategy that integrates meaningful community service with instruction and reflection to enrich the learning experience, teach civic responsibility, and strengthen communities. "Service learning is an organizational expression of our commitment to social responsibility," says Marla E. Salmon, ScD, RN, FAAN, dean of the nursing school and director of the Lillian Carter Center for International Nursing (Comeau, 2005).

Fuld Fellowship Program

Funded through a $5 million endowment from the Helene Fuld Health Trust, the Fuld Fellowship program is awarded to second-career nursing students committed to improving care for vulnerable populations. Fellows are enrolled through the Emory Nursing Segue option for non-nurses with degrees in other fields. Students in the program receive a bachelor's and then a master's degree in nursing.

One of the unique strengths of the Fuld program is its blending of academics and leadership training with hands-on provision of health care to vulnerable populations from inner-city residents to rural migrant workers. Fellows volunteer at Café 458, a restaurant for the homeless in downtown Atlanta. Guests order from a menu, sit at small tables with volunteers, and receive counseling, social services, and legal services. The innovative café, which provides not only delicious food but also dignity to its patrons, was founded by A. B. Short and his wife, Ann Connor. Ann is a clinical assistant professor at the School of Nursing and coordinates the Fuld program (Loftus, 2005).

Other community outreach activities available for the Fuld Fellows are MedShare International, which collects and recycles surplus medical supplies and equipment for distribution to other countries; Joe's Place, which offers a foot care clinic for the homeless; Project Open Hand, which provides meals and nutrition services to people with symptomatic HIV/AIDS, homebound seniors, and others with critical illnesses or disabilities; and the International Rescue Committee, a refugee resettlement agency (Loftus, 2005):

> "Through the IRC [International Rescue Committee], I was introduced to a newly arrived family from Kabul, Afghanistan, and have developed a strong relationship with the parents and their children," says Jordan, a senior who intends to work in international health. "I witnessed the birth of the fifth child and felt thankful to share that precious moment with them."

Fuld Fellows gain a global nursing perspective through involvement with the school's Lillian Carter Center for International Nursing and the exchange program with Emory and Yonsei University in South Korea. Students also have traveled to Cuba, Mexico, the Bahamas, and Jamaica to study healthcare systems abroad (Loftus, 2005).

Says faculty mentor Connor, "The expectation is that they're going to change the profession of nursing. They're already changing the school. With their backgrounds, they are coloring the water in some marvelous ways. They are all going in wonderful directions. I'm not leading them. I'm kind of a sheepdog, guiding and nudging them and giving support from the sidelines. I'm tremendously excited about these amazingly talented people coming into nursing" (Loftus, 2005, pp. 2, 5).

Dean Salmon echoes the high regard for these innovative and creative leaders: "These master's-prepared students will re-enter their careers with a deep working knowledge of health issues for vulnerable people in the United States and internationally, coupled with a strong sense of direction and mission for addressing these problems realistically" (Loftus, 2005, p. 4).

Global Government Health Partners Forum

Both undergraduate and graduate students are exposed to international and national health leaders when they volunteer to assist in the Global Government Health Partners Forum and/or the Government Chief Nursing Officers' Institute and Networking meeting, which precedes the Forum. Although perhaps not technically service learning, the experience is a powerful one for students, many of whom already have international experience or intend to work internationally.

This biennial forum, initiated in 2001, brings together chief nursing officers, chief medical officers, and ministers of health from over 100 developed and developing countries to address worldwide health issues such as the shortage of healthcare professionals, bioterrorism, and pandemic diseases. They meet with leaders from the World Health Organization, Centers for Disease Control and Prevention, Pan American Health Organization, the Carter Center, Emory University's Woodruff Health Sciences Center, the Claus M. Halle Institute for Global Learning, and others under the auspices of the nursing school's Lillian Carter Center for International Nursing.

"Partnerships between government medical and nursing leaders are critical," notes Dean Salmon, founder of the forums. "Many key partnerships, built at our first global conference, continue to bring significant results to the world of global health as will the new working relationships built at this forum" (Comeau, 2004, p.1). Notes staff member and graduate student Rebecca Wheeler, "It was amazing to think that we had some of the most important people in governments from around the world and that our GGHP was one of the only opportunities they had to come together and discuss their efforts to overcome international problems. I felt like we were providing a true service to global health" (personal communication, January 19, 2007).

Farm Worker Family Health Project

Georgia's migrant farm workers travel across the country and work up to 18 hours per day harvesting tobacco, fruits, and vegetables and working at packing houses. They have no primary physician or health insurance and virtually no time or resources to attend to their health needs and those of their children. According to Judith Wold, PhD, RN, who has directed the Emory program since it moved from Georgia State University in 2002, "Agriculture is one of the most dangerous occupations in the U.S. and the migrant farm workers are terribly at risk" (Comeau, 2006, p. 1).

For the past 14 years the Farm Worker Family Health Program, based in rural Georgia, has provided a 2-week intensive health service delivery initiative each June to care for over 1,000 migrant farm workers and their families. The most common conditions treated are muscle strains, back problems, foot fungus, urinary tract infections, parasitic infections, skin rashes, eye and ear infections, anemia, hypertension, and diabetes (Comeau, 2006). Undergraduate student nurses in their community health rotation and family nurse practitioner, adult nurse practitioner, family nurse midwife, pediatric nurse practitioner, and women's health nurse practitioner students provide screening, episodic care, and educational and counseling services.

The program is coordinated by the School of Nursing in conjunction with the Ellenton Rural Health Clinic, a part of the Georgia Division of Public Health in Colquitt County. Other partners have included Kennesaw State University (nursing), Georgia State University (psychology and physical therapy), Clayton State University and College (dental), Darton College in Albany (dental), the Colquitt County Board of Education, the Southern Pine Migrant Education Agency, the Atlanta and SOWEGA (Southwest Georgia) Area Health Education Centers, and the owners of farms and packing houses in the Colquitt, Brooks, Cook, and Tift County areas. Support has been provided by the Charles and Mary Grant Foundation, the Stahl Family Foundation, the Georgia Health Foundation, the Georgia Division of Public Health, Emory alumni, and churches and other community organizations in both Atlanta and South Georgia.

Students begin their long day at elementary schools or summer camps, where they perform a variety of preventive and assessment services. The children are given health, developmental, and psychological assessments. Nurse practitioner students refer them to the Ellenton Clinic, if needed. The dental hygiene students apply sealants and provide fluoride treatments, referring those needing additional intervention to the evening clinic if a dentist is available or to the Ellenton Clinic. Dental caries/conditions are the number one problem in both children and adults in this population (Auchmutey, 2003). In the process each child's school health record is updated on a database that was created by a student majoring in nursing leadership and administration.

In the afternoons undergraduate students each present a seminar on topics related to migrant health. Sometimes they accompany county outreach workers as these nurses visit their family caseload. Some students battle the southern Georgia heat and humidity to observe and actually conduct some field screening on the workers as they work. A few have tried their hand at harvesting alongside the workers and discovered firsthand how arduous this work is.

By evening the students and faculty have set up tents, tables, and supplies in the front yard of a church, camp, neighborhood, or mobile home park. At sunset, about 9:00 p.m., workers come in from the fields to be seen, along with children referred earlier in the day from the school screening. Undergraduate nursing students check in and screen farm workers and family members, while nurse practitioner students supervised by faculty provide episodic care services in the Ellenton Clinic van (a mobile clinic) for those who need them. Separate tents offer physical therapy and dental care with volunteer dentists providing tooth extractions and other dental services. Volunteers from the community assist with setup and serve as interpreters.

Caring for these families has a profound effect on students. "Before the trip, I was scared to death," confesses Rebecca, MSN03. "I was afraid I would be so lost, but I wasn't. I was hoping to come away with a little more knowledge. I came away with the world" (Auchmutey, 2003).

Alternative Spring Break

During spring break many students opt for the international experiences available to them. Depending on what activities they do, they may receive course credit in community health. They have gone to the British Virgin Islands, the Bahamas, Haiti, and Jamaica.

Their activities include physical assessments, health needs assessments, home visits with the public health nurse, and health fairs. A major role is teaching families, teachers, and community groups about topics such as nutrition, exercise, drug abuse prevention, HIV/AIDS, and other topics relevant to the needs of the population they are serving. They also visit hospitals, health clinics, and wellness centers. Some students used these opportunities to study the relationship between faith and health. They accompanied visiting nurses who, in addition to providing care, would often share scripture or a prayer. "I found it incredibly rejuvenating" said Emily, "We were singing and praying with them. It was a wonderful way to connect with them" (Auchmutey, 2005, p. 1).

In Jamaica students work with Missionaries of the Poor, a Jesuit community staffed by brothers from around the world. Presently in Kingston, Jamaica, the works of Missionaries of the Poor include housing and total care of over 450 destitute homeless, including children and AIDS patients; distribution of food and clothing to poor families in inner-city communities; spiritual and pastoral care of the poor and needy; and community building among the homeless residents, religious brothers, lay volunteers and staff, and the general public.

In Their Own Words: Impact of Service Learning on Students

Each baccalaureate student at Emory's School of Nursing has multiple opportunities to volunteer, some of which are related to their course requirements. For several years the author taught an undergraduate policy course that had a service learning component. Students were allowed to choose a vulnerable population, interact with the population, identify a political or policy issue that affected their population, and advocate with state or federal legislators on behalf of their population. Just the simple act of interacting with vulnerable populations and becoming personally involved in actions on their behalf is a life-altering event for students. Students were encouraged to reflect on their experiences and to record their reflections in a journal. Their journal reflections, cited with their written permission, of the impact of service learning made the case far better than any narrative written by faculty.

Students interacted with vulnerable populations in a variety of ways, volunteering with the American Red Cross, the State Council on Maternal and Infant Health, the State Nurses' Association School Health Task Force, children's shelters, food banks, Planned Parenthood, the Salvation Army, refugee programs, the State Council on Aging, AIDS outreach programs, and various agencies serving the homeless with shelters, health clinics, treatment centers for addiction, and educational programs.

Volunteer activities were challenging and rewarding. One student reported on her day building a house with Habitat for Humanity volunteers: "We had to dance around large families of baby mice. We made walls until all the prepared materials were gone. This was inside an unheated warehouse but we kept on swinging those hammers. . . . We got pretty good! My family all want to come another time and try it."

After coaching a blind young woman about interviewing for jobs over the phone, a student reported, "By the fourth call, she was amazing! She had poise and confidence that surprised both of us. Needless to say, she made several appointments for job interviews. It made me feel incredibly good to have made such a difference in this young lady's job search."

Another student who worked in a mobile healthcare clinic that visits shelters and places where homeless people congregate observed, "I've begun to recruit my friends into volunteering with the Task Force (for the Homeless). I laugh to myself at the crusader I've become."

Some activities led students to move out of their comfort level. A female student volunteering at the Atlanta Union Mission, which serves the homeless, wrote, "When I walk into that building I feel so AFRAID. I can't imagine what the people feel like who have to live out there on those streets." One of the biggest eye openers was the plight of the homeless. "Last year I began working in the homeless clinic to meet a class requirement. This was my first introduction to the homeless. I began to realize that these men and women were individuals much like me." A student wrote, "How can this situation we call homelessness but includes joblessness, hopelessness, nutritionessless [sic] and respectlessness [sic] be happening in what is supposed to be the greatest country in the world? It is mind-boggling and heart-wrenching and irrational."

Students welcome the opportunity to be advocates. Using service learning, especially with vulnerable populations, is an effective way to teach advocacy and to expose students to experiences that will affect the way they look at vulnerable clients and the way they practice nursing. An additional benefit is the recognition by students that political awareness and activism is a critical part of the nurse advocacy role. Transforming professional nurses into professional nurse advocates not only promotes learning but has a ripple effect that can transform their lives and those of others.

References

Aikens, C. A. (1916). *Studies in ethics for nurses.* Philadelphia: Saunders.

American Nurses Association (ANA). (1950). A code for nurses. *American Journal of Nursing, 50*(4), 196.

American Nurses Association (ANA). (1986). *Code for nurses with interpretive statements.* Kansas City, MO: Author.

Annas, G. (1974). The patient rights advocate: Can nurses effectively fill the role? *Supervisor Nurse,* 5(7), 21–25.

Annas, G. (1975). *The rights of hospital patients: The basic ACLU guide to a hospital patient's rights.* New York: Discus.

Auchmutey, P. (2003, Spring). Powerful lessons. *Emory Nursing.* Atlanta, GA: Emory University.

Auchmutey, P. (2005, Winter). Spring break alternatives. *Emory Nursing.* Atlanta, GA: Emory University.

Comeau, A. (2004, June 5). *Global government health partners met in Atlanta; Discussed emerging biological threats and forged partnerships* [Press Release]. Atlanta, GA: Emory University.

Comeau, A. (2005, November 4). *Emory's School of Nursing receives $60,000 for service learning program* [Press Release]. Atlanta, GA: Emory University.

Comeau, A. (2006, May 30). *Emory nursing students provide care for migrant workers and their families* [Press Release]. Atlanta, GA: Emory University.

Davis, A. J., & Aroskar, M. A. (1978). *Ethical dilemmas and nursing practice.* New York: Appleton-Century-Crofts.

Goodrich, A. W. (1932). *The social significance of nursing.* New York: Macmillan.

International Congress of Nursing. (1953). International code of nursing ethics. *American Journal of Nursing, 53*(9), 1070.

Kolb, D. A. (1984). *Experiential learning: Experience as the source of learning and development.* Englewood Cliffs, NJ: Prentice Hall.

Knowles, M. (1984). *The adult learner: A neglected species.* Houston, TX: Gulf Publishing.

Letter to the editor. (1910). Where does loyalty to the physician end? *American Journal of Nursing, 10*(1), 274, 276.

Loftus, M. (2005, Winter). Making bigger beds. *Emory Nursing.* Atlanta, GA: Emory University.

Mueller, C., & Norton, B. (1998). Service learning: Developing values and social responsibility. In D. M. Billings & J. Halstead (Eds.), *Teaching in nursing education.* Philadelphia: Saunders.

Parsons, S .E. (1916). *Nursing problems and obligations.* Boston: Whitcomb & Barrows.

Pellietier, S. (1995). The quiet power of service learning: Report from the National Institute on Learning and Service. *The Independent, 95*(2), 6.

Winslow, G. R. (1984). From loyalty to advocacy: A new metaphor for nursing. In *The Hastings Center Report* (pp. 32–40). Hastings-on-Hudson, NY: The Hastings Center.

Designing a Model for Predicting or Working with Vulnerable Populations Based on Graduate Fieldwork

Jane W. Peterson, Heather Andersen, Jennifer U. Mercado, Julia F. Shellhorn, Justin Speyer, and Lakshmi Thiagaraj

The excerpts in this chapter are taken from the final written assignments of graduate students in *NURS 502: Vulnerability, Nursing, and Culture* taught by the first author. The class is much as described in the first edition of this book (Phillips & Peterson, 2005). However, the written assignments emphasized the creation of a model for predicting or working with the vulnerable populations with whom the students did fieldwork. The fieldwork inspired the following models that represent a beginning stage of critically grappling with concepts in the literature that influence vulnerability.

Vulnerability Assessment Model (Andersen)

I developed an assessment model for assessing vulnerability (Figure 40-1) based on my fieldwork with children who lived in a low-income area of the city. The model could be used in medical offices to determine the presence and extent of vulnerability of different clients. The model asks 14 yes or no questions with a score attached to each "no" answer. An individual with a sum of 12 or more is considered to be "vulnerable." Scores between 6 and 10 are deemed "moderately vulnerable," and scores of 5 or less indicate individuals who are most likely to be "not vulnerable."

The weights for each "no" answer are based on how vulnerable each response makes an individual in comparison with the other "no" responses. Questions relating to adequate food and shelter are heavily weighted so that individuals without these basic needs (Maslow, 1968) are automatically labeled as vulnerable. Additionally, a variety of combinations of others factors can qualify an individual as vulnerable. For example, Campos-Outcult et al. (1994) suggested three criteria for assessing vulnerability in a

	No
1. Do you feel that you have adequate family or social support?	3
2. Do you have enough money to choose the food you want or need?	6
3. Are you a single parent household?	2
4. Do you have adequate shelter?	6
5. Do you have access to a primary care provider?	4
6. Do you have health insurance?	4
7. Do you feel like you can successfully use the health care system?	4
8. Are you able to read and write well in the dominant language?	3
9. If unemployed, are you unemployed by choice?	3
10. Do you feel like you could change your employment if you wanted to?	2
11. Do you feel safe in your neighborhood?	2
12. Could you change your living situation if you needed to?	2
13. Are you able to practice your cultural traditions?	2
14. Do you have the ability to get where you need to?	2
Total	_____

Figure 40-1 Vulnerability Assessment Model

This is an assessment model for vulnerability based on fieldwork with children who lived in a low-income metropolitan area.

population—lack of access of care, fragmentation of care, and lack of cultural competence—that I integrated into my model. "No" answers on all three of the corresponding questions in my model add up to 12, indicating vulnerability. I wanted my model to be comprehensive enough to capture the multitude of factors that contribute to vulnerability but not so much as to label everyone as vulnerable.

A large range of scores indicates moderate vulnerability. In these instances each area that contributes to vulnerability should be addressed and clients should be connected with the appropriate and available resources in their respective communities. Hence, the model can be used not only to identify vulnerable populations but also to highlight areas of concern.

	Highest Risk	Higher Risk	Moderate Risk	Lower Risk
	Check the Box That Best Describes the Client			
Self-actualization				
Do you feel your life has purpose?	❏ Never or rarely	❏ Sometimes	❏ Often	❏ Almost always
You feel you are able to reach your potential	❏ Never or rarely	❏ Sometimes	❏ Often	❏ Almost always
Esteem				
Are you satisfied with your achievements?	❏ Never or rarely	❏ Sometimes	❏ Often	❏ Almost always
Do you feel respected by others?	❏ Never or rarely	❏ Sometimes	❏ Often	❏ Almost always
Do you feel accepted by others?	❏ Never or rarely	❏ Sometimes	❏ Often	❏ Almost always
Love/belonging				
Do you feel you are loved by others?	❏ Never or rarely	❏ Sometimes	❏ Often	❏ Almost always
How often do you feel lonely?	❏ Almost always	❏ Often	❏ Occasionally	❏ Never or rarely
How often do you feel depressed?	❏ Almost always	❏ Often	❏ Occasionally	❏ Never or rarely
Family support networks	❏ No support	❏ Little support	❏ Some support	❏ Strong support
Friend support networks	❏ No support	❏ Little support	❏ Some support	❏ Strong support
Community support networks	❏ No support	❏ Little support	❏ Some support	❏ Strong support
Family status	❏ Single/divorced/ widowed			❏ Married/partner

(continues)

Figure 40-2 Vulnerability Assessment Tool Utilizing Maslow's Hierarchy of Needs

This tool is used to predict vulnerability that incorporates both visible and nonvisible risk factors based on volunteer fieldwork at a local soup kitchen.

	Highest Risk	Higher Risk	Moderate Risk	Lower Risk
	Check the Box That Best Describes the Client			
Safety				
Do you feel safe in your community?	❏ Never or rarely	❏ Sometimes	❏ Often	❏ Almost always
Do you feel safe in your home?	❏ Never or rarely	❏ Sometimes	❏ Often	❏ Almost always
Physical/sexual abuse	❏ Ongoing abuse	❏ Past abuse	❏ Female: no prior abuse	❏ Male: no prior abuse
Employment status	❏ Unemployed	❏ Inadequate work	❏ Insecure employment	❏ Adequate and secure
Financial resources	❏ Less than poverty level	❏ 100% + poverty level	❏ 200% + poverty level	❏ 300% + poverty level
Access to health care services	❏ No access	❏ Unreliable access	❏ Somewhat reliable access	❏ Reliable access
Access to preventive health services	❏ No access	❏ Unreliable access	❏ Somewhat reliable access	❏ Reliable access
Health insurance	❏ No health insurance	❏ Medicaid/ Medicare	❏ Medicare and supplementary	❏ Private insurance
Health status	❏ HIV/AIDS	❏ Terminal/ chronic disease	❏ Managed chronic illness	❏ Good/excellent health
Physical disability	❏ Disability: dependent	❏ Disability: requires assistance	❏ Disability: independent	❏ No disability

Figure 40-2 Vulnerability Assessment Tool Utilizing Maslow's Hierarchy of Needs

This tool is used to predict vulnerability that incorporates both visible and nonvisible risk factors based on volunteer fieldwork at a local soup kitchen. (*continued*)

Check the Box That Best Describes the Client

	Highest Risk	Higher Risk	Moderate Risk	Lower Risk
History of mental health (MH)	☐ Untreated MH issue	☐ Poorly controlled MH issue	☐ Well controlled MH issue	☐ No MH issue
Substance addiction/abuse in household	☐ Addiction/overuse ongoing	☐ Occasional overuse	☐ Prior addiction/overuse	☐ No abuse/addiction
Housing	☐ Homeless/shelter/car	☐ Friends/family	☐ Insecure/inadequate housing	☐ Secure housing
Access to transportation	☐ No access	☐ Occasional access	☐ Usually have access	☐ Always have access
Access to telephone	☐ No access	☐ Occasional access	☐ Usually have access	☐ Always have access
Education level completed	☐ Less than high school	☐ High school	☐ Some college	☐ College graduate
Citizenship/immigration status	☐ Illegal immigrant	☐ Legal immigrant	☐ Naturalized citizen	☐ Native-born citizen
Language as a communication barrier	☐ Almost always	☐ Often	☐ Occasionally	☐ Never or rarely
Literacy level	☐ Grades 0–4	☐ Grades 5–8	☐ Grades 8–12	☐ Grades 13+
Race/ethnicity/sexual orientation	☐ Minority			☐ Nonminority
Age	☐ Frail elderly; <age 6	☐ >Age 65; <age 18		☐ Adult
Gender	☐ Transgender		☐ Female	☐ Male

(*continues*)

Figure 40-2 Vulnerability Assessment Tool Utilizing Maslow's Hierarchy of Needs

This tool is used to predict vulnerability that incorporates both visible and nonvisible risk factors based on volunteer fieldwork at a local soup kitchen. (*continued*)

	Highest Risk	Higher Risk	Moderate Risk	Lower Risk
	Check the Box That Best Describes the Client			
Physiological				
Food and nutrition	☐ Food insecure with hunger	☐ Food insecure: malnutrition	☐ Food secure: malnutrition	☐ Secure: good nutrition
Adequate warmth (clothing and heat)	☐ Poor	☐ Barely adequate	☐ Adequate	☐ More than adequate
Adequate sleep and rest	☐ Rarely adequate	☐ Sometimes adequate	☐ Usually adequate	☐ Almost always adequate
Air quality at home/work	☐ Poor	☐ Fair	☐ Good	☐ Excellent
Water quality	☐ Poor	☐ Fair	☐ Good	☐ Excellent
Sanitation/hygiene	☐ Poor	☐ Fair	☐ Good	☐ Excellent
Assessment of level of vulnerability	Score 1 point for each item checked above	Score 2 points for each item checked above	Score 3 points for each item checked above	Score 4 points for each item checked above

Note: Although the aggregate score may be useful in evaluating someone's overall risk, each factor must also be considered independently. One response at a highest or high level of risk may indicate vulnerability.

Lower risk for vulnerability   = 160

Moderate risk for vulnerability   = 140

High risk for vulnerability   = 120

Figure 40-2 Vulnerability Assessment Tool Utilizing Maslow's Hierarchy of Needs

This tool is used to predict vulnerability that incorporates both visible and nonvisible risk factors based on volunteer fieldwork at a local soup kitchen. (*continued*)

Vulnerability Assessment Tool Using Maslow's Hierarchy of Needs (Shellhorn)

My volunteer fieldwork was at a local soup kitchen serving members of the community whose basic physiological need for food is insecure. In designing a tool to predict vulnerability, I wanted to incorporate both visible and nonvisible risk factors for vulnerability. I used Maslow's (1968) hierarchy of needs as a frame for my model (Figure 40-2). I could then address identity and specific exposures, including physical, social, resource, and environmental driven factors that influence vulnerability.

In the model basic human needs are categorized according to Maslow's (1968) hierarchy. Building on a foundation of basic physiological needs are needs associated with safety, love, esteem, and self-actualization. Partially met or unmet human needs are associated with increasing vulnerability. Physiological needs are evaluated in terms of nutrition and environmental health risks such as air pollution, impure water, and poor sanitation that impact health (World Health Organization, 2004). Safety is evaluated in terms of existing physical and mental health issues, disability, adequate housing, and threats to safety, including domestic violence, crime, and substance abuse. This section also addresses the ability to meet basic needs and issues related to vulnerability based on identity such as immigrant status. Finally, strength of connectedness to others, self-esteem, and self-actualization provide a measure of psychological and emotional vulnerability (de Chesnay, 2005).

The model successfully captures most risk factors for hunger as well as many of the associated problems facing families with food insecurity. However, it is important to note that while risk factors increase one's chance of becoming vulnerable to hunger, many of those who are actually vulnerable to hunger do not come from these higher risk groups. According to a report on local food security (Mathematica Policy Research, Inc., 2006) more than 40% of those relying on food programs in western Washington are employed, nearly half have some form of postsecondary education, and about one-third have high school diplomas.

Balancing the Tower of Vulnerability (Speyer)

Vulnerability is a complex state that is not easily quantified. A series of circumstances that make one person vulnerable may not be enough to make another person vulnerable. I did fieldwork with an after-school program for children in a low-income neighborhood that has a large immigrant population. To visualize the vulnerable state I chose a model (Figure 40-3) based on the game Jenga®. In the game a standard stack of wood blocks is built, and then one by one blocks are removed and placed on top of the stack. As more blocks are removed the tower becomes both taller and less stable, until eventually it collapses. No two attempts are ever the same. I believe this represents both the complexity of vulnerability and the unpredictable nature of the individual. A given tower can easily be constructed and the vulnerabilities presented to give a visual gauge of the individuals risks and strengths.

My model assigns roles to each block in the tower, and although the specific location of a given factor may vary, they are all present in some capacity and provide strength or induce weakness in the tower. Factors that can be present in varying degrees are represented by more blocks, such as money and education, whereas factors that are either present or absent, such as illegal drugs or health insurance, are more limited. We might, for

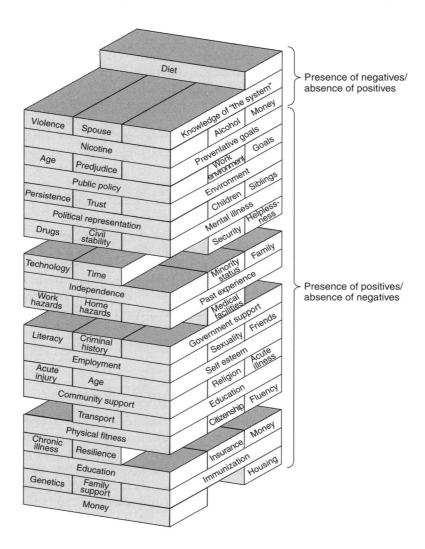

Figure 40-3 Balancing the Tower of Vulnerability

This model of vulnerability uses a woodblock stacking game that was developed after completing fieldwork with an after-school program for children in a low-income neighborhood with a large immigrant population.

example, start with our tower, remove three money blocks and the drugs block, and place them on top. In doing so we have created a model representing the presence of drugs and the relative absence of money. Although other factors still provide strength for the tower, it is certainly weaker than an unadulterated model. The more factors that move from "advantages" in the tower's base to "disadvantages" on the tower's summit, the more at risk the individual. A child who has little home support, no access to out-of-home support, a single parent, and little money has had several supports removed. This child's tower is now more vulnerable to small risks. Such risks may not have their own block but instead may simply "rock the tower," leading to its collapse.

Small risks may be missed days of school, forgetting a small assignment, an injury, or negative feedback from a teacher. The unmeasurable ability of a given individual to resist these small changes may be best characterized by the concept of resilience or one's "ability to 'bounce back' in spite of significant stress or adversity" (Place, Reynolds, Cousins, & O'Neill, 2002; Stewart, Reid, & Mangham, 1997). Although it may not be the expected normal response, some individuals do rise above circumstances that have dragged down many of their peers. For many individuals their tower is incomplete based on unalterable factors. Genetic predisposition and being part of a nondominant culture are examples of factors that make an individual more vulnerable regardless of the other factors at work in their tower.

Because minority groups tend to be marginalized despite education and income (de Chesnay, 2005), we would expect blocks to be absent from such a person's tower regardless of the rest of their circumstances. It is also completely plausible that a minority child who speaks English as a second language with no insurance and little money could be very successful. In this case the removal of blocks representing insurance, money, dominant culture, and fluency have not compromised the tower critically and stability remains. The child is certainly more vulnerable than if these supports were in place, but the child has not "collapsed." The individual circumstances and the individual him- or herself determine much of the outcome, just like every attempted tower.

The Vulneracycle Model (Thiagaraj)

The Vulneracycle Model (Figure 40-4) was derived from the 20 hours of interacting with a community at a family center. The people who attended the center's sessions and programs were from all around the world, but they all had one thing in common: They were all immigrants. This population consisted of women, men, and children of all ages who had emigrated from China, Mexico, Vietnam, Peru, Thailand, Russia, and Somalia. Immigrants can be considered as vulnerable according to de Chesnay (2005) because of their limited access to health care. The vulneracycle bicycle represents the immigrants in this community and the factors that contribute to their vulnerability.

The front tire of the bicycle represents the nonmodifiable risk factors of this community, such as age and race. Although these factors impact the level of vulnerability, they

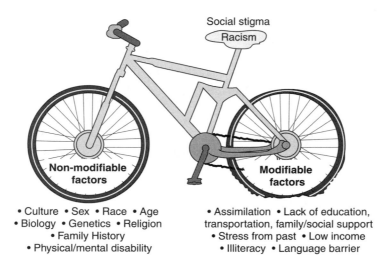

Social stigma
Racism

Non-modifiable factors

Modifiable factors

• Culture • Sex • Race • Age
• Biology • Genetics • Religion
• Family History
• Physical/mental disability

• Assimilation • Lack of education,
transportation, family/social support
• Stress from past • Low income
• Illiteracy • Language barrier

Figure 40-4 The Vulneracycle Model

This model was developed after extended interaction with a multicultural immigrant community.

cannot be changed, so an inflated tire represents these factors. The deflated rear tire represents the modifiable risk factors of this community, such as language barrier and unemployment. This tire can only be inflated if the individuals modify their risk factors. Without inflating the rear tire, the bicycle will not work efficiently and the immigrants will continue to be vulnerable.

The immigrants at the center were always enthusiastic to learn, not only about America but also about one another. Of the many challenges listed in the rear tire, their inability to speak English and their lack of transportation were the most challenging. Attending English as a second language classes regularly and attempting to speak English gave them the opportunity to start inflating the rear tire. Although many of the immigrants had no mode of transportation, most of them still managed to attend the family center daily. Some walked many blocks, even miles in the rain, to attend their classes. Their dedication and interest in attending their classes also contributes to inflating the tire and moving forward in life.

Racism had an impact on almost all the immigrants at the center. During an "Undoing Institutional Racism" seminar, many people tearfully shared stories of how they experienced racism in America. Racism and social stigmatization are both represented on the bicycle seat. If immigrants experience high levels of racial and social stigmatization, their seat will be higher than normal, making it difficult to ride the bicycle. Because undoing racism and social stigmatization are an ongoing process, the immigrants need to adjust their seat by not allowing these negative experiences to discourage them from becoming successful in life.

Shields and Berhman (2005) noted that immigrant families tend to assimilate with people from their same country of origin. This concept was represented in the rear tire because the Chinese women at the family center would sit together and speak in their native language, whereas the Latino women did the same on the other side of the room. During the children's tutoring session, the Muslim children sat on one side of the classroom and the African-American children sat on the other side of the room. People sat and interacted with others from their own country because it gave them a sense of comfort, but adjusting to mainstream society may be more challenging as a result.

Barbell Framework of Vulnerability: The Heavy Burden of Vulnerability (Mercado)

I worked at a secondary bilingual education program in a public school for immigrants (ages 12–20) who needed to gain greater command of the English language before entering mainstream schools. My framework for predicting or working with a vulnerable person or group is derived from the image of a barbell that would be used in a weightlifting competition. It is called "the barbell framework for vulnerability: the 'heavy' burden of vulnerability" (Figure 40.5). The three main components of this framework are the bar and the weights that can be added to the bar, both of which contribute to the overall weight and risk for vulnerability, and the weightlifter, who is expected to have the strength to lift the barbell. The principle that governs the barbell framework of vulnerability is that vulnerability increases with the increasing weight of the barbell and decreases with decreasing weight or increasing strength of the weightlifter.

The minimum amount of weight the weightlifter can be expected to lift is the bar alone. Using this idea, each person is given a "bar" to start with based on their age, gender, genetics, race, and ethnicity, social status factors according to Aday (2001). These factors cannot change; the bar cannot be exchanged for another one of lighter or heavier weight. The differences in the starting weights of the bar convey two very important ideas: everyone begins with some amount of weight (risk), so zero risk is not possible, and some, by virtue of non-negotiable factors, begin at a higher level of risk for vulnerability than others.

The weights represent factors that can change throughout a person's life to affect their vulnerability status. There are four different categories of weights that include factors that may or may not be relevant for each person or population. To use this framework, only the weights relevant for the person or population being studied are selected for consideration. There are personal "weights" (family, social network, language, religion, culture, literacy, education, health insurance, income, level of assimilation), community "weights" (demographics of their home community, housing, access to and quality of schools, employment, socioeconomic status, healthcare access), psychological health "weights" (self-esteem, depression, profound

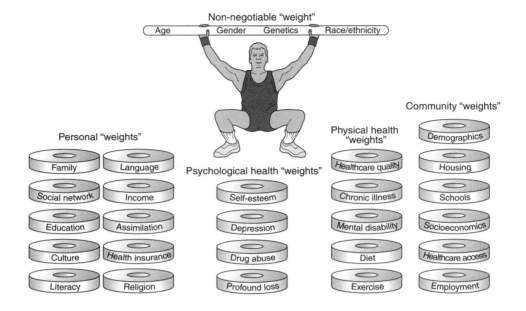

Figure 40-5 The Barbell Framework of Vulnerability: The Heavy Burden of Vulnerability
This model was developed after working at a public school for immigrants to improve English skills before entering mainstream schools.

loss, drug abuse), and physical health "weights" (healthcare quality, chronic illness, mental disability, diet, exercise). Each of these weights can be added either to the bar to signify increasing vulnerability or as "muscle" to the "weightlifter" to offset vulnerability depending on the character of the factor in the individual's life. For example, low literacy, unemployment, lower self-esteem, and lack of exercise would increase risk for vulnerability and be added to the bar to make it heavier, whereas high literacy, steady employment, high self-esteem, and regular exercise would decrease risk for vulnerability and empower the weightlifter.

Some factors, such as family, culture, religion, and language, can be sources of risk as well as sources of strength to allay other risks. For example, some cultures value family over the individual, which ensures a solid support system and decreased risk for vulnerability, but this value can also lead people to choose working to provide for their family over education despite the increased risk for vulnerability attributed to lower education. In these cases weight must be added to the bar and to the weightlifter's strength.

Implications for Advanced Nursing Practice

As a result of developing a model for predicting or working with vulnerable populations based on fieldwork, graduate nursing students learned several important lessons:

1. Using a model to identify risk factors of vulnerability for clients helps the nurse begin a dialogue about possible solutions and connections to available resources. In addition, provider awareness of these factors is important when designing an appropriate and effective treatment regimen and when making recommendations for life-style changes, referrals, and follow-ups.

2. Awareness of potential and existing vulnerability in communities and clients is important for nurses. Vulnerability directly threatens clients' health and well-being; therefore identifying vulnerability is essential to providing quality and holistic nursing care.

3. An important point to carry from a model into nursing practice is the individual nature of every patient. Despite identical risk factors and even seemingly near identical genetics, two individuals may cope with life's experiences differently, experience different problems, and achieve different goals. Although a model predicts well what might be expected from a given set of circumstances by highlighting the precariousness induced by these circumstances, it cannot account for the ability of a person to rise above his or her circumstances even against horrendous odds.

4. A model can demonstrate that because everything is linked, addressing any part of the model has an impact on the entire model and can lead to a change in a client's risk factors. A model can also show that vulnerability presents itself in many different ways and is not just limited to those who are poor and uneducated.

5. Some models work well with immigrant populations, especially when they understand the risk factors that need to be modified. Change is of course easiest when immigrant populations want to assimilate, which is to change. Even for those immigrants who are unwilling to make a change, a model can depict the common nonmodifiable and modifiable risk factors within the immigrant population and can still guide advanced nurse practitioners on how to provide health care for the immigrant population as a whole.

6. A model reminds nurses to focus on things that are negotiable to decrease vulnerability. A model can present two possible ways to decrease vulnerability: eliminate the risk factors (e.g., replace low self-esteem with high self-esteem) or combat the risk factors by drawing on other aspects (strengths) of a person's life to increase their ability to thwart vulnerability (e.g., religion can help people deal with profound loss). Both of these strategies can be used to increase health.

7. There is an extensive variation on healthcare perspectives, specifically the role of the individual and spirituality in sickness, decision making, health maintenance, and mentality. In this sense an advanced nurse practitioner is the accompanist who empowers those seeking help, respecting their needs and wants.

Overall, students learned that a model provides valuable guidance in collecting and assessing data on risk factors that can predict or confirm vulnerability in individuals and populations. Models constructed from what is familiar to the individual or group has a much better chance of producing accurate information. Students have glimpsed how they might use these data to plan interventions and evaluate health outcomes. Using a model of vulnerability constructed from a population's way of life has the potential to decrease health disparities and improve health outcomes for that population more so than a more generalized model.

References

Aday, L. A. (2001). *At risk in America: The health and health care needs of vulnerable populations in the United States* (2nd ed.). San Francisco: Jossey-Bass.

Campos-Outcult, D., Fernandez, R., Hollow, W., Lundeen, S., Nelson, K., Schuster, B., et al. (1994). *Providing quality care to vulnerable populations.* Retrieved September 17, 2007, from http://www.primarycaresociety.org/1994d.htm

de Chesnay, M. (2005). Vulnerable populations: Vulnerable people. In M. de Chesnay (Ed.), *Caring for the vulnerable: Perspectives in nursing theory, practice, and research* (pp. 3–12). Sudbury, MA: Jones and Bartlett.

Maslow, A. H. (1968). *Towards a philosophy of being* (2nd ed.). New York: Van Nostrand Reinhold.

Mathematica Policy Research, Inc. (2006). *Hunger in America 2006: Local report prepared for Food Lifeline.* Princeton, NJ: Mathematica Policy Research, Inc.

Phillips, D. A., & Peterson, J. W. (2005). Graduate studies approach to vulnerability. In M. de Chesnay (Ed.), *Caring for the vulnerable: Perspectives in nursing theory, practice, and research* (pp. 385–394). Sudbury, MA: Jones and Bartlett.

Place, M., Reynolds, J., Cousins, A., & O'Neill, S. (2002). Developing a resilience package for vulnerable children. *Child and Adolescent Mental Health, 7*(4), 162–167.

Shields, M., & Behrman, R. (2005). Children in immigrant families. *InFocus, 1.* Retrieved September 17, 2007, from http://www.healthinschools.org/News-Room/InFocus/2005/Issue-1.aspx

Stewart, M., Reid, C., & Mangham, C. (1997). Fostering children's resilience. *Journal of Pediatric Nursing, 12*(1), 21–31.

World Health Organization. (2004). *Water, sanitation and hygiene links to health.* Retrieved September 17, 2007, from http://www.who.int/water_sanitation_health/publications/facts2004/en/

Chapter 41

Vulnerable Populations: A Model for a Web-Enhanced Doctoral-Level Course

Angeline Bushy

This chapter provides an overview of a doctoral core course program entitled "Vulnerable Populations" offered at the University of Central Florida, College of Nursing. One of the first courses in the program of study, the format consists of 50% face-to-face class seminars in a traditional classroom setting and 50% online web-based class seminar assignments. An electronic course (e-course) makes education more accessible to professional nurses with multiple personal and professional responsibilities. The information herein could serve as a model for other faculty who are considering a fully web-based online course or a web-enhanced course, which is partially face-to-face and partially online.

Background and Rationale

Historically, the principle components of the educational process have been a teacher, student, content, and context. Obviously, students are those who seek content, the instructor is the person who disseminates the information, and the content varies with the subject matter being taught. In respect to the context, traditionally this has been a group of learners (class) who meet face-to-face with a teacher in a fixed facility "bricks-and-mortar" classroom. The teacher was expected to disseminate content to the student while the latter passively absorbed the lectured didactic content. Adult learning theory changed what was known about students' learning preferences and appropriate teaching strategies. That is to say, the teacher and learner came to be viewed as partners in the educational process that meshes with needs and preferences of the mature student (Knowles, 1980).

With the advent of the Internet and electronic communication technology, the context of where learning takes place was dramatically changed as well. In other words, with e-courses learning opportunities and access to relevant content occurs outside of a formal classroom setting. Metaphorically, an online web-based course can be viewed as a context (setting) without physical boundaries (i.e., in cyberspace) in which extensive information (content, experts) is readily available to both the learner and the teacher, from which is created new knowledge.

Telecommunication technology expanded educational opportunities for consumers and healthcare providers alike; as with most things, there are both benefits and challenges associated with it. On the one hand, along with allowing for greater student diversity and more immediate access to educational offerings, online classes can reduce actual student "seat time" in a formal classroom and reduce or even eliminate commuting to teach or attend classes. These are definite benefits in a resource-driven environment in light of the costs of constructing university buildings, traveling time and vehicle-related expenditures, and the multiple personal and professional responsibilities of adult learners, in this case nurses. Conversely, students who enroll in an online course must be self-directed and motivated, whereas the teacher may feel less in control of the learning environment. Also, some question whether online courses are of similar quality as conventional classroom offerings. However, the literature reported quality is comparable for the two delivery modalities, and a discussion of this issue is beyond the scope of this chapter (Bushy, 2003).

Lexicon for Online Courses

With the emergence of technology, traditional educational concepts assume broader connotations and a somewhat new lexicon. For example, *distributive learning* is used in lieu of more conventional terms such as outreach or distance education and correspondence courses. *Community of learners* has a broader contextual dimension without regard to space or time. Essentially, *distributive learning* is used in reference to the relative nature of time and the multiple sites (virtual cyberspace classroom) where learners can access course materials and content. A *virtual classroom* can be accessed by learners at any time and from almost any place on the globe. *Logging on* involves accessing/connecting into a specific site on the World Wide Web (Internet). As for dialogue among the learning partners in a virtual classroom, discussions can be *synchronous* (real-time discussions such as a chat room) and *asynchronous* (posting comments on the Internet to be available, read, and commented on by peers, around the clock, 7 days a week; Little, Passmore, & Schullo, 2006). *Posting* entails submitting a written comment in a designated site on the Internet; subsequently, that information is available for others who log on to view on their computer screen.

The technology and software used to teach an online course varies from one institution to another and from student to student. Lack of standardization is one of the most significant challenges for the instructor and students enrolled in a course. Most educational institutions have recommendations regarding minimum technology requirements and computer proficiencies for students and faculty (Bushy, 2003; Tilley, Boswell , & Cannon, 2006). Table 41-1 suggests minimum requirements for access, capability, and usage for online courses based on the author's experiences.

TABLE 41-1   **Minimum Technology and Behavioral Proficiencies for Teaching Online Coursess**

Equipment	Behavioral Proficiencies
Instructional design capability within the university; faculty/student development program for e-learning	Flexible attitude about teaching–learning; open to new ideas regarding uses of technology in education; self-directed about learning opportunities
Desktop/laptop computer/printer less than 3 years old	Proficiency in use of computer/printer/ Microsoft Office software functions; ensuring Internet security
Recent version of Microsoft Office (word processing, e-mail, presentation tool, web browser, spreadsheet); Internet security systems	Know when/whom to contact when telecommunications are down/slow
Fastest commonly available modem, Ethernet, or other connection for Internet access (greater bandwidth than provided by telephone modem)	Know how to access/use course management system of sponsoring institution
Institutional instructional design "help desk" capacity sufficient to respond within 1 hour 24/7 to instructor/students (phone, e-mail)	Know when, how, and whom to ask for help (e.g., help desk personnel, peers, student assistants)
No personal usage fees for accessing databases and library services	Access/identify/use online library services/ databases; know when/how to ask librarian for assistance

Development of the Online Component of Vulnerable Populations

In many ways designing the doctoral-level online course, "Vulnerable Populations," was similar to developing one for the traditional classroom using the following process (Bushy, 2003; Parker & Howland 2006):

- Planning the course
- Setting the stage
- Guiding and managing the discussion
- Problem solving and trouble shooting
- Evaluating the process and outcomes

Developing a course is not a linear process. Rather, an instructor progresses forward and then revisits content, assignments, and activities based on new insights about the topic area. Keys to successfully integrating online teaching–learning strategies are keeping an open mind about teaching–learning processes and having a willingness to assess various technologies to determine "best fit" with unique content, course objectives, and student learning needs. For the instructor it is of the utmost importance when developing an online course to become comfortable with the classroom management software that is being used at their institution. Table 41-2 summarizes information to take into consideration when planning an online course.

At first, teaching an online course can be daunting; most faculty who develop a doctoral-level course probably have taught in a conventional classroom setting. Rarely is there a need to develop an online course without having access to course management software specifically designed for this purpose. Course management systems (CMS) software facilitates instructor management and student experience in e-learning situations. Terms used in reference to CMS include, among others, managed learning environment, learning management system, virtual learning environment, learning management system, learning content management system, and learning support system. Popular CMS used within academic settings include WebCT/Blackboard and others. Essentially, CMS allows for instructor creativity while controlling the layout, colors, texts, and graphics for the course in creating lesson plans, specific assignments, student discussion, e-mail capabilities, online testing, and chat room capabilities.

Metaphorically, CMS software is comparable with the architectural structure of a school building in that it provides consistency for online courses. The CMS software used by the University of Central Florida allows the College of Nursing to standardize the format for its online courses, including the home page of all nursing courses (screens), which has similar graphics and content arrangement. For instance, on the home page button-type links are located on the left side of the screen for students to access the course syllabus, learning modules/assignments with corresponding discussion topics, examinations, and course evaluations. The CMS software can be used to monitor, evaluate, and respond to individual students. For instance, CMS software allows an instructor to track the first, last, and total number of times a student logged on to the course along with the number of postings. Progressive e-tracking does not indicate the quality or appropriateness of a student's response or even if he or she reads the materials. Rather, it is an indicator of an individual's level of class activity, or lack thereof, to which an instructor might consider follow-up either to encourage or reinforce student behavior.

Posted responses and proffered student questions can offer insights about the quality of an individual's understanding of course materials. It is therefore imperative that the instructor read student postings and then, as appropriate, intersperse questions to individuals either via course e-mail or to the group as a whole. Such strategies reinforce or redirect class discussions and can enhance the quality of content submitted in student postings.

TABLE 41-2 General Considerations for Faculty Developing an Online Course

Consideration	Questions to Ask
Determine appropriateness of technology (best fit) to achieve course/instructional goals	Have you taught the course before?
	What are course goals/objectives/outcomes? Essential content areas?
	Which areas do students tend to have difficulty?
	What are possible solutions using technology?
	What technology/software is available at your university/school? How familiar are you with it?
Know your students	How proficient are students with the computer/Microsoft Office software?
	Have they taken other web-based courses?
	How comfortable are they with the Internet, search, and library resources?
	Have students attended a university/department-sponsored orientation class for online learning?
	What are specific critical competencies needed to be successful in an online course? How can these be addressed in your course?
	Do students have access to the required computer/hardware/Internet/software and hardware for taking an online course?
	Does their Internet service provider allow for extended time usage without disconnecting?

(continues)

TABLE 41-2 General Considerations for Faculty Developing an Online Course (continued)

Consideration	Questions to Ask
Be familiar with institutional/other resources (technology/support)	What support (technical/instructional) is available to faculty/students within your university?
	How familiar are you with the services?
	Do you know how to access these services? How to refer students?
	How familiar are you with online library resources for teaching web-based courses?
Develop the course	Are you able to use institutional course management/design software?
	What course content should be included? How should it be organized?
	What features of the CMS software can be used to meet your course objectives?
	How can a community of learners be developed among students enrolled in the course?
Assess quality and measure outcomes	How do students believe they benefit by taking an online course?
	While teaching the course/upon completion evaluate process and outcomes. What worked? What course modification could promote more effective learning?
	How should the course/technology be adapted/revised to make learning more successful in the future?
	How can university/college evaluation protocols/findings be integrated into the course?
	What potential areas of research can you identify to pursue related to the course/personal experiences?
	Is it feasible to participate in faculty teaching peer review?

Vulnerable Populations Course Format

Regardless of the context, be it in a traditional classroom or an e-course, ideally an instructor of a doctoral-level course facilitates comprehensive critiques of the research and professional literature and fosters development of new knowledge relative to phenomenon of interest to each learner. Subsequently, precise articulation, in both the oral and written word, is a proficiency that needs to be developed in doctoral students. With those educational precepts in mind, the Vulnerable Populations course was organized into 10 learning modules. Of these, five modules occurred in a traditional classroom seminar and the remaining five modules entailed web-based online seminars. Students are expected to actively participate in *all* seminar discussions by sharing insights gleaned from outside readings (textbooks, professional/research articles) coupled with personal and professional experiences related to the topic under discussion. Each student is expected to write and post substantive responses along with supporting documentation within a specified time frame. Students subsequently propose relevant questions for future class seminars.

Two other course requirements are writing a scholarly "publishable" paper that examines in-depth a vulnerable population of particular interest to the student and a formal 20-minute oral class presentation. Students are required to have their paper reviewed by two randomly assigned classmates using criteria commonly used by peer-reviewed journals. Microsoft Word "track changes" tool is used for the peer-review process. All student-generated documentation is submitted to the instructor along with the final version of a student's paper. In a face-to-face seminar near the end of the semester, each student presents key points of his or her paper using PowerPoint software. As with the scholarly paper, each oral presentation is reviewed by all classmates using a rating rubric. Given space constraints, it is not possible to describe the entire course in this chapter. Table 41-3 shows four modified exemplars of class module/learning units from that course.

Lessons Learned

Using prescribed university and college tools, the process and outcomes of the course were evaluated. Overall, this course is highly rated by students. Along with the content being informative to them, they noted that the scholarly paper and oral presentations were valuable learning experiences. Although the chosen textbook was deemed appropriate, Internet resources proved to be the best source for current information relative to topics under discussion. Based on the instructor's personal experience and anecdotal comments from students, the following sections highlight lessons learned for others who are considering developing an online course (Bushy, 2003; Pullen, 2006; Tilley et al., 2006).

Building Community of Learners

Establishing rapport is critical to building a learning community, whether it is in the traditional or virtual classroom. Regardless of the delivery modality, it is critical for the

TABLE 41-3   Online Vulnerable Population Exemplars: Four Course Modules
Exemplar: Module A

Unit Objective:

Upon completion of this Module the student will define vulnerability and identify specific at-risk populations.

Unit Content:

Introduction to vulnerability

- Define vulnerability
- Identify specific vulnerable populations
- Precursors for vulnerability

Demographics related to vulnerable populations:

- What data are needed
- Places to find data
- Data interpretation

Required Reading:

Select textbook chapters
Search databases and the Internet to become familiar with literature on vulnerable populations. Select/focus on population of interest to you

Assignment (Web):

1. Define vulnerability in your own words, before completing the next question (short paragraph).
2. Read/analyze an article that focuses on a vulnerable population of interest to you in light of the information that is provided in your assigned readings. Respond to the following questions. (*No duplication of articles please.*)
   a. Post an annotated bibliographic citation for the article, highlighting the target population (250–300 words).
   b. Defend your position as to why you believe this is a "vulnerable" group.
   c. How does your analysis of this article fit with your preliminary definition of "vulnerability"?
3. Based on the designated course objectives and your readings develop at least one question for the topic under discussion in class next week.
4. Post your responses in the designated Discussion site.

I look forward to a spirited discussion about vulnerable populations of interest to you.

Preparation for next face-to-face class:

Each student should come to class prepared to discuss the content relative to the Class Objective and *all of the student generated* (posted) questions for this Module. Please bring full text versions of the article(s) to class with you next week.

TABLE 41-3 **Online Vulnerable Population Exemplars: Four Course Modules** (continued)

Exemplar: Module B

Unit Objective:

Upon completion of this Module the student will apply various theoretical perspectives to select vulnerable populations.

Unit Content:

Theoretical perspectives related to vulnerability
Nursing theories
Theories from other disciplines

Required Reading:

Select textbook chapters
Relevant articles from the professional literature

Weekly Assignment (Web):

1. Each student will be responsible to synthesize and analyze two articles. (*No duplication of articles please.*)

   • The first should be a research/evidence-based article focusing on student-selected vulnerable population that includes a nursing theory.

   • The other should be a research article from another discipline that includes a relevant theory from that discipline.

   • Post an annotated bibliographic citation for each article, focusing on the application of theory (250–300 words each).

2. Select a conceptual framework/model that fits the vulnerable populations of interest to you. Justify your choice.

3. Based on the designated course objectives and your readings, develop at least one question for the topic under discussion in class next week.

4. Post your response in the designated Discussion site.

I look forward to a spirited discussion about vulnerable populations of interest to you.

Preparation for next face-to-face class:

Each student should come to class prepared to discuss the content relative to the Class Objective and *all of the student generated* (posted) questions for this Module. Please bring full text versions of the article(s) to class with you next week.

(continues)

TABLE 41-3 Online Vulnerable Population Exemplars: Four Course Modules (continued)

Exemplar: Module C

Unit Objective:

Upon completion of this Module the student will analyze trending data as they relate to various vulnerable populations in this geographical region of the state.

Unit Content:

Microperspectivies of vulnerability (vulnerable populations in local/region area)
Specific vulnerable populations and trending data on:

- Impoverished
- Children
- Adolescents
- Elderly women
- Ethnic/racial minorities
- Disenfranchised groups
- Physically and mentally ill
- Disabled
- Other

Required Reading:

Select textbook chapters
Select research articles from the literature

Weekly Assignment (Web):

1. Each student will be responsible to synthesize/analyze one research/evidence-based article related to a student-selected vulnerable population in the Central Florida Region. Post an annotated bibliographic citation for the article focusing on the demographic data, health statistics, life-style trends, and risk factors (250–300 words). (*No duplication of articles please.*)

2. Based on the designated course objectives and your readings develop at least one question for the topic under discussion in class next week.

3. Post your response in the designated Discussion site.

I look forward to a spirited discussion about your findings related to vulnerable populations in this region of the state.

Preparation for next face-to-face class:

Each student should come to class prepared to discuss the content relative to the Class Objective and *all of the student generated* (posted) questions for this Module. You must bring a copy of the full text version of your article to refer to in class.

TABLE 41-3 **Online Vulnerable Population Exemplars: Four Course Modules**
(continued)

Exemplar: Module D

Unit Objective:

Upon completion of this Module the student will analyze the influence of social, cultural, political, and economic factors on health care.

Unit Content:

Macro-perspectives of vulnerability: Global perspectives
Risk and risk factors associated with vulnerability within and among nations of the world (global society)

Required Reading:

Select textbook chapters
Select research articles from the literature

Weekly Assignment (Web):

1. Each student will be responsible to synthesize/analyze the international research literature relating to his or her vulnerability of interest. In your summary response focus on what you have gleaned (i.e., similarities/differences in the areas of social, cultural, political, and economic factors). Prepare an annotated bibliographic report (250–350 words each) for two articles. *(No duplication of articles please.)*

2. Compare/contrast two international reports with a comparable U.S. population, for example, demographic profile, methodologies, findings, implications, health status/disparities, etc.

3. Based on the designated course objectives and your readings develop at least one question for the topic under discussion in class next week.

I look forward to a spirited discussion about vulnerable populations in this region of the state.

Preparation for next face-to-face class:

Each student should come to class prepared to discuss the content relative to the Class Objective and *all of the student generated* (posted) questions for this Module. Please bring full text versions of the article(s) to class with you next week.

instructor to stay in contact with students and to respond to individual needs. Achieving these outcomes can be difficult when meeting in a face-to-face seminar but pose even greater challenges in the virtual classroom. Along with course e-mail, for the Vulnerable Populations course three discussion sites were dedicated to facilitate communication, much like traditional classroom bulletin boards. One, "Instructor Notes to Students," was a site for the instructor to disseminate information important to all in the course in a consistent and timely manner. Another, "Student Notes to Instructor," was a place for students to post questions or comments relating to the course content in general and technology-related concerns in particular. "Espresso Café" allowed for other types of sidebar discussions indirectly relevant or not related at all to the course, such as notices of conferences, local newsworthy items, or policy-related issues (Tilley et al., 2006).

Grading and Assignments

Active participation in the form of attentiveness and insightful discussion are features of courses taught both in the conventional classroom and in the online seminar class. At the outset of the course, expectations must be clearly communicated by the instructor, for example:

- What are the instructor's protocols for web courses?
- How should a student present him- or herself online and in front of the world?
- What topics are included in the discussion for a particular learning module?
- Should students only post original contributions?
- How/when should citations be included?
- Where and when are replies to be posted?
- What rubrics are used to grade and evaluate student responses and assignments?

Facilitating meaningful participation among students in an online course is an art in itself, and with experience most instructors become more proficient in the process. In brief, for the Vulnerable Populations course, discussion questions were constructed in such a way to allow students to share and defend their positions relative to the topic under discussion.

Course Evaluations

Evaluation focused on process and outcomes of the course along with an assessment of student learning and course effectiveness. Ultimately, the instructor is responsible for determining students' final grades. Timely and objective evaluation can be awkward, especially after students are encouraged to generate and elaborate on ideas. Self-evaluation coupled with peer feedback can create an atmosphere that encourages a high level of learning among a community of learners. Self-evaluation infers that one critically examines and then reexamines his or her contributions to online discussions and, further, knows, understands, and is allowed to apply criteria put forth by the instructor for assignments. In the Vulnerable Populations course peer reviews of the scholarly paper along with the formal presentations validated and offered insights that enhanced individuals' learning and the quality of their work.. Students were expected to complete College of Nursing course evaluations and University Perception of Instructor Evaluations that were available online at a designated time near the end of the semester.

Delineating Student–Instructor Roles and Responsibilities

Regardless of the course or level of the offering, understanding the roles of the instructor and students is critical to successfully building a community of learners. Optimum learning is associated with the instructor allowing students to set the tone and pace of the discussion. Students in the Vulnerable Populations course, on the one hand, understand they are responsible for generating and elaborating on ideas related to the assigned topic and course materials. The instructor, on the other hand, is responsible for guiding and facilitating student interactions about the course content and encouraging creative ways of organizing information.

Modeling Appropriate Behaviors

Instructor modeling of appropriate class participation can show students how to express ideas appropriately, critically, and effectively online. An opportune time for the instructor to join in and perhaps lead the discussion is in the beginning of the course. For the Vulnerable Populations course, by the second or third assignment the instructor's role evolved from active participant to a less obtrusive facilitator. Supportive modeling can motivate a reserved student or guide a student with minimal computer experience as well as improve the overall quality and quality of student discussions.

Facilitating Active Student Participation

Student participation, in the form of assignments and class discussions, is a critical component in building a community of learners. Through online discussions, students learn vicariously from each other as they share experiences, build consensus, and learn new content. A carefully worded question can facilitate in-depth analysis of the topic being studied. Questions posed by students, as well as the instructor, can be used to validate, amplify, clarify, and, in some cases, refute an idea. For the Vulnerable Populations course sometimes there is a common understanding among a segment of the class that conflicts with one or more students' viewpoints. In turn, the processes of reflection, discussion, and debate led to better understanding of the course material.

Modifying Strategies to Fit the Technology

When adapting a course to an online modality, established teaching–learning practices may need to be modified. For example, for the Vulnerable Populations course both synchronous and asynchronous were used, with benefits and trade-offs with each. One advantage of synchronous discussion is that it occurs in real time. In other words, at a specified time and place students, the instructor, and an expert or guest lecturer can log into a virtual classroom to discuss a particular topic in a chat room. Considering the multiple personal and work-related schedules of adult learners, one drawback of synchronous discussion is coordinating a meeting time. However, similar problems arise when trying to organize a mutually agreeable meeting time among a group of students in a conventional class. Likewise, technological problems arise at the most inconvenient times, and Murphy's Law seems to go into effect during a synchronous discussion. For example, one or more participants have problems logging on to the course, computers crash, and Internet service providers could not be operating at that particular time.

Obviously, technological glitches create stress, more so for some than for others, which can hinder building a learning community. To reiterate, asynchronous discussions do not occur in real time and, hence, there is both a benefit and downside to this modality. The benefit is that students are able to complete assignments and post responses at their convenience, whether it is late at night, early morning, or the weekend. Likewise, if technological glitches occur, assignments can be completed after these are resolved. Suffice it to say, instructor flexibility goes a long way to reduce the stress among the learning community in an online course.

Clearly Defining Course Expectations

Doctoral students are highly motivated in their educational pursuits. Willingness to participate actively in discussion tends to be directly related to the grade allocated to it. Sometimes, though, the instructor's criteria are vague; for instance, "for an 'A' grade your posted messages should have substance." In turn, a student's perception of "substance" may not be congruent with the instructor's. Standards for participation should be clearly articulated. If not, students will revert to previous practices and define their own level of performance. For example, the teacher can clarify expectations for participation by

- Specifying expectations for assignment postings
- Explaining how posted comments are evaluated and by whom (i.e., the instructor, a teaching assistant, or peers)
- Being explicit regarding the format, spelling, grammar, and length of the message; the forum in which it should be posted; and the assignment deadlines
- Overall expectations from the class such as avoiding duplication of articles and approval of student questions

In brief, questions should be put forth that require analysis, synthesis, and evaluation to meet the learning objectives along with clearly delineated criteria (rubric) for grading the assignment. Conventional classroom contexts allow for verbal and nonverbal exchanges that must be communicated in the written form for an online course.

Addressing Issues Related to Security, Confidentiality, and Privacy

Internet security is of utmost concern for all. Therefore the instructor must reiterate the importance of current and reliable antivirus protection. Reinforce this requirement with a penalty of some sort when a virus is attached to a student's electronic submission. Anyone participating in an e-course must be knowledgeable about the information technology security systems provided by their sponsoring institution. At the outset of any course, students must demonstrate proficiency in maintaining Internet security and also provide evidence of security maintenance on personal computers. Privacy and confidentiality also are important considerations when designing an online course and establishing rapport among the learners. Before sharing personal ideas, a student must have a certain level of rapport with the teacher and classmates. For this reason class discussions should be restricted to enrolled students and the instructor or, on occasion, a guest speaker. Without respect for privacy, the quality and quantity of individuals' participation will also suffer.

Conclusion

This chapter presents an overview of a doctoral-level partially online course at the University of Central Florida, College of Nursing. Successfully integrating teaching–learning approaches to an online course include having an open mind and willingness to assess various technologies to determine best fit with unique content, course objectives, and learners' educational needs, in this case students enrolled in the Vulnerable Populations course.

References

Bushy, A. (2003). Issues in rural health: Model for a web-based course. In M. H. Oermann & K. T. Heinrich (Eds.), *Annual Review of Nursing Education* (Vol. 3, pp. 245–266). New York: Springer.

Knowles, M. (1980). *The modern practice of adult education: From pedagogy to andragogy.* Englewood Cliffs, NJ: Cambridge/Prentice-Hall Regents.

Little, B., Passmore, D., & Schullo, S. (2006). Using synchronous software in web-based nursing courses. *Computer Informatics in Nursing, 24*(6), 317–325.

Parker, E., & Howland, C. (2006). Strategies to manage the time demands of online teaching. *Nurse Educator, 31*(6), 270–274.

Pullen, D. (2006). An evaluative case study of online learning for healthcare professionals. *Journal of Continuing Education in Nursing, 37*(5), 225–232.

Tilley, D., Boswell, C., & Cannon, S. (2006). Developing and establishing online student learning communities. *Computer Informatics in Nursing, 24*(3), 144–149

Unit Seven

"Use your political and economic power for the community and others less fortunate."

■ ■ ■

Marion Wright Edelman

POLICY IMPLICATIONS

Public Policy and Vulnerable Populations

Jeri A. Milstead

Government policies that target vulnerable populations may seem like an oxymoron. On the one hand, vulnerable populations may be difficult to define. On the other hand, vulnerable populations may not have much of a voice to articulate their plight. How and to whom in government do "populations" direct their pleas? Agencies? Programs? The purpose of this chapter is to define vulnerable populations, examine the policy process, and consider issues inherent in linking the two. Examples are provided as to how nurses can work within the policy process to the benefit of vulnerable populations.

Definitions

The term *vulnerable populations* is a latecomer to nursing literature and did not appear until the 1990s as a descriptor in the *Cumulative Index to Nursing and Allied Health Literature* (Marcarian & Burns, 2002). Users of the term often refer to low socioeconomic status (the poor and those out of work), the underserved (i.e., those who lack healthcare insurance or lack access to healthcare delivery), disease categories (e.g., diabetes, congestive heart failure), chronic illness (arthritis, AIDS), or those at risk for developing disease or illness. These terms are not really interchangeable, that is, all diabetics may not be poor, and low socioeconomic status may not indicate the presence of chronic disease. These terms may not reflect either vulnerability or populations.

Flaskerud et al. (2002) defined vulnerable populations as "social groups who experience health disparities as a result of a lack of resources and/or increased exposure to risk" (p. 75). The *Cumulative Index to Nursing and Allied Health Literature* carries a category of vulnerability that is defined by Marcarian and Burns as "the state of being at risk or more susceptible physically, mentally or socially" (2002, p. 405). The two major concepts appear to be the degree of risk and the experience of health problems without access to resources. However, a full understanding of vulnerable populations requires a deeper look.

Flaskerud et al. (2002) noted the evolution of knowledge about vulnerable populations from the 1950s to the early 2000s through a study of articles published in *Nursing Research*.

Although the study was not comprehensive in that writings from other journals or other sources were excluded, the researchers chronicled terms that were used in investigating groups or aggregates. In the 1950s only one study was published regarding chronically ill aged adults. Group identity was based in the 1960s on socioeconomic status, education, occupation, gender, or race. The 1970s noted "race, ethnicity and gender" (p. 76), and the beginning of research at this time focused on high-risk parents, infants, women, and immigrants. The concept of culture and its effect on the delivery of health care came into the literature in the 1980s (Leininger & McFarland, 2002). Reported as an "influence" in outcomes of social groups, culture became the context for studying a variety of societal problems that were not limited to health or health care.

The concept of health disparities did not surface until late in the 1990s, and the term reflected differences in health care and outcomes among many groups, such as adolescents and the elderly, women and infants, and low- and middle-income families. Ethnic groups also were studied as groups, often with a focus on the quality (or lack thereof) of health and health care. Quality was approached through professional accountability (vis-à-vis ethics and standards), marketing accountability (as evidenced in informed choices), and regulatory accountability (as reflected in government action) (Taub, 2002). Although the marketing method seemed prominent, the regulatory scheme used the Health Plan Employer Data and Information Set, hospital discharge data from the now-defunct Health Care Financing Administration, and information on the quality of managed care organizations from the National Committee for Quality Assurance. Today, Medicare assesses "a nationally representative sample of aged, disabled, and institutionalized Medicare beneficiaries" through the Medicare Current Beneficiary Survey (U.S. Department of Health and Human Services, n.d.).

In the early years of the 21st century, many terms surfaced that referred to vulnerable populations. "Uninsured" became a blanket term for poor or low-income people, regardless of their gender, ethnicity, or employment status. Researchers discovered that the uninsured, which included the working poor, had more health problems than those who carried insurance. The homeless, as a group, were uninsured (often because they also were unemployed) and exhibited many physical and mental health problems. The range of health disparities was great. Migrants were considered "disadvantaged" (Ward, 2003), and African-Americans (Plowden & Thompson, 2002; Richards, 2000) and Latinos (Campinha-Bacote, 2002) experienced much inequity related to health care. The disabled were identified as having social and physical barriers to health (Harrison, 2002). Those who lived near hazardous waste sites were considered at-risk for serious health problems (Gilden, 2003). Finally, the term "vulnerable populations" evolved to include whole populations, not just aggregates of individuals, as identifiable groups.

A major concern today is the international migration of nurses from country to country. Developed countries recruit nurses to fill local shortages, which creates scarcities in underdeveloped or developing countries, leaving those countries to poach nurses from yet other countries. The International Council of Nurses created an International Centre for Human Resources in Nursing in November 2006. "The Centre is an innovative initiative aimed at informing policy-making . . . " (Communique de presse, 2006, p. 1). Through a ground-breaking electronic resource, the International Council of Nurses expects to address global workforce issues that will ultimately result in the education, retention, and distribution of more nurses.

Migration also is noted internationally from rural areas to urban areas. Nurses often are the key care providers in rural areas, and resettlement from farm to city, although providing greater opportunity for jobs and larger salaries, results in a serious lack of health-care services for the rural underserved population (Buchan, 2006).

Policy Process

Many people think of legislation and/or laws when they hear the term *policy*. Although legislation may be the most recognizable component, there are many other elements to the policy process. When discussing public policy (as opposed to private-sector policy), it is the process of taking problems to government and obtaining a response that is being referenced. Within this broad approach four major aspects are evident: agenda setting, government response, program and/or policy implementation, and program and/or policy evaluation.

The process is not linear or sequential. That is, one does not always start with agenda setting and move to government response. A nurse may initially become involved during program implementation after a law has been signed. A garbage can model of organizations (Cohen, March, & Olsen, 1982) provides a foundation for considering the process of making public policy as the interweaving of streams of problems, policies, and politics. These streams mingle in government circles, often joining and breaking apart as ideas and solutions are considered, rejected, or reconsidered (Kingdon, 1995). At times, a solution hooks up with a problem, and a window of opportunity opens that results in a program that addresses the difficulty. A brief discussion of each component of the policy process will reveal opportunities for becoming involved.

Agenda Setting

The agenda is a list of items to which the president and his advisors (known as the Administration) attend. Agenda setting is the activity in which problems are brought to the attention of the Administration. If the president is not interested in a problem, it has little chance of being addressed. The issue is how to get the president's attention (Furlong, 2004). Crises can propel an issue onto the national agenda. For example, the attacks of September 11, 2001, brought immediate attention to the issue of terrorism, and funding was made available for projects and programs such as Homeland Security.

One of the issues in agenda setting is defining a problem so that it is palatable to the Administration and to the public. When HIV/AIDS was first discovered, it was defined as a problem of intravenous drug users and homosexuals. The Administration believed that the public would not support funding for research into the cause or treatment of the disease, and little funding was forthcoming. When children like Ryan White and heterosexual nondrug users began to get the disease (most often from infected blood products), the disease was redefined as a community health problem, and funding was made available. Nurses are experts at choosing words and scenarios to describe problems. Creative use of language may not be necessary in alerting an Administration to a problem, but one should know how to use key words to advantage. The point in defining a problem is to pique the interest of the Administration so that a solution can be found. Knowing that the public will scrutinize funding options is part of the context of defining the difficulty.

Government Response

The government may respond to a problem in several ways. The three most common responses are the enacting of a law, a regulation, or a program. Policy experts develop these activities in policy communities. Policy communities are loose groups of people who can provide expertise about an issue and who, for the most part, work in government agencies. Policy experts often know one another through professional associations, the literature or other media exposure, or prior experience with each other. Often legislative aides, who serve as staff in the offices of legislators, are good contacts for nurses who want to connect with "insiders." Experts discuss problems, suggest solutions, and exercise their opinions about the relative political worth of issues. Legislative aides in one legislator's office often talk informally with legislative aides in other legislators' offices and with staff in government agencies, faculty in university settings, and members of special interest groups to establish a priority list and to consider alternative solutions. Nurses who have cultivated relationships with government policy staff have a golden opportunity to be recognized as experts who are sought out to consider problems (Wakefield, 2004).

Laws are made in legislative sessions that last 2 years. Bills (potential laws) are introduced throughout the session, but bills introduced early have a better chance of action. The "how a bill becomes a law" page that can be found in nearly every basic government or political science textbook provides a simplified overview of the steps for moving a bill from introduction to signature by the president. Neither legislators nor their aides are expected to know about the myriad issues brought to them. Issues range from health to transportation to economy to defense and beyond. Nurses have a wonderful opportunity to serve as experts about many health issues. A nurse can provide a one-page overview of a problem, a summary of relevant research in ordinary language, and phone or e-mail information to pave the way for a serious contact.

Seasoned nurses understand the importance of informal processes—political processes. Many nurses shun the idea of politics, believing this is a tainted process that skews judgment and biases legislators. On the contrary, the political process is merely the exercise of persuasion and education to one's perspective. What nurse has not spoken informally to others before a decision was made in an effort to gather support, challenge a conclusion, or talk out a problem? The same communication techniques are used with legislators and their staffs or anyone in the policy community. Reflection, active listening, and clarification are therapeutic communication skills that are integral to how nurses approach others. The art of using talents in this way should be natural for nurses.

The legislative process must be followed carefully, and nurses must be vigilant for amendments that will help or hurt their causes. Developing strong positive relationships with legislators, staff, and other interested parties results in a network that leads to "inside" information. Working at the subcommittee level is a more efficient use of time than letting a bill get to the committee level, but it is important to stay with a bill through passage by both houses of congress and, in many instances, a conference committee where final negotiations are completed. Nurses may recommend language for inclusion in drafting a bill or an amendment and must be cognizant of amendments that could derail or inhibit passage.

Once a bill becomes a law that establishes a program, the program is assigned to a government agency for implementation. The choice of which agency is very political. Not all health programs go to agencies in the Department of Health and Human Services. Some may go to the Department of Defense (for piloting by the military), the Department of Education (school health programs), the Department of the Treasury (drug enforcement programs), or other departments and agencies. The choice may be based on past experience with similar programs, the chance for an infusion of new funding needed by an agency, rejection of a program due to lack of time or expertise, or many other reasons.

Agencies must write regulations or rules that interpret the law and provide for smooth implementation (Loquist, 2004). The regulatory process is similar to the legislative process in that legislative action is required. However, the regulatory process is governed by the Administrative Procedures Act, which dictates a specific format and course. All proposed rules require notification of the public, an established time for public comment, and public announcement of the final rule. The *Federal Register* is the vehicle for publishing information on federal issues. Public comment can be in the form of letters, e-mail messages, phone calls, or in-person visits to the appropriate agency. All comments must be considered before the final rule is adopted. This is a particularly easy way for nurses to involve themselves in expressing their opinions about potential rules. Communication should be brief, focused, and identifiable (i.e., the rule on which you are commenting). Arguments should be stated clearly and prefaced by whether you are for or against the issue or section of the rule. Solutions are welcomed.

Implementation

Implementation is a fluid process that involves getting a program up and running. Agency staff may need assistance in determining eligibility. That is, who is entitled to participate? Who is excluded from participation? What are the criteria, and who monitors participation? Nurses can suggest policy tools, such as incentives (waivers, coupons), educational brochures, posters advertising a program, or learning tools (training sessions) to assist staff in operating a program (Smart, 2004).

Nurses should confer with agency personnel, known as street-level bureaucrats, who are putting the programs into operation. These street-level bureaucrats often use ideas from the participating public about how to streamline programs or make them more efficient or user friendly. Nurses may provide tips about the population being served or thoughts about how a program could be conducted. Sometimes programs can be expanded to include broader involvement or shrunk to remain within the legislative intent and purpose. Nurses can provide concrete assistance and guidance by recommending ideas about how to alter the provision of a program.

Bardach (1977) identified games that are played by agency personnel during the implementation phase of a program. Many of the games have to do with budget, policy goals, and administrative control. For government agencies, spending funds early and requesting additional funding later is one way to increase a budget. Encouraging overspending, known as boondoggling, can be seen when consultant fees exceed the budget. Inflating costs estimated for a program is a way of padding a budget so that some of the funds can be used later (e.g., as discretionary funds) or in a way different from original intent.

Nurses study implementation to determine to what extent programs meet original policy goals (Wilken, 2004). They investigate any modifications that were made and seek explanations for changes. Researchers examine the level of difficulty or "tractability" of the initial problem and whether technology was accessible to address the problem. The range of services provided by a program may produce variation in program performance such that many services might dilute operations negatively. On the other hand, successful programs can become a target for piling on additional objectives. The idea is to be part of a thriving program, but too many extra activities may result in program failure.

Evaluation

Evaluation is rarely conducted and usually is not part of an original program plan, despite literature that recommends appraisal. Evaluation should be both formative and summative. Formative data can help bureaucrats determine progress during implementation. They can provide information for decisions about whether or not to continue to function as usual or to change direction. Formative data can also indicate whether resources are adequate and are being distributed appropriately.

Summative data can be useful for evaluating public programs for effectiveness or outcomes, not just efficiency or outputs. That is, what difference does it make to the public good if thousands of poor women are offered free mammograms? Has this screening method resulted in significant prevention or early treatment of breast cancer? This is not to say that efficiency is not worth assessing; a poorly run program wastes tax dollars.

Evaluative reports should be provided to agency personnel, legislators, and the public. Charts and other visual media can be used to present aggregate data, identify trends, and track progress. Reports may contain recommendations for adjusting goals and objectives or implementation strategies.

Linking the Policy Process and Vulnerable Populations

Agenda Setting

Nurses can propel issues of vulnerable populations onto the national agenda by defining needy groups, serving as a voice for vulnerable populations, and alerting legislators to problems that affect the public health. For example, the homeless usually are not organized in any formal way and have little voice as a group. Their worries about health care go unheard unless someone, known as a policy entrepreneur, makes available his or her reputation, money, or other resources on their behalf. A nurse can serve as an entrepreneur or can mobilize the media to take up a cause. Issues of social justice are political issues. Discrimination against marginalized populations and against people based on health status, income, employment status, or type of disease or disability is unethical and unjust and may be illegal in the United States. The distribution and allocation of resources is a political process. The choice of which problems get on the national agenda is very political, and nurses are skilled in political interaction. Nurses must take up the mantle of social problems, especially health problems, for those who cannot or do not speak for themselves.

Nurses can help bureaucrats define problems in ways that help the public understand and value them. Drug users often are unemployed or financially poor and are disenfranchised in the public eye because of related crimes. (In contrast, employed drug users often go undetected by the general public and escape bias [Milstead, 1993].) Legislators ignore or shun known drug users as a group, often because officials perceive that the "druggies" create violence, do not vote, and are not organized politically. Social activists (including nurses) in the 1980s formed groups such as the Association for Drug Abuse Prevention and Treatment and the AIDS Coalition to Unleash Power. Members recognized the link between gay men, intravenous drug users, and HIV/AIDS, and a few created needle exchange programs and served as policy entrepreneurs. These volunteers changed the definition from drug "addict" to drug "user" as one way to change the public's perception of a vulnerable group. Volunteers in Tacoma, Washington, and New York City educated legislators, bureaucrats, and public health officials about HIV transmission and the need for research on diagnosis and treatment (Milstead, 1993). Communications techniques such as consciousness raising and the use of sound bites were developed to a high level. Policy entrepreneurs may take years to attain their goals, and some of the first group of volunteers are still staffing exchange programs on the streets and working the state legislature to obtain legitimacy for their programs. Most needle exchange programs in the United States are still operating—and are still illegal—despite the sustained efforts of volunteers to change the laws and a legal opinion that "possession of needles was a 'medical necessity' that was intended to prevent a greater societal harm, AIDS" (*New York Times,* 1991).

Government Response

Laws are composites of language that reflect the wishes and priorities of those who craft them. Laws often are the result of negotiation and compromise among many people with disparate philosophies and values. Nurses can help shape laws by means of their expertise in health care and healthcare delivery. Congressional representatives usually do not know much about diseases such as diabetes or tuberculosis. A nurse who has nurtured relationships with elected officials by becoming a contact for health issues and providing understandable explanations of medical terminology has a great opening to contribute to language as a bill is being constructed. A nurse's knowledge of current issues can be a tremendous help to a legislator or the staff. Nurses also bring anecdotes to the policy community that put a personal face on an issue.

The elderly are often considered a vulnerable population. The designation may be confusing because the term does not necessarily refer to low socioeconomic status, the underserved, or disease categories. "Elderly" cuts across all types of categories, and as a vulnerable population there is inference of risk and lack of resources for health care, specifically in relation to an increased danger of suffering disease or disability and a lack of resources because of fixed incomes. The elderly have a strong organized lobby through the American Association of Retired Persons (AARP). During the early years of the 21st century, the AARP waged a campaign in the U.S. Congress to create protection for members (aged 50 years or older) in the form of a program for funding prescription drugs.

The Medicare Prescription Drug, Improvement, and Modernization Act of 2003 amended Title XVIII (Medicare) of the Social Security Act to add a new part D (Voluntary Prescription Drug Benefit Program) under which each individual who is entitled to benefits under Medicare part A (hospital insurance) or Medicare part B (supplemental medical insurance) is entitled to obtain qualified prescription drug coverage. The law was passed by both the House of Representatives and the Senate and became public law 108-173 on December 8, 2003. Many people found that prescription costs soared under this law, and vulnerable populations that were to have been helped were hampered when they could not afford needed medications.

Nurses, physicians, and other healthcare providers participated in a focused assault on legislators in an effort to affect this law. Senators and representatives held hearings, met with lobbyists and AARP members, talked with constituents, and discussed issues within the policy community. The issue evolved into a hotly debated partisan battle, but compromise language created a bill that was acceptable enough to pass the Republican-dominated House and Senate. Herein lies a caveat: Although the bill has been signed into law, there are many changes that must be made as the program continues to be implemented. Nurses have an occasion to become knowledgeable about the current law and can peruse the law and how it came into being online (http://www.ustreas.gov/offices/public-affairs/hsa/pdf/pl108-173.pdf). The Medicare prescription plan is an example of how the streams of agenda setting, government response, and implementation interconnect.

During efforts to move the issue of prescription costs onto the national agenda, work already was in process to determine alternative solutions, and the basic rudiments of a program were already being conceived.

Implementation

An example of a purely symbolic policy action is the Stewart B. McKinney Act of 1987. Vladeck (1990) studied the homeless: characteristics, causes of homelessness, and health status. He chronicled the evolution of a joint initiative between the Robert Wood Johnson Foundation and the Pew Charitable Trusts that became a model for a program that would provide federal support for the homeless. Even though there was agreement among policymakers that homelessness was a problem worthy of government intervention, authorization of funding did not eliminate the problem or even address most of the social, economic, health care, and other issues.

A brief search for initiatives about the homeless in the 108th Congress shows a plethora of attempts in which bills were introduced but stalled in committee or subcommittee. These attempts include House of Representatives (HR) 1941, a bill to convert the voucher system to state-administered block grants to help low-income families find safe and affordable housing; HR 1256, to place memorials (e.g., wreaths) at the graves of homeless or indigent veterans; HR 2897, to end homelessness in the United States; HR 3459, to improve the health of minorities; and Senate (S) bill 100, to expand access to affordable health care and make more services available in rural and underserved areas. Symbolic efforts are important and may keep an issue from fading from the agenda. Symbolism is important because it is just that—symbolic or representative or illustrative that someone or some agency hears pleas for help. This "splinting" (Ebersole, 2002) helps to keep up spirits and encourages perseverance, especially when the effort expended has not produced an implementable program.

Evaluation

Evaluation of health policy that affects vulnerable groups does not occur often at the program level. Rather, policy itself has been evaluated through research. Nurse-led studies in the 1990s and the early 2000s reported in *Nursing Research* (Flaskerud et al., 2002) evaluated resources available for Hispanics, Cubans, African-Americans, Filipinos, lesbians and other women, men, low-income families and age-related groups, and the homeless. Disease categories included mental illness (including depression), chronic illness, addictive disease, pregnancy, injuries, and specific populations with asthma, hypertension, HIV/AIDS, lung and heart disease, sexually transmitted diseases, and tuberculosis. The discovery of health disparities between vulnerable groups and the general population indicated levels of risk and lack of access to healthcare providers and resources.

Research uncovered problems in defining vulnerable populations, specifically in relation to issues of race and ethnicity. The Institute of Medicine challenged the National Institutes of Health to replace the term *race* with *ethnic group* (Oppenheimer, 2001). The Office of Management and Budget sets policy about which racial and ethnic classes are to be referenced by any federal agency, although the Office of Management and Budget recognizes that these terms are based on ill-defined social or political types, not scientific categories. The American Anthropological Association approves the concept of race/ethnicity as an interim combined term until race is eliminated in the next census. Researchers need to take care to define race or ethnicity clearly as they study various groups. Vulnerable groups will be subject to scrutiny, and federal agencies that authorize programs, initiate policies, and appropriate funds must take into consideration the legal, governmental, cultural, and historic implications of terms.

Sudduth (2004) asserted that nurses "are not strangers to evaluation" (p. 194). She urged advanced practice nurses to transfer the skills they use to determine outcomes in a healthcare setting to evaluation of government programs. "Social programs are public policy made visible" (p. 197), and nurses are well equipped to determine the worth, efficacy, and efficiency of many programs.

Conclusion

Nurses work with vulnerable populations in the provision, administration, and evaluation of health care. Public officials design policies in response to problems that rise to the agenda-setting attention of the president and his advisors. The policy community is involved in defining problems, prioritizing their value, and seeking and considering alternative solutions. Legislators, their staff, interest groups, and others in the community of interest draft government responses to the problems, often in the form of laws, regulations, and programs.

Nurses must integrate political knowledge and skill into their professional lives. Nurses can identify problems, bring them to the Administration, keep them from fading, suggest redefinitions, and propose alternative solutions. Nurses must persevere throughout the process by using their expertise to help legislators choose policy tools and implement and evaluate programs and policies. Public officials are not accustomed to nurses participating actively in the process of policymaking; therefore nurses must initiate the contacts, provide information that a lay person can understand, and acknowledge those legislators or bureaucrats who respond positively and move government to action.

Nurses are experts in the provision of health care, especially for the vulnerable. Not only do nurses have an ethical obligation to inform policymakers on issues for which at-risk populations have little or no voice, as professionals we will cede our societal accountability if we do not.

References

Bardach, E. (1977). *The implementation game: What happens after a bill becomes a law.* Cambridge, MA: MIT.

Buchan, J. (2006). The impact of global nursing migration on health services delivery. *Policy, Politics, & Nursing Practice, 7*(3), 16S–25S.

Campinha-Bacote, J. (2002). The process of cultural competence in the delivery of healthcare services: A model of care. *Journal of Transcultural Nursing, 13*(3), 181–184.

Cohen, M., March, J., & Olsen, J. (1982). A garbage can model of organizational choice. *Administrative Science Quarterly, 17*, 1–25.

Communique de presse. (2006, November). Launch of the International Centre for Human Resources in Nursing. Geneva, Switzerland: Author.

Ebersole, P. (2002). Situational vulnerability. *Geriatric Nursing, 23*(1), 4.

Flaskerud, J. H., Lesser, J., Dixon, E., Anderson, N., Conde, F., Kim, S., et al. (2002). Health disparities among vulnerable populations. *Nursing Research, 51*(2), 74–85.

Furlong, E. A. (2004). Agenda setting. In J. A. Milstead (Ed.), *Health policy and politics: A nurse's guide* (2nd ed., pp. 37–66). Sudbury, MA: Jones and Bartlett.

Gilden, R. C. (2003). Community involvement at hazardous waste sites: A review of policies from a nursing perspective. *Policy, Politics, & Nursing Practice, 4*(1), 29–35.

Harrison, T. C. (2002). Has the Americans with Disabilities Act made a difference? A policy analysis of quality of life in the post-Americans with Disabilities Act era. *Policy, Politics, & Nursing Practice, 3*(4), 333–347.

Kingdon, J. W. (1995). *Agendas, alternatives, and public policies* (2nd ed.). New York: Harper Collins.

Leininger, M., & McFarland, M. R. (2002). *Transcultural nursing: Concepts, theories, research and practice* (3rd ed.). New York: McGraw-Hilll.

Loquist, R. S. (2004). Government regulation: Parallel and powerful. In J. A. Milstead (Ed.), *Health policy and politics: A nurse's guide* (2nd ed., pp. 89–127). Sudbury, MA: Jones and Bartlett.

Manhattan Criminal Court Judge Laura E. Drager. (1991, June 26). *New York Times*, p. 1.

Marcarian, S., & Burns, K. (Eds.). (2002). Vulnerability. In *Cumulative Index to Nursing and Allied Health Literature: CINAHL Subject Headings* (Vol. 47-A, p. 405). Glendale, CA: CINAHL Information Systems.

Milstead, J. A. (1993). *The advancement of policy implementation theory: An analysis of three needle exchange programs.* Doctoral Dissertation, University of Georgia, Athens.

Oppenheimer, G. M. (2001). Paradigm lost: Race, ethnicity, and the search for a new population taxonomy. *American Journal of Public Health, 91*(7), 1049–1054.

Plowden, K. O., & Thompson, L. S. (2002). Sociological perspectives of Black American health disparity: Implications for social policy. *Policy, Politics, & Nursing Practice, 3*(4), 325–332.

Richards, H. (2000). And miles to go before we sleep: Rising to meet the challenges of ending health care disparities among African-Americans. *Journal of National Black Nurses Association, 11*(2), 2.

Smart, P. (2004). Policy design. In J. A. Milstead (Ed.), *Health policy and politics: A nurse's guide* (2nd ed., pp. 129–160). Sudbury, MA: Jones and Bartlett.

Sudduth, A. L. (2004). Policy evaluation. In J. A. Milstead (Ed.), *Health policy and politics: A nurse's guide* (2nd ed., pp. 193–228). Sudbury, MA: Jones and Bartlett.

Taub, L.-F. M. (2002). A policy analysis of access to health care inclusive of cost, quality, and scope of services. *Policy, Politics, & Nursing Practice, 3*(2), 167–176.

U.S. Department of Health and Human Services. (n.d.). *Medicare current beneficiary survey.* Retrieved October 5, 2007, from http://www.cms.hhs.gov/MCBS/

Vladeck, B. (1990). Health care and the homeless: A political parable for our time. *Journal of Health Politics, Policy and Law, 15*(2), 305–317.

Wakefield, M. (2004). In J. A. Milstead (Ed.), *Health policy and politics: A nurse's guide* (2nd ed., pp. 67–88). Sudbury, MA: Jones and Bartlett.

Ward, L. S. (2003). Migrant health policy: History, analysis, and challenge. *Policy, Politics, & Nursing Practice, 4*(1), 45–52.

Wilken, M. (2004). Policy implementation. In J. A. Milstead (Ed.), *Health policy and politics: A nurse's guide* (2nd ed., pp. 161–192). Sudbury, MA: Jones and Bartlett.

Health Care for Some Borne on the Backs of the Poor

Elizabeth Furlong

In this chapter we discuss the factors in society and in the healthcare system that cause and/or contribute to people's poverty, their diminished health status, and their lack of access to health care. Examples are given from both developed and developing countries. This chapter is based on the premise that the poor are "needed" by the middle and upper class groups for the latter to enjoy their economic life-styles. Rather than viewing the poor as a problem in society, this chapter theorizes that society and the healthcare system perpetrate poverty. The chapter closes with proposed solutions that are based on a justice ethic.

Contributing Factors

Four factors are discussed in terms of the way they contribute to the causes of poverty, the diminished health status of the poor, and the lack of access to health care: (1) a life course of cumulative advantage or disadvantage, (2) inequality in social classes and nations, (3) use of language to diminish poor people, and (4) public policies at all levels: local, state, regional, national, and international.

Factor 1: Life Course

The first factor, that of the model of cumulative advantage or disadvantage, has been studied by Crystal and Shea (1990) in a population of the elderly. This model is based on the hypothesis that individuals "who are initially advantaged . . . are more likely to receive a good education, leading to good jobs, leading to better health and better pension coverage, leading to higher savings and better postretirement benefit income" (p. 437). Their research demonstrated this hypothesis, even given the benefit of the Social Security program. They found that as people aged, the percentage of inequality among people increased. Although the Social Security program has been an important public policy for providing a base of financial security, postretirement income sources are mainly determined by preretirement economic experiences, which in return result from earlier cumulative advantage factors such as good education, a good job, good benefits, and so on.

For example, if one has the ability to purchase a home rather than rent one, this has cumulative economic benefits. Another example is the cumulative advantage from education and the type of job worked, which affects benefits and salary. For example, a teacher may have received health insurance benefits during her lifetime, whereas a construction worker may have had the same salary history but no health insurance benefits; thus he may have postponed seeking medical care.

Crystal, Shea, and Krishnaswami (1992) summarized this study with this finding: "stratification established early in the life course continues at least as sharply in the later years" (pp. S220-S221). However, although Social Security has been an advantage for many, it was not effective for many African-Americans. When this legislation was passed in the 1930s, it was because of the power of the southern democrats who controlled important congressional committees (Albelda, Folbre, & The Center for Popular Economics, 1996). Passage of this bill, which excluded agricultural and domestic workers (most of whom are African-American), helped to keep a low-wage workforce in the southern states. "Black exclusion was the price, President Roosevelt believed, of getting the law [Social Security] through Congress" (Albelda et al., 1996, p. 108).

Crystal et al. (1992) stressed the importance of looking at many factors other than strict salary compensation when studying the life course of individuals and their cumulative advantages/disadvantage. For example, they noted the importance of education. The assets of an educated individual include access to better jobs and higher pay; increased income from these better jobs in the years preceding retirement, which heavily influence postretirement income; better employment security and less risk; and the ability to work longer because of the fewer risks to health, thereby enhancing the educated individual's cumulative disadvantage. The converse—cumulative disadvantage—is what happens to poor people.

The importance of education to one's life course can also be seen in two other examples. A study showed the correlation between level of education, adherence to complex medical regimens, and health outcomes (Reed, 2002). Those who had a better education had higher adherence levels to complex treatment regimens and therefore had better health outcomes. This study is important in the current health environment because of changes in the health system, such as the move from inpatient to outpatient treatment (with the patient increasingly responsible for care) and the increased complexity in treatment and/or medication regimens. A second example is the societal structure found in many southern states relative to the low tax base and availability of funds to spend on public education (Kreiger, 1999; S. Kay, personal communication, July 15, 2002). Although southern states complied with civil rights laws and integrated public schools, it can be argued that they undermined this directive by simply not proportionately raising property taxes and also by spending relatively little on public education. Thus there was a minimal amount of money to allocate to educate African-Americans. Because southern states—the ones with relatively high proportions of black residents—had a low tax base and spent relatively less on public education, illiteracy in these states was also high among their white counterparts (Kreiger, 1999, p. 330). Therefore the results of having received poor or no education in one's early life leads to cumulative lifetime disadvantages.

Ehrenreich (2001) reported on current research into poor individuals attempting to make it in the United States today but without success. The disparity in income is increasing when comparing college-educated individuals with high school–educated individuals. In 1979 the differential in income was 38% higher for college-educated individuals. In 2006 the differential was 75% in income. This disparity is noted by Federal Reserve Chairman Ben Bernanke (personal communication, R. Withem, February 9, 2007). The importance of education for one's health status has been reiterated by recent research by James Smith, a RAND Corporation economist. His research demonstrated education as a major social variable for having a longer life (Kolata, 2007).

Factor 2: Inequalities

A second factor that contributes to poverty and diminished health status is the concept of inequality among people within a society and the inequality among countries. Recent publications in both the United States and Great Britain have addressed these concerns (Government Report: Whites get better quality health care, 2002; Marmot & Wilkinson, 2001). There has been extensive professional and lay publicity of these income and health disparities in the United States. The Institute of Medicine's report, "Unequal Treatment: Confronting Racial and Ethnic Disparities in Health Care," has raised an alarm within the health sector (Government Report: Whites get better quality health care, 2002). A major concern from this study is that even when the variables of insurance status, income, age, and severity of conditions are compared, racial and ethic minorities still receive lower quality health care. Other examples of inequality are the following statistics: in 1960 chief executive officers made 12 times what the average factory workers made; by 1980, chief executive officers in the largest companies made 42 times what the average factory worker made; and in 2001, that ratio had changed to chief executive officers making 411 times the average worker's compensation (Albelda et al., 1996; Goodman, 2002).

Several other economic indicators of concern have been noted. One indicator of income disparity is a 2005 statistic that the top 20% of Americans earn 50% of the nation's income (Michaels, 2006). In the United States there are more children living in poverty now compared with 1969. In 1969 one in every seven children was poor; today, even though there is more wealth, one in every sixth child is poor (Krugman, 2006). Thirteen percent of Americans live in poverty (Filteau, 2007).

In Great Britain there has been decreased absolute mortality; however, the mortality disparities have increased: "there is a strong relationship between mortality and income inequalities. People living in countries with greater income inequality have a shorter life expectancy . . . a similar relationship has been found for geographical areas within countries" (Marmot & Wilkinson, 2001, p. 1223). These authors postulated the additive effect of psychosocial pathways on the negative health status of poor persons, in addition to the direct negative influence of decreased material living standards. Marmot and Wilkinson discussed the psychosocial effects of relative deprivation, which includes loss of control over life, anxiety, insecurity, depression, and decreased social affiliation in helping to explain decreased health status. Hemingway and Marmot's (1999) review article synthesized the research studies that demonstrated a correlation between many of these psychosocial effects and coronary heart disease. Many other research studies showed the relationship in animals of social status, with this experiencing downward mobility showing resultant increased atherosclerosis.

To concretize and emphasize the importance that some of the these factors may have, as opposed to strictly the deprivation of material goods, Marmot and Wilkinson (2001) compared the income and life expectancy of African-American men in the United States and Costa Rica in 1996. The median income for U.S. African-American men was $26,522 per year, and life expectancy was 66 years. For men in Costa Rica, the income was $6,410, and their life expectancy was 75 years. The authors argued that the discrepancy in life expectancy was due to the psychosocial effects of relative deprivation versus the direct effects of fewer material conditions (i.e., education disadvantage, racism, gender discrimination, social and family disruption, and fear of crime) (p. 1235).

Navarro (1999) wrote about global inequalities among countries because of the increased globalization of commerce, investments, and finance, which then has direct and indirect effects on all policies, including health policy. He argued that individual national governments are increasingly restricted in their ability to set their own national policies because the economy is becoming increasingly competitive internationally.

In continuing with the theme of inequalities raised by Marmot and Wilkinson (2001), Navarro (1999, p. 126) gave the example that the net worth of the world's richest 358 people is equal to the combined income of the poorest 45% of the world's population (i.e., 2.3 billion people). Another way of understanding the inequalities is that 20% of people in high-income countries account for 86% of private consumption, and the poorest 28% of the globe consume 1.3% of the world's materials (p. 219). Navarro postulated that the inequalities within countries and among countries are because of three factors: (1) the unprecedented growth in wealth and income from capital as opposed to labor, (2) the growing polarization of wages with a great increase in wage dispersion, and (3) decreased redistributive effect of the welfare state and the rapid deterioration of public infrastructures (p. 216). Of all countries, those in Latin America are the worst in terms of inequalities among individuals. Navarro raised concerns about globalization as isolationist, xenophobic, and protectionist. Navarro's concern is that such international organizations (whether public, private, nonprofit, governmental, or corporate) wrap their language and arguments in scientific and technical discourse with the belief that their proposals are value free. However, he sees an absence of analysis of power and politics in the policies they propose and how this contributes to poverty and decreased health status and health care for those in poverty.

An example of Navarro's (1999) analysis of changes is the for-profit health insurance sector in Third World countries. Navarro noted that the World Health Organization, the World Bank, the Pan American Health Organization, and U.S. Agency for International

Development "are actively promoting managed care and managed competition in Latin America" and other countries (p. 221). This integrates with the provisions of the General Agreement on Trade in Services agreement. While consulting in Armenia, a newly independent state of the former USSR, I observed the promotion of private for-profit managed care companies. The inequalities referenced by Navarro were obvious in this country: minimal public healthcare infrastructure and morbidity and mortality indicators of concern. Yet this aspect of Western healthcare financing was being promoted for the small cohort of Armenians who might be able to pay for it. Navarro (1999, p. 222) argued, "class relations through the political, economic, and cultural institutions, are at the root of our understanding of current realities." Navarro compared and contrasted developed capitalist countries according to the power of capital and labor. He noted in the 35-year period from 1960 to 1995 the northern European countries, which have had a strong commitment to equity, have scored better on many indicators: greater economic growth, lower unemployment, better health indicators, and fewer inequalities (p. 223).

In other research, Navarro and Shi (2001) studied the impact of political parties in determining the level of equalities or inequalities in a country. They cited the example of the state of Kerala in southern India, which has been extensively studied for the past 40 years because that state has been noteworthy for a major reduction in inequalities and for the improved health status of its population. As a Peace Corps volunteer serving in the contiguous state of Mysore from 1966 to 1968, I was well aware of Southern Indians frequently discussing the better social indicators of individuals in Kerala State compared with all other states of India. Navarro and Shi (2001) critiqued the literature because it is rare when writers report on the positive indicators being a result of the public policies implemented by Kerala's governing party, the Indian Communist Party. It is this absence of analysis, or perhaps denial, that Navarro and Shi also alluded to when discussing that many international organizations (World Health Organization, World Bank, U.S. Agency for International Development, corporations, etc.) omit such analysis when they promote globalization. Thus Navarro and Shi (2001) posited that political parties, as well as the policies they implement, make a difference in determining the equalities or inequalities in a country. They ascribed these indicators to the policies implemented by these political parties. In the Christian democratic countries, poverty in general and in children specifically was greater than in social democratic countries. Furthermore, life courses and cumulative advantages and disadvantages were heavily influenced by gender roles. Caregiving was viewed as a heavier family responsibility, with fewer women employed outside the home than in social democratic countries. Thus the male breadwinner's income and pension were especially important.

Earlier content in this article by Crystal et al. (1992) on the model of cumulative advantage and disadvantage can easily be applied here by observing what happens to poor people over a lifetime. The greatest inequalities in the European Union occurred in the fascist countries (Crystal et al. 1992, p. 18). Navarro and Shi (2001) also listed a fourth category of liberal countries, that is, the United States, Canada, Ireland, and Great Britain. This group consists of the Anglo-Saxon countries where labor has been particularly weak and the capitalist class particularly strong. These countries have been governed for the most part by parties clearly committed to a full expression of market forces, with little interference from the state as possible (Navarro and Shi, 2001, p. 18). These countries shared the following traits: they had the largest inequalities, and they had low public healthcare expenditures. Also, the United States and Ireland had the lowest percentage of population covered by health care compared with all the liberal countries studied. Navarro and Shi argued that the reduction of inequalities is a precondition for economic efficiency and economic growth.

Krieger (1999) also wrote about inequalities and asserted that the research on discrimination as a determinant of population health is just in its infancy. Such research is especially necessary because of the changed focus in the healthcare delivery system on population health status versus individual health status. Discrimination occurs when people are treated as second-class citizens because of their race, gender, sexuality, disability, and/or age. Krieger applies the model of ecosocial theory, which integrates the relationships among discrimination, inequality, and health. This theory can be summed up as follows: "taken literally the notion of 'embodiment,' this theory asks how we literally incorporate biologically—from conception to death—our social experiences and express this embodiment in population patterns of health, disease and well being" (p. 296). She posited that the casual components of social arrangements of power—ownership of property, patterns of production and consumption, the constraints of biology, and ecological history of populations—structure the inequalities in the exposure and susceptibility to pathogenic processes and options for resisting these process across the life trajectories of populations of people.

Because this chapter is focused on poverty, emphasis is given to the example Krieger (1999) gave of the embodiment of inequality in health status when the form of discrimination is social class (i.e., there is a socioeconomic gradient in morbidity and mortality with the poor at greatest risk). This is an epidemiographic finding that has been noted for decades. However, Krieger gave examples of how inequalities in health status embody other kinds of discrimination: race, gender, sexuality, disability, and age. She noted that many times people experience multiple forms of discrimination. For example, I attended a national nursing convention where the lecturer spoke to the issue of having three strikes against her: she was black, a woman, and old. Furthermore, when people experience discrimination, it can run the gamut from "everyday" discrimination to particularly horrible life-transforming events. Finally, discrimination can be obvious in an interpersonal manner or visible and perpetuated via an institutional manner.

The value of Krieger's writing is to challenge researchers to study this area because there is a paucity of research on the effect of discrimination on health status. A lack of research may reflect the dominant power structure of the healthcare system. When attending a hospital seminar 30 years ago on increased hypertension among African-Americans, I was struck by the fact that the seminar's only focus was on the physiological aspects and that no attention was given to social racism as a causative factor. Kuczewski's (2006) recent ethical case study of end-of-life care decisions for an older African-American woman is one of many examples that demonstrate the need for far more education and cultural humility and competence on the part of dominant white health providers.

Forbes (2000) saw societal structural forces as antecedents of health inequalities. He noted that power relationships and both relative and absolute economic disadvantage contributes to health status. When analyzing the social class differences in the United Kingdom, he noted that the mortality rate in social class I (highest of a V class social class) decreased 50% in the last 20 years but only decreased 10% for those in social class V. He also wrote that those most in need of health care may not receive it, that is, "the so-called inverse care law" (p. 610).

Factor 3: Language

A third factor that has contributed to the diminished health status of poor people is how society has used language negatively against them. "Many pundits and politicians in this country [the United States] are making careers out of demonizing poor people" (Albelda et al., 1996, p. 8). Numerous authors have written of how language is used against the poor (Albelda et al., 1996). The language phenomenon is not new; Carlson (2001) mapped out the use of language from biblical times of how the unfit are perceived and classified with derogatory language. Gans (1995) wrote extensively of how journalists, policymakers, experts, and others have contributed to the derogation of the poor by their choice of language in writing about the poor, policies affecting the poor, and so on. For example, one frequently reads of welfare policies for the poor but less frequently reads of welfare policies for farmers in the form of subsidies and of welfare policies for corporations in the form of "bailouts." In addition to his analysis of the use of language in American society, Gans analyzed the psychological needs of Americans (and others) to "blame the victim" instead of studying the larger context of society and to understand people in that structural perspective. Furthermore, he advocated for programs that educate Americans on not stigmatizing the poor. He saw this as an indirect way to improve the health of the poor.

Factor 4: Public Policy Influence

This chapter has included several examples of private and public policy at the local, state, regional, national, and international levels that have an impact on people's lives. Such policies have made differences in people's life courses, have contributed to inequalities within and among groups both nationally and internationally, and have been parts of the language used to derogate and diminish poor people.

Proposed Solutions

"Politics is 'public health in the most profound sense'" (Navarro & Shi, 2001, p. 20). Anyone interested in committing oneself to "the preferential option for the poor," which is advocated by Catholic social teaching, has to be involved in policymaking. As noted in this chapter, many past and proposed policies have been harmful to the poor and have facilitated their poverty and diminished health status and lack of access to health care. One's activism in policymaking can run the gamut from discussion of issues with family, friends, and colleagues; to voting; to putting a policy on the agenda or blocking a policy proposal; to being a candidate oneself. One policy implication from the research of Crystal and Shea (1990) on the elderly using the cumulative advantage/disadvantage model is to seriously evaluate the proposed policy of privatization of Social Security. If people are living hand-to-mouth during their working years, it is questionable that they would initiate such savings. It must also be recognized that the current tax policy, which creates incentives for private pensions, salary deferral programs, individual retirement accounts, Keogh programs, and so on, are, in effect, major subsidizations in which poor people do not participate and that contribute to their cumulative disadvantage.

A second policy implication is taken from Crystal et al.'s (1992) research on the importance of education for poor people. Promotions of state and national policies for public education are imperative. The currency of this issue is noted by debate in the Nebraska Unicameral of how best to meet the current state deficit. State cuts in public postsecondary education have been made (Unicameral Update, 2002a). Cuts in this area can have a negative impact on the life course of many poor Nebraskans.

A third policy implication can be seen from the writing of Marmot and Wilkinson (2001). One needs to recognize the societal structures that perpetuate inequalities in and among countries that lead to health disparities: racism, policies that create educational disadvantages, sexism, classism, and so forth. This is the antithesis of blaming the victim. If policymakers are unable to see and understand all these connections that create and contribute to poverty and diminished health status for people, they may want to follow the easy route and blame individuals for their poverty. The knowledge base of educated people calls us to do better than that.

A fourth policy change stems from Navarro's (1999) concern about globalization. As an example, a candidate for the U.S. Congress as raised concerns about the recent passage of a bill that allows President Bush to engage in fast-track negotiations to create a North American Free Trade Agreement–style corporate trading zone to include almost all countries in the Western Hemisphere (D. Deichman, personal communication, July 29, 2002). Current Congressman Bernie Sanders, an independent from Vermont, has said, "When you have bad policy, why would you want to extend it?" He notes the $346 billion trade deficit of the United States and the erosion of 10% of our country's manufacturing base in the last 4 years. Rep. Sanders raised the question "When will you catch on? When all of our kids are flipping burgers?" (D. Deichman, personal communication, July 29, 2002). Many representatives have been concerned at the rapidity with which this agreement passed and the manner in which it was done. Because of the rapidity, representatives did not have time to study it well. This is but one example of policy, national in this case, in which global policy has an effect on the life course of individuals. This U.S. national policy that was enacted will have global implications, especially for those workers in the Western Hemisphere. In the United States the phrase "flipping hamburgers" is code for a low-status minimum wage job with no benefits. This kind of job for large cohorts of Americans can result in cumulative disadvantage over a lifetime and can be a contributing factor to poverty.

A fifth action stemming from Navarro's (1999) research is the importance of studying power relationships and the effects of class, gender, and race domination and exploitation as it affects inequalities within and among countries. His research provides the global context to help one understand many factors contributing to poverty and decreased health status and health care. He advocated for such research as " we owe it to the millions of people who do not have health and remain voiceless" (p. 225). Further, students and practitioners need to be knowledgeable of the first of the UN's 8 Millennium Development Goals, that is, to eradicate extreme poverty and hunger (Winker, 2006). In 2000 there were 189 countries of the United Nations who voted on this.

A sixth policy strategy is to be knowledgeable of public policy: how issues get on the formal and informal agendas, who has the power in affecting agendas, the importance of action via coalitions, and so forth. There are many current examples in the United States that reflect negative economic conditions and negative stereotypes of the poor. At the national level, President Bush has criticized the Senate Welfare Bill (President criticizes Senate welfare bill, 2002). For example, one could analyze his criticisms (not appropriating as much money as requested to promote marriage, giving too much money for child care, and providing educational opportunities) as putting forth constraints on the realistic ability of people on welfare to transition to a working nonpoverty life course. Because of this proposed legislation, many poor people may experience the lived experience of cumulative life disadvantages described by the research of Crystal and Shea (1990). At the state level, governments (because of state constitutions that mandate balanced budgets) implemented Special Sessions during Summer 2002 to problem solve budget deficits (Lutey, 2002; Reed, 2002). Although both Montana and Nebraska proposed cutting funding to education, a larger concern in Nebraska was the proposed cuts to Medicaid (Kaiser Network, 2002). Nineteen thousand individuals have been dropped from the Medicaid program in Nebraska (Unicameral Update, 2002b). This is an exemplar case of needed budget cuts affecting the most vulnerable and, again, negatively affecting their course and cumulative disadvantage.

An educational strategy for health science students and practicing health professionals is to teach the impact of poverty on people's health status and to determine their role in moving societies to reduce poverty. Some believe reduction of poverty may be the more important strategy in reducing the burden of illness. When teaching students, I believe the more appropriate way to teach the epidemiographic aspects of disease is from a social class perspective rather than from that of a specific illness. A resource for educators to use is the Poverty Coalition (J. G. Chamberlin, personal communication, August 5, 2002). This is a group of multidisciplinary educators from universities across the United States who are interested in better educating students on the issues and problem-solving strategies of poverty.

A communicative strategy to decrease poverty is to be critically aware of language used by oneself and by others and to be sure that such language does not condemn the poor. Although it is beyond the scope of this chapter to expand on this area, I believe this to be an extremely important area. Gans (1995) performed a critical analysis of how language has been used by citizens, policymakers, journalists, health professionals, and others to condemn the poor.

For individuals working out of religious and spiritual traditions, a strategy to decrease poverty and to improve health status outcomes for all emanates from their beliefs and church doctrines. For example, for Roman Catholics there is an emphasis on social justice, a preferential option for the poor, stewardship, working for the common good, and solidarity (U.S. Catholic Conference, 1993). As stated by the U.S. Catholic Conference of Bishops in 1993, "The existing patterns of health care in the United States do not meet the minimal standard of social justice and the common good" (p. 1). Catholics can live out these beliefs in a number of ways, such as participation in problem solving, communicative, and education strategies and participation in organizations that address the challenges of poverty and health status inequalities. For example, the Bread for the World organization has many antipoverty initiatives (Bread for the World, 2002). Over the last several years, many cities have initiated and passed Living Wage ordinances (Amour, 2002). Passage of the ordinance in Omaha, Nebraska, was a result of the multifaith multiethnic community development organization, Omaha Together One Community. Although it was passed for city employees, Omaha is one of only a few cities where the law was rescinded. However, there are now 80 communities where poor people are benefiting from this measure (Armour, 2002). When payroll taxes and earned income tax credits are calculated, this can mean an increase in earnings of about $5,000 more per year for someone. Citizens can be a part of furthering this ordinance in their respective cities.

At the international level, one could participate in the International Society for Equality in Health (N. Barton, personal communication, November 2, 2001). As the name suggests, health professionals from around the globe belong to this organization and are committed to decreasing health inequities. In late Fall 2006 there were raids on six Swift & Company meat processing plants to arrest illegal immigrant employees. These raids captured much national attention and, in particular, much attention in the Midwest because of raids in central Iowa, central Nebraska, and in Colorado. However, there was minimal media coverage of how corporations have benefited from discounted salaries such employees earn. For example, in 1980 such employees earned about $19 an hour. However, these plants then moved to rural nonunionized areas and the salary then became $9 an hour (Harrop, 2006). For the individual and family crises that these raids created, nurses and many other community citizens responded with immediate crisis interventions to meet needs of families. Although changing policy is the ultimate long-term solution, such immediate interventions are also important for nurses to be involved in.

Conclusion

In this chapter we addressed the cause of poverty and how this leads to decreased health status and lack of access to health care for poor people. More importantly, we identified strategies that various individuals can take to decrease poverty and increase the health status and access to health care for poor people. Such strategies are necessary for a just society and world: "social justice is the foundation of public health" (Krieger, 1999, p. 296).

References

Albelda, R., Folbre, N., & The Center For Popular Economics. (1996). *The war on the poor, a defense manual.* New York: New York Press.

Armour, S. (2002, July 23). Living-wage movement takes root across nation. *USA Today,* p. 18.

Bread for the World. (2002). *Working from poverty to promise. Bread for the World's 2002 offering of letters* [Pamphlet]. Washington, DC: Author.

Carlson, E. A. (2001). *The unfit.* Cold Springs Harbor, NY: Cold Springs Harbor Laboratory Press.

Crystal, S., & Shea, D. (1990). Cumulative advantage, and inequality among elderly people. *The Gerontologist, 30*(4), 437–443.

Crystal, S., Shea, D., & Krishnaswami, S. (1992). Educational attainment, occupational history, and stratification: Determinants of later-life economic outcomes. *Journal of Gerontology: Social Sciences, 47*(5), S213–S221.

Ehrenreich, B. (2001). *Nickel and dimed: On (not) getting by in America.* New York: Henry Holt.

Filteau, J. (2007, January 19). U.S. poverty called major moral and policy challenge. *The Catholic Voice,* p. 10.

Forbes, A. (2000). Community health issues: A community-health nurse-led project to tackle health inequalities. *British Journal of Community Nursing, 5*(12), 610–618.

Gans, H. J. (1995). *The war against the poor.* New York: BasicBooks.

Goodman, E. (2002, July 20). Bush Inc. blames everyone. *Omaha World Herald,* p. A21.

Government report: Whites get better-quality health care. (2002). *RN, 65*(5), 16.

Harrop, F. (2006, December 22). The poor lose out in wage wars. *Omaha World Herald,* p. 7B.

Hemingway, H., & Marmot, M. (1999). Psychosocial factors in the aetiology and prognosis of coronary heart disease: Systematic review of prospective cohort studies. *British Medical Journal, 318*(1), 460–467.

Kaiser Network. (2002). *Nebraska Governor Johanns announces plans that would change Medicaid eligibility rules, end coverage for about 19,000.* Retrieved October 5, 2007, from http://www.kaisernetwork.org/daily_reports/rep_index.cfm?hint=3&DR_ID=12524

Kolata, G. (2007, January 3). *A surprising secret to a long life: Stay in school.* Retrieved October 5, 2007, from http://www.iht.com/articles/2007/01/03/healthscience/web.0103aging.php

Kreiger, N. (1999). Embodying inequality: A review of concepts, measures, and methods for studying health consequences of discrimination. *International Journal of Health Services, 29*(2), 295–352.

Krugman, P. (2006, December 28). *Omaha World Herald,* p. 7B.

Kuczewski, M. G. (2006). Our cultures, our selves: Toward an honest dialogue on race and end-of-life decisions. *American Journal of Bioethics, 6*(5), 13–17.

Lutey, T. (2002, July 25). University R & D funds targeted for cut backs. *Bozeman Daily Chronicle,* p. 19.

Marmot, M., & Wilkinson, R. (2001). Education and debate, psychosocial and material pathways in the relation between income and health: A response to Lynch et al. *British Medical Journal, 322,* 1233–1236.

Micheals, W. B. (2006, December 15). Why identity politics distracts us from economic inequalities. *The Chronicle of Higher Education, 53*(17), B10–B13.

Navarro, V. (1999). Equality, health, and international relations, health and equity in the world in the era of "globalization." *International Journal of Health Services, 29*(2), 215–226.

Navarro, V., & Shi, L. (2001). The politics of policy, the political context of social inequalities and health. *International Journal of Health Services, 31*(1), 1–21.

President criticizes Senate welfare bill. (2002, July 30). *Bozeman Daily Chronicle,* p. 2.

Reed, L. (2002, August 3). 60 new hires in Medicaid plan. *Omaha World Herald,* p. B1.

Study links education, health care. (2002, July 23). *Omaha World Herald,* p. 4.

Unicameral Update. (2002a, July 30–August 15). Nebraska Legislature's Weekly Publication.

Unicameral Update. (2002b). Legislature passes Medicaid changes. XXV(17), 7.

U.S. Catholic Conference. (1993, June 18). *A framework for comprehensive health care reform, protecting human life, promoting human dignity, pursuing the common good. A resolution of the Catholic Bishops of the United States.* Washington, DC: Author.

Winker, M. A. (2006). Theme issue on poverty and human development call for papers on interventions to improve health among the poor. *Journal of the American Medical Association, 296,* 2970–2971.

Resolving Disparities in Elder Care: Clinical Quality, Translational Science, and the Clinical Doctorate

Mary K. Walker

Changes in the healthcare industry in the United States mirror two major phenomena of our time: movement from the age of industrialization to the age of technology and globalization of the economy in virtually every sector of the free market. Instantly, it seems, we reallocated services from a cottage-industry healthcare delivery system, with stand-alone "mom and pop" hospitals, medical centers, and fee-for-service pricing, to integrated systems positioned through merger to maximize the continually evolving healthcare environment. All along, we witnessed and participated in the characteristics of an industry ripe for change: heavy regulation, old-guard stakeholders, well-entrenched interests, intractable class divisions, and resistance to anything that threatened the established order (Fuhrer & Moore, 1995). Ramifications of these constructs were evident in our daily practice lives: casted systems of care, maldistribution of clinical services, and anticompetitive barriers that stymied the full range of practice by healthcare providers.

Forty-four million Americans, the "working poor," did not have access to health care at all. Additionally, the working poor were typically employed in positions that did not offer health insurance as a benefit, yet they made too much money to qualify for federal and state programs such as Medicaid and were unable to purchase health insurance for themselves. We came to understand that, even now, no systemic safety net exists to provide services for these individuals (Walker, 2005).

We watched as the gross domestic product attributable to health care reached an alarming projection of 21% by 2010 (Austin, 2006). We puzzled over how we could be spending so much money on health care when patient days in high-intensity environments had decreased by 33% during the preceding 10 years (Reinhardt, 1997). We struggled with understanding the differences, sometimes not so subtle, between high costs and rising costs attributable to health care and technological advancement.

Indicators of rapid, deep, and permanent change were in the environment (Day & Schoemaker, 2004). When changes came, however, we were not prepared for them—either as they transformed our thinking from illness encounter to illness episode or as they affected new and sometimes revolutionary roles for registered professional nurses. In a very real sense, Hurricane Katrina hit the levees of our healthcare system and our infrastructure could not sustain it. Rather, rapid changes occurring in systems of care themselves propelled us, eventually, to explore alternative and emerging roles for nurses and to engage in the fierce conversation of adaptive change.

Advanced practice nurses, including nurse practitioners, nurse anesthetists, and nurse midwives, received renewed preference in legislative, political, and professional discussions in the mid to late 1990s. Massive media campaigns by organized nursing resulted in consumers of care, politicians, legislators, policymakers, and other key stakeholders becoming aware of the capabilities of advanced practice nurses to diagnose and treat illness (Government Accounting Office, 1993, 1996; Brown and Grimes, 1993). Similarly, a renewed understanding on the part of healthcare executives regarding the abilities of advanced practice nurses to produce positive health outcomes led to their incorporation as providers in practice networks and health plans (Mundinger, 2000).

Funding streams were redirected toward illness prevention rather than treatment. "Primary care" became watchwords of the industry, as if they had just been invented. Foundations such as the Pew Health Professions Commission (1995) predicted that we would lose between 200,000 and 300,000 acute care beds in this country; thus we would require 200,000 to 300,000 fewer registered professional nurses. These dire predictions prompted much dialogue in the discipline relative to how we should position nursing and the nurse workforce for the future (Aiken, Clarke, & Sloane, 2002; Aiken, Clarke, Cheung, Sloane, & Silber, 2003; Clarke and Aiken, 2003). At the end of the day the pundits could, or would, neither predict our movement into an era of profound nursing shortage nor light the way to resolving yet a deeper shortage, the shortage of professional nursing practice.

In this chapter we explore the intense dialogue surrounding the movement toward clinical doctoral preparation for advanced specialty nursing practice. This discussion is one of many that occurred over the last 10 years as a result of reconfiguring care systems and realigning professional priorities. It is noteworthy that such dialogue occurred within the rubric of social and economic changes in the healthcare industry, whereas acknowledging that the term "healthcare industry" serves as a placeholder, of sorts, for profound economic and social migration in our culture and around the globe.

Further, in this chapter we address what these roles mean for the patients, elders among them, that nurses serve. We examine evidence that supports the complexity of care requirements and healthcare quality as well as the need for nurses who can navigate the vagaries of multiple care systems and structures while leveraging the environment to meet patient need. Finally, we will come to understand that in emerging systems of care, providing the expertise to create healing organizations and ensure that our efforts toward healthcare quality are realized set the occasion for nursing practice in this country now.

Systems Integration and Patient Care Requirements: The 1990s

Theoretically, integrated service delivery systems were intended to facilitate continuity of care across service system levels. In 1996 the term "seamless integration" was proposed as one outcome of rapidly (e)merging healthcare systems. Seamless integration referred to the relationships crafted between newly articulated stand-alone care systems. For example, systems were represented as vertically and/or horizontally integrated. "Vertical integration" referred to the relationships existing between primary care networks, such as home healthcare agencies, and secondary and tertiary providers, such as community hospitals and academic health science centers. "Horizontal integration," on the other hand, referred to the cooperative relationships existing between different types of primary care agencies: home health care, ambulatory care, public health, and hospice, to name a few. In the new economy of health care, strategic relationships between maximally similar and maximally different provider types arose, as much in search of economic viability as in search of better ways to ensure quality in patient care.

The challenge of seamless integration from a clinical perspective included addressing the caring imperative across episodes of acute and chronic illness and managing both transitions between settings and the settings themselves. The processes associated with seamless integration required guiding individuals and populations through experiences associated with lifelong changes in health status. Economic incentives to reduce the amount of care, as well as other issues that impact care delivery, included care access, affordability, acceptability, accuracy, and appropriateness (Haas & Walker, 2001).

Such considerations amplified both clinical and economic anticipatory needs with regard to aging, chronicity, and vulnerability. Nursing roles expanded to include the nurse case manager, the "watchful eye" during episodes of acute illness as well as during periods of exacerbation and remission. Although nurse case managers optimized certain aspects of horizontal integration, integration in the absence of reproducible outcomes was fundamentally flawed. To date, there are as many studies that support cost increases from the use of nurse case managers as there are studies to suggest cost savings (Levine, 2006), testimony to the notion that quality care can be made more efficient but can never be done cheaply. Additionally, the decade of the 1990s saw erosion of the clinical nurse specialist role in favor of emphasizing nursing roles that optimized the relationship of the organization with funding streams. In so doing, staff nurses lost valuable allies in their continuing work to improve the quality of patient care. From an evolutionary perspective, then, is it any wonder that we are now considering a migration of advanced practice nursing to the clinical doctoral level?

This latest migration to a policy proposal for clinical doctoral preparation acknowledges that optimizing systems of care does not, in and of itself, provide or promote a healing environment or ensure quality. Rather, it maximizes the relationship of the patient to the organization at the expense of complex care consultation to staff nurses in the environments in which they work and in which care is delivered. The following data are provided as one example of "optimization" waiting to happen.

Complicating Factors in Patient Management: Severity of Illness and Comorbidity in Elders with Cardiac Illness

Acutely and critically ill individuals often have multiple, overlapping, healthcare needs that defy management by any one element of the healthcare system, such as acute care, alone. De la Loge and Arnould (2005) distinguished at least two domains of clinical, or patient, outcomes: condition specific and treatment specific. *Condition-specific* outcomes included signs, symptoms, and sensations of illness. Prevention of disease through population-focused health promotion is included as well as epidemiological trending of the consequences of illness. Such trending data include costs, because decisions of direct providers impact not only insurance claims but out-of-pocket expenses for those within their care. *Treatment-specific* outcomes included documenting gains and risks associated with proposed or prevailing treatment modalities as well as evaluating usefulness of one specific course of clinical action over another. Four overarching goals for contemporary providers and systems of care emerged from these considerations: (1) prevention of symptom occurrence; (2) alleviation, modification, or cure of the symptom experience; (3) prolonging the symptom-free period; and (4) improving quality of life, particularly health-related quality of life.

Glessner and colleagues (Glessner, Shermer, Roser, & Walker, 1999; Glessner & Walker, 2003), in an outcomes management study, examined condition-specific (acute and chronic illness) and treatment-specific (coronary artery bypass grafting [CABG]) outcomes in an elderly population requiring CABG. In this study two standardized features of patient evaluation were assessed for their capacities alone and together to predict elder outcome after CABG: *a severity of illness model*, the Acute Physiology and Chronic Health Evaluation (APACHE III) severity scoring system (Wong & Knaus, 1991), and a comorbidity measure, the Charlson Comorbidity Index (Charlson, Pompei, Ales, & McKenzie, 1987).

The challenge of evaluating care in contemporary systems is often as simple as how the word *severity* is defined and used within a given organization. Iezzoni (2003) defined illness severity in the APACHE system as the "risk of dying among ICU [intensive care unit] patients." Other severity scoring systems, such as patient management categories, defined severity as "intensity of care or costs that a specific patient incurs" (Iezzoni, 2003). One definition emphasized the status of the patient and the other, the status of the organization.

By definition, then, illness severity relates to intrinsic characteristics of both patient and treatment that impact mortality, cost, and disposition at discharge. In severity models such as the APACHE system, treatment utilization becomes a proxy measure for severity. Severity is inferred in this model because, all other things being equal, a given patient consuming large numbers of resources and not improving is, by definition, deteriorating. However, in the absence of a common definition, collapsing data across care systems or engaging in benchmarking practices is virtually impossible.

Comorbid conditions, on the other hand, are known to complicate intraoperative risk and set the occasion for postoperative complications. Thus they contribute to but do not define illness severity. Lezzoni et al. (1994) identified that preexisting chronic conditions significantly increased the likelihood of death for all patients, even those admitted for low-mortality problems. Further, patients admitted for high-risk problems died more often as a result of chronic conditions (e.g., congestive heart failure, chronic obstructive pulmonary disease, cancer).

In the instance of subjects in the study series cited previously, a secondary analysis of existing data was undertaken to identify the common and unique predictive capabilities of both severity of illness and comorbidity relative to outcomes for individuals who had undergone CABG. The two clinical indicators, illness severity and comorbidity, were analyzed with respect to four dependent measures in 100 post-CABG subjects: mortality, intensive care unit and hospital lengths of stay, and disposition at discharge.

Mortality and disposition at discharge were identified as clinical outcomes, whereas intensive care unit and hospital lengths of stay were identified as organizational outcomes (proxy measures of cost). Seventy-eight men and twenty-two women comprised the subject sample. The mean age of subjects was 61 years, and the average number of bypass grafts per subject was three. Only two subjects had no evidence of comorbidity at the time of surgery.

On average, subjects presented for surgery with 3.4 comorbid conditions that could possibly influence surgical outcome. Of the 100 subjects, 4 died subsequent to the procedure. Those who died averaged three to six comorbid conditions. APACHE III scores for these subjects ranged from 19 to 86, with a mean score of 50.2 (on a scale of 0–299), suggesting that the APACHE system captured acuity but not chronicity. APACHE III data alone, however, predicted which subjects were alive at the time of discharge ($p < 0.02$) and narrowly missed predicting outright mortality ($p < 0.06$). Additionally, the APACHE data were able to predict actual disposition at discharge, differentiating subjects sent home, sent to a rehabilitation or stepdown facility, or sent to long-term care. Chronological age of subjects had no predictive capability in this data set. That is, 80-year-olds did just about as well as 60-year-olds when undergoing the procedure.

On the other hand, the Charlson Comorbidity Index demonstrated strong predictive capability, $p < 0.003$ and $p < 0.002$, respectively, for determining hospital and intensive care unit lengths of stay. Charlson scores did not predict disposition at discharge or mortality. In subsequent multiple regression analyses, comorbidity scores accounted for 12% and 14%, respectively, of explained variance in intensive care unit and hospital length of stay. APACHE III predicted only disposition at discharge. There were no interaction effects. That is, attempting to combine these two instruments to enhance predictive capability of outcome measures was futile. Clean breaks in the data indicated that the APACHE and Charlson Index were predicting different features of patient and organizational outcome.

In two subsequent prospective studies, the investigators (Glessner et al., 1999) contacted the sample of 100 subjects to determine community-based outcomes of CABG procedures. These studies emphasized postoperative quality of life and explored whether elderly subjects had additional physical and behavioral health needs not being addressed by the system. We contacted subjects at three additional time periods: 3 months, 6 months, and 1 year after surgery. Of the 100 subjects, at the 3- and 6-month time frames 70 and 65 subjects, respectively, returned quality of life surveys: the Medical Outcomes Study Short Form-36 Health Survey (Sherbourne & Stewart, 1991; Ware & Sherbourne, 1992). Both physical and mental health after CABG surgery improved across the measurement time frames. At 3 months subjects reported significant needs for health professionals' guidance in resuming physical activities, work (role functioning), exercise (energy/fatigue issues), diet, and intimate activities within the structure of their primary relationships. Subjective reports of physical and mental health peaked at 6 months after the procedure.

These reports led us to believe that all was well and that surgical bypass contributed significantly to improved physical, functional, social, and behavioral health outcomes in these elderly CABG subjects. At 1 year after surgery, however, we again surveyed the 100 subjects. We again mailed the Medical Outcomes Study Short Form-36 survey and included a Center for Epidemiologic Studies–Depression instrument (Radloff, 1977) to more explicitly capture behavioral or mental health issues experienced by the subjects. Fifty-two subjects returned the instruments. Of these, 33 subjects reported some affective disturbance, and 17 subjects (one-third of those returning surveys) met clinical criteria for depressive affect. Subjective reporting of physical health had declined as well, with increased reports of bodily pain and inability to sustain reentry into social and role functions. There were statistically significant correlations of depression that accompanied bodily pain and failure to resume social and role functions, suggesting that untreated depression after surgery may adversely affect the gains achieved by surgical intervention in the population.

Data suggest that systematic covariation of depression and cardiac illness is not taken seriously by providers. Rather, depression is described as an "understandable" reaction in elders to physical and functional loss, serving as a predictor of noncompliance with therapeutic regimen (DiMatteo, Leppe, & Croghan, 2000). A review of recent cardiovascular literature and best practice studies revealed a paucity of reference to the systematic covariation of depression and heart disease in the medical, surgical, geriatric, or critical care literature. Further, features of physical illness superimpose unique difficulties in diagnosing depression in that symptoms of medical conditions often overlap those of affective disorder. Symptom presentation of both cardiovascular illness and depression in elders is reported as "atypical" by clinicians (Musselman, Evans, & Nemeroff, 1998), suggesting that clinicians and scientists alike must be sensitive to the broad range of symptomatic presentations and varying severities of both mood and medical disorder if accurate treatment is to occur. Older persons are more apt to suffer from coexisting illness, to be functionally impaired, or to receive medication that can lead to symptoms of depression or mask existing depression (Cahalan, 1996).

A review of neuropsychiatric literature, on the other hand, revealed consistent concern related to the covariation of cardiac and depressive illness. In their seminal reviews, Rabins, Harvis, and Koven (1985), Rabins (1988), and Tresch, Folstein, Rabins, and

Hazzard (1985) found that 75% of elders who were depressed died within 1 year of index admission for cardiovascular disease. Further, although mechanisms are poorly understood, depression constituted a major risk factor for mortality from ischemic heart disease in a Centers for Disease Control and Prevention study (1998) of over 2,800 subjects aged 45–77. Subjects, derived from the National Health Examination Follow-up Study, had no history of ischemic heart disease or serious illness at baseline. There were 189 cases of fatal ischemic heart disease during follow-up. After adjusting for demographic and risk factors, depressed affect was related to fatal ischemic heart disease (relative risk = 1.5; 95% confidence interval = 1.0–2.3), as was hopelessness. Depressed affect and hopelessness, further, were associated with increased risk of nonfatal ischemic heart disease. Data were interpreted to indicate that depressed affect and hopelessness may play a causal role in the occurrence of both fatal and nonfatal ischemic heart disease.

This Centers for Disease Control and Prevention study supports the earlier premise of this section of the chapter—that the needs of elders with chronic lifelong health problems defy management in a single sector of the healthcare system. Indeed, it is the definition of what constitutes quality care and healing across the episode of illness rather than clinical specialization alone that must compel us in our discussion of treatment outcomes. The data, in fact, have important implications not only for patient outcome but also for expanding and sustaining new roles for geriatric and gerontological nurses in an effort to produce an environment of quality and maximize therapeutic gains and healing.

In summary, for consumers of health care, failure to address the entire illness episode impacts physical, functional, and psychological health. Indeed, for persons with cardiac disease, emphasis on the physical features of illness to the exclusion of psychiatric comorbidity results in diminished quality of life and premature death. For healthcare organizations, failure to address illness as a multidimensional experience results in disproportionate resource consumption and recidivism. Certainly, treatment decisions that address only a portion of the illness experience often result in prolongation of an episode of illness and failure to achieve optimal health outcomes. Such considerations advance the thesis that clinical doctoral preparation for advanced practice nurses is long overdue, if data integration and application (elements of the broader construct of "handoff") are suggested as mechanisms to ensure quality in health care.

Crossing the Quality Chasm: Healing Environments and Emerging Nursing Roles

O'Malley (2005), in his investigation of optimal healing environments, suggested that the climate in health care is "harsh," citing that healthcare environments are not truly integrated with respect to the predictability of resources and processes across aspects of the care system. In reality, the processes and resources for both quality and healing have never been predictable, save for the presence of registered professional and advanced practice nurses. The literature of the 1990s (Brannon, 1994; Brown and Grimes, 1993; Friss, 1994) focused on "tasks" of emerging nursing roles, such as that of case manager. In this day and time the potential impact of preparing doctorally prepared clinicians suggests that it is the outcome of creating healing environments and emphasizing quality care through translational research that serves as the best measure of role effectiveness.

Hall (2005), in her award-winning book, *The Art of Becoming a Nurse Healer,* suggested that organized nursing and nurses themselves become trapped in the notion of "role" to the exclusion of understanding that role entrapment can, and often does, become a barrier to the healing relationship. We believe, for example, that nurse scientists generate new knowledge for practice. That belief is fundamental to PhD education in nursing. Further, our literature suggests that we, then, select nurse educators and clinicians as individuals responsible for the "science of application" (Boyer, 1991). For most of us these are theoretical distinctions because at this time PhD-prepared nurses in academic settings have no true or consistent clinical counterparts in health care.

Nursing at the Quality Chasm

In advancing the argument for clinical doctoral preparation, it is useful to learn from our past. Fagin (1994) and other investigators provided evidence that the lag time from the generation of new nursing knowledge until its full incorporation into direct nursing practice is about 14 years. Fagin and her colleagues provided no information regarding timelines for incorporation of new nursing knowledge into health policy. At this time our discipline defers to the National Institute of Nursing Research to make judgments and advancements in this arena. It is hardly inappropriate to suggest that, in a time of sophisticated communication and instructional technology, we might and can do better. The new area of "translational research" is expected to back-fill this provider knowledge application lag, even as the generation and circulation of new knowledge becomes more rapid and competitive and its implementation into policy more nimble. However, institution of programs of translational research begs the question, Who, in the clinical arena, is remotely prepared to provide support to staff nurses and others as they attempt such translation?

Leeman, Jackson, and Sandelowski (2006) indicated that an essential feature of accurate and complete research application is making all information from a given investigative activity available to clinicians. At this point in time, they argued, the way research is reported in clinical and investigative journals is a potential barrier to using research in practice. Specifically, they suggested that the implications for practice are not made clear (McCleary & Brown, 2003). Essential features of application include "how to" directives from principal investigators, cost and cost-effectiveness data, and clear explication of outcomes (Leeman et al., 2006; Titler et al., 2001). Leeman et al. (2006) suggested four domains of "practice utility" applicable to the use of nursing science in practice: relative advantage, compatibility, complexity, and implementation (p. 176 and distilled from earlier work of Davidson et al., 2003).

Of interest is the fact that Leeman et al. do not address another, equally important, translation—the translation of research into health policy. Thus we persist in turning our quality gaze toward the patient–provider interface alone, suggesting a lack of recognition that data must undergird health policy if meaningful changes toward bridging the quality chasm are to occur. Recently, Asch et al. (2006) reported that just over 50% of healthcare interventions delivered in the United States are defensible through evidence. We are left to assume that remaining interventions are remnants persisting in our educational and clinical practice from the oral history and wisdom of those who have gone before us.

Asch et al. (2006) advanced the thesis that individual characteristics (of subjects), often exerting protective effect, do not shield most people from deficits in quality of care. Pierson (2006) suggested that our healthcare systems (and, parenthetically, the barriers imposed on care delivered in them) represent a single form of social organizing and that current subsystems contribute to health quality failures through suboptimization. His arguments are testimony to our collective failures, ostensibly from misadventures in the 1990s, in which care systems replaced nurses and other healthcare providers with the organization in the patient–provider dyad.

Lessons from the "Front"

In the 1990s advanced practice nurses and nurse care managers (now subsumed in the nursing literature as clinical nurse leaders) complemented generalist nursing services by managing the care of groups (e.g., selected case types) both within and across agencies (Walker & Sebastian, 1996). In addition to the traditional brokering, care, and teaching functions of staff nurses, case managers, and traditionally prepared advanced practice nurses, there was indeed an emphasis on shortening lengths of stay. Clapp (2006) suggested that despite tangible benefit, nurse case managers were never able to penetrate the nurse–patient dyad. Thus there is suggestion that nurse case managers were organizationally aligned around fiscal realities, positioned not so much to impact the quality of care as its efficiency.

Swanson (personal communication, 2006) suggested that such an environment was "corrosive." Her terminology was predicated on the notion that healthcare systems in the 1990s confused low-cost task-oriented staffing ratios with quality care. In the process we risked patient safety on the one hand and relationship-centered caring on the other. Further, she noted that optimal care was compromised under conditions of poor staffing, too little time, and intense workloads, contributing to staff nurse burnout and profound job dissatisfaction. Wagner et al. (2005) framed the dilemma as "finding common ground between patient-centeredness and evidence-based chronic illness care" (p. S-7).

The thesis of this chapter supports the American Association of Colleges of Nursing position that role expansion toward clinical doctoral preparation is necessary to achieve full continuity of care for groups of individuals who are chronically ill, vulnerable, or frail, such as the elders who provided data for the CABG studies. Translational research can position nurse clinicians with contemporary science that, in turn, can impact outcomes. However, just as Tripp-Reimer (1984) noted almost 20 years ago, there needs to be an individual who can stand between the emic and etic positions of such translation. That is, we now need doc-torally prepared advanced practice nurses to bridge the growing divide between the patients' need for healing and the rigors of the scientific enterprise and quality demands of the care delivery system. Is the clinical doctorally prepared nurse that person? Is there a relationship between quality of care and level of nursing preparation?

Aiken et al. (2003) suggested that the outcomes of acute care in at least 10 diagnostic categories were improved when a preponderance of nurse staffing was provided by bac-calaureate-prepared nurses. A closer look at the proposal to migrate advanced practice nursing to the clinical doctoral level illustrates very well the holes in the healthcare system that require remedy for us to advance the quality agenda. For example, the CABG data indicate that a fundamental flaw in "the system" is dichotomization between the patient and provider relationship on the one hand and the patient and organization relationship on the other. That is, although we speak strongly about the "illness episode," we still actu-alize "illness encounter" through parallel processes that are not formally connected and, in fact, have little to do with one another. Indeed, between these two relational worlds is a third world in which there is minimal staffing "coverage"—that is, the world of the patient traversing the broad expanse of "healthcare delivery" alone in search of healing.

These staffing and competency shortfalls, if you will, support migration of specialty practice to the clinical doctoral level. Sawyer et al. (2002) offered a few examples of current competencies missing from contemporary nursing advanced practice programs but that are necessary to support quality measurement and organizational transparency:

- Retrofitting and modifying data
- Validity and reliability of clinical indicators
- Uniform application and relevance of clinical indicators
- Risk stratification/risk adjustment, including measures of severity
- Providing the context for interpretation/identification of true outliers
- Strategic definitional work to allow interinstitutional comparisons
- Accurate interpretation of data by type
- Transforming data into information
- Demonstrated causality or dynamics whenever possible
- Data display that supports the analytic goal
- Notations of data source, problems with data or method
- Physical display of the most fundamental measurement characteristics, such as means and some measure of variation
- Financial data
- Assessment of change implying comparison of costs between baseline and new targets

- Demonstrated means and standard deviations
- Representation of financial data against time, adjusted for inflation
- Report standardization
- Demonstrated cause–effect relationships
- Use of models to represent data
- Use of organizational data to support migration and adjustment of care processes

These competencies represent contemporary processes of care and support the role of clinical doctoral preparation as one mechanism for achieving full integration of these competencies into care systems. But if one outcome is to include creation and support of a healing environment, it becomes evident that Hall's (2005) thesis is accurate: It is possible to become so enamored with new roles that we lose sight of the outcomes we are trying to create in the first place, namely, reconnecting nurses and patients around a quality and a healing agenda.

Vision for the Clinical Doctorate

The creation of the clinical doctorate is an attempt to reconnect nursing not with its power base but with its passion base. That is, a dialogue of nursing roles and the appropriate educational preparation to support them begs the question of how such roles, in turn, contribute to the quest of refining and improving patient outcome. The consistent rush to "role" as one mechanism of garnering clinical power for nursing suggests that the healing passion of nursing has been overlooked and undervalued in the last two decades. Yet the 2.6 million U.S. nurses are well aware that their mission is to heal those who need them. Their frustration, represented in increased unionization activity, springs from the fundamental reorganization of health care—a reorganization that emphasizes the patient–organizational relationship at the expense of the patient–nurse relationship. In nursing's rush to representation at "the table" in a time of intense systemic change, nursing embraced roles posited on organizational health. Indeed, as we look back at the healthcare system of the 1990s, it is only too clear that we marred the nature of the healing relationship and, in so doing, contributed to safety and quality shortfalls.

The national clinical doctorate proposal makes explicit that to translate research systematically, nurses need not only advanced clinical specialization but substantive academic preparation to amplify science in care. The Essentials for Practice Doctorate Programs (American Association of Colleges of Nursing, 2004) indicate the areas of emphasis:

- Scientific underpinnings for practice
- Advanced nursing practice
- Organization and system leadership/management, quality improvement, and system thinking

- Analytic methodologies related to the evaluation of practice and the application of evidence for practice
- Use of technology and information for the improvement and transformation of health care
- Health policy development, implementation, and evaluation
- Interdisciplinary collaboration for improving patient and population health outcomes

A cursory review of these essentials suggests that both content and process competencies are identified as components of clinical doctoral preparation. It is argued that moving clinical specialty competencies to the doctoral level ensures that nurses, along with their clinical counterparts in physical therapy and pharmacy, are prepared with a terminal clinical degree. Thus the proposal produces standardization of clinical competencies both within and across practice disciplines.

Educational standardization occasioned by the terminal degree provides a commonality in specialty preparation that does not currently exist in our educational preparatory structure. Again, the quality and healing agendas of nursing are supported by systematically advancing the preparation of specialty practitioners while proceeding cautiously with the preemption of the healing agenda by a rush to define advanced practice "roles" according to mechanistic and conventional biomedical models (Agdal, 2005).

Wagner and colleagues (Wagner, Austin, & Von Korff, 1996; Wagner et al., 2005) noted that a more cogent concern is whether evidence-based medicine's impetus to standardize care (and, by extension, clinician competencies) conflicts with patient-centered medicine's emphasis on individualizing treatment. Eddy (2005) argued for integration of two dominant views or paradigms: safety and effectiveness and contextualization of care. Perhaps Eddy's suggestion begins to bridge the divide between mounting evidence and common sense.

Assumptions and Analysis

It is striking that within this nursing rubric of specialty migration to the clinical doctoral level, there is the presumed ability of advanced practice nurses to stand between and integrate the new emic and etic perspectives: the healing nature of the nurse–patient relationship on the one hand and the leading edge of science and technological application to ensure quality on the other. Agdal (2005) noted that science itself relies on images and metaphors to inform theoretical application, whereas Western biomedical theory, based in mechanistic models, refers to literal objects. She goes on to suggest that metaphors and culture-bound conceptual systems influence the perception of the body itself and thereby dictate what is considered specific knowledge and suitable interventions for the caring disciplines—that is, culture-bound conceptual systems that mitigate against healing and quality in favor of regulatory frames.

Indeed, as Jonas and Chez (2003) and McNutt (2004) recognized and Chez and Jonas (2005, pp. S3–S5) specifically identified:

> Helping the patient attain healing must become one of the essential goals of care . . . all patients seeking care have spoken and unspoken expectations, needs, and preferences. The challenge for the provider is to solicit them, define them, understand them and respond appropriately to them.

Conclusion

Clinical doctoral education positions advanced practice nurses with higher order capability to integrate clinical care requirements with scientific information. Indeed, the individuals who graduate from such programs are the new disciplinary partners of nurse scientists. In a sense the proposal forges an agenda for alliance and change in the tacit relationship between nurse scientists on the one hand and nurse clinicians on the other. Such change represents the move to the next developmental level for nursing, even as we debate the roadmap to full implementation.

Further, for those who pursue preparation in executive leadership, appropriate data application preserves and advances the health outcomes of a given patient population, such as elders, while maintaining the fiscal viability of organizations. In the book of "lessons learned," the clinical doctorate proposal represents our ability as a practice discipline to confront our shortcomings, to learn from them, and to move in a direction consonant with our social contract (American Nurses Association, 1995).

I end this chapter with a final thought from Margaret Stacey:

> The kinds of society we invent and particularly the way we handle issues of life, health, suffering, and death arise from the way . . . we perceive this essential part of our humanness. And how we perceive it, how we behave in relation to the biological base, also affects our destiny as social beings. For there is no doubt about the social creation of illness and suffering as well as the social construction of the knowledge about it.

References

Agdal, R. (2005). Diverse and changing perceptions of the body: Communicating illness, health, and risk in an age of medical pluralism. *Journal of Alternative and Complementary Medicine, 11*(Suppl. 1), S67–S75.

Aiken, L. H., Clarke, S. P., Cheung, R. B., Sloane, D. M., & Silber, J. H. (2003). Education levels of hospital nurses and patient mortality. *Journal of the American Medical Association, 290,* 1617–1623.

Aiken, L. H., Clarke, S. P., & Sloane, D. M. (2002). Hospital staffing, organizational support, and quality of care: Cross-national findings. *International Journal for Quality in Health Care, 14,* 5–13.

Alexopoulos, G. S., Vrontou, C., Kakuma, T., Meyers, B., Young, R., Klausner, E., et al. (1996). Disability in geriatric depression. *American Journal of Psychiatry, 153,* 877–885.

American Association of Colleges of Nursing. (2004). *Position statement on the practice doctorate in nursing.* Washington, DC: Author.

American Nurses Association. (1995). *Nursing's social policy statement, 1995.* Washington, DC: Author.

Asch, S. M., Kerr, E., Keesey, J., Adams, J., Setodji, C., Malik, S., & McGlynn, E. (2006). Who is at greatest risk for receiving poor-quality health care? *The New England Journal of Medicine, 354,* 2617–2619.

Austin, J. (2006). *Dealing with uncertainty.* Swedish Medical Center Board Retreat, Seattle, WA.

Boyer, E. L. (1991). Ready to learn: A mandate for the nation. Princeton, NJ: Carnegie Foundation for the Advancement of Teaching.

Brannon, R. L. (1994). *Intensifying care: The hospital industry, professionalization, and the reorganization of the nursing labor process.* New York: Baywood.

Brown, S. A., & Grimes, E. D. (1993). *A meta-analysis of process of care, clinical outcomes, and cost-effectiveness of nurses in primary care roles: Nurse practitioners and certified nurse-midwives* (pp. 1–86). Washington, DC: American Nurses Publishing.

Cahalin, L. P. (1996). Heart failure. *Physical Therapy, 75,* 516–533.

Centers for Disease Control and Prevention. (1998). Changes in mortality from heart failure— United States, 1980–1995. *Morbidity and Mortality Weekly, 47,* 633–667.

Charlson, M. E., Pompei, P., Ales, K. L., & McKenzie, C. R. (1987). A new method of classifying prognostic comorbidity in longitudinal studies: Development and validation. *Journal of Chronic Diseases, 40,* 373–383.

Chez, R. A., & Jonas, W. B. (2005). Challenges and opportunities in achieving healing. *Journal of Alternative and Complementary Medicine, 11*(Suppl, 1), pp. S3–S6.

Clapp, C. (2006). *The clinical nurse leader: A paradigm for change.* Presentation to the Washington State Nurses Association Practice Council, Tukwila, Washington.

Clarke, S. P., & Aiken, L. H. (2003). Registered nurse staffing and patient and nurse outcomes in hospitals: A commentary. *Policy, Politics, & Nursing Practice, 4,* 104–111.

Day, G. S., & Schoemaker, P. J. H. (2004). Driving through the fog: Managing at the edge. *Long Range Planning, 37,* 127–142.

Davidson, K.W., Goldstein, M., Kaplan, R., Kaufman, P., Knatterud, G., Orleans, C., et al. (2003). Evidence-based behavioral medicine: What is it and how do we achieve it? *Annals of Behavioral Medicine, 26,* 161–171.

De la Loge, C., & Arnould, B. (2005, November 6–8). *The use of composite end points: A review of the regulators' perspective and methodological issues.* Presented at the International Society for Pharmacoeconomics and Outcomes Research, Annual European Congress, Florence, Italy.

DiMatteo, M. R., Leppe, H., & Croghan, T. (2000). Depression is a risk factor for noncompliance with medical treatment. *Archives of Internal Medicine, 160,* 2102–2107.

Eddy, D. M. (2005). Evidence-based medicine: A unified approach. *Health Affairs, 24,* 9–17.

Fagin, C. M. (1994). Cost-effectiveness of nursing care revisited: 1981–1990. In C. Harrington & C. L. Estes (Eds.), *Health policy and nursing: Crisis and reform in the U.S. health care delivery system* (pp. 313–330). Sudbury, MA: Jones and Bartlett.

Friss, L. (1994). Nursing studies laid end-to-end form a circle. *Journal of Health Politics, Policy, & Law, 19,* 597–663.

Fuhrer, J., & Moore, G. (1995). Inflation persistence. *Quarterly Journal of Economics, CX,* 127–160.

Government Accounting Office. (1993). *Health care access: Innovative programs using non-physicians* (HRD 93-128). Washington, DC: Author.

Government Accounting Office. (1996). *Nonphysician specialists.* HEHS-96-135R. Washington, DC: Author.

Glessner, T., Shermer, E., Roser, L., & Walker, M. K. (1999). Coronary artery bypass surgery: Outcomes and explanations. Presented at the 13th Annual Southern Nursing Research Society, Charleston, SC.

Glessner, T., & Walker, M. K. (2003). Standardized measures: Documenting processes and outcomes of care for patients undergoing coronary artery bypass grafting. *MEDSURG Nursing, 10,* 23–30.

Haas, S., & Walker, M. K. (2001). *Developing collaborative models of master's education: The Jesuit model.* Presented at the AACN Master's Conference, Denver, Colorado.

Hall, B. A. (2005). *The art of becoming a nurse healer.* Orlando, FL: Bandido Books.

Jonas, W. B., & Chez, R. A. (2003). The role and importance of definitions and standards in healing research. *Alternative Therapies in Health and Medicine, 9,* A5–A9.

Leeman, J., Jackson, B., & Sandelowski, M. (2006). An evaluation of how well research reports facilitate the use of findings in practice. *Journal of Nursing Scholarship, 38,* 171–177.

Lezzoni, L. I. (2003). *Risk adjustment for measuring healthcare outcomes* (3rd ed.). Chicago: Health Administration Press.

Lezzoni, L. I., Heeren, T., Foley, S., Daley, J., Hughes, J., & Coffman, G. (1994). Chronic conditions and risk of in-hospital death. *Health Services Research, 29*(4), 435–460.

Levine, M. (2006, June 14). Commentary. Governor's Chronic Care Management and Long-term Care Task Force, Olympia, Washington.

McCleary, L., & Brown, G. T. (2003). Barriers to pediatric nurses' research utilization. *Journal of Advanced Nursing, 42,* 364–372.

McNutt, R. A. (2004). Shared medical decision making: Problems, process, progress. *Journal of the American Medical Association, 292,* 2516–2518.

Mundinger, M., Kane, R., & Lenz, E. (2000). Letter to the editor. *Journal of the American Medical Association.*

Musselman, D. L., Evans, D. L., & Nemeroff, C. B. (1998). The relationship of depression to cardiovascular disease. *Archives of General Psychiatry, 55,* 580–592.

O'Malley, P. G. (2005). Studying optimal healing environments: Challenges and proposals. *Journal of Alternative and Complementary Medicine, 11,* S17–S22.

Pew Health Professions Commission. (1995). *Critical challenges: Revitalizing the health professions for the twenty-first century.* San Francisco: University of California at San Francisco Center for the Health Professions.

Pierson, M. (2006, June 14). *Pursuing perfection (P2) in chronic and complex conditions.* Platform Presentation to the Governor's Chronic Care and Longterm Care Task Force, Olympia, Washington.

Rabins, P. V. (1988). Co-morbidity and mental health in later life. *Aging and Mental Health, 2,* 262–263.

Rabins, P. V., Harvis, K., & Koven, S. (1985). High fatality rates of late-life depression associated with cardiovascular disease. *Journal of Affective Disorders, 9,* 165–167.

Radloff, L. S. (1977). The CES-D scale: A self-report depression scale for research in the general population. *Applied Psychological Measurement, 1,* 385–401.

Reinhardt, U. E. (1997). Spending more through "cost control": Our obsessive quest to gut the hospital. *Nursing Outlook, 45,* 156–160.

Sawyer, L. M., Berkowitz, B., Haber, J. E., Larrabee, J. H., Marino, B. L., Martin, K. S., et al. (2002). Expanding ANA's quality indicators to community-based practices. *Outcomes Management for Nursing Practice, 6,* 53–61.

Sherbourne, C. D., & Stewart, A. L. (1991). The MOS social support survey. *Social Science & Medicine, 32,* 705–714.

Titler, M. G., Kleiber, C., Steelman, V., Fakel,, B., Budreau, G., & Everett, L. (2001). The Iowa model of evidence-based practice to promote quality care. *Critical Care Nursing Clinics of North America, 13,* 497–550.

Tresch, D. D., Folstein, M. F., Rabins, P. V., & Hazzard, W. R. (1985). Prevalence and significant of cardiovascular disease and hypertension in elderly patients with dementia and depression. *Journal of the American Geriatrics Society, 33,* 530–537.

Tripp-Reimer, T. (1984). Reconceptualizing the construct of health: Integrating emic and etic perspectives. *Research in Nursing and Health, 7,* 101–109.

Wagner, E. H., Austin, B. T., & Von Korff, M. (1996). Organizing care for patients with chronic illness. *Milbank Quarterly, 74,* 511–544.

Wagner, E. H., Bennett, S. M., Austin, B. T., Greene, S. M., Schaefer, J. K., & Von Korff, M. (2005). Finding common ground: Patient-centeredness and evidence-based chronic illness care. *Journal of Alternative and Complementary Medicine, 11*(Suppl. 1), S7–S15.

Walker, M. K. (2005). Forward. In M. de Chesnay (Ed.), *Caring for the vulnerable: Perspectives in nursing theory, practice, and research* (pp. xix–xx). Sudbury, MA: Jones and Bartlett.

Walker, M. K., & Sebastian, J. (1996). Complementarity of advanced practice nursing roles in enhancing health outcomes of the chronically ill: Acute care nurse practitioners and nurse case managers. *Series on Nursing Administration, 9,* 170–190.

Ware, J. E., & Sherbourne, C. D. (1992). The MOS 36-item short form health survey (SF-36). I. Conceptual framework and item selection. *Medical Care, 30,* 473–483.

Wong, D. T., & Knaus, W. A. (1991). Predicting outcome in critical care: the current status of the APACHE prognostic scoring system. *Canadian Journal of Anaesthesia, 38,* 374–383.

Global Nursing Migration: Issues in Social Justice and Vulnerability

Barbara A. Anderson

The World Health Organization (WHO) identified the global shortage of healthcare professionals and the high attrition of health professionals from developing nations to high-income countries as the *most critical factor* affecting the dissemination of health care and the implementation of public health programs in low-income countries. Aggressive marketing by high-income nations contributes to the severe personnel shortages in low-income countries. WHO is addressing this crisis as a key agenda item in the next decade. *The Decade of Workforce Shortage* (WHO, 2006) is a call for study and implementation of solutions to the problem. In 2006 WHO released a major report, "Why the Workforce Is Important," calling for nations to cooperate in the planning and management of human resources in the health professions. This report proposes a "roadmap" that addresses the preparation of healthcare workers, the maintenance of competencies, and the retention of human resources, focusing particularly on the needs of low-income nations (WHO, 2006) (Table 45-1).

TABLE 45-1   WHO Plan for Workforce Sustainability

Entry: Preparing the Workforce	Workforce: Enhancing Performance	Exit: Managing Migration and Attrition
Build strong institutions	Provide adequate supervision	Manage migration
Ensure educational quality	Ensure fair and reliable compensation	Accommodate the needs of female workers
Revitalize recruitment capabilities	Develop critical support systems	Ensure safe work environments
	Offer lifelong learning	Provide retirement planning

Source: World Health Organization. (2006). *Why the workforce is important.* Retrieved November 12, 2006, from www.who.int/whr/2006/overview/en/print.html

Background

According to the WHO, there is a deficit of 4 million health professionals (doctors, nurses, midwives, and public health professionals) across 57 nations, mostly in very poor regions of the world. Sub-Saharan Africa, with the devastation of HIV/AIDS, carries 24% of the global burden of disease but has only 3% of the world's health professionals (Chaguturu & Vallabhaneni, 2003; Poaching nurses, 2006). In this region there is an estimated shortage of 620,000 nurses, the greatest deficit across all the health professions. In Kenya and Ghana alone, 50% of nursing positions are unfilled because of a lack of adequate numbers of nurses (Chaguturu & Vallabhaneni, 2003). Compounding the problem is the high attrition of health professionals, especially nurses, from low-income nations to high paying affluent nations. The World Bank estimates that 23,000 health professionals migrate from Africa every year, further eroding a limited pool of human resources (Cholanda, 2003). The effects are not only on poor nations. With 126,000 currently unfilled nursing positions in the United States and a projected deficit of 1 million by 2020, the issue of adequate numbers of healthcare workforce, especially nursing, is clearly a crisis. The projected impact of workforce shortage on the health of nations, regardless of economic status, is daunting (Buchan, 2006; Buerhaus, Staiger, & Auerbach, 2000; Chaguturu & Vallabhaneni, 2003; Spacracio, 2003).

Migration: The Perspective of Low-Income Countries

Concurrent to workforce shortage, populations in the developing world are growing. Birth rates are high and populations are aging. Poor nations often have "hourglass" population pyramids with large losses in early to mid-adulthood, frequently due to HIV/AIDS mortality and workforce migration. Healthcare services are not expanding, and many nations are closing health facilities because of lack of available personnel, especially nurses (Cholanda, 2003; Ross, Polsky, & Sochalski 2003; Spacracio, 2003). As an example, key health leaders in the Philippines predict the collapse of the healthcare system within 5 years if the current patterns of emigration continue (Migration threatens health systems, 2003; Spacracio, 2003). I have personally witnessed the closing of the pediatric hospital in Kingston, Jamaica, because of widespread migration of the nursing workforce to the United States. In Guyana, South America, I have observed the nursing shortage in healthcare facilities resulting from migration.

Public health systems, likewise, are stressed and collapsing by the shortage of healthcare workforce, especially nursing personnel (Poaching nurses, 2006; Spacracio, 2003). Although the Global Fund and other major funders are providing huge amounts of money for public health programs (e.g., antiretroviral drugs), implementation is crippled by lack of available human resources to deliver the programs and the services (Buchan, 2006; Clark, Stewart, & Clark, 2006; Dugger, 2006; Internation Council of Nurses [ICN], 2001; Kamal-Yanni, 2006).

The ministries of health in many low-income nations are stretched as they attempt to expand health professional education, especially nursing, to provide minimal staffing domestically. They, effectively, subsidize nursing education for First World nations. The response by the ministries has been to attempt to increase the numbers of students, particularly nursing students, to counter the migration flow. Laws prohibiting migration and requiring national service before migration have, for the most part, been ineffective (ICN, 2006).

On the other hand, the migration of health professionals from low-income nations provides a significant source of remittances to poor nations, a consistent flow of "hard" currency (e.g., U.S. dollars, British pounds, or Japanese yen) that can be used on the international monetary market. In addition, family units within developing countries often benefit and frequently survive on the cash flow coming from their emigrated family member (Abyad, 2003; Ross et al., 2003). Some low-income nations plan the preparation of health professionals, especially nurses, for employment in high-income nations as a strategy for obtaining remittances (Eastwood et al., 2003; ICN, 2006; WHO, 2006). Yet their own people lack sufficient access to health care.

Migration: View from the First World

Populations in high-income nations are also growing, mostly from immigration and aging. There are severe shortages of healthcare professionals, most acutely in nursing (Green, 2006; ICN, 2006; Migration threatens health systems, 2003; O'Dowd, 2003). Health professionals in high-income nations, in tandem with the general demographics of these regions of the world, are an aging population (Buerhaus et al., 2000; Health Resources and Services Administration, 2004; Pond & McPake, 2006). The pool of younger health professionals are not at a replacement level (ICN, 2006). Further, the nursing shortage in the United States is driven by limited access to nursing education programs. In 2005, 150,000 *qualified* applicants were denied admission into U.S. nursing programs; 32,000 of these denials were to BSN programs (Dugger, 2006; ICN, 2006; Ross et al., 2003; Yordy, 2006). Admission to nursing programs are capped, not because of lack of interested students but rather because of the severe shortage of nursing faculty linked to disparity in educator salaries compared with clinician salaries and the availability of faculty prepared at the graduate level (American Academy of Nursing, 2006; ICN, 2006; Ross et al., 2003; Yordy, 2006). One solution to the nursing shortage in First World nations is active recruitment of nurses from less-developed countries. Incentives include high salaries, opportunities for job and educational advancement, and good working conditions (Riley, Anderson, Noguchi, & Vindigni, 2005; Ross et al., 2003; WHO, 2006; Xu & Zhang, 2003).

Social Justice and the Migration of Nurses

While affirming the right of healthcare professionals, including nurses, to seek economic and personal security and to practice their professions in varying settings, the WHO and the ICN have asked high-income nations to desist from aggressive marketing techniques

- Effective human resource planning and development
- Credible nursing regulation
- Access to full employment
- Freedom of movement
- Freedom from discrimination
- Good faith contracting
- Equal pay for work of equal value
- Access to grievance procedures
- Safe work environment
- Effective orientation, mentoring, and supervision
- Employment trial periods
- Freedom of association
- Regulation of recruitment

Figure 45-1   ICN Ethical Nurse Recruitment Position Statement: Key Principles (ICN, 2001)

and to abide by the key principles (Figure 45-1) outlined in the ICN Ethical Nurse Recruitment Position Statement (ICN, 2001, 2006; Spacracio, 2003; WHO, 2006).

Ethical concerns have been raised about recruitment efforts by high-income nations that subsequently undermine the efforts of low-income nations to establish viable health-care systems for their peoples (Clark et al., 2006; Eastwood, et al., 2003; Green, 2006; ICN, 2006; McElmurry et al., 2006; Poaching nurses, 2006; Spacracio, 2003; Xu & Zhang, 2003). The debate is heated with charges of "outsourcing" nursing education (Dugger, 2006) and directives to low-income nations to increase numbers of workforce trained, improve retention plans, and implement migration restrictions (Abyad, 2003; Kamal-Yanni, 2006; McElmurry et al., 2006; Padilla, 2006; Ross et al., 2003; Xu & Zhang, 2003).

OXFAM and Physician's for Human Rights, two leading global organizations promoting human rights, have called for high-income nations who practice active recruitment to work collaboratively with low-income nations. They recommend subsidizing professional education, providing resources for continuing education, and assisting with infrastructure development (Kamal-Yanni, 2006). Meanwhile, the National League for Nursing asks why, in the midst of the nursing workforce crisis in the United States, the U.S. government is proposing a funding cut of up to 44 million U.S. dollars for Nursing Workforce Development authorized by Title VIII of the PHS Act (Klestzick, 2007).

Vulnerability of Migrating Nurses

Nurses who have migrated from low-income nations to seek employment in high-income countries are recognized as a vulnerable population. The principles of the ICN Position Statement on Ethical Nurse Recruitment (Figure 45-1) as described below outline a standard of support to decrease vulnerability (ICN, 2003).

Effective Human Resource Planning and Development

This standard calls for planning on the global level to ensure a balance in the supply and demand in nursing resources. Neglecting this planning puts both individual nurses and populations at significant risk, creating situations of inadequate staffing in the care of individual clients and in the provision of public health programs. A key example is the difficulty in implementing HIV/AIDS programs in low-income countries where there is a critical shortage of nurses.

Credible Nursing Regulation and Regulation of Recruitment

Nurses who migrate for employment frequently do so for economic reasons. In a foreign country and under economic constraints, a nurse could easily be coerced into practicing at a level beyond established competency. Regulation of scope of practice is essential to protect the individual nurse and the needs of the general population (Jeans, 2006; Yan, 2006). Further, the ICN recommends government oversight and policy regulation of recruiting agencies and the levying of sanctions on agencies that practice unethically, for example, presenting employment opportunities under false pretenses (McElmurry et al., 2006).

Freedom of Movement, Freedom of Association, and Freedom from Discrimination

Nurses recruited from low-income nations should be assured the right to move between their natal countries and nations of employment. They should receive fair and equitable treatment on the job. There are recorded cases of discriminatory practices perpetrated against "foreign" nurses that make these points of the ICN document essential (African nurses report, 2005; O'Brien-Pallas, 2006; Poaching nurses, 2006)

Good Faith Contracting, Equal Pay for Work of Equal Value, and Access to Grievance Procedures

Based on ethical standards of informed consent and social justice, migrating nurses have the right to expect equity in their contracts compared with nationals in the country of employment. Because of the nature of their foreign status and their economic need, migrating nurses are very vulnerable to abuses in these areas and may be reluctant to pursue grievance procedures. Oversight through regulatory bodies and policy is essential.

Safe Work Environment; Effective Orientation, Mentoring, and Supervision; and Employment Trial Periods

Migrating nurses are particularly vulnerable to coercion or abuse (Poaching nurses, 2006) and may be reluctant to report incidents (e.g., sexual harassment, inadequate supervision, or orders to practice beyond competency). Therefore the principles outlined by the ICN need to be well integrated into the nursing regulations of hiring countries.

Conclusion

Although both the WHO and the ICN acknowledge the significant value of cross-cultural exchange and the right of individuals to choose their working environment, these policy bodies lead the world in raising awareness about the vulnerability of migrating healthcare professionals, their families, and their nations. Recruitment of nurses from low-income countries places poor nations in the position of subsidizing nursing education and patient care in First World settings. This issue is particularly germane where high-income countries actively recruit nurses from poorer nations while concurrently ignoring solutions to workforce shortages in their own countries. In addition, without providing leaders in low-income nations with compensation, infrastructure support, and assistance in the development of systems, high-income nations are creating disruption and even collapse of healthcare systems (Chaguturu & Vallabhaneni, 2003). Low-income nations are vulnerable, frequently not in a position of political power to speak against practices of high-income nations. George Cordero, President of the Philippine Nurse Association, stated, "The Filipino people will suffer because the U.S. will get all our trained nurses. But what can we do?" (Dugger, 2006, p. 1). Justice compels the profession of nursing to recognize the vulnerability of poor nations and their migrating nurses and to advocate for policy and practices that promote distributive justice and equitable solutions to the global shortage of healthcare workforce, particularly in the nursing profession.

References

Abyad, A. (2003). Effect of the migration of health professionals: Brain drain or brain gain? *Long-Term Care Interface, 6*, 22–28.

African nurses report unfair treatment [Editorial]. (2005). *Nursing Times, 101*, 4.

American Academy of Nursing Expert Panel on Global Nursing and Health. (2006). White paper on global nursing and health: A brief. *Nursing Outlook, 32*, 111–113.

Buchan, J. (2006). The impact of global nursing migration on health services delivery. *Policy, Politics and Nursing Practice, 7*(Suppl.), 16S–25S.

Buerhaus, P., Staiger, D., & Auerbach, D. (2000). Implications of an aging registered nurse workforce. *Journal of the American Medical Association, 281*, 2928–2932.

Chaguturu, S., & Vallabhaneni, B. (2003). Aiding and abetting—Nursing crises at home and abroad. *New England Journal of Medicine, 131*, 1761–1761.

Cholanda, A. (2003). Nurse migration from Zimbabwe: Analysis of recent trends and impacts. *Nursing Inquiry, 12*, 162–172.

Clark, P., Stewart, J., & Clark, D. (2006).The globalization of the labor market for health-care professionals. *International Labor Review, 145,* 37–64.

Dugger, C. (2006, May 24). U.S. plan to lure nurses may hurt poor nations. *The New York Times.* Retrieved February 12, 2007, from http://topics.nytimes.com/top/reference/timestopics/people/d/celia_w_dugger/index.html?inline=nyt-per

Eastwood, J., Conroy, R., Naicker, W., West, P., Tutt, R., & Plange-Rhule, J. (2003). Loss of health professionals from sub-Sahara Africa: The pivotal role of the UK. *The Lancet, 163,* 1891–1900.

Green, A. (2006). Nursing and midwifery: Millennium development goals and the global human resource crisis. *International Nursing Review, 31,* 11–13.

Health Resources and Services Administration. (2004). *National sample survey of registered nurses.* Retrieved February 26, 2007, from http://www.bhpr.hrsa.gov/healthworkforce/reports/rnpopulation/preliminary findings.htm

International Council of Nurses (ICN). (2001). *Position statement: Ethical nurse recruitment.* Retrieved October 5, 2007, from www.icn.ch/psrecruit01.htm

International Council of Nurses (ICN). (2006). *The global nursing shortage: Priority areas for intervention.* Geneva, Switzerland: International Council of Nurses.

Jeans, M. (2006). In-country challenges to addressing the effects of emerging global migration on home care delivery. *Policy, Politics, and Nursing Practice, 7*(Suppl.), 58S–61S.

Kamal-Yanni, M. (2006). *Health worker crisis-international networks demand funding for African health workers.* Retrieved August 16, 2006, from www.oxfam.org.uk

Klestzick, K. (2007, February 5). *President's budget unacceptable in the face of nurse and nurse educator shortages* [National League for Nursing Press Release]. Retrieved October 8, 2007, from http://www.nln.org/newsreleases/pres_budget2007.htm

McElmurry, B., Solheim, K., Kishi, R., Coffia, M., Woith, W., & Janepanish, P. (2006). Ethical concerns in nurse migration. *Journal of Professional Nursing, 22,* 226–235.

Migration threatens health systems in developing countries [Editorial]. (2003). *Australian Nursing Journal, 11,* 10.

O'Brien-Pallas, L. (2006). Innovations in health care delivery: Responses to global nurse migration—A research example. *Policy, Politics, and Nursing Practice, 7*(Suppl.), 49S–57S.

O'Dowd, A. (2003). The looming nurse recruitment crisis. *Nursing Times, 101,* 20–22.

Padilla, P. (2006). Breakthrough to nursing: nurse migration and the nursing shortage. *Imprint 31,* 18, 20–21.

Poaching nurses from the developing world [Editorial]. (2006). *The Lancet, 167,* 1791.

Pond, B., & McPake, B. (2006). The health migration crisis: The role of four organizations for economic cooperation and development countries. *The Lancet, 367,* 1448–1455.

Riley, P., Anderson, B., Noguchi, L., & Vindigni, S. (2005). Caring for global caregivers: A call to action. *The Journal of Midwifery and Women's Health, 50,* 265–267.

Ross S., Polsky, D., & Sochalski, J. (2003). Nursing shortages and international nurse immigration. *International Nursing Review, 32,* 231–262

Spacracio, D. (2003). Winged migration: International nurse recruitment—Friend or foe to the nursing crisis? *Journal of Nursing Law, 10,* 97–111.

World Health Organization (WHO). (2006). Why the workforce is important. Retrieved October 8, 2007, from www.who.int/whr/2006/overview/en/print.html

Xu, Y., & Zhang, J. (2003). One size doesn't fit all: Ethics of international nurse recruitment from the conceptual framework of stakeholder interests. *Nursing Ethics, 12,* 371–381.

Yan, J. (2006). Health services delivery: Reframing policies for global nursing migration in North America—A Caribbean perspective. *Policy, Politics, and Nursing Practice, 7*(Suppl.), 71S–75S.

Yordy, K. (2006). *The nursing faculty shortage: A crisis for health care.* Princeton, NJ: Robert Wood Johnson Foundation.

Passionate Global Public Health Champions Needed

Barbara Hatcher, PhD, RN

Director, Center for Learning and Global Public Health, and Secretary General, the World Federation of the Public Health Association

For to be free is not merely to cast off one's chains, but to live in a way that respects and enhances the freedom of others.

—Nelson Mandela

Of all forms of inequality, injustice in health care is the most shocking and inhumane.

—Rev. Martin Luther King, Jr.

Over the last several decades public health professionals have launched a variety of interventions and advocated for policies designed to improve the health and health care of vulnerable populations. However, vulnerable populations have not achieved the same level of improved health status as the general population in spite of applying the best evidence-based interventions. Vulnerable populations continue to have less access to health resources and get sicker and die earlier than wealthier and/or more privileged groups. Although it is commonplace to designate very different groups as vulnerable, what is similar about these groups is that they believe they cannot comfortably or safely access and use standard resources. Although there is enough knowledge and technologies to improve the health of vulnerable populations, there seems to be a lack of the will and political commitment to make it happen.

One key area that has received limited attention is health communication and its impact on vulnerable populations. Health communication is the dissemination of understandable and usable information that concerns itself with health. It is a fundamental ingredient in virtually every form of medicine and health (Rogers, 1996). The importance of health communication has been best captured by Calderón & Beltrán (2004, p. 9), who define it as follows:

> [I]nterlacing of government healthcare policy (strategic plans, laws, fiscal commitment, judicial enforcement), institutional directives (healthcare equality and quality oversight), healthcare structure (geographic distribution and access to care, professional education and training, and research priorities), healthcare process (distribution of services, information and its dissemination venues, targeted patient education campaigns, and interpersonal and intergroup encounters) and ethnosocial realities (linguistics, health beliefs, socioeconomic status, and literacy) that influences healthcare utilization, satisfaction, compliance, and public health status at the national and community levels.

The major benefit of health communication is enabling persons to increase control over and improve their health. Despite having the greatest need, vulnerable populations are least likely to benefit from health communications, and the barriers to useful health information contribute to the disproportionate burden of disease they continue to experience in their health and health care (Weiss, Hart, McGee, & D'Estelle, 1992). Studies document the existence of language barriers and limited proficiency in both English and Spanish. Although limited English proficiency typically characterizes those who speak other languages (U.S. Department of Health and Human Services and the Office of Minority Health, 2001), this may be a faulty concept (Calderón, & Beltrán, 2004). Nationally, educational attainment is worse for vulnerable populations who speak English; therefore they are also limited in their proficiency in the use of the English language as well. The result of not turning this evidence into action is that limited and ineffective health communication campaigns targeting vulnerable populations are everywhere (Cavis, Crouch, & Wills, 1990; Clarence, 1998).

An important drawback in health communication policy at all levels, including the recently proposed Health Equity and Accountability Act of 2007, is that its language uses the term "linguistically appropriate" as meaning "language translation." As such, directives do not address the importance of linguistics per se (readability, word choice, syntax, and idiomatic variation within languages) in health communication but target only the translation of information into other languages. Further, there have been no evidence-based mandates to provide comprehensible health information set forth by law, accrediting and oversight agencies, and healthcare delivery systems (Calderón & Beltran, 2004).

The health information provided to vulnerable people, including the growing body of web-based information (Birru et al., 2004; Kaphingst, Zanfini, & Emmons, 2006)—blogs, podcasts, viral videos, and websites—just do not match the literacy and health literacy skills of vulnerable people. As previously stated, this mismatch not only relates to language but to syntax and to comprehension as well. For example, the readability levels of English- and Spanish-language websites and most available health information have been found to require 10th- to 14th-grade levels, higher than the estimated 6th-grade reading level of the general population (Davis et al., 1990; Jubelirer, 1991). Further, vulnerable persons are often unable to afford Internet services and personal computers and thus have no access to the information largely provided in web-based formats.

The benefit of health communications has been less striking for vulnerable populations because much of the available information is unusable. Researchers have determined that the lack of comprehensible and usable written and spoken language is a major barrier to health communication targeting primary and secondary disease prevention and is a major contributor to the misuse of health care, patient noncompliance, rising healthcare costs (Calderón & Beltrán, 2004; Weiss & Palmer, 2004).

Unusable health communication negatively impacts vulnerable populations. As Dervin and Huber (2005) suggested, there is a need to change the health communication paradigm from the current emphasis on the top-down transmission of expert information to one that envisions communication as the reception of information by multiple interpreters. With the goal of reaching vulnerable populations with the health information they need, the researchers provide the following evidence-based propositions (Dervin & Huber, 2005):

1. Reaching target audiences or users with health information is tough; bridging the gap between information and behavior is even tougher.

2. One-way information transmission works best with people who are similar to the information providers.

3. Too often, top-down information transmission rests on a host of faulty assumptions about target audiences.

4. Too often, top-down information transmission has ignored the experiential realities of lay persons' lives; too often, it blames the victims and is received as irrelevant at best and as prejudicial and oppressive at worst.

5. The information environment is increasingly marked by decreasing trust in expert and institutional sources.

6. Lay people are increasingly wise about how information is tied to vested interests.

7. The growing complexity of the information environment is making information dissemination more difficult.

8. The volatility of the information environment makes the professionals' jobs harder.

9. When it comes to expertise, all nonexperts are vulnerable.

10. One-way information transmission can backfire.

11. Information is rarely enough.

12. Information is not sufficient, but it is necessary.

13. Tinkering with information presentation strategies can make a big difference, but there is a big caveat: The difference depends on where the recipient is coming from.

14. The biggest increases in campaign effectiveness have come from reconceptualizing campaign design away from information transmission to multistage communication intervention.

15. Communication interventions must be communicative; if they revert to transmission they will fail.

16. Communication-based interventions necessarily involve community context; the most common route has been cultural, in the hope of addressing lived experiences and societal circumstances.

17. The culture or·community route to communicating is not a quick fix.

18. Although target group memberships may define policy aims, they are not the best way of defining information dissemination purposes.

19. Recipient readiness is, in fact, the best predictor of information receptivity.

20. Recipient readiness is predicted best phenomenologically and situationally, not in terms of a priori demographic or expert system categories.

21. Alternative research approaches have shown that what was formerly seen as chaotic behavior is in fact patterned information seeking and use.

22. Focusing on information seeking and use situationally and contextually decreases the variability that information disseminators must cope with.

23. Focusing on the verbs of information seeking and use provides even greater capacity to predict and explain.

24. Treating people as human works best.

25. Communication's most basic fundamental is the quid pro quo.

There is an opportunity to improve the health and well-being of our most vulnerable populations through good public health. Effective health communication is good public health. Good public health relies on lessons learned from several fields of experience—human rights, church and church-based efforts, community economic development, youth development, and new social movements. The most notable of these—the human rights approach—seeks to promote and protect the societal-level prerequisites for human well-being in which each individual can achieve his or her full potential (Mann et al, 1999). The lessons from this and other experiences previously mentioned can help nurses and other public health professionals design a new approach to helping vulnerable populations that builds on the accomplishments documented in this text while addressing the pitfalls of current approaches as outlined above. To reach this, we need passionate global public health champions committed to providing and advocating health for all. For health is, indeed, according to Michael Marmot (World Health Organization, 2006), a measure of the degree to which society delivers a good life to its citizens.

References

Birru, M., Monaco, V., Charles, L., Drew, H., Njie, V., Bierria, T., et al. (2004). Internet usage by low-literacy adults seeking health information: An observational analysis. *Journal of Medical Internet Resources, 6*(4), 25.

Calderón, J., & Beltran, R. (2004). Pitfalls in health communication: Healthcare policy, institution, structure, and process. *MedGenMed, 6*(1), 9.

Cavis, T., Crouch, M., & Wills, G. (1990). The gap between patient reading comprehension and the readability of patient education materials. *Journal of Family Practice, 31*, 533–537.

Clarence, B. (1998). Advancing the cause of informed consent: Moving form disclosures to understanding. *American Journal of Medicine, 105*, 354–355.

Davis, T., Crouch, M., Willis, G., Miller, S., & Abdehou, D. (1990). The gap between patient reading comprehension and the readability of patient education materials. *Journal of Family Practice, 31*(5), 533–538.

Dervin, B., & Huber, J. (2005). Libraries reaching out with health information to vulnerable populations. *Journal of the Medical Library Association, 93*(4, Suppl.), 74–80.

Health Equity and Accountability Act of 2007. Retrieved May 26, 2007, from http://mailman1.u.washington.edu/pipermail/cbpr/attachments/20070509/53656d8e/20070509SummaryofDraftDisparitiesBill.doc

Jubelirer, S. (1991). Level of reading difficulty in educational pamphlets and informed consent documents for cancer patients. *West Virginia Medical Journal, 87*(12), 554–557.

Kaphingst, K., Zanfini, C., & Emmons, K. (2006). Accessibility of websites containing colorectal cancer information to adults with limited literacy. *Cancer Causes and Control, 17*(2), 147–151.

Mann, J., Gostin, L., Gruskin, S., Brennan, T., Lazzarini, Z., & Fineberg, H. (1999). Health and human rights. In J. Mann (Ed.), *Health and human rights reader* (pp. 7–20). New York: Routledge.

Rogers, E. M. (1996). Health communication: Up-to-date report. *Journal of Health Communication, 1*, 15–33.

U.S. Department of Health and Human Services and the Office of Minority Health (2001). Recommended standards for culturally and linguistically appropriate health care services. Retrieved May 30, 2007, from http://www.omhrc.gov/clas/cultural1a.htm

Weiss, B., Hart, G., McGee, D., & D'Estelle, S. (1992). Health status of illiterate adults: Relation between literacy and health status among persons with low literacy skills. *Journal of the American Board of Family Practice, 5*(3), 257–264.

Weiss, B., & Palmer, R. (2004). Relationships between health care costs and very low literacy skills in a medically needy and indigent Medicaid population. *Journal of the American Board of Family Practice, 17*, 44–47.

World Health Organization. (2006). *Commission on social determinants of health*. Retrieved October 5, 2007, from http://www.who.int/social_determinants/en/

INDEX